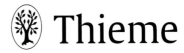

Caries Management—
Science and Clinical Practice

Univ.-Prof.
Dr. Hendrik Meyer-Lueckel, MPH
Department of Operative Dentistry,
Periodontology, and Preventive Dentistry
Rheinisch-Westfälische Technische Hochschule
(RWTH) Aachen
Aachen, Germany

Priv.-Doz. Dr. Sebastian Paris, DDS
Clinic for Operative Dentistry
and Periodontology
Christian-Albrechts-Universität zu Kiel
Kiel, Germany

Assoc. Prof. Kim R. Ekstrand, DDS, PhD
Vice Dean and Chair
Section for Cariology, Endodontics,
Pediatric Dentistry, and Clinical Genetics
Department of Odontology
Faculty of Health and Medical Sciences
University of Copenhagen
Copenhagen, Denmark

Managing Editor:
Dr. Susanne Effenberger
Manager Clinical Research
DMG Dental-Material Gesellschaft mbH
Hamburg, Germany

With contributions by

Mohammad Alkilzy, Bennett T. Amaechi, Uwe Blunck, Wolfgang Buchalla, Brian H. Clarkson,
Agata Czajka-Jakubowska, Christof Doerfer, Hafsteinn Eggertsson, Roland Frankenberger,
Rainer Haak, Leandro Augusto Hilgert, Soraya Coelho Leal, Stefania Martignon,
Vera Mendes Soviero, David Nigel James Ricketts, Ulrich Schiffner, Christian Andres Schneider,
R. Peter Shellis, Christian H. Splieth, Svante Twetman, Martin J. Tyas, Cornelis van Loveren,
Bart Van Meerbeek, Michael Jochen Wicht, Yasuhiro Yoshida, Domenick T. Zero

409 illustrations

Thieme
Stuttgart · New York

Library of Congress Cataloging-in-Publication Data is available from the publisher.

RK
331
.C375
2013

Illustrators: Christine Lackner, Ittlingen, Germany; Eva M. Reinwald, Copenhagen, Denmark (portraits in preface)

© 2013 Georg Thieme Verlag KG
Rüdigerstrasse 14, 70469 Stuttgart,
Germany
http://www.thieme.de
Thieme Medical Publishers, Inc., 333 Seventh Avenue,
New York, NY 10001, USA
http://www.thieme.com

Cover design: Thieme Publishing Group
Translation: Dolphin Translations, Stuttgart, Germany
Typesetting by primustype Robert Hurler GmbH, Notzingen,
Germany
Printed in Italy by L.E.G.O., Vicenza

ISBN 978-3-13-154711-8
eISBN 978-3-13-169381-5

Preface

Dental caries is still one of the most common diseases in human beings, causing smaller or larger problems to millions of people around the world every day. As dental professionals we have to help people to understand the disease to enable them to prevent caries by themselves (self-management). When more severe decay is diagnosed, we, together with the patient, should manage the caries disease in a minimally interventional way.

This introductory chapter will present some general thoughts about caries and where we come from in cariology. Moreover, we will explain why we think it is important to have another book about cariology and will describe the concept of the book, which is presented in two main parts: science and practice.

Caries—Important but Preventable

Dental caries is the term used for pathoanatomical changes of the dental hard tissues. These changes are caused by acids that are created in the dental plaque (biofilm) covering the affected tooth surface, when certain microorganisms ferment sugars, which in turn demineralize the dental hard tissues. Thus, the disease, which professionals perceive as changes of the dental hard tissues, in fact reflects activities within the overlying dental biofilm. If these unfavorable biofilm activities are occurring frequently, the signs of the caries process on the dental hard tissues will become more easily detectable. Nonetheless, the caries "scar" starts with signs that are only visible with high magnification in the laboratory but end up with clinically visible alterations of the tooth surface integrity. Thus, caries is a term which actually covers changes in the dental hard tissue from the time the first mineral ion leaves the tissue to when no mineral is left. This development takes several years, fortunately, giving the dental professional and the patient time to act. In the clinically nonvisible stages we can adopt a risk-related approach to intervene noninvasively; in the early visible stages of the disease, we can intervene noninvasively or microinvasively. Later stages of the disease need invasive intervention that aims to preserve the tooth as much as possible.

Where We Come From...

Numerous individuals or groups of scientists have contributed to our understanding of caries over time. In the following we have selected a few of the many contributors and taken the liberty to sketch their faces and make a small note about their contribution. We have not included those who are still among us. The figure captions will give the reader a good idea of the history and development of cariology including adhesive dentistry.

Do We Need Another Book about Cariology?

Nowadays the dental professional has to face an overwhelming amount of **information** concerning dental caries and its clinical management, which is derived from various "traditional" sources such as pre- and postgraduate courses at dental schools and from continuing educational programs. In addition, the Internet updates current knowledge not only for dental professionals, but also for their patients. As with everything else, when a variety of goods is on offer, the choice becomes more difficult!

From a researcher's perspective this also holds true for the increasing variety of scientific journals that provide us with evidence on related issues for dental caries and allied topics such as tooth wear. Thus, the choice and assessment of scientific information are becoming more difficult compared with former years, although this process has been formalized and professionalized in the form of **evidence-based dentistry**. Here, systematic reviews or even meta-analyses about a certain topic should help to inform the professional, being based on relevant science. Nonetheless, this systematic approach is not always feasible, either because there is not much clinical evidence available or the subject matter is quite complex. For the dental practitioner systematic reviews might even be too impracticable to provide clinical guidance in the daily grind.

In this area of conflict a textbook may be of help. Although, it cannot and need not be as objective as a scientific paper, the format of a book is capable of summing up the most relevant points in a readable manner, and is thus still an important tool in teaching. This is what we have aimed for, together with over 20 other authors from more than 10 countries, who are all experts in their respective fields of cariology.

Proposal to Read the Book

The **target groups** for this book are those studying or working within dentistry: dental hygienists, dental students, graduates, and dentists whether working in the public dental service or in private practice. Dental assistants who would have their working arena extended within the field of cariology may also benefit from reading parts of this book.

The book is divided into two parts: science and clinical practice. The **science part** is divided into five main subparts. Starting from oral ecology merging to etiology and (clinical) pathogenesis of caries and noncarious defects, the first subpart (Chapters 1–4) is rounded off by a more philosophical approach on how caries can be seen from a "modelling aspect." The second subpart (Chapters 5–9) is about clinical and radiographic detection of caries and assessment at the tooth surface level, as well as taking into account the individual level, meaning caries risk assessment. After a brief introduction to epidemiological

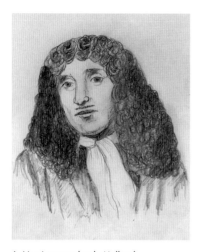

A. Van Leeuwenhoek, Holland
As far back as the 1650s Van Leeuwenhoek observed small animals in dental plaque, by using simple microscopes which he had made himself.

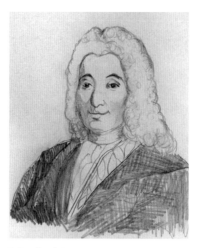

P. Fauchard, France
Around 1710, Fauchard asserted that sugar-derived acids like tartaric acid were responsible for dental decay. He also introduced dental fillings as treatment for dental caries.

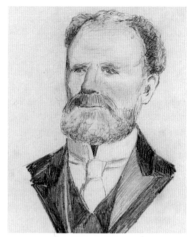

W.D. Miller, USA
In the 1870s Miller observed that a multitude of microorganisms could produce acid. He suggested *the chemoparasitic caries theory*, which is still valid today.

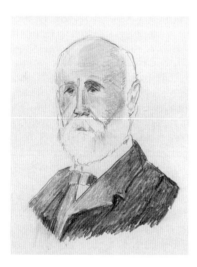

G.V. Black, USA
From the 1860s onward Black organized, among other things, Black's classification system for caries lesions (Class I, II, III, VI, V) and principles of tooth preparations for fillings.

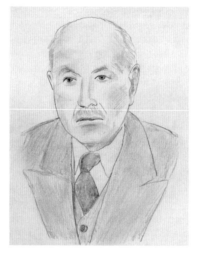

F.S. McKay, USA
In the 1930s McKay described the phenomenon of Colorado stained teeth, which later became synonymous with dental fluorosis.

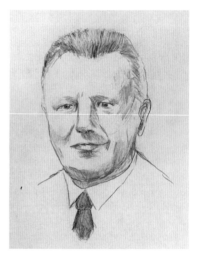

H.T. Dean, USA
In the 1930s and 40s Dean observed an inverse relationship between dental fluorosis and dental caries.

matters on the topics of the book, the second subpart concludes with a proposal of how to transfer the knowledge about the caries process and its clinical assessment into clinical action. The noninvasive strategies (biofilm, diet, and mineralization modification) of how to deal with the caries process are described in the third subpart (Chapters 10–13) and possible ways of implementation in individualized and community-based dentistry are presented. The fourth subpart (Chapters 14–19) of the scientific section deals with microinvasive and minimally invasive caries treatment. This includes adhesion technology, sealing and infiltration, caries removal, and tooth-coloured direct restorations. The fifth subpart (Chapters 20–22) focuses on decision-making in treating caries in general as well as on special aspects of the presented concept in children. The scientific part concludes with some thoughts on future aspects in cariology.

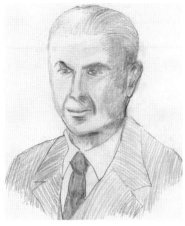

H. Klein, USA
In the late 1930s, Klein and co-workers introduced the DMF index for recording caries in the United States, where D corresponds to decayed teeth/surfaces, M to missing teeth/surfaces due to caries, and F to filled teeth/surfaces due to caries.

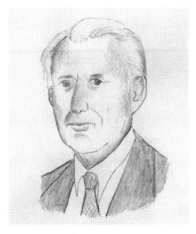

B. Krasse, Sweden
In the 1950s, Krasse and co-workers showed that the caries increment in mentally handicapped people (Vipeholm caries study) increased if sugar was consumed between meals in a form that was retained in the mouth for a long time. In contrast, no caries increment was seen if the diet did not contain sugar.

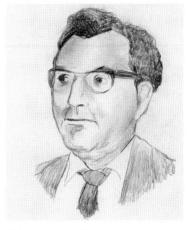

M.G. Buonocore, USA
In the mid-1950s Buonocore introduced a method for increasing the adhesion of acrylic filling materials to enamel surfaces, which was necessary for realizing the concept of sealing in caries.

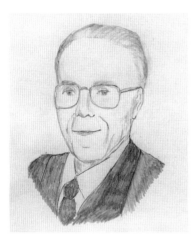

R. Bowen, USA
In the 1950s and 60s Bowen devised Bowen's resin, a forerunner for the majority of the composite materials that dentists have used for fillings ever since.

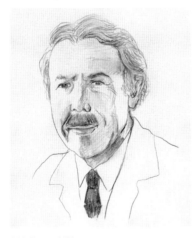

P.H. Keyes, USA
In the 1960s Keyes described the etiology of caries by means of three overlapping circles.

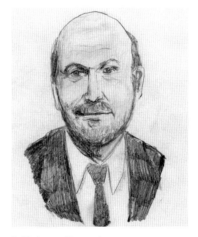

A. Thylstrup, Denmark
In Denmark during the 1980s, Thylstrup and co-workers disagreed with the principle of caries resistance as being due to embedment of fluoride in the dental hard tissue, but instead explained that the effect of fluoride on caries was related to its presence in small concentrations in the plaque fluid.

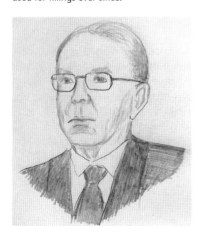

D. Bratthal, Sweden
During the 1980s and 90s Bratthal introduced the caries risk assessment program, CARIOGRAM.

The **clinical practice** part describes step-by-step clinical processes as well as clinical cases, for which treatment decisions are reflected on and the treatment outcomes shown.

As the target readership for this book is very broad, the different groups within the dental profession will probably read the book differently. The best advice we can give a reader before tackling a chapter is to read the introduction, the headings, the fact boxes, and the concluding summary. Then it is time for detailed study of the chapter. Enjoy!

Hendrik Meyer-Lueckel
Sebastian Paris
Kim Ekstrand
The Editors

Contributors List

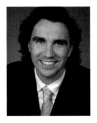

Univ.-Prof. Dr. Hendrik Meyer-Lueckel, MPH
Department of Operative Dentistry,
Periodontology, and Preventive
Dentistry
Rheinisch-Westfälische Technische
Hochschule (RWTH) Aachen
Aachen, Germany

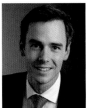

Priv.-Doz. Dr. Sebastian Paris, DDS
Clinic for Operative Dentistry
and Periodontology
Christian-Albrechts-Universität zu Kiel
Kiel, Germany

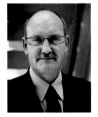

Assoc. Prof. Kim R. Ekstrand, DDS, PhD
Vice Dean and Chair
Section for Cariology, Endodontics,
Pediatric Dentistry, and Clinical Genetics
Department of Odontology
Faculty of Health and Medical Sciences
University of Copenhagen
Copenhagen, Denmark

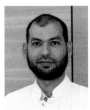

Dr. Mohammad Alkilzy
Department for Preventive and Pediatric
Dentistry
University of Greifswald
Greifswald, Germany
Department of Pediatric Dentistry
University of Aleppo
Syria

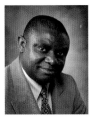

**Prof. Bennett T. Amaechi,
BS, BDS, MS, PhD**
Department of Comprehensive Dentistry
University of Texas Health Science Center
at San Antonio
San Antonio
Texas, USA

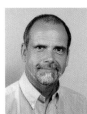

Dr. Uwe Blunck
Department for Conservative Dentistry
and Preventive Dentistry
Charité – Universitätsmedizin Berlin
Berlin, Germany

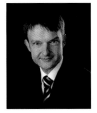

Prof. Dr. Wolfgang Buchalla
Department for Preventive Dentistry,
Periodontology, and Cariology
University of Zurich
Zurich, Switzerland

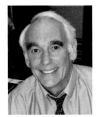

**Prof. Brian H. Clarkson,
BCHD, LDS, MS, PhD**
Department of Cariology, Restorative
Sciences, and Endodontics
School of Dentistry
University of Michigan
Ann Arbor
Michigan, USA

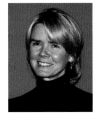

**Dr. hab. n. med.
Agata Czajka-Jakubowska**
Department of Conservative Dentistry
and Periodontology
Poznan University of Medical Sciences
Poznań, Poland

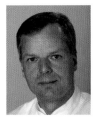

Univ.-Prof. Dr. Christof Doerfer
Clinic for Operative Dentistry and
Periodontology
Christian-Albrechts-Universität zu Kiel
Kiel, Germany

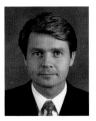

**Dr. Hafsteinn Eggertsson,
DDS, MSD, PhD**
Honorary Research Fellow
University of Iceland
Associate Dentist
Willamette Dental Eugene
Oregon, USA

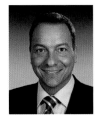

Univ.-Prof. Dr. Roland Frankenberger
Department for Conservative Dentistry
Philipps-Universität Marburg
Marburg, Germany

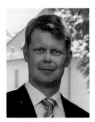

Univ.-Prof. Dr. Rainer Haak, MME
Department for Conservative Dentistry
and Periodontology
Universität Leipzig
Leipzig, Germany

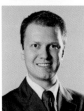

Prof. Leandro Augusto Hilgert
Department of Dentistry
Faculty of Health Sciences
University of Brasília
Asa Norte
Brasilia, Brazil

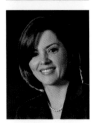

Profa. Soraya Coelho Leal
Department of Dentistry
Faculty of Health Sciences
University of Brasília
Asa Norte
Brasilia, Brazil

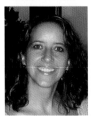

Prof. Stefania Martignon, PhD
Caries Research Unit UNICA
Universidad El Bosque
Bogotá, Colombia

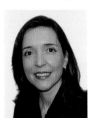

Profa. Dr. Vera Mendes Soviero
Department of Preventive and
Community Dentistry
Faculty of Dentistry
University of the State of Rio de Janeiro
Rio de Janeiro, Brazil

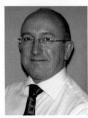

Prof. David Nigel James Ricketts
Professor of Cariology and Conservative
Dentistry
Honorary Consultant in Restorative
Dentistry
University of Dundee Dental School
Dundee, UK

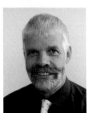

Prof. Dr. Ulrich Schiffner
Department of Restorative and
Preventative Dentistry
Universität Hamburg
Hamburg, Germany

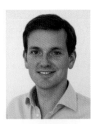

Dr. Christian Andres Schneider
Clinic for Operative Dentistry
and Periodontology
Christian-Albrechts-Universität zu Kiel
Kiel, Germany

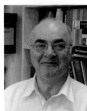

Dr. R. Peter Shellis, MSc, PhD
School of Oral and Dental Sciences
University of Bristol
Bristol, UK

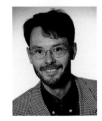

Univ.-Prof. Dr. Christian H. Splieth
Department for Preventive
and Paediatric Dentistry
Greifswald University
Greifswald, Germany

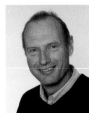

Prof. Svante Twetman
Section for Cariology, Endodontics, Pe-
diatric Dentistry, and Clinical Genetics
Faculty of Health and Medical Sciences
University of Copenhagen
Copenhagen, Denmark

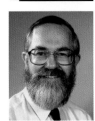

Prof. Martin J. Tyas
Professorial Fellow
Melbourne Dental School
The University of Melbourne
Melbourne, Australia

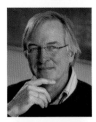

Prof. Dr. Cornelis van Loveren
Department of Cariology,
Endodontology, Pedodontology,
Microbiology
Academic Centre for Dentistry
Amsterdam (ACTA)
Amsterdam, The Netherlands

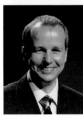

Prof. Dr. Bart Van Meerbeek
Department of Conservative Dentistry
BIOMAT Research Cluster
Catholic University of Leuven
Leuven, Belgium

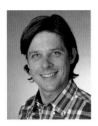

Priv.-Doz. Dr. Michael Jochen Wicht
Department of Conservative Dentistry
and Periodontology
University of Cologne
Cologne, Germany

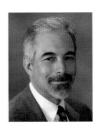

Prof. Domenick T. Zero, DDS, MS
Department of Preventive
and Community Dentistry
Indiana University School of Dentistry
Indianapolis, USA

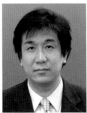

Prof. Yasuhiro Yoshida
Department of Biomaterials
Graduate School of Medicine,
Dentistry, and Pharmaceutical Sciences
Okayama University
Okayama, Japan

List of Abbreviations

ACP	amorphous calcium phosphate
APF	acidulated phosphate–fluoride
API	approximal plaque index
BEWE	basic erosive wear examination
BMP	bone morphogenic protein
BW	bitewing
CAR	caries adjacent to restorations
CCOG	Calgary–Cambridge Observation Guide
CHAP	carbonate modified hydroxyapatite
CHX	chlorhexidene
CPP	Casein phosphopeptides
Dd	Diagnodent value
DDE	developmental defects of dental enamel
DMF(T,S)	decayed, missing, filled (teeth, surface)
dmft	decayed, missing, filled teeth (primary dentition)
DVT	digital volume tomograph
EDJ	enamel–dentin junction
EPS	extracellular polysaccharides
FAP	fluorapatite
FHAP	fluoride hydroxy apatite
FOTI	fiberoptic transillumination
GPDM	glycerophosphoric acid dimethacrylate
HAP	hydroxyapatite
HEMA	2-hydroxyethyl methacrylate

ICDAS	International Caries Detection and Assessment System
IPS	intracellular polysaccharides
MDP	methacryloyloxy decyl dihydrogenphosphate
MFP	monofluorophosphate
MHAP	magnesium modified hydroxyapatite
MIH	molar–incisor hypomineralization
mPBI	modified periodontal bleeding index
MTCP	magnesium containing β-tricalcium phosphate
MWH	magnesium whitlockite
NNT	number needed to treat
PF	prevented fraction
PSI	periodontal screening index
QHI	Quigley Hein index
RCI	root caries index
RI	refractive index
ROC	receiver operating characteristics
SEM	scanning electron microscopy
SSFR	stimulated saliva flow rate
TACT	tuned aperture computed radiography
TEM	transverse electron microscopy
TFI	Thylstrup–Fejerskov index
TMR	transverse microradiography
TSIF	tooth surface index of fluorosis

Table of Contents

Part 1: Caries—Science

The Disease

8 Epidemiology of Caries and Noncarious Defects

Ulrich Schiffner

9 From Diagnostics to Therapy

Sebastian Paris, Kim R. Ekstrand, Hendrik Meyer-Lueckel

Noninvasive Therapy

10 Caries Management by Modifying the Biofilm

Sebastian Paris, Christof Doerfer, Hendrik Meyer-Lueckel

Adhesion

14 Basics in Adhesion Technology

Bart Van Meerbeek, Yasuhiro Yoshida

Microinvasive Therapy

15 Fissure Sealing

Hafsteinn Eggertsson

Treatment Decision

20 Decision-Making in Managing the Caries Process

Hendrik Meyer-Lueckel, Martin J. Tyas, Michael J. Wicht, Sebastian Paris

Special Aspects in Children and the Young

21 How to Maintain Sound Teeth: an Individualized Population Strategy for Children and Adolescents

Kim R. Ekstrand

22 Individualized Caries Management in Pediatric Dentistry

Christian H. Splieth, Mohammad Alkilzy

A Glimpse into the Future

23 Future Trends in Caries Research
Brian H. Clarkson, Agata Czajka-Jakubowska

Part 2: Caries—Clinical Practice

24 Diagnostics, Treatment Decision, and Documentation
Sebastian Paris, Rainer Haak, Hendrik Meyer-Lueckel

25 Minimal Interventional Treatment of Caries in the Permanent Dentition: Clinical Cases
Hendrik Meyer-Lueckel, Sebastian Paris, Christian A. Schneider, Leandro A. Hilgert, Soraya Coelho Leal

Part 1 Caries—Science

Ecology of the Oral Cavity

Kim R. Ekstrand, Domenick T. Zero

1

In simplified terms, dental caries develops because certain bacteria in the oral cavity ferment carbohydrates (sugars) into organic acids,[1] which in the case of lactic acid may result in dissolution of dental hard tissue.[2] However, in reality the etiology and pathogenesis of caries are much more complex and will be comprehensively discussed in the following chapters. All oral tissues, especially the dental hard tissues, microorganisms, and the saliva interact not only in the physiology of the oral cavity, but also in the caries process. Therefore it is important to know their composition, structure, and functions to understand the caries process.

This chapter will deal with basic knowledge about the oral cavity focusing on the teeth, saliva, and oral microbiology, primarily from the perspective of caries disease. The subsequent chapters will build further on this knowledge. Age-related changes in dental hard tissue as well as in the salivary glands will also be touched on, as will related diseases and conditions other than caries.

In particular this chapter will cover:
- the structure of teeth,
- the functions of saliva,
- changes in the dental hard tissues and saliva with aging,
- dental plaque and its role in caries, and
- the interaction between tooth structure, saliva, and plaque in the oral cavity.

Teeth

The structure of the coronal part of the teeth is as follows.[3] The **enamel** is the outermost layer covering the **dentin**, which in turn covers the **pulp** (**Fig. 1.1**). In the roots the outer layer consists of **cementum**, covering the dentin, which covers the pulp.

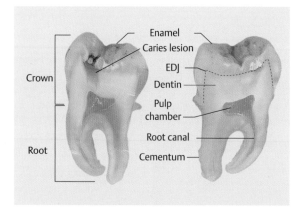

Fig. 1.1 Hemi-sectioned molar showing the major components of the tooth. The dentin forms the bulk of the tooth and encloses the pulp chamber and root canals. The enamel covers the dentin in the coronal part of the tooth and the cementum covers the dentin in the roots. EDJ: enamel–dentin junction.

Tooth Development and Tooth Emergence

Human beings have two sets of teeth: those belonging to the primary dentition, and those belonging to the permanent dentition. The conditions influencing the start of mineralization of the individual teeth, when the crowns are formed, the time for eruption, and when the roots are fully formed were mapped during the first half of the last century.[4] Teeth start to develop late in embryonic development. The first tooth type to erupt is most commonly a primary incisor in the lower jaw, which normally happens when the child is 6–8 months old (**Fig. 1.2a**). All teeth in the primary dentition are fully erupted when the child is about 2½ years old,[6] and approximal contact between first and second primary molars is seen about 1 year later.[7]

The first permanent teeth to erupt are either the central incisors or the first molar teeth; this happens in about 90% of children between 5 and 6 years of age.[8] The last permanent tooth to erupt is the third molar, which happens at the age of around 18 years. Thus, during a period of 18 years, different teeth erupt into the oral cavity, and between the ages of 5–6 and 12 years the child has a mixed dentition consisting of primary as well as permanent teeth (**Fig. 1.2b**).

Macromorphological Terms

Professionals know where caries develops: in the primary dentition it develops mainly on the approximal and occlusal surfaces and occasionally on smooth surfaces along the gingival margin; in the permanent dentition it develops primarily on the occlusal surfaces, foramen cecum, and later, on approximal surfaces. In the elderly, caries also develops on root surfaces. The following paragraph will describe macromorphological terms related to these caries-prone sites of the teeth.

Occlusal Surfaces

In a simple model, Carlsen (1987) suggested dividing the crowns of teeth into **lobes**—from one (e.g., incisors) to five (e.g., some molars) in number.[3] Often molar teeth have five lobes, each with an essential cusp. Three of them (**Fig. 1.3a**) are the facial lobes, namely the mesiofacial, centrofacial, and distofacial lobes, which are separated on the occlusal surface by the mesiofacial and distofacial interlobal grooves. These interlobal grooves run down to the facial surface. In particular, the mesiofacial interlobal groove can end cervically in a (sometimes deep) tract called the **foramen cecum**.

The remaining two lobes are placed lingually: the mesiolingual and distolingual lobes separated on the occlusal surface by the lingual interlobal groove. The facial lobes are separated from the lingual lobes by the mesial and distal interlobal grooves. Where the interlobal grooves meet, a tract called the **fossa** arises. Thus molar teeth often have at least three fossae: the mesial, central, and distal

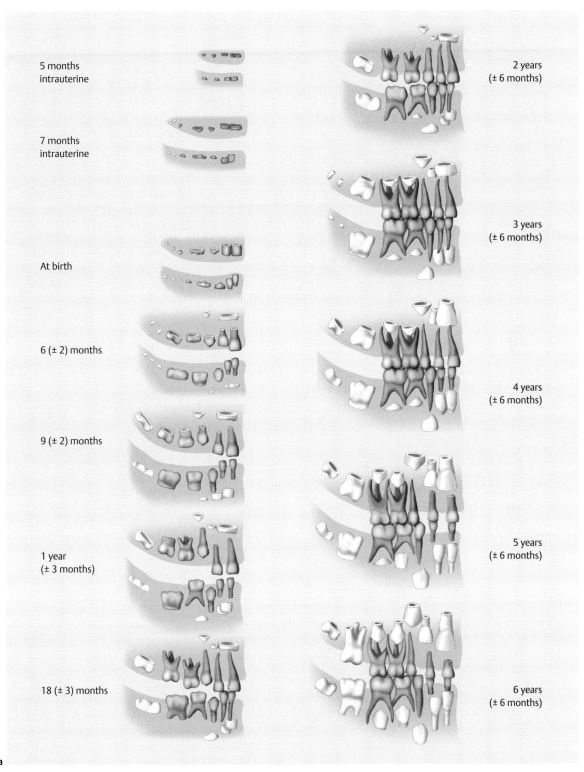

5 months
intrauterine

7 months
intrauterine

At birth

6 (± 2) months

9 (± 2) months

1 year
(± 3 months)

18 (± 3) months

2 years
(± 6 months)

3 years
(± 6 months)

4 years
(± 6 months)

5 years
(± 6 months)

6 years
(± 6 months)

a

Fig. 1.2a,b Development and growth patterns of the teeth in both dentitions.[5]

Fig. 1.2b ▷

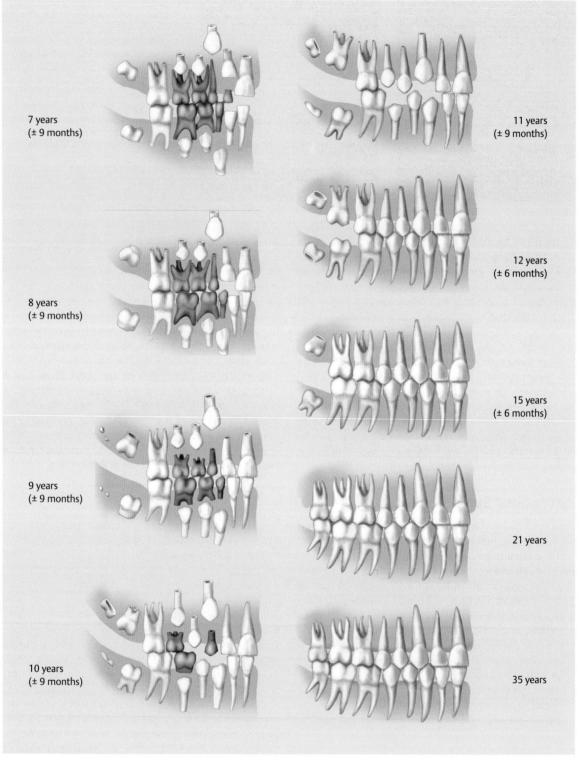

7 years
(± 9 months)

8 years
(± 9 months)

9 years
(± 9 months)

10 years
(± 9 months)

11 years
(± 9 months)

12 years
(± 6 months)

15 years
(± 6 months)

21 years

35 years

b

Fig. 1.2 (Continued)

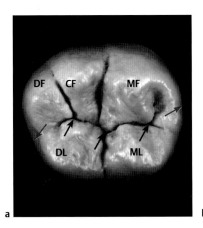
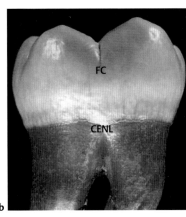

Fig. 1.3a,b
a Occlusal aspect of a permanent first molar. MF, CF, and DF are the mesiofacial, centrofacial, and distofacial lobes. The ML and DL are the mesiolingual and distolingual lobes. Black arrows point to fossae areas and red arrows point to margino-segmental grooves.
b Lingual aspect of a first permanent molar. The cervical enamel line/cemento-enamel junction separates the crown from the root. FC: location of foramen cecum.

fossae (**Fig. 1.3a**). On each lobe there are also several **intersegmental grooves**. On the marginal ridge, particularly in molars, grooves termed **margino-segmental grooves** run downward along the approximal surface. Premolars have normally two lobes, one buccal and one lingual, separated by the mesiodistal interlobal groove.

The total number of grooves, intersegmental grooves, and fossae on the occlusal surface are termed the "**groove–fossa system**," replacing the classical term "**pits and fissure system**." To build a bridge between the two classification systems, it has been suggested that the groove–fossae systems can be fissurelike or groovelike, where "fissurelike" is defined as an area where the bottom of the groove–fossa system is not clinically visible. On the occlusal surface, caries most often develops in wide fissures and in the fossae areas.[9]

Approximal Surfaces

On approximal surfaces at least three macromorphological features can influence the development of caries and must be taken into consideration:
- The width and location of the approximal contact area. That is, approximal surfaces on tooth types with narrow contact points (front teeth) have less caries than approximal surfaces of tooth types with wide approximal surface contact areas (molar teeth).[10,11]
- The curvature of the approximal surfaces. Certain molars in both dentitions show a degree of concavity on the approximal surfaces.[3]
- The margino-segmental grooves (**Fig. 1.3a**) may contribute to an uneven contact with the adjacent tooth, and the grooves can be both fissurelike and groovelike.

The Cervical Enamel Line and the Roots

The cervical enamel line (**Fig. 1.3b**) is also termed the cemento-enamel junction and is the boundary line between the anatomical crown and the anatomical root complex.[3] In patients with healthy gingiva, the line/junction is at the same level as the marginal gingiva. This line/junction is irregular and rough, so microorganisms can adhere easily to this area of the tooth.

Apart from some grooves on the roots of particular teeth, there are no macromorphological structures which promote caries development in the roots. Rather, the gingiva around the neck of the tooth promotes stagnation of microorganisms, eventually developing into plaque. In the case of gingival recession, new plaque stagnation areas are formed where root caries can develop.

NOTE

Caries usually develops in specific locations in the teeth: these are the occlusal surfaces, the approximal surfaces, and along the gingival margin.

Enamel

The enamel is formed by **ameloblasts** in three consecutive steps. Initially, the ameloblasts secrete proteins in such a way that the final form of the tooth is developed; simultaneously, a part of the protein is replaced by mineral. This is the **secretory phase** of amelogenesis.[12] The majority of the protein is, however, replaced by mineral during the **maturation stage** of amelogenesis, which takes place over several years. The amelogenesis ends at the time for emergence of the tooth when the reduced ameloblast fuses with the epithelium cells. More details can be found in Mjör and Fejerskov.[12]

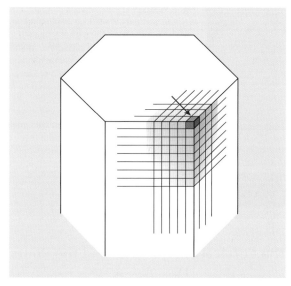

Fig. 1.4 Illustration showing the structure of a hydroxyapatite crystal. The smallest repeating entity of the crystal in enamel (arrow) has in its purest form the formula $Ca_5(PO_4)_3(OH)$.

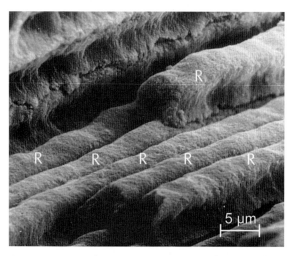

Fig. 1.5 Scanning electron microscopic images of enamel rods (R) built up by crystals.

Chemical Composition and Structure of Apatite Crystals

The inorganic content of mature enamel amounts to 96%–97% by weight; the remainder is organic material and water. On the basis of volume around 86% is mineral, 12% is water, and 2% is organic material.[12]

Owing to its hardness, enamel is difficult to cut for histological examinations used to study its structure. Therefore different approaches have been considered to describe its nature. One way to do this is at the crystalline level. In material science, a crystal is a solid substance in which the atoms, molecules, or ions are arranged in an orderly repeating pattern extending in all three dimensions. The crystals made by the ameloblasts consist of calcium phosphate, and the smallest repeating entity of the crystals in enamel has, in its purest form, the formula $Ca_5(PO_4)_3(OH)$, which is termed **hydroxyapatite** (HAP) (**Fig. 1.4**). The crystals are approximately hexagonal in cross-section, with a diameter of ca. 40 nm. The length of the crystals is difficult to assess, but today it is assumed that the length is between 100 nm and 1000 nm.[13]

At the chemical level, several substitutions of the ions in HAP can and do occur (resulting in impure forms of HAP)—for example, substitution with fluoride giving **fluoride hydroxyapatite** (FHAP); with carbonate, **carbonate-modified hydroxyapatite** (CHAP); and with magnesium, **magnesium-modified hydroxyapatite** (MHAP). **Fluorapatite** is a crystal where (nearly) all of the OH^- ions in HAP are replaced by fluoride, and which has a lower solubility than HAP; this, however, is not that common in human enamel.[14] More commonly, the OH^- ions are only partially replaced by fluoride, and FHAP is formed. These crystals also have a lower solubility than HAP, which again has lower solubility than CHAP.[15–17] These chemical conditions have great influence on the caries process and will be highlighted in Chapters 2 and 3.

The individual crystals are arranged in rods (or prisms) (**Fig. 1.5**) extending from the enamel–dentin junction to the surface, with an average diameter of about 4–5 μm. The crystals in the rods all align in the same direction except at the periphery, where the crystals change direction from those in the core of the rod. Thus, the space between the crystals or intercrystalline spaces (also called the pore volume which is filled with air, water, or proteins) is larger at the periphery of the rod than at the core. As the periphery of one rod meets other peripheries of other rods, the pore volume between rods is relatively large and much larger than in the core of the rod (**Fig. 1.6**). This is important for caries formation as acid and other products more easily penetrate through areas of enlarged pore volume (see also Chapter 3).

Due to this uniform structure of the enamel with tightly packed crystals, **light** penetrates through the enamel and is reflected or absorbed in the dentin. Well mineralized, permanent enamel is translucent, and it is the underlying dentin which, eventually, gives the tooth its color (**Fig. 1.7**). If the **pore volume** in the enamel increases, the light is scattered and reflected in the enamel which results in a white color. Primary teeth (see **Fig. 1.7**), which show a greater pore volume than the erupting permanent enamel, appear therefore whiter than permanent teeth.

Macroscopically/clinically the enamel generally looks smooth and even (**Figs. 1.3, 1.7**); however, at high magnification the surface enamel is full of **developmental defects** such as pits, cracks, and fissures[18,19] as well as normal anatomical features such as Tomes' process pits corresponding to the head of the ameloblasts (**Fig. 1.8**). Thus, there are numbers of surface irregularities on enamel where the microorganism can shelter.

In some parts of the surface enamel, and particularly in teeth of the primary dentition, the enamel is covered by crystals which are not organized as rods, but the direc-

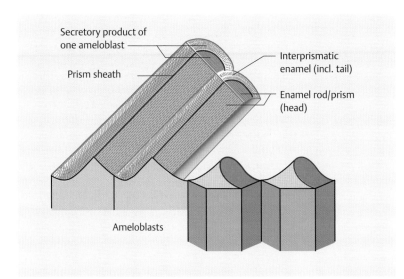

Fig. 1.6 Schematic illustration of three-dimensional arrangement of enamel crystallites within the rods (prisms) resulting from their formation by ameloblasts. Note the in the prism periphery, the crystal orientation changes abruptly, resulting in enlarged intercrystalline spaces in the prism boundaries.[45]

Labels: Secretory product of one ameloblast; Prism sheath; Interprismatic enamel (incl. tail); Enamel rod/prism (head); Ameloblasts

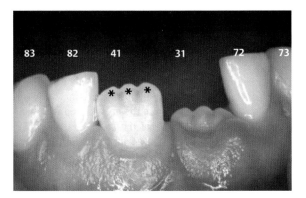

Fig. 1.7 Mandibular front teeth of a 6-year-old child, with erupting permanent first incisors. They appear more yellowish than the adjacent more opaque deciduous teeth, owing to the color of the underlining dentin. * protuberances.

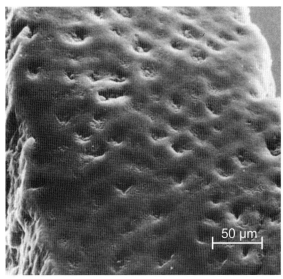

Fig. 1.8 Scanning electron microscopic view of an enamel surface showing developmental defects as Tome's process pits, large enough for microorganisms to shelter in them.

tions of the individual crystals are oriented perpendicular to the surface. This layer is called aprismatic enamel[12] and can present problems when etching enamel for sealing/bonding procedures (see below).

NOTE

Enamel is the hardest tissue in the human body; however, it is still soluble in acid with a pH below 5.5. The inorganic content of enamel is hydroxyapatite (HAP), fluoride hydroxyapatite (FHAP), carbonate-modified hydroxyapatite (CHAP), and magnesium-modified hydroxyapatite (MHAP). FHAP is less soluble than HAP, which is less soluble than CHAP or MHAP.

The Dentin–Pulp Organ

The dentin and the pulp (see **Fig. 1.1**) are closely related developmentally and functionally. The odontoblasts, which are the cells responsible for the formation of the dentin, are separated from the pulp cells only by a cell-free zone.

In contrast to the enamel, dentin continues to be formed after crown formation is complete. This is called secondary dentin formation, which over time results in reduction of the size of the pulp chamber.

The dentin consists of about 70 wt% inorganic material, 18 wt% organic material, and 12 wt% water.[12] As in the enamel, the inorganic material consists of HAP crystals (20 nm in length, <20 nm in width, and 3.5 nm in thickness) which are smaller than those in enamel. As in enamel, the ions in dentin HAP can also be substituted by other ions, for example, fluoride. About 90% of the organic material consists of collagen. The structure of dentin includes dentinal tubules holding the odontoblast process, surrounded by the periodontoblastic spaces, the peritubular dentin, and the intertubular dentin. The mineral content varies in these different parts of the dentin, with the highest mineral level in the peritubular dentin. Dentin is a vital tissue that reacts to a stimulus such as caries by further dentin formation, in particular tubular sclerosis but also reparative dentin (see Chapter 3).

The pulp consists of 25 wt% organic material and 75 wt% water. The organic content is connective tissue cells (fibroblasts), fibers (collagenous in nature), and ground substances (proteoglycans and fibronectin).[12] Arterioles and venules enter and leave the pulp through the apical foramen and accessory root canals. The pulp is richly vascular; however, this changes with age. The nerves follow the course of the blood vessels and often a triad of artery, vein, and nerves is found scattered around the pulp. Extensions of nerve fibers in the pulp are seen along with the odontoblast process in the dentin.

Sensations in the pulp and in the dentin are limited to pain reactions irrespective of the factor initiating the reaction. Pulpal pain is usually dull, throbbing and lasts for some time, dentinal pain is sharp, stabbing, and short-lived.

The Cementum

Cementum made by cementoblasts is the least mineralized of the three dental hard tissues, consisting of about 65 wt% HAP/FHAP or other impure forms of HAP. As with dentin, the majority of the organic matrix (~23%) is composed of collagen. Cementum is a part of the attachment apparatus of the tooth to the alveolar bone. Cementum plays no major role in caries disease as it is often abraded at predilection sites in elderly patients.

NOTE

In contrast to enamel, dentin is a vital tissue, with less inorganic content, and is therefore more soluble in acid than enamel. Cementum often abrades before caries initiates.

Saliva

Saliva Production, Salivary Glands

Saliva is produced mainly by three large pairs of glands: the parotid glands, the submandibular glands, and the sublingual glands (**Fig. 1.9**). The amount of saliva secreted per day is **0.7–1.5L**.[20] Without stimulation, an average of

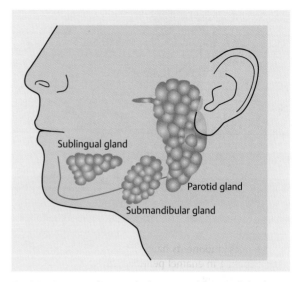

Fig. 1.9   Overview showing the location and names of the three large glands producing >90% of the daily production of saliva.

0.25 mL per minute is produced, while in stimulated conditions an average **0.7 mL per minute** is produced. The saliva covers all surfaces in the mouth with a thin film. The parotid gland secretes thin, watery saliva rich in amylase (an enzyme that breaks down starch into sugar). The submandibular glands secrete viscous, slimy saliva rich in mucin (a protein lubricant that also protects body surfaces). The sublingual glands produce viscous saliva. Without stimulation, two-thirds of the total saliva is secreted by the submandibular glands. Some 50% of stimulated saliva is secreted by the parotid glands and 35% comes from the submandibular glands. On viewing reflected light, one will notice that the floor of the mouth is always wet. About 10% of the daily volume of saliva comes from the minor salivary glands in the tongue, lips, and palate.

Function of Saliva

More than 99% of saliva is water, the rest is electrolytes and organic components including proteins, glycoproteins, and enzymes. The functions of saliva concerning caries are related to all three types of constituent.

The **water** in the saliva contributes to the following:
- Rinsing effect of the mouth (clearance rate)
- Solubilization of food substances
- Facilitation of bolus formation
- Facilitation of food and bacterial clearance
- Dilution of detritus
- Lubrication of oral soft tissues
- Facilitation of mastication, swallowing, and speech

The **electrolytes** have the following functions:
- Maintaining supersaturated calcium and phosphate concentrations in saliva with regard to HAP
- Neutralization of acid by buffering actions

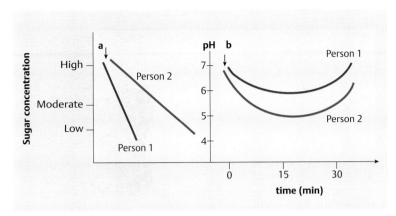

Fig. 1.10a, b
a Simplified illustration of sugar clearance of two persons after sugar intake (arrows); person 1 eliminates sugar faster than person 2.
b Consequently person 2 has a lower pH for a much longer time than person 1. Under such circumstances person 2 will likely develop caries faster than person 1.

The **organic components** have the following functions:
- Participating in enamel pellicle formation
- Mucosal coating
- Antimicrobial defense
- Digestive actions

Clearance rate. Oral clearance can be defined as the dilution and elimination of substances in the oral cavity, which can be fast or slow.[21] **Figure 1.10a** illustrates diagrammatically two persons with different saliva clearance rates,[21] person 1 with a fast clearance and person 2 with a slower clearance. The curves in **Fig. 1.10b** are the corresponding pH variations in plaque (see definition below) following the elimination of the sugar lump. This figure aims to show that a slow clearance may result in a pH drop in the saliva and/or plaque that will be lower and remain so for a longer period, which may be more harmful to the teeth than a faster clearance. It is the salivary flow rate and volumes of saliva in the mouth before and after swallowing that affect the clearance rate. Thus, stimulating saliva secretion by using chewing gum will increase the clearance rate.

Electrolytes. From the caries disease angle, the most important electrolytes are calcium, inorganic phosphate, bicarbonate, and fluoride. The concentration of the various salivary electrolytes is strongly dependent on the salivary flow rate[22,23] (**Fig. 1.11**). It appears that when the flow rate increases, the concentration of the electrolytes increases, apart from inorganic phosphate. The pH of unstimulated and stimulated saliva is between 6 and 7. At this level the relevant ions in saliva are supersaturated, which actually should result in precipitation of the electrolytes resulting in development of mineral on the tooth surface. Why this is not a common phenomenon is explained below.

Buffers. Saliva also has systems which buffer acids from the sugar-fermenting oral microorganisms. A buffer in this context is a substance which, to a certain degree, resists changes in pH. In the development of caries disease the two following buffer systems are important:

- The phosphate system
- The bicarbonate system

The form of phosphate in saliva is influenced by its pH. At pH 7.5–6.0 most of the phosphate is present as dihydrogen ($H_2PO_4^-$) and monohydrogen (HPO_4^-) phosphate, which exchange H^+ ions according to the following reaction:

$$H^+ + HPO_4^{2-} \rightleftarrows H_2PO_4^-$$

When the pH value decreases, that is, the H^+ concentration increases, hydrogen phosphate binds a hydrogen ion and changes to a dihydrogen phosphate ion. Thus, if there is sufficient monohydrogen species to react with H^+, the pH will not drop further.

The bicarbonate system works at a lower pH than the phosphate system (around 6) and takes up H^+ according to the following reaction:

$$H^+ + HCO_3^- \rightleftarrows H_2CO_3 \rightleftarrows CO_2 + H_2O$$

This system works best with stimulated saliva, because the concentration of HCO_3^- increases with increasing flow rate (**Fig. 1.11**).[22–24] The release of carbon dioxide gas (CO_2) from saliva further boosts the buffering capacity of the system as the reaction shifts toward the right.

The organic components of saliva. Table 1.1 presents the most important proteins and enzymes in the saliva and their known functions. It appears that several of them—lysozymes, agglutinins, and antibodies—have a strong antimicrobial function. Of note among the phosphoproteins found in saliva is **statherin**, which is rich in the amino acid tyrosine and is indirectly very important in the caries process. As mentioned above, neutral pH saliva is supersaturated with respect to the ions of HAP, which is the main inorganic component of tooth enamel. Phosphoproteins contain sequences of phosphorin that bind calcium very strongly, thereby maintaining the supersaturated state and at the same time preventing random crystallization from occurring.[25] Statherin is so far the only salivary protein currently known to inhibit both the primary and secondary precipitation of HAP in the supersaturated environment of the saliva. As statherin and

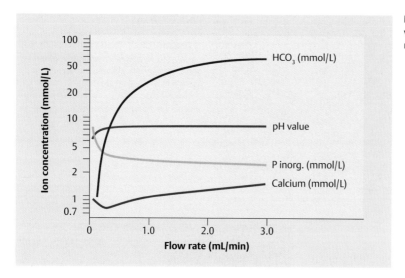

Fig. 1.11 Concentrations of important salivary electrolytes depend on the salivary flow rate (modified from Dawes 2004).[23]

Table 1.1 Organic components in the saliva and their possible roles

Organic component	Function
Amylase	Degradation of starch
Lysozyme	Antimicrobial activity by destruction of bacterial cell membranes
Lactoferrin	Antimicrobial activity by high affinity for iron
Peroxidase	Antimicrobial activity and protection against H_2O_2
Agglutinin	Antimicrobial activity by agglutination of bacteria to large aggregates
Statherin	Inhibits spontaneous precipitation
Antibodies	IgA/IgG, IgM inhibition of adhesion, enhancement of phagocytosis

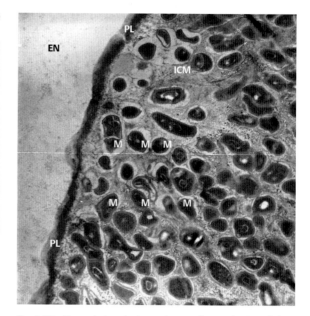

Fig. 1.12 Transmission electron microscopic examination of dental plaque consisting of microorganisms (M) and intercellular substances (ICM) lying next to the pellicle (PL) which in turn is lying next to the enamel (EN), which in this case has been removed artificially.

other inhibitors are proteins, they are subject to microbiological degradation, in particular caused by acids in the plaque.

Pellicle

The pellicle is a thin, bacteria-free layer covering the teeth (**Fig. 1.12**). It is formed by the adsorption of salivary proteins, for example, glycoproteins, which have high affinity for the mineral in the surface of the tooth.[26] The positively charged HAP crystals will attract negatively charged organic components from the saliva. If the pellicle is removed, for example, by the dentist during a professional cleaning, it will start forming again within seconds. The thickness of the pellicle varies in different areas of the

teeth, generally ranging from 1 µm to 10 µm. However, it can be thicker and it can become discolored due to the staining from foods and/or tobacco.

The pellicle plays an important role in protecting the dental hard tissue against mechanical and chemical damage: mechanically, so it is not worn away, and chemically because the pellicle serves as a permselective diffusion barrier,[27] limiting what can pass through it, including plaque acids.

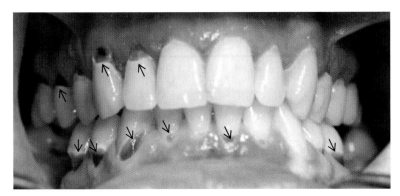

Fig. 1.13 Example of a patient who suffers from hyposalivation (unstimulated flow rate of 0.05 mL/min) and xerostomia due to the use of antidepressants. The oral mucosa is dry and caries (arrows) is seen located primarily along the gingival margin.

Hyposalivation

Hyposalivation is a diagnosis made when the unstimulated salivary flow rate is less than 0.1 mL/min and/or when the stimulated flow rate is less than 0.7 mL/min.[28]

The following conditions can influence the flow rate and lead to hyposalivation:

- Medications—for example, antidepressants, diuretics, antihistamines, antihypertensives, antiemetics, narcotics
- Radiation
- Autoimmune diseases, AIDS, diabetes mellitus
- Menopause
- Eating disorders
- Salivary gland stones

Xerostomia is the subjective feeling (symptom) of a sensation of oral dryness, which often impairs oral function and even the overall quality of life. A salivary flow rate below 0.16 mL/min increases the risk of developing caries[29] (**Fig. 1.13**), which is related to the reasons mentioned above (low clearance rate, less supersaturation with respect to important electrolytes).

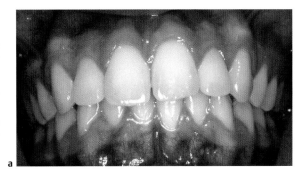

a

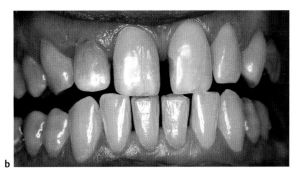

b

Fig. 1.14a, b Dentition of a young (**a**) and old (**b**) person. Wear is a natural aging process that only turns pathologic if it is excessive for the respective age and results in clinical symptoms.

> **NOTE**
>
> Saliva is the liquid of the oral cavity and reduces dissolution of the dental hard tissue by its clearance ability, by means of its content of electrolytes, and its content of antimicrobials. Hyposalivation therefore increases the risk of caries development.

Changes in Teeth and Saliva with Aging

Most tissues in the human body have a physiological turnover of their components. The rate of turnover varies from tissue to tissue; in the pulp tissue the turnover is considered to be high, while it is limited for the dentin and cementum. Tooth enamel is a tissue with no biological turnover after it is formed. Alteration of enamel during a lifetime is thus physico-chemically related. Wear will cause loss of incisal protuberances, perikymata, and imbrication lines resulting in a flattening of the teeth with age (cf. **Fig. 1.14a, b**). At the crystal level, old enamel has a higher content of fluoride,[30] the reason for which will be covered in Chapters 2 and 12.

At least two age-dependent changes take place in the dentin; namely physiological dentin formation and gradual obturation of the dental tubules. The former is referred to as **secondary dentin** formation, to differentiate it from primary dentin formation which occurs until the tooth is fully formed, while the latter is referred to as **dentin**, or **tubular sclerosis**. The changes in the dentin during a lifetime have some clinical and cosmetic implications[31]; thus the diminishing size of the pulp chamber due to the secondary dentin formation may prevent pulp reaction and pulp exposure, but may also complicate pulp treatment. Tubular sclerosis results in a   reduction in the sensitivity and permeability of dentin, although the latter may prevent ingress of toxic agents deeper into the dentin. The sum effect of changes in the dentin (condensation) influences the color of the teeth, thus owing to the translucence of the enamel, the color of older teeth is more yellow than younger teeth (**Fig. 1.14b**).

The most striking age-related change in the cementum is that its width nearly triples with age. To the best knowledge of the authors this has no clinical implication.

The pulp changes with age—in general from a cell-rich and fiber-poor tissue to a cell-poor and fiber-rich tissue.[31] These changes are important from a clinical point of view, as the reactivity of an old pulp is different from the young one. This must be taken into consideration when choosing between different treatment options.

As described above, more than 99% of saliva is water, thus less than 1% is electrolytes and organic components. What happens to these components with age? Most data[32,33] indicate that there are changes in the structure of the salivary glands due to age, but it seems that these changes are not sufficient to significantly influence the three components (water, electrolytes, and organics) in such a way that the tendency for developing caries increases. Instead of relating the increasing prevalence and incidence of caries seen in elderly people to age-related disorders of the salivary glands, we should rather consider age as a possible contributory factor to increasing patient vulnerability.[33]

Dental professionals should be able to differentiate between signs of natural aging/wear and signs of pathological processes. However, it should be kept in mind that the transition between "natural aging" and "disease" is mostly fluid, and the definition of what is "disease" is often controversial.

Dental Plaque or Dental Biofilm?

Definition. Dental plaque is a general term for the complex microbial community found on the tooth surface embedded in a matrix of polymers of bacterial and salivary origin.[34] The term "**dental plaque**" has been used by the dental profession since G.V. Black (see Preface) defined it at the end of the 19th century. Professionals use it clinically for describing **visible accumulations of microorganisms on teeth**. More recently the term "**dental biofilm**" has been used to describe dental plaque. Biofilms are defined as "3-D accumulations of interacting microorganisms attached to a surface, embedded in a matrix of extracellular polymers."[35] Biofilms are also found on other, water-covered surfaces, for example, the waterlines in dental units and in aquariums. Throughout this book the

authors will use both terms for visible accumulations of microorganisms on the teeth.

> **NOTE**
>
> In the context of caries, dental plaque or dental biofilm is the same—meaning visible accumulation of microorganisms mixed with intercellular substance on the teeth.

Classifying Oral Microorganisms

The Dutchman Antonie van Leeuwenhoek was the first to discover small organisms in dental plaque by means of simple microscopy. Actually what he saw was microorganisms of differing morphology—some small and round, some quite long, some lying still, and some moving. Since then, microorganisms in the oral cavity have been examined using simple and more complex light microscopes; sometimes the microorganisms are colored, other times not so (e.g. **gram+** or **gram−**) (**Table 1.2**). The microorganisms have also been examined by means of electron microscopy, cultivation on different media, and more recently by means of genetic methods. Today, more than 700 different species have been identified in oral biofilms. The composition of species varies between individuals and various tooth sites, and even within different locations of the plaque.

Table 1.3 shows the overall **biological classification hierarchy** of two of the most studied microorganisms relating to caries disease, namely *Streptococcus mutans* and *Lactobacillus acidophilus*. Both are Bacteria (Kingdom) and have a gram-positive cell wall structure (Firmicutes). *S. mutans* is a coccus and *L. acidophilus* a rod (Class), and the major metabolic end product of carbohydrate fermentation is lactic acid, making them *Lactobacillales* (Order); they belong to the families of Streptococcaceae and Lactobacillaceae, respectively. Microbes of the genus *Streptococcus* (**Table 1.3**)—which make up the majority of the microorganisms in the oral cavity and include the species *S. mutans*—are thus facultative anaerobic gram-positive cocci occurring in chains, which do not move or produce spores (**Table 1.2**). Microbes of the genus *Lactobacillus*, of which *L. acidophilus* is a member (**Table 1.3**), are mainly facultative anaerobic gram-positive rods, which do not move or produce spores (**Table 1.2**).

Differentiation within the individual species can be seen, for example, by means of the growth pattern on a range of selective and nonselective agar plates (**Table 1.2**). Concerning the streptococci, *S. mutans* can be differentiated from *S. sanguinis* by the pattern of colony formation when cultivated on Mitis Salivarius Agar. *S. mutans* appears as slimy granulated colonies, while *S. sanguinis* appears as small, firmly adhering colonies. Biochemical tests show in addition that *S. mutans* metabolizes sorbitol while *S. sanguinis* does not.

Table 1.2 Traditional way to classify oral microorganisms, with examples

Feature	Parameter value	Streptococci	Lactobacilli
Cell morphology	Cocci, rods, filaments, etc.	Coccoid	Rod
Gram (dye) coloring of micro-organisms	Positive or negative	Positive	Positive
Cell arrangement	Single or chains	Chains	Random, but often in chains
Movements	yes/no	no	no
Spore	yes/no	no	no
Oxygen tolerance	Aerobe, facultative anaerobe and strict anaerobe	Facultative anaerobe	Facultative anaerobe
Catalase	Positive or negative	Negative	Negative
Carbohydrate metabolism	Homo- or hetero-fermentation	Both	Both

By the use of other techniques introduced in the 1980s such as serological and genetic testing methods (checkerboard DNA–DNA hybridization, polymerase chain reaction),[36,37] it has been suggested that *S. mutans* can be subdivided into subgroups, such as serotypes a–h, where the original *S. mutans* consists of serotypes c, e, and f. Serotypes d and g are called *S. sobrinus*. This differentiation is important because some serotypes produce more acid from sucrose than *S. mutans*.[38]

Colonization of the Mouth in the Newborn

When a child is born his or her mouth is usually sterile, but will very quickly become colonized by microorganisms, particularly from the mother, but also from other sources such as milk, food, water, etc. The first microorganisms to colonize the mouth of a newborn are termed **pioneers**.[34] Further development or microbial succession is dependent on the conditions offered to or changed by these pioneers, for example, nutrition and local pH. Eventually, a **climax community develops**, which is a stable, complex microbial community of great species diversity. In the period before the first teeth appear, the microflora consists mainly of Streptococcus and in particular *Streptococcus salivarius*. However, plaque development does not occur on oral soft tissues in the same way as on teeth, owing to the continual shedding of the outer cells harboring the microorganisms. When the first teeth appear, a change in the microflora is noted, as types which can adhere to dental hard tissues such as *S. mutans* and *S. sanguini* become established.

Table 1.3 Biological classification of the *Streptococcus mutans* and *Lactobacillus acidophilus*

	Streptococcus mutans	Lactobacillus acidophilus
Kingdom	Bacteria	Bacteria
Division/Phylum	Firmicutes	Firmicutes
Class	Bacilli (coccoid)	Bacilli (rod)
Order	Lactobacillales	Lactobacillales
Family	Streptococcaceae	Lactobacillaceae
Genus	Streptococcus	Lactobacillus
Species	*Mutans, salivarius*, etc.	*Acidophilus, casei*, etc.

Plaque: Development and Metabolic End Products

Professional cleaning as well as tooth brushing, if done properly, removes plaque and the pellicle on the teeth leaving the enamel naked. When saliva moistens the teeth a new pellicle will start to form. During the first couple of hours after the cleaning procedure microorganisms in the saliva will adhere to the **pellicle** on the teeth by means of weak biological as well as electrostatic forces such as van der Waal's interaction.[39] Such microorganisms are also called **pioneers**, as mentioned above, when a newborn child's mouth is colonized. The pioneers are mostly *Streptococcus sanguinis*, *S. oralis* and *S. mitis* biovar 1, but genera such as *Actinomyces*, *Haemophilus*, and *Neisseria* are also present.[40] The mechanism of this initial adherence of microorganisms to the pellicle is complex and not fully

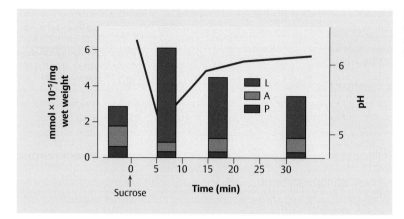

Fig. 1.15 Acidic metabolic end products and change of pH in dental plaque before and after intake of a lump of sugar [2]. L: lactic acid; A: acetic acid; P: propionic acid.

understood. However, it seems that microorganisms have a kind of recognition system in their cell membrane which fits to receptors in the pellicle.[39] In addition, microorganisms can shelter in development defects and in the groove–fossa system without physicochemical interactive forces.[18,19]

The microorganisms need energy for their survival and replication. They can use many different methods for obtaining energy, which is influenced by the substrate available in the mouth that comes from saliva and the host's diet. The pioneers accumulated on the teeth after 3–6 hours are arranged in a **monolayer**. The pioneers, which primarily are aerobes or facultative anaerobes, will most likely use oxygen from the surrounding salivary film, which enters via the cell membrane, and the tricarboxylic acid cycle of Krebs (see Ref. [1] or other biochemical textbooks) to get intracellular energy. The end products leaving the cells are CO_2 and water, which are not harmful to the teeth.

Through multiplication of the pioneers and arrival of newcomers, over the next few hours a rapid increase in the number of microorganisms accumulating on the teeth is seen (6–12 h). Thus, the monolayer of microorganisms is replaced by **multiple layers**.[40] As the thickness of the layers increases (at a certain stage it becomes visible, and thus, as plaque), the oxygen tension in the inner layer (against the tooth surface) will drop, and the microorganisms in that layer will shift their metabolism and become more facultative anaerobic or strictly anaerobic.

In the case of no access to dietary sources of nutrition, the microorganisms get energy primarily from the glycoproteins in the saliva. Under such conditions, the by-products of metabolism by microorganisms on the teeth are evenly distributed among lactic acid, acetic acid, and propionic acid (**Fig. 1.15**). The concentration and strength of these acids do not harm the teeth, mainly owing to the action of the buffering systems. In the case of access to fermentable carbohydrates, the pH will drop in the liquid phase of the plaque within 3 minutes, and it takes about 20–30 minutes for the pH to return to normal. The reason for the pH drop is that some microorganisms are able to convert the available sugar—which due to its very high

concentration enters the cell membrane passively—via the glycolytic pathway and metabolize it to lactate[1] (**Fig. 1.16**). The fraction of lactate increases eightfold[2] during the first couple of minutes after starting to eat breakfast. This process requires that the microorganism has a system of constitutive enzymes, and in this case it is the **lactate dehydrogenase** that enables the microorganism to transform pyruvate to lactate, which then is released through the cell membrane (lactate gate) to the environment[1] (**Fig. 1.16**). During the metabolic process energy in the form of ATP is created. The microorganisms use the energy from ATP mainly for cell functions and replication. Microorganisms that do not possess lactate dehydrogenase may die, caused by substrate (sugar) killing. Some microorganisms can also synthesize intracellular polysaccharides to be used as "fuel" when there is no sugar in the surroundings to be metabolized.[1] Finally, some microorganisms also have constitutive enzymes, such as glucosyltransferases and fructosyltransferases, which can convert sucrose to glucans and fructans (extracellular polysaccharides), respectively. Glucans serve to glue the microorganisms together, and fructans are easily metabolized and can act as a reserve source of nutrients.[1]

NOTE

Microorganisms in cariogenic plaque have the following characteristics[35]:
- Anaerobe or facultative anaerobe
- Acidogenic (produce acid, mainly lactic acid)
- Aciduric (can survive under low pH conditions)
- Produce intracellular polysaccharides
- Produce extracellular polysaccharides

Plaque Stagnation Areas

Plaque development can only happen on areas of the teeth where there is no mechanical or chemical disturbance.[9,34,35,41] Examples of mechanical disturbance on the teeth are movements of the tongue and lips, and oral hygiene practices such as tooth brushing, flossing, etc.

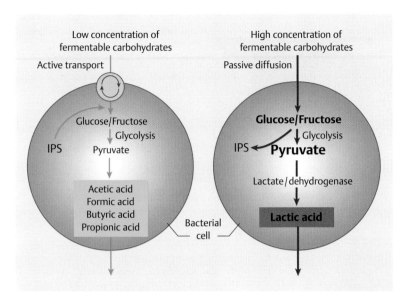

Fig. 1.16 Schematic illustration of how polysaccharides and disaccharides (carbohydrates) enter into the cells of the microorganism and are broken down into monosaccharides (glucose and fructose), which are used to create energy by glycolysis or to create intracellular polysaccharides (JPS) as an energy reservoir. The end products of fermentation are acids which the microorganism excretes. When carbohydrates are present in high concentration, lactic acid is created which can demineralize the dental hard tissues.

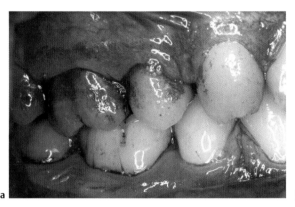

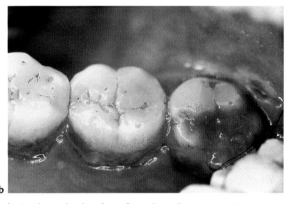

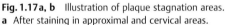

Fig. 1.17a, b Illustration of plaque stagnation areas.
a After staining in approximal and cervical areas.

b On the occlusal surface of a molar without antagonist.

Due to mechanical disturbance from chewing, we don't see plaque accumulation on the incisal third of the incisors. **Functional wear and tear is limited** along the marginal gingiva, below or above the contact points between approximal surfaces and on the entire occlusal surface including the cusp areas during the eruption period of molar and premolar teeth, and after full occlusion is established the groove–fossa system of these teeth, while plaque will accumulate in these locations (**Fig. 1.17**) if it is not removed by oral hygiene methods. These locations are called plaque stagnation areas in dentistry. Interestingly, it is exactly in these areas that caries can develop.[9,41]

Plaque Composition and Structure in Stagnation Areas

Different methods, including light and electron microscopy (**Fig. 1.18**) as well as cultivation studies, have been used to examine the composition and structure of plaque in stagnation areas, from which it is clear that the composition and structure of plaque vary in different locations.

In fissure parts of the groove–fossa system, on smooth surfaces, and on approximal surfaces the microorganisms are arranged in palisades perpendicular to the tooth surface and composed of many dividing cells[40,42] (**Fig. 1.18 d**). This indicates a vital flora.[42] In contrast, the content in the bottom part of the fissures consists of an unorganized material of dead microorganisms, with inter- as well as intracellular evidence of minerals[40] (**Fig. 1.18 e**). This arrangement of the microflora in the fissures suggests that the unfavorable conditions for bacterial growth deep in the fissures account for the findings that caries in fissures develops at the entrance to the fissures.[42–44]

Chapter 2 will cover the diversity of the oral microflora in more detail.

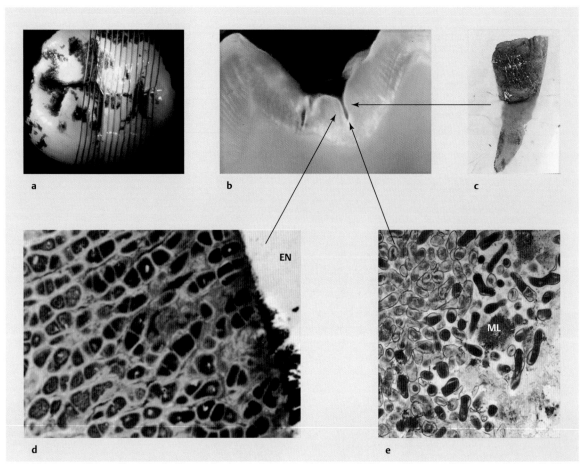

Fig. 1.18a–e   An example of how to examine microorganisms in the groove–fossa system. Just after extraction the tooth was serial-sectioned (**a, b**). The hard tissue was removed leaving the plaque of which semi-thin sections were prepared (**c**). Ultrathin sections were prepared and examined in a transmission electron microscope (**d, e**). At the entrance many dividing microorganisms are seen and they are arranged perpendicular to the enamel surface (EN) (**d**). In the lower zone few cell divisions, no structure, and areas of mineralization (ML) are visible (**e**).

SUMMARY

Physiological Interaction Between the Three Systems in the Oral Cavity

Teeth consist of enamel, dentin, cementum, and the pulp tissue. Microorganisms in the mouth will adhere to the tooth surface and grow if not removed by physiological functions or by oral hygiene measures. When the teeth are clean and in direct contact with saliva with a pH around 7 (**Fig. 1.19a**), saliva is supersaturated with respect to the minerals found in the dental hard tissue, which is mainly hydroxyapatite. According to the Le Chatelier law, the hydroxyapatite should be precipitated; however, due to various proteins in the saliva, such as statherin, this does not take place. In the case that microorganisms accumulate, and metabolize carbohydrates, different kinds of acid are produced and consequently the pH will drop somewhat (**Fig. 1.19b**).

The buffering systems in the saliva will initially neutralize the acids. If mature (cariogenic) plaque is developed, the microorganisms will primarily secrete lactic acid when they metabolize carbohydrates, which will lead to an undersaturation of relevant ions in the saliva and this will result in demineralization of the dental hard tissues (**Fig. 1.19c**). The undersaturated condition in the saliva, relative to calcium, phosphate, and the hydroxyl ions, occurs when the pH is lower than 5.5. What happens when the pH returns to normal, and how fluoride and statherin interact with these processes, will be covered in Chapters 2 and 3. Besides the electrolytes in the saliva, the clearance rate is very important in the caries process, as a high clearance rate, for example, by masticating chewing gum, will cause the pH drop to be less than if the clearance rate were suboptimal, or even compromised as seen in cases of hyposalivation (**Fig. 1.20**).

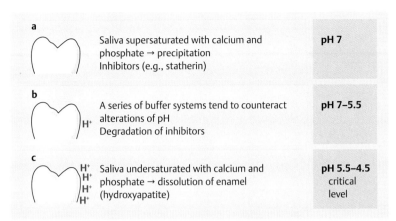

a

Saliva supersaturated with calcium and phosphate → precipitation Inhibitors (e.g., statherin)

pH 7

b

A series of buffer systems tend to counteract alterations of pH Degradation of inhibitors

pH 7–5.5

c

Saliva undersaturated with calcium and phosphate → dissolution of enamel (hydroxyapatite)

pH 5.5–4.5 critical level

Fig. 1.19a–c Schematic illustration of the relation between acid (H^+), pH drop, and the interaction of the buffers in the saliva.

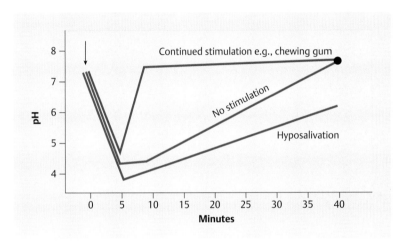

Fig. 1.20 Schematic diagram showing the relationship between pH drop after sugar intake (arrow) and the function of saliva with stimulation, without stimulation, and in hyposalivation. It appears that with stimulation the pH returns much faster to its normal level.

REFERENCES

1. Cole AS, Eastoe JE. Biochemistry and Oral Biology. Bristol: John Wright and Sons; 1977

2. Geddes DA. Acids produced by human dental plaque metabolism in situ. Caries Res 1975;9(2):98–109

3. Carlsen O. Dental Morphology. Copenhagen: Munksgaard; 1987

4. Krogh-Poulsen W. Tændernes morfologi. 3rd ed. Copenhagen: Munksgaard; 1967

5. Schour I, Massler M. Studies in tooth development. The growth patterns of human teeth. J Am Dent Assoc 1940;27:1778–1793, 1918–1931

6. Lysell L, Magnusson B, Thilander B. Time and order of eruption of the primary teeth. A longitudinal study. Odontol Revy 1962;13: 217–234

7. Kurol J, Rasmussen P. Occlusal development, preventive and interceptive orthodontics. In: Koch G, Poulsen S, eds. Pediatric Dentistry. Copenhagen: Munksgaard; 2001:321–349

8. Helm S, Seidler B. Timing of permanent tooth emergence in Danish children. Community Dent Oral Epidemiol 1974;2(3): 122–129

9. Carvalho JC, Ekstrand KR, Thylstrup A. Dental plaque and caries on occlusal surfaces of first permanent molars in relation to stage of eruption. J Dent Res 1989;68(5):773–779

10. Ekstrand KR, Martignon S, Christiansen ME. Frequency and distribution patterns of sealants among 15-year-olds in Denmark in 2003. Community Dent Health 2007;24(1):26–30

11. Nielsen LA. Cariesprogression i det primære tandsæt fra 3-til 7 års-alderen. Tandlaegebladet 2001;105:704–711

12. Mjør IA, Fejerskov O, eds. Human Oral Embryology and Histology. Copenhagen: Munksgaard; 1986

13. Wang L, Guan X, Yin H, Moradian-Oldak J, Nancollas GH. Mimicking the self-organized microstructure of tooth enamel. J Phys Chem C Nanomater Interfaces 2008;112(15):5892–5899

14. Young RA. Implications of atomic substitutions and other structural details in apatites. J Dent Res 1974;53(2):193–203

15. Larsen MJ. Dissolution of enamel. Scand J Dent Res 1973;81(7): 518–522

16. Ten Cate JM, Featherstone JDB. Physicochemical aspects of fluoride-enamel interactions. In: Fejerskov O, Ekstrand J, Burt BA, eds. Fluoride in Dentistry. Copenhagen: Munksgaard; 1996: 252–272

17. Shellis RP, Duckworth RM. Studies on the cariostatic mechanisms of fluoride. Int Dent J 1994; 44(3, Suppl 1)263–273

18. Fejerskov O, Josephsen K, Nyvad B. Surface ultrastructure of unerupted mature human enamel. Caries Res 1984;18(4): 302–314

19. Ekstrand K, Holmen L, Qvortrup K. A polarized light and scanning electron microscopic study of human fissure and lingual enamel of unerupted mandibular third molars. Caries Res 1999;33(1): 41–49

20. Ferguson DB. The salivary glands and their secretions. In: Ferguson DB, ed. Oral Bioscience. Edinburgh: Churchill Livingstone; 1999:118–150

21. Bardow A, Hofer E, Nyvad B, et al. Effect of saliva composition on experimental root caries. Caries Res 2005;39(1):71–77

22. Dawes C. The effects of flow rate and duration of stimulation on the condentrations of protein and the main electrolytes in human parotid saliva. Arch Oral Biol 1969;14(3):277–294

23. Dawes C. The effects of flow rate and duration of stimulation on the concentrations of protein and the main electrolytes in human submandibular saliva. Arch Oral Biol 1974;19(10):887–895

24. Dawes C. Factors influencing salivary flow rate and composition. In: Edgar M, Dawes C, O'Mullane D, eds. Saliva and Oral Health. London: BDJ Books; 2004:32–49

25. Moreno EC, Varughese K, Hay DI. Effect of human salivary proteins on the precipitation kinetics of calcium phosphate. Calcif Tissue Int 1979;28(1):7–16

26. Lendenmann U, Grogan J, Oppenheim FG. Saliva and dental pellicle—a review. Adv Dent Res 2000;14:22–28

27. Zahradnik RT, Moreno EC, Burke EJ. Effect of salivary pellicle on enamel subsurface demineralization in vitro. J Dent Res 1976; 55(4):664–670

28. Nederfors T. Xerostomia and hyposalivation. Adv Dent Res 2000;14:48–56

29. Bardow A, Lagerlöf F, Nauntofte B, et al. The role of saliva. In: Fejerskov O, Kidd E, eds. Dental Caries. The Disease and its Clinical Management. Oxford: Blackwell Munksgaard; 2008: 190–207

30. Brudevold F. Aldersforandringer I tandnemaljen. Nor Tandlægeforen Tid 1957;67:451–458

31. Mjør IA. Changes in the teeth with aging. In: Holm-Pedersen P, Löe H, eds. Textbook of Geriatric Dentistry. Copenhagen: Munksgaard; 1996:94–102

32. Scott J. Degenerative changes in the histology of the human submandibular salivary gland occurring with age. J Biol Buccale 1977;5(4):311–319

33. Baum BJ. Changes in salivary glands and salivary secretion with aging. In: Holm-Pedersen P, Löe H, eds. Textbook of Geriatric Dentistry. Copenhagen: Munksgaard; 1996:117–126

34. Marsh PD, Martin M. Oral microbiology. 3rd ed. London: Chapman and Hall; 1992

35. Marsh PD. Microbial ecology of dental plaque and its significance in health and disease. Adv Dent Res 1994;8(2):263–271

36. Sibley CG, Ahlquist JE. The phylogeny of the hominoid primates, as indicated by DNA-DNA hybridization. J Mol Evol 1984;20(1): 2–15

37. Smith M. Nobel lecture. Synthetic DNA and biology. Biosci Rep 1994;14(2):51–66

38. de Soet JJ, Nyvad B, Kilian M. Strain-related acid production by oral streptococci. Caries Res 2000;34(6):486–490

39. Gibbons RJ. Bacterial adhesion to oral tissues: a model for infectious diseases. J Dent Res 1989;68(5):750–760

40. Nyvad B, Kilian M. Microbiology of the early colonization of human enamel and root surfaces in vivo. Scand J Dent Res 1987;95(5):369–380

41. Thylstrup A, Bruun C, Holmen L. In vivo caries models—mechanisms for caries initiation and arrestment. Adv Dent Res 1994; 8(2):144–157

42. Ekstrand KR, Bjørndal L. Structural analyses of plaque and caries in relation to the morphology of the groove-fossa system on erupting mandibular third molars. Caries Res 1997;31(5): 336–348

43. Carvalho JC, Thylstrup A, Ekstrand KR. Results after 3 years of non-operative occlusal caries treatment of erupting permanent first molars. Community Dent Oral Epidemiol 1992;20(4): 187–192

44. Ekstrand KR, Kuzmina IN, Kuzmina E, Christiansen ME. Two and a half-year outcome of caries-preventive programs offered to groups of children in the Solntsevsky district of Moscow. Caries Res 2000;34(1):8–19

45. Wakita M, Kobayashi S. The three-dimensional structure of Tomes' processes and the development of the microstructural organisation of tooth enamel. In: Suga S, ed. Mechanisms of Tooth and Enamel Formation. Berlin: Quintessenz;1983:165

Etiology and Pathogenesis of Caries

Peter Shellis

2

As described in Chapter 1, teeth are continuously bathed in saliva, one of the main functions of which is to minimize mineral dissolution and precipitation within the mouth[1,2]: both can be harmful to the teeth and other oral tissues. Saliva can ameliorate the effects of challenges that tend to dissolve tooth tissue, such as consumption of acidic foods, because it has an approximately neutral pH, is reasonably well buffered, and contains mineral ions. In dental caries, this homoeostasis is overcome by acid-generating metabolic processes in localized accumulations of bacteria. This in turn causes loss of mineral from the hard tissues, which destroys their integrity and eventually impairs their function.

Most of the surface of a tooth is kept free of bacteria by friction from the tongue, cheeks, and foodstuffs. However, bacteria colonize areas of the surface protected from these frictional forces (plaque stagnation areas) and form a film of closely packed bacteria known as **dental plaque**[3,4] within which is created a unique microenvironment, partly isolated from the saliva and immediately adjacent to the tooth surface. The human diet includes a variety of easily-fermentable carbohydrates: monosaccharides such as glucose and fructose; disaccharides such as sucrose and maltose; and oligosaccharides such as those found in honey. In this chapter, these will be collectively referred to as 'sugar' and specific carbohydrates will be named. On each occasion when sugars are ingested, they are metabolized by plaque bacteria and this results in the accumulation of organic acid end products and hence causes a temporary reduction in plaque pH. Such an episode can pose a "**cariogenic challenge**" since, if the plaque pH falls low enough, mineral within the underlying dental hard tissue can dissolve. The progressive loss of mineral through dissolution by plaque acid (**demineralization**) during repeated cariogenic challenges is the primary process in dental caries.

This basic etiology is summarized by the well-known Venn diagram of Keyes[5] (**Fig. 2.1**), which illustrates the interaction of the three factors "tooth," "bacteria," and "diet." While the combination of two factors will produce a contribution (e.g., bacteria + tooth → plaque; bacteria + diet → acid), the interaction of all three is required for caries initiation. Lesions are initiated only at sites where plaque accumulates. In economically developed populations, primary caries lesions are initiated in children on the enamel surface: most commonly in occlusal pits and fissures, less often on approximal surfaces, and rarely on smooth surfaces. In young adulthood, approximal caries increases. In older people, root surfaces exposed by gingival recession are sites for new primary lesions, and the margins of restorations are sites for secondary or recurrent caries lesions.[6]

Caries tends to progress relatively slowly (over months or years) and in the early stages demineralization produces subsurface lesions which can in principle be arrested or reversed. Between cariogenic challenges, plaque pH returns toward "resting" levels which are approximately neutral, and this allows the possibility that mineral ions in

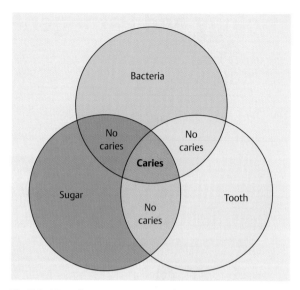

Fig. 2.1   Venn diagram summarizing the etiology of caries. The diagram demonstrates that caries requires both the presence of acidogenic bacteria and availability of a diet from which the bacteria can produce acid, in conjunction with acid-susceptible dental tissues.[5]

plaque can contribute to re-deposition of mineral within the caries lesion: a process known as **remineralization**. Thus, the caries process is not one-directional but involves a dynamic process of mineral loss and regain[7] (**Fig. 2.2**). If the balance between these processes favors demineralization, caries lesions progress and ultimately the damage to the tissue, due to mechanical breakdown (enamel) or to bacterial action (dentin), becomes irreversible. Restoration or extraction then becomes the only treatment option.

Despite this apparently simple etiology, caries is regarded as a multifactorial disease, for two main reasons. First, despite much research, it has not been proven whether it is caused by one specific pathogen or by several bacteria. Second, the risk of caries occurrence, and the rate at which the disease progresses, are influenced by a large number of factors.[6,8] These form a hierarchy at individual, behavioral, and social levels:

- **Individual factors**: the oral bacterial flora; the solubility of tooth mineral; hard tissue structure; salivary flow rate and composition
- **Behavioral factors**: frequency with which foods containing fermentable carbohydrate are consumed; frequency and effectiveness of oral hygiene; pattern of dental check-ups
- **Social factors**, such as level of education and socioeconomic status, influence aspects of individual behavior which impinge on caries. Caries incidence in children is strongly influenced by the level of care provided by those looking after them, especially with respect to diet, attention to oral hygiene, and attendance at the dentist. Care provision is in turn influenced by the caregiver's background.

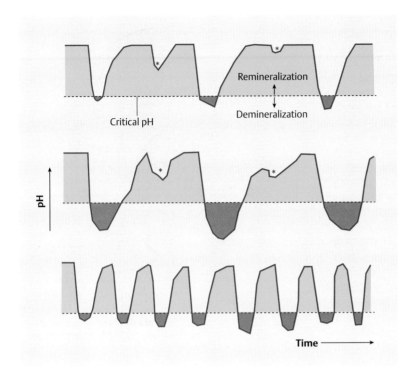

Fig. 2.2 The demineralization–remineralization balance in caries etiology. During the course of a day, intakes of sugar lead to episodes of reduced plaque pH. Not all present a threat to the tooth tissues (asterisks): only those in which pH falls below the critical pH can induce demineralization (shaded areas). Where sugar intake is infrequent and limited (top), the proportion of time spent below the critical pH is small and the resulting demineralization is compensated by remineralization during periods when plaque pH is approximately neutral. However, the demineralization–remineralization balance is tipped in favor of demineralization if increased amounts of sugar are ingested leading to deeper, more prolonged pH falls (middle), or if sugar is ingested more frequently (bottom). In both cases, the proportion of time when plaque conditions favor demineralization is increased at the expense of time when remineralization could replace the lost mineral.

Caries is profoundly influenced by exposure to **fluoride**, which reduces demineralization and enhances remineralization.[7,9] As fluoride is most often delivered in the form of toothpaste, social and behavioral influences on oral hygiene habits take on a special significance (see Chapter 13).

The aims of this chapter are to outline the relevant biological and chemical factors, and to describe their interactions in caries initiation and progression. In particular this chapter will cover:

- **Microbiology**: changes in plaque flora associated with caries
- **Chemistry of dental minerals**: concepts of solubility, dissolution and crystal growth; properties of tooth minerals; the effects of fluoride
- **The cariogenic challenge**: properties of dental plaque; acid production from sugar and its effect on pH; factors influencing severity of the cariogenic challenge
- **Chemistry of caries**: physicochemical processes controlling lesion formation and arrest

Caries is not the only demineralization-related oral disease. **Dental erosion,** caused by direct action of acids on tooth surfaces without bacterial action, results in increased wear.[10] A brief discussion of dental erosion concludes the chapter.

Microbiology of Caries

In his chemo-parasitic theory (1890), Miller postulated that caries was caused by acids produced in the mouth by bacteria metabolizing dietary carbohydrate in food particles retained between the teeth.[68] Until the 1960s lactobacilli were favored as the likely pathogens because they are highly **acidogenic** (capable of rapidly converting sugar to acid) and **aciduric** (capable of withstanding low-pH conditions). Then, from a series of classic experiments with rodents, it was concluded that caries was an infectious, transmissible disease[11] and attention shifted to streptococci, especially *Streptococcus mutans*, first isolated in 1928. Besides being acidogenic and aciduric, *S. mutans* synthesizes an insoluble, sticky extracellular polysaccharide from sucrose which promotes adhesion of the organism. Since the 1960s, an enormous body of research on the microbiology of caries has accumulated and many observational, longitudinal, and intervention studies have provided strong evidence for an association of *S. mutans* with caries.[12] Indeed, many workers have concluded that *S. mutans* is the sole pathogen involved in caries. Usually, this is extended to include other members of the taxonomic group to which *S. mutans* belongs—the mutans streptococci (see Chapter 1)—particularly *S. sobrinus*, which is also isolated from cariogenic plaque of humans, although less frequently and in smaller numbers than *S. mutans*. The hypothesis that caries is caused by infection with *S. mutans* or the mutans streptococci, is known as the **specific plaque hypothesis**.[13]

However, *S. mutans* usually makes up only a very small proportion of the plaque flora, is not always detectable in plaque associated with caries, and can occur in plaque without caries developing.[14] Further, while *S. mutans* is particularly acidogenic and aciduric, these properties are also exhibited to some extent by a variety of plaque bacteria. These include not only *S. sobrinus* but several "low-pH" members of the Streptococcaceae, such as strains of *S. oralis*. Other acidogenic/aciduric plaque bacteria include strains of *Actinomyces*, such as *A. israelii and A. gerencseriae*, bifidobacteria, and lactobacilli. Recognition of this fact underlies the **nonspecific plaque hypothesis**, which suggests that acidogenic, acid-tolerant bacteria besides *S. mutans* contribute to the caries process and, in the absence of *S. mutans*, could be the sole agents of caries initiation.[14,15]

A third hypothesis, the **ecological plaque hypothesis**, emphasizes the importance of the oral environment in determining the composition and properties of the plaque microflora.[16] According to this hypothesis (**Fig. 2.3**), in the mouths of persons consuming a low-sugar diet the plaque bacteria would derive their energy predominantly from slow breakdown of complex salivary and dietary molecules, so would experience only small and infrequent drops in pH. An increased frequency of sugar intake disrupts the homoeostasis of such a plaque because it favors growth of acidogenic, aciduric bacteria and hence promotes low-pH conditions. Bacteria which are sensitive to low pH grow less well under these conditions and are selected against. Thus an increased availability of sugar causes an **ecological shift** in the plaque microflora which establishes caries-conducive conditions. Since bacteria are selected solely on the basis of their ability to produce acid and to withstand low pH, this process is nonspecific and the bacteria which increase in a high-sugar environment can include a range of species, as noted above. However, if *S. mutans* has colonized the mouth its growth will certainly be favored, especially under conditions of very high sugar intake, which will result in the creation of extremely acidic conditions which give this species a competitive advantage. Such a sugar-rich, low-pH environment would also favor colonization by lactobacilli and by the fungus *Candida*.

The ecological plaque hypothesis is supported by considerable evidence. The microflora of plaque from the approximal region is complex and dominated by Gram-positive, rod-shaped bacteria (mainly *Actinomyces*) and streptococci, of which the most abundant is typically *S. sanguinis*, with smaller proportions of other bacteria, such as *Bacteroides, Neisseria, Veillonella, Fusobacterium, Rothia*, and *Lactobacillus*. However, the composition of the flora varies considerably between different sites on the tooth surface. An increased sugar intake results in a higher proportion of acidogenic/aciduric bacteria,[17] and increases in *S. mutans, Lactobacillus*, and others have been observed, along with a decrease in the less acid-tolerant *S. sanguinis*[18] (**Fig. 2.4**). Plaque from caries-active people has a higher proportion of acidogenic bacteria than that from caries-free people: these changes affect plaque in general,

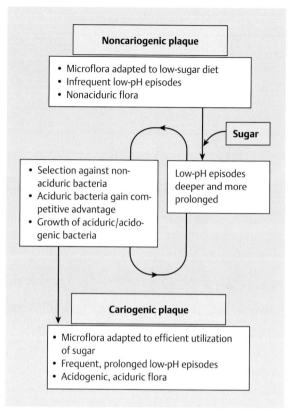

Fig. 2.3 Ecological plaque hypothesis: conversion of noncariogenic plaque (low-sugar diet) to cariogenic plaque (frequent sugar intake). Increased sugar intake causes plaque pH to fall to low levels more frequently or more deeply. If sugar intake is maintained, this leads to a positive feedback loop in which the more acidic plaque environment drives ecological selection of acidogenic, aciduric bacteria and this in turn increases the acidity of the plaque environment. Ultimately the ecological shift favors conditions acidic enough for caries to be initiated.

not just on surfaces on which lesions form.[19] Changes in the plaque flora can be difficult to identify because of extensive intra- and inter-individual variation, but in caries-active people the proportion of *S. sanguinis* and of *Actinomyces naeslundii* typically fall. During the initial stages of caries, the abundance of *S. mutans, S. oralis*, acidogenic actinomyces, such as *A. gerencseriae*, and lactobacilli increase. In advanced (cavitated) lesions, there may be moderate increases in *S. mutans*, but the flora is dominated by lactobacilli, *Bifidobacterium*, and *Prevotella*.[20,21]

Proponents of the specific plaque hypothesis recognize the powerful ecological effect of dietary sugar in determining the composition of plaque microflora, but would argue that only the increases in abundance of *S. mutans* are etiologically significant. However, while there is little doubt that *S. mutans* is a major agent of caries initiation,[22] it is very likely that other acidogenic/aciduric bacteria play important roles in both initiation and progression of lesions.[14,15]

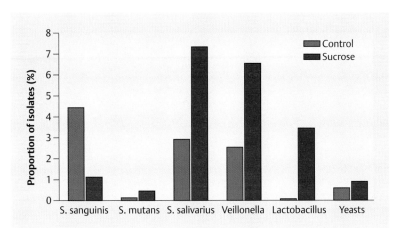

Fig. 2.4 Selected examples of population shifts in the microflora of plaque formed in situ, as a result of exposure to sucrose. "Sucrose" plaques were rinsed with 10% sucrose 6 times a day for 7 days while control plaques were exposed to equivalent numbers of saline rinses. Sucrose exposure results in reduced numbers of the nonacidogenic species, *Streptococcus sanguinis*, but increases in numbers of acidogenic species and of lactate-utilizing *Veillonella*. (Data from ref.[18].)

NOTE

Caries is probably not a "classical" infectious disease, that is, one caused by a specific bacterium not normally found in the body. Instead, it is probably due to over-growth of acid-producing, acid-resistant members of the normal oral flora, driven by excessive consumption of sugars. However, some species, especially *Streptococcus mutans*, do have a prominent, well-documented role in caries etiology.

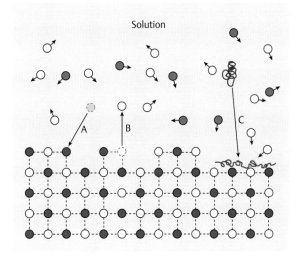

Fig. 2.5 Crystal growth (A) and dissolution (B) as surface processes of exchange of ions/molecules between a solid surface and the bathing solution. On the right (C) is shown adsorption of a macromolecule, which blocks transfer of ions between the solid surface and the solution.

Chemistry of Dental Minerals

Solubility, Dissolution, and Crystal Growth

The processes underlying the phenomena of demineralization and remineralization in caries are crystal dissolution and precipitation. In caries, the latter process is usually manifested as re-growth of partly-dissolved crystals, although precipitation of new crystals can occur. Dissolution and crystal growth are both surface-related processes. At the surface of a solid immersed in an aqueous solution (e.g., enamel crystals bathed in saliva), ions are constantly detaching from the surface and entering the solution and other ions are following the reverse path to become incorporated into the solid (A and B in **Fig. 2.5**). When the rates of these processes are equal, the solid is in equilibrium with the solution and no net dissolution or crystal growth will occur. In this situation, the solution is said to be "saturated" with respect to that particular solid. The concentration of dissolved solid in a saturated solution is a measure of the solid's **solubility**. When the solution contains less than the equilibrium concentration of dissolved solid it is said to be **undersaturated** and when the concentration of dissolved solid in solution is greater than at equilibrium, the solution is **supersaturated**. When

in contact with an undersaturated solution, the rate of ions leaving the solid will tend to exceed that of ions leaving the solution. This means that the solid will tend to dissolve and that crystal growth is not possible. In a supersaturated solution, crystal growth will tend to occur, as more ions leave the solution and are added to the surface of the solid, but the opposite process of dissolution cannot take place. In this description, the use of "will tend to" rather than "will" is deliberate. The reason is that in the complex environment of the mouth, both dissolution and crystal growth can be heavily influenced by another surface-related process: adsorption to the crystal surface of ions or molecules that inhibit movement of ions between the solid and the solution (C in **Fig. 2.5**). Inhibitory substances, including macromolecules such as peptides and proteins (e.g., statherin) and low-molecular-weight substances such as the pyrophosphate ion, abound in biological fluids,[23] including saliva[1,2] and the interstitial fluid of plaque.

In the foregoing an empirical definition of solubility is given. This is adequate for understanding the basis for demineralization and remineralization in caries, but it is important to understand that there exists a more sophisticated approach, based on fundamental principles of physical chemistry.[24] This approach is more generalized and allows predictions about dissolution and crystal growth in complex systems to be made. For example, it is possible to define quantitatively the state of a given solution with respect to dissolution and crystal growth of all possible solids by calculating for each one the **degree of saturation** (DS). This has a value of 1 in saturated solutions, >1 in supersaturated and <1 in undersaturated solutions. Furthermore, the greater the difference between the DS and the value of 1, the greater the potential chemical driving force for the respective process. However, it is difficult to exploit this approach fully because of uncertainties in defining the solubilities of the impure minerals found in dental tissues.

NOTE

Dental minerals are impure forms of a calcium phosphate—hydroxyapatite. They become rapidly more soluble as the pH of the aqueous environment falls. Hence, teeth lose mineral in response to pH falls due to acid production in plaque and can gain mineral when the pH rises again. Fluoride reduces solubility and dissolution of tooth mineral and promotes hydroxyapatite crystal growth, so exerts powerful preventive effects on the caries process.

Minerals of Dental Tissues

Dental hard tissues are composite materials in which crystals of mineral are intimately associated with an organic matrix. The mineral is a form of **hydroxyapatite**, a type of calcium phosphate which in its pure form has the formula $Ca_5(PO_4)_3OH$, and is the least soluble nonfluoridated calcium phosphate at neutral pH.[24] Hydroxyapatite belongs to a family of minerals (**apatites**) which share a similar crystal structure that is remarkable for its capacity for accepting substitutions of one ion for another.[25,26]

The composition of hydroxyapatite in dental hard tissues is altered by incorporation in the crystal structure of several **"impurity" ions**, especially magnesium, sodium, and carbonate (**Fig. 2.6**; **Table 2.1**), which originate from the tissue fluids during tooth formation. Impurity ions differ—in charge, size or both—from the Ca^{2+}, PO_4^{3-}, or OH^- ions which they replace (**Fig. 2.6**). These misfits disturb crystal structure and this in turn increases solubility. The exception to this rule is the fluoride ion, which both improves crystallinity and reduces solubility (see below). Enamel mineral contains fewer impurities than the min-

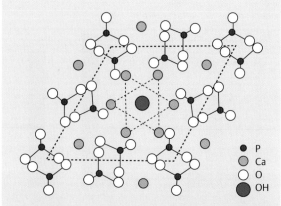

Lattice ion	Radius (pm)	Substituent ion	Radius (pm)
Ca²⁺	99	Mg²⁺	65
		Na⁺	95
PO₄³⁻	238	CO₃²⁻	185
OH⁻	140	F⁻	133
		CO₃²⁻	185

Fig. 2.6   In crystalline substances, the constituent ions or atoms are arranged in a regular, repeating array, which can be thought of as being made up of numerous basic units (**unit cells**). The diagram above shows the arrangement of calcium, phosphate, and hydroxyl groups in hydroxyapatite, as if looking down the long axis of a crystal. The outline of one unit cell, which has the formula $Ca_{10}(PO_4)_6(OH)_2$, is marked by a bold dashed line. The dotted triangles in middle mark groups of three Ca^{2+} ions which are rotated 60° in successive layers of the structure, forming a "channel" in which lie the OH^- ions (cf. **Fig. 2.8**). The remaining calcium ions form two columns of single ions. For clarity, the ions are not shown to scale. In reality, the oxygen atoms would be much larger and would fill most of the space within the structure. (Modified from Brown WE, et al: Ann Rev Mater Sci 1976;6:213–235.) The table compares lattice ions and impurity ions that can take their place, to show the disparities in charge and size (except for fluoride).

eral of dentin or cementum, the crystals are larger and more perfectly formed. Accordingly, enamel is only slightly more soluble than pure hydroxyapatite, while dentin is significantly more soluble,[27] although a reliable solubility has yet to be established.

The solubility of a particular form of calcium phosphate, as defined by the concentration of dissolved solid in a saturated solution, is not constant but varies according to the solution composition. The dominant factor in calcium phosphate chemistry is pH: the solubility of all calcium phosphates increases as the pH falls below 7. The solubility of hydroxyapatite increases particularly rapidly with pH, by a factor of ca.10 per pH unit fall (**Fig. 2.7**).

Table 2.1 Major constituents of the mineral component of enamel and dentin (weight %) compared to hydroxyapatite[26]

Constituent	Hydroxy-apatite	Enamel	Dentin
Calcium	39.9	37.6	40.3
Phosphorus	18.5	18.3	18.6
Carbonate		4.1	6.5
Sodium		0.7	0.1
Magnesium		0.2	1.1
Fluoride		0.01	0.07

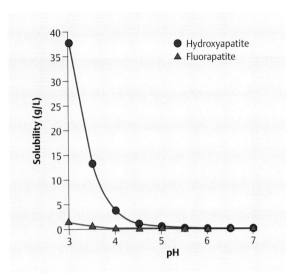

Fig. 2.7 Variation of solubility of hydroxyapatite and fluorapatite with pH.

Fluoride and Calcium Phosphate Chemistry

Fluoride has profound effects on solubility of hydroxyapatite and dental minerals. It is readily incorporated into the apatite structure because F^- ions can replace OH^- ions. **Fluorapatite**, in which all OH^- is replaced by F^-, is less soluble than hydroxyapatite at pH 7 or below (**Fig. 2.7**). In hydroxyapatite crystals, OH^- ions are located within channels formed by triangular groups of Ca^{2+} ions, but lie between the triangles[25,26] (A in **Fig. 2.8**). In fluorapatite, the slightly smaller F^- ion fits within the triangles (B in **Fig. 2.8**) and this is associated with a denser, more stable crystal structure. Partial substitution of F^- for OH^- produces **fluorhydroxyapatites**, which are thought to be stabilized by hydrogen-bonding between adjacent F^- and OH^- ions[24] (C in **Fig. 2.8**).

Important though they are, the effects of fluoride on crystal structure are probably much less significant than the reactions which take place between crystal surfaces of apatites and fluoride dissolved in the bathing liquid. If fluorhydroxyapatite, or even pure hydroxyapatite—which of course contains no fluoride ions—is placed in an acidic solution containing low concentrations of fluoride, the rate of dissolution is lower than in one that is fluoride-free[28,29] (**Fig. 2.9**). This phenomenon is due to replacement of OH^- ions by F^- ions at the crystal surfaces, probably not much deeper than one unit cell thickness.[30] The F^- ions stabilize the surrounding Ca^{2+} ions.[30] Regions of the crystal surface in which F^- has replaced OH^- are in effect converted into fluorapatite, so are much less soluble than nonfluoridated regions.[28,31,32] When exposed to acidic conditions, nonfluoridated regions of the crystal surfaces dissolve at the rate normal for hydroxyapatite, while the fluoridated regions will dissolve more slowly or not at all. The overall rate of dissolution is therefore slower than in the absence of fluoride, and the higher the concentration of fluoride in the ambient solution the greater the effect, because a greater proportion of the crystals surfaces is converted to fluorapatite. Thus, disso-

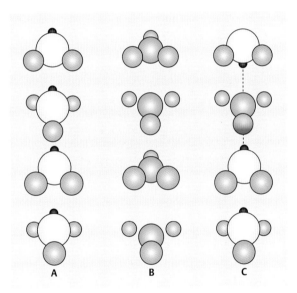

Fig. 2.8 The crystal lattice of hydroxyapatite (see **Fig. 2.6**) contains channels formed by stacked triangles of Ca^{2+} ions (orange), with successive triangles being rotated by 60°. In hydroxyapatite (A), the OH^- ions (large white circles representing the oxygen + small black circle representing the hydrogen) are too large to fit within the Ca triangles. In fluorapatite (B), the F^- ions (green) fit within the triangles, because they are smaller than the OH^- ion, and a more compact structure results. In fluorhydroxyapatites (C), F^- ions occupy some of the OH^- sites and can form hydrogen bonds with adjacent OH^- ions (dashed lines); this helps to stabilize the structure.

lution of tooth mineral can be partly or wholly prevented by low concentrations of fluoride in the environment of the tooth. A similar effect is thought to be responsible for the reduced solubility of fluorhydroxyapatites in fluoride-free acid.[33] Here, partial dissolution of the solid produces

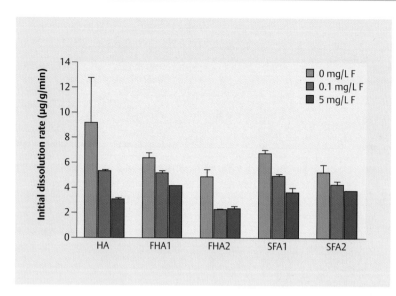

Fig. 2.9 Effects of fluoride (F) on hydroxy-apatite (HA) dissolution. HA and hydroxy-apatites modified with fluoride (FHA, SFA) were added to acetate buffer, pH 5.0, containing 0, 0.1, or 5 mg/L of F. The dissolution process was followed by measuring the release of Ca with time. FHA1 and FHA2 contained, respectively, 44 and 602 mg/g F *in the crystal lattice*, whereas SFA1 and SFA2 were samples of HA powder that had been treated with F solution and contained respectively 60 and 706 mg/g F, which was *concentrated at the crystal surfaces*. The results show, first, that fluoride incorporated in the crystal structure or adsorbed to the crystal surfaces reduces dissolution rate, since the rates of FHA and SFA in fluoride-free buffer were lower than that of HA; and second, that the presence of fluoride in solution reduced dissolution rate, even that of HA, which contained no fluoride at all. (Data from ref. [29].)

enough fluoride ions to convert the crystal surfaces to fluorapatite.[32]

The lower solubility of fluorapatite also affects crystal growth. If fluoride ions are available in a solution supersaturated with respect to hydroxyapatite, crystal growth is accelerated. The solid that forms will not be hydroxyapatite but fluorapatite or a fluorhydroxyapatite, depending on how much fluoride is available, so the product of remineralization in the presence of fluoride tends to be less soluble than the mineral which had been lost.[7]

If teeth are exposed to high concentrations of fluoride, for example, by treatment with fluoride varnish, a form of **calcium fluoride** (CaF_2), probably combined with phosphate, may be precipitated on the tooth surfaces.[31] The Ca^{2+} ions required for precipitation of the CaF_2-like material are derived from the tooth mineral, so more of the precipitate is formed at lower pH. Although its formation removes Ca^{2+} ions from the tooth surface, CaF_2-like material could have a beneficial effect: since it is relatively soluble, it can act as a fluoride reservoir, maintaining raised concentrations of Ca^{2+} and F^- ions in the tooth environment.

On the basis of this evidence, the prevailing current opinion is that strategies for caries prevention using fluoride should be aimed at maintaining low but sufficient concentrations of fluoride ions in the environment of the tooth, rather than at increasing the fluoride concentration in the tooth mineral.[31] This is achieved by topical methods of fluoride administration such as toothpastes, mouth rinses, varnishes, and also by water fluoridation which, even though originally intended to reduce solubility of tooth mineral, has a significant topical effect[34] (see Chapter 12).

The Cariogenic Challenge

Dental plaque is an example of a biofilm, a film of microorganisms adhering to a solid surface. Biofilms exist in a wide variety of types adapted to different habitats. Life in a biofilm requires physiological adaptations on the part of the constituent microorganisms and also provides several advantages, for instance, protection against antimicrobial agents.[35] The structure of biofilms varies widely, but in the case of dental plaque the constituent bacteria are closely packed together, occupying ca. 75% of the volume.[36] The remaining volume is made up of a matrix comprising proteins, carbohydrate polymers, and other substances (**Fig. 2.10**). Many matrix components, such as extracellular polysaccharides, are largely of bacterial origin, but others, including several proteins, originate from saliva and gingival crevicular fluid.

Because of the dense structure of dental plaque, movement of nutrients and metabolic end products between the oral cavity and plaque, and within plaque, is mediated by **diffusion**, which is a relatively slow process (**Fig. 2.11 a**). One consequence is that availability of nutrients or antibacterial substances will not be uniform but will vary with depth. For instance, when a nutrient is ingested, a gradient will be set up within the plaque (**Fig. 2.11 b**), with the concentration falling toward the interior, and bacterial metabolism will steepen this gradient because utilization near the outer surface will make less nutrient available for inward diffusion (**Fig. 2.12**). This phenomenon has important effects on plaque ecology. For instance, most plaque bacteria are anaerobic (surviving only in the absence of oxygen), such as *Veillonella* or facultative (preferring to live in absence of oxygen), such as streptococci and *Actinomyces*, probably because oxygen is consumed by aerobic bacteria such as *Neisseria* at the plaque surface, and none reaches the inner plaque.[3] A similar process probably limits exposure of plaque bacteria to antimicrobial

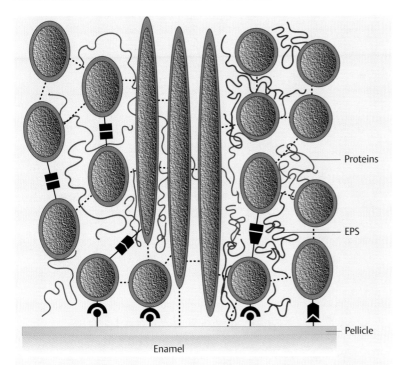

Fig. 2.10 Diagram to represent some aspects of plaque structure. Tooth surfaces exposed to saliva are covered by an acquired pellicle consisting of adsorbed salivary proteins. Initial bacterial colonists attach to the pellicle, and the plaque increases in bulk and complexity by attachment of further bacteria to the initial colonists. Attachment is mediated by specific receptors on bacterial surfaces (indicated by geometrical lock-and-key shapes). However, plaque cohesion is further enhanced by nonspecific interactions (dotted lines), e.g., calcium bridging, and by interactions between polymers forming the plaque matrix: proteins and extracellular polysaccharides (EPS) such as glucans.

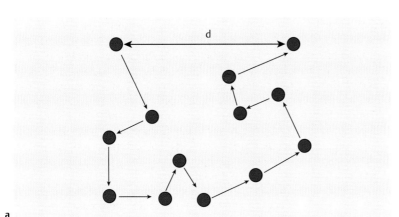

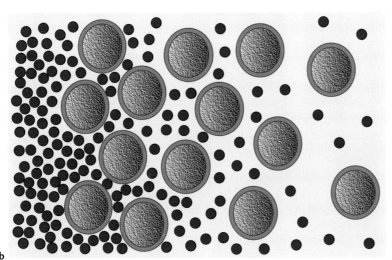

Fig. 2.11a, b Diffusion.
a A single molecule (small red circle) in solution makes frequent small 'jumps' (single arrows). Even though each jump is in a random direction, a series of jumps results in net movement of the molecule (double arrow,
d = net distance moved).
b Since more molecules move from regions of high concentration into regions of low concentration than vice versa, there is net transfer of molecules down gradients of concentration. This is illustrated for molecules diffusing from saliva (left) into plaque, via the plaque fluid.

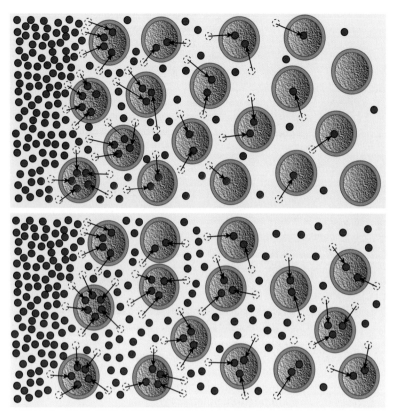

Fig. 2.12 Diffusion-with-reaction in plaque. Molecules of a nutrient such as sugar or oxygen (small red circles) diffusing into the surface of the plaque (left) are utilized immediately by superficial bacteria and this leaves less to diffuse deeper into the plaque. This results in a much steeper fall in concentration than in the case of simple diffusion (cf. **Fig. 2.11**). If metabolism is rapid, little or no nutrient will reach the deepest parts of the plaque. In plaque containing little extracellular polysaccharide (EPS) (above), the bacteria are closely packed and quickly utilize sugar molecules diffusing in from the saliva, allowing little to reach the interior. If EPS is abundant (below) the bacteria are more widely spaced, more sugar can diffuse into the interior and bacteria near the tooth surface can produce acid, which causes a greater pH drop in the environment of the tooth mineral.

agents, because such agents will be immobilized by strong interaction with bacteria in the outer plaque, and the concentration reaching the inner plaque may be too low to be effective. Metabolic end products clear slowly from plaque because their movement is similarly regulated by diffusion. These phenomena are central to the process of dental caries because they control the different phases of the cariogenic challenge.

The interstitial fluid bathing the matrix, referred to as **plaque fluid**, is the component of plaque in direct contact with the tooth surface and is therefore the medium for the flux of H^+ ions and mineral ions during the caries process. Analysis of plaque fluid isolated by centrifugation shows that its electrolyte composition differs markedly from that of saliva[37] (**Table 2.2**), mainly because exchange of ions between the two fluids is diffusion-dependent and slow. Thus, the elevated potassium concentration is due to slow clearance of K^+ ions released by bacterial lysis. In plaque that has not recently been exposed to nutrients, the predominant organic acid is acetic acid (**Table 2.2**), which is an end product of metabolic pathways that derive the maximal ATP from the low amounts of available carbohydrate[3].

A **cariogenic challenge** is initiated by exposure to fermentable carbohydrate, which provokes a characteristic pattern of change in plaque pH, known as the **Stephan curve**[3,4] (**Fig. 2.13**), which can be recorded by micro-electrodes inserted into the plaque. The duration of a Stephan curve varies, but is typically 30–60 minutes. The curve can

be divided into two phases: an initial rapid pH fall from the resting value (approximately pH 7), followed by a slower recovery of pH. These phases reflect the underlying pattern of bacterial metabolism. In the initial phase, the high intra-oral sugar concentration typical of confectionery or sweetened drinks drives diffusion of sugar into the plaque, where it is rapidly metabolized to produce energy. The main metabolic pathway is conversion of sugar by **glycolysis** to pyruvic acid and then directly to lactic acid (see Chapter 11), which reduces the pH within the plaque fluid[3] (**Table 2.2**). The rate of pH fall is slowed by combination of H^+ ions with plaque buffers, made up mostly of macromolecules associated with the bacterial cell walls. Simple sugars are cleared from the mouth by saliva within 1–2 minutes but the pH fall in plaque lasts for somewhat longer because the bacteria continue to metabolize the sugar that diffused inward initially. Eventually the sugar is used up and acid production ceases, so the initial phase of the Stephan curve comes to an end. The minimum local pH during a Stephan curve is about 4.0, which represents the lowest value at which even the most aciduric bacteria can produce acid, but average values will be higher than this.

Although plaque pH is lower than under "resting" conditions for the whole duration of a Stephan curve, only part of it represents the cariogenic challenge. At neutral pH, plaque fluid is actually supersaturated. This means that the pH must fall to a certain value before the plaque fluid becomes just saturated with respect to the dental

Table 2.2 Comparison of electrolyte compositions of saliva (unstimulated) and plaque fluid, and changes in plaque fluid composition during a cariogenic challenge

| | Saliva | Plaque fluid | |
		Resting	3 min after sucrose
pH	6.8	6.66	5.37
Calcium, total	1.43	3.16	5.47
Phosphate, total	5.10	11.0	9.4
Chloride	23.2	45.2	24.1
Sodium	10.1	29.4	23.0
Potassium	22.7	66.4	62.8
Ammonium	4.35	21.6	12.4
Magnesium	0.21	2.3	1.7
Acetate	–	22.5	15.6
Lactate	–	5.6	33.1
DS(HA)*	–	8.85	1.50

Columns 2 and 3 compare electrolyte concentrations (mmol/L) in unstimulated mixed saliva and in "resting" plaque fluid from subjects who had not eaten overnight. Columns 3 and 4 show changes in mean electrolyte concentrations in plaque fluid either resting or 3 min after a 1-min exposure to 5% sucrose solution for a group of caries-active subjects. The degree of saturation with respect to hydroxyapatite falls, but although local undersaturation might have been reached, it is not reflected in this sample of the whole plaque.
* Degree of saturation with respect to hydroxyapatite.
  Source: Refs [37,67].

mineral. This pH is called the **critical pH**.[24] For enamel mineral, this is calculated from analyses of plaque fluid to be 5.2–5.5. Dentin mineral is known to be more soluble than enamel mineral,[27] so the critical pH must be higher than for enamel, but as the solubility of dentin is not accurately known a good estimate has yet to be made. Once the pH of plaque fluid falls below the critical pH, demineralization can occur. Conversely, once the pH of plaque fluid rises above the critical pH, dissolution will cease. Therefore, only the fraction of the Stephan curve between the critical pH and the minimum pH represents a cariogenic challenge (see **Figs. 2.2** and **2.13**).

During the second phase of the Stephan curve, pH returns to the resting value, but this typically takes longer than the pH fall in the first phase of the curve. During this phase, H^+ ions are released from the immobile buffers associated with the bacterial cell walls and diffuse slowly outward into the saliva. H^+ ions are also removed from plaque by mobile buffers—small, diffusible ions such as phosphate and bicarbonate—which act as H^+ "carriers" between the plaque fluid and the saliva[38] (**Fig. 2.14**). During the second phase of the Stephan curve, the pH will rise above the critical pH and precipitation of mineral will become possible. This can occur either as crystal growth within the caries lesion—where it will help to replace lost mineral (remineralization)—or as precipitation within the plaque (calculus formation).

Acids are not the only products of sugar utilization by plaque bacteria. In particular, many plaque bacteria synthesize **polysaccharides** from dietary sugar (see Chapter 11). These include extracellular polymers of glucose (glucans) or fructose (fructans) and intracellular glycogen-like storage polysaccharides. All are relevant to the caries process. **Intracellular polysaccharides (IPS)** can be utilized for energy between intakes of sugar, as can soluble extracellular fructans, and the resulting acid production may

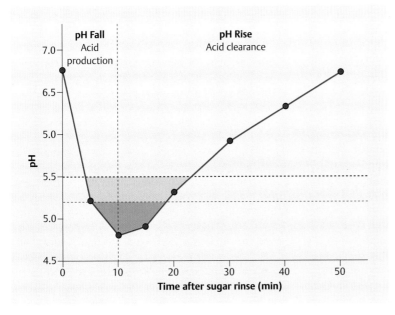

Fig. 2.13 Stephan curve. The dashed horizontal lines indicate the range for the critical pH. The shading indicates the period of the cariogenic challenge, when the plaque fluid is undersaturated with respect to enamel mineral. The denser shading below the lower estimate of critical pH indicates the increasing severity of the challenge with falling pH (see **Fig. 2.7**).

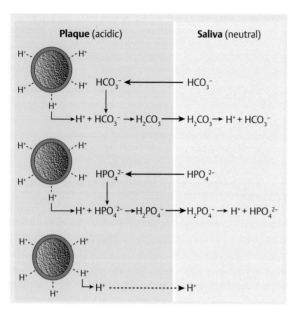

Fig. 2.14 Clearance of H⁺ ions from plaque during the second phase of the Stephan curve. H⁺ ions released from fixed (nondiffusible) buffers associated with bacterial cell walls (left) diffuse out slowly (dashed arrow, bottom). Clearance is accelerated by diffusible buffers from saliva—bicarbonate (top) and phosphate (middle)—which act as H⁺-transporters.

$$\text{—COOCa}^+ + H^+ \leftrightarrow Ca^{2+} + HOOC\text{—}$$

$$\text{—COO–Ca–OOC—}$$

$$\text{—O}\diagdown\text{OPOCa}^+ + H^+ \leftrightarrow Ca^{2+} + HOPO\diagup\text{O—}$$

Fig. 2.15 Release of calcium ions bound to bacteria during a cariogenic challenge. At neutral pH, Ca^{2+} ions are bound to carboxyl groups (top left) and phosphate groups (bottom left), associated with bacterial cell walls. When plaque pH falls, Ca^{2+} ions are displaced by H⁺ ions (top right, bottom right). The resulting fall in H⁺ ion concentration and the rise in Ca^{2+} concentration raise the degree of saturation of the plaque fluid and hence ameliorate the cariogenic challenge. Some Ca^{2+} ions act as bridges between neighboring plaque bacteria (middle) and increase plaque cohesion; these bridging Ca^{2+} ions are also released under acidic conditions.

extend the recovery phase of the Stephan curve. IPS-producing bacteria are more abundant in the plaque of caries-active individuals, owing to the selection pressure of frequent sugar ingestion.[19] **Extracellular glucans** tend to be insoluble and are not utilized for energy. The insoluble, sticky glucans synthesized by *S. mutans* are important in the adhesion of these bacteria to tooth surfaces and in their retention in plaque. They may also increase the cariogenicity of plaque in another way. In plaque with abundant extracellular glucans, the number of bacteria per unit volume is reduced. Consequently, sugar diffusing into plaque at the start of a cariogenic challenge is utilized

less rapidly and so can diffuse further into the plaque. This brings acid production closer to the tooth surface, thereby creating a more cariogenic environment[39] (see **Fig. 2.12**). Sucrose might induce other alterations in plaque matrix composition which lead to depletion of mineral ions.[39]

The overall severity of a cariogenic challenge is influenced by several factors. It is mainly the overall **concentration of sugar** in a food item that determines how far the pH will fall in a single exposure, so high-sugar foods pose a greater challenge (see **Fig. 2.2**). Similarly, the more frequently sugar is consumed, the longer the plaque pH can remain below neutrality, so that the potential for remineralization is reduced (see **Fig. 2.2**). As predicted by the ecological plaque hypothesis, **frequent exposure to sugar** causes selection for acidogenic, aciduric bacteria and for bacteria producing intracellular polysaccharides, which will intensify the cariogenic challenge (greater, more prolonged pH fall). If the main sugar to which the plaque is exposed is sucrose (the most abundant sugar in sweetened foodstuffs), the plaque cariogenicity will be increased as explained above. Although complex dietary carbohydrates, such as starch, are thought to be relatively noncariogenic, starch probably increases the stickiness of sugar-rich foods, thereby retaining them close to the tooth surface and prolonging the cariogenic challenge.[40]

Some members of the plaque flora mitigate the effects of lactic acid production. *Veillonella*, which is consistently found in plaque, derives energy from metabolizing lactic acid to acetic and propionic acids. As these are weaker acids than lactic acid, they will remove H⁺ from the plaque fluid and thus tend to raise pH.[3] Other bacteria can produce ammonia from nitrogen-containing substances—amino acids, for example—and this will tend to raise the pH. Plaque bacteria bind appreciable quantities of calcium[41] and when the pH falls, Ca^{2+} ions are released (**Fig. 2.15**; **Table 2.2**) in exchange for H⁺ ions. This will increase the degree of saturation.

The main host factors influencing the cariogenic challenge are the flow rate and buffering capacity of saliva.[1,38] The pH rise in the second phase of the Stephan curve is facilitated by good salivary flow, as this helps to clear H⁺ ions away from the plaque. A mitigating factor in the caries process is that consumption of foods stimulates salivary flow and this is accompanied by increased salivary bicarbonate concentration: both enhance H⁺ ion removal from the plaque.

NOTE

The presence of dental plaque, made up of densely-packed bacteria, on sheltered regions of the tooth prevents flow of oral fluids over the tooth surface, so exchange of substances between the tooth surface or plaque and the oral fluids occurs by the slow process of diffusion. Consequently, metabolism of sugar by plaque bacteria results in accumulation of acid, and a fall in plaque pH, followed by a pH rise as H⁺ ions are cleared into the saliva. The pattern of rapid pH fall and slower pH recovery in plaque is called the "Stephan curve." An episode when plaque pH is below the "critical pH" (~5.2–5.5 for enamel) constitutes a cariogenic challenge, when the tooth can lose mineral. The severity of the cariogenic challenge is influenced by many factors, including diet (especially sugar consumption), the plaque flora, the flow rate and buffering properties of saliva.

Table 2.3 Depths of lesions created in vitro by 21 days' exposure to lactate buffer + carboxymethylcellulose, pH 4.5, in specimens of enamel from deciduous and permanent teeth. Also shown are the proportion of the enamel structure made up of the more porous interprismatic enamel, and the specific surface area of the prism boundaries, which are the sites of the largest pores in enamel. All differences between the two types of enamel are statistically highly significant[45]

	Lesion depth (µm)	Inter-prismatic fraction (%)	Prism boundary specific surface area (m^2/g)
Deciduous	199 ± 39	30.2 ± 5.2	0.27 ± 0.02
Permanent	115 ± 27	23.1 ± 3.6	0.23 ± 0.03

Chemistry of Caries

Lesion formation is controlled by two processes: dissolution of mineral and diffusion of acid into the hard tissues (and of mineral ions outward).

Enamel Lesion Formation

The solubility, and therefore the rate of dissolution, increases from the surface to the enamel–dentin junction[27,42] (see also Chapter 3), in correlation with a similar gradient in the concentrations of carbonate and magnesium.[43] At a smaller scale, the mineral at the prism boundaries (intraprismatic mineral) is significantly more soluble than that in the prism cores[27] and is the first part of the enamel structure to be attacked at the advancing front of a lesion (translucent zone). The prism boundaries contain the largest enamel pores, and they are further enlarged by this loss of mineral to form preferential **pathways of diffusion** during further lesion progress, when demineralization occurs within the prisms.[44]

The overall rate of lesion advance is governed by diffusion, which means that the lesion progresses more slowly the further it penetrates into the tissue,[45] although this may be modified by the inward gradient of increasing solubility. Lesions progress faster in enamel of deciduous teeth than in that of permanent teeth[46] (**Table 2.3**). This seems to be due mainly to quantitative differences in pore structure (**Table 2.3**) rather than to differences in mineral solubility.[27,46]

A prominent feature of caries lesions of enamel is a **surface layer** which retains much more mineral than the underlying body of the lesion. Numerous mechanisms by which the surface layer could retain so much mineral have been proposed.[45] The theory that seems to be best supported by the available evidence, is that inhibitors dissolved in the aqueous environment of the tooth adsorb to crystals in the surface layer and inhibit dissolution, so that this layer is spared while underlying tissue remains vulnerable and continues to dissolve (**Fig. 2.16**). The inhibitors involved could include such substances as proteins and pyrophosphate but fluoride is likely to play an especially important part.[45,47] In-vitro experiments under reasonably realistic conditions suggest that in the absence of

fluoride enamel surfaces are simply demineralized, whereas in the presence of fluoride at low concentrations, for example, 0.1 mg/L, a surface layer is formed instead.[47,48] Fluoride ions probably also promote precipitation of fluorhydroxyapatite on crystals in the surface layer and this would account for improved crystallinity observed in this layer.[49] **In vivo**, a surface layer does not form immediately, possibly because of the low fluoride concentrations available.

In-vitro experiments suggest that progress of enamel lesions is slowed by proteins derived from the tooth milieu,[50] which presumably adsorb to crystals surfaces and inhibit dissolution within the lesion.

NOTE

Demineralization is the central process in caries but varies at the tissue level and histological level. The relatively intact surface layer characteristic of enamel caries probably owes its existence to the effect of inhibitors of demineralization, especially fluoride. Quite low concentrations of fluoride in the tooth environment during a cariogenic challenge inhibit caries progression and during periods when pH is neutral can promote remineralization. Lesions can become arrested: a state which implies cessation of cariogenic conditions and inhibition of remineralization.

BACKGROUND

Mineral Precipitation in Caries

Beside hydroxyapatite, there exist many other calcium phosphates, with different compositions and solubility properties, and some have, or might have, a role in caries. **Brushite** ($CaHPO_4 \cdot 2H_2O$) is more soluble than hydroxyapatite at neutral pH but, because its solubility varies less with pH, it becomes less soluble than hydroxyapatite at approximately pH 4. It has been suggested as an intermediate in formation of the surface layer of the caries lesion but there is no direct evidence for this.[45]

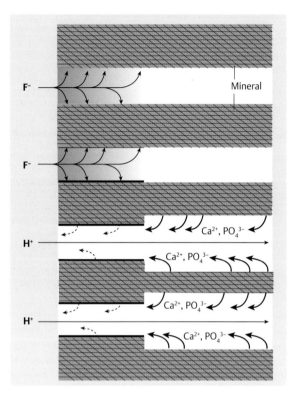

Fig. 2.16 Hypothesis for role of inhibitors (e.g., fluoride) in formation of a surface layer on caries lesions.[45] The mineral phase is patterned. Fluoride, dissolved in plaque fluid, diffuses into enamel pores and adsorbs to the mineral forming the pore walls (top), thereby reducing its solubility (depicted by heavy lines at the mineral surface). Because the concentration of available fluoride is low, it is depleted within the outer enamel (indicated by the shading within the pores), so the solubility of the inner enamel is not reduced. Consequently, during a cariogenic challenge, acid diffusing into the enamel dissolves only small quantities of mineral from the surface layer and more from the inner enamel, resulting in increased porosity.

Two mixed calcium-magnesium salts—**magnesium whitlockite** [MWH; $Ca_9Mg(HPO_4)(PO_4)_6$] and **magnesium-containing β-tricalcium phosphate** [MTCP; $(Ca,Mg)_3(PO_4)_2$—are often referred to indiscriminately as whitlockite. MWH is more soluble than hydroxyapatite at neutral pH but in plaque fluid it becomes less soluble than either hydroxyapatite or brushite at about pH 5.5. During enamel lesion formation, small crystals, probably of MWH, are formed at the prism boundaries,[44] probably in association with release of magnesium, calcium, and phosphate from labile mineral at the advancing front. The intra-tubular mineral formed during dentin sclerosis may be needlelike hydroxyapatite or coarser crystals of MTCP or MWH.[51-53]

Dentin Lesion Formation

In agreement with the higher concentration of impurities, lower crystallinity, and smaller crystal size of the mineral, in situ studies suggest that lesions in (root) dentin pro-

gress more than twice as fast as in enamel.[54] Demineralization of dentin exposes the abundant organic matrix and this then becomes vulnerable to the action of bacterial proteases and to nonenzymic chemical processes which alter dentin matrix irreversibly and impair its capacity to remineralize. Mineral usually precipitates within tubules in a narrow band between the lesion and the pulp: a phenomenon referred to as **dentin sclerosis**.[52,53] This plays a vital role in retarding the progression of bacteria from the lesion to the pulp. It is usually assumed that sclerosis is due to odontoblast activity but physicochemical dissolution–reprecipitation processes might play a large part[54] (for further elaboration, see Chapter 3).

Fluoride and Lesion Formation

Fluoride in the aqueous tooth environment diffuses into the lesion and slows down demineralization. In-vitro experiments show that the concentration required to affect mineral loss is inversely related to pH, but 2 mg/L fluoride in the pH range 4.0–5.5 seems to be sufficient to prevent lesion formation in enamel.[47,48] Much higher fluoride concentrations (5–10 times) are required to obtain equivalent inhibition of lesions in dentin.[55] In vivo, dissolved fluoride in the oral environment is derived mainly from fluoride toothpaste, mouth rinses, or fluoridated water but the immediate source for the lesion is the plaque. Fluoride diffusing into plaque—for example, after toothbrushing— is bound by two mechanisms: by binding to bacterial surfaces by way of Ca^{2+} ions[56] (**Fig. 2.17**), and possibly by precipitation of calcium fluoride-like mineral. Both reactions are reversible and provide a source of F⁻ ions as the plaque fluoride concentration falls. Release is accompanied by release of Ca^{2+} ions and is greater at lower pH. These processes exert a considerable caries-preventive action. Fluoride is also taken up by other intra-oral "reservoirs," for example, the oral mucosa and the tooth surfaces. However, the special effectiveness of the plaque fluoride storage is demonstrated by the fact that one hour after a fluoride rinse (1000 mg/L, ~1000 ppm), the concentration of dissolved fluoride in the plaque fluid is not only higher than in saliva but is still at a level which in-vitro experiments indicate can prevent lesion formation[57] (**Fig. 2.18**).

Remineralization and Lesion Arrest

The progression of a caries lesion can be slowed or halted if the severity or frequency of cariogenic challenges is reduced, for example, by **plaque control** or **restriction of sugar** intake, by a reduced frequency of ingestion of sugar, or by **loss of an adjacent tooth**, which exposes a previously inaccessible approximal surface to the cleansing and buffering action of saliva. Such changes favor remineralization over demineralization, especially when fluoride is available. However, in-situ experiments suggest that, even when the cariogenicity of the tooth environment is reduced, not all lesions remineralize and some continue to

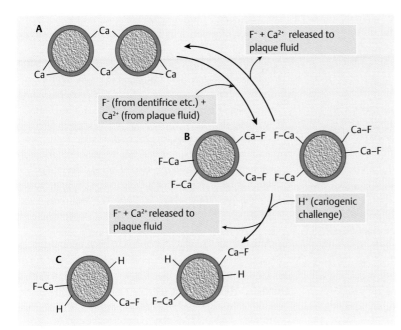

Fig. 2.17 Fluoride binding and release in plaque. **A**: Before exposure to fluoride, plaque bacteria bind calcium ions, some of which act as bridges between adjacent cells (cf. **Fig. 2.15**). **B**: After exposure to high concentrations of fluoride (e.g., dentifrice, mouth rinse) fluoride ions form complexes with bound calcium ions. Because each fluoride ion uses only one of the calcium valencies, further sites for calcium and fluoride binding are created. With time, the reverse process occurs, fluoride and calcium being slowly released, so that the fluoride concentration in plaque fluid remains elevated for a prolonged period. **C**: A rapid fall in pH, as during a cariogenic challenge, causes calcium ions to be displaced from binding sites on bacterial surfaces. This results in a rapid release of both calcium and fluoride ions to the plaque fluid.

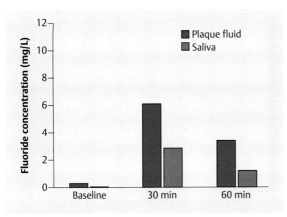

Fig. 2.18 Fluoride in plaque fluid and saliva at baseline and at 30 and 60 minutes following a rinse with 1000 mg/L sodium fluoride. (Data from ref.[57].)

progress. The fate of a lesion seems to depend on intra-oral factors such as saliva flow rate and composition.[58]

Lesions take up **proteins** from the oral fluids[59] and these tend to inhibit crystal growth.[1,2,60] Under some circumstances, such protein might actually enhance the effect of fluoride, by inhibiting mineral crystal growth in the surface layer of enamel lesions, so that remineralization can occur in the subsurface part of the lesion.[60] However, continuing accumulation of protein would eventually inhibit remineralization in all parts of a lesion. Sealing of a lesion by complete remineralization of the surface layer, or inhibition of crystal growth within the lesion by proteins could explain the observation that lesions that have been in existence for a long time (6 months or more) seem to be resistant to fluoride treatment.[61]

NOTE

Remineralization is a fundamental part of pH cycles (pH drop and a subsequent rise) and happens primarily when the pH returns, say, from 5.5 to 7.0. Caries arrest is when no nett loss of ions happens over time.

Dental Erosion

In erosion there is a direct effect on all exposed tooth surfaces by acidic substances, without the mediation of bacteria, so the damage extends over a wide area and is not localized as in caries lesions. However, approximal and gingival areas seem to be spared, probably because of the high buffer capacity of plaque. The acids responsible for erosion can be endogenous or exogenous.[62] **Endogenous acid** consists of gastric juices entering the mouth by reflux, as in bulimia or in gastro-esophageal disorders. **Exogenous acid** may be industrial or occupational in origin, for example, acidic industrial vapors, or may be contained in foods (e.g., pickles) or drinks (e.g., wines, soft drinks, fruit juices).

The challenge posed to the tooth surface by exposure to an acidic substance is typically much more severe than a cariogenic challenge. In a cariogenic challenge, the milieu (plaque fluid) is partly saturated with respect to tooth mineral and the pH rarely falls as low as 4.0, whereas erosive substances typically contain little or no calcium or phosphate and the pH can be as low as 2.4.[63] The pH/solubility curve for HA (see **Fig. 2.7**) shows that at such low pH values dissolution is extremely high. Moreover, whereas transport of dissolved mineral away from the

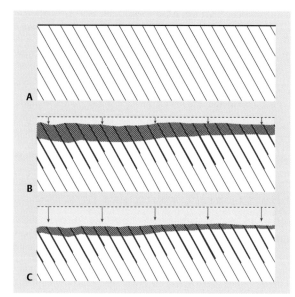

Fig. 2.19a–c Softening and abrasion in erosive tooth wear. **a**: Cross-section of sound enamel with prism boundaries marked as oblique lines. **b**: Enamel after exposure to erosive liquid. At the outermost surface, some enamel has been dissolved completely (original surface marked by dashed line). Beneath this zone, acid has diffused into the enamel and produced a "softened" zone (stippled), in which there is partial demineralization. Demineralization extends deepest along the prism boundaries (marked by heavy lines), because of the raised solubility of the mineral at these sites. **c**: If the surface in **b** is exposed to abrasive forces (e.g., toothbrushing), the outer, more heavily demineralized, part of the softened layer is worn away, resulting in further loss of tooth surface.

tooth during a cariogenic challenge is diffusion-controlled and slow, clearance is much faster in erosion, especially where the erosive agent is a liquid. Thus, even though an erosive challenge is typically short (1–2 minutes for a soft drink[64]), the rate of demineralization is very much faster than in caries.

The primary lesion in enamel erosion is **partial demineralization** ("softening") of a layer extending some micrometers below the surface, created by acid diffusing into the submicroscopic pores of the tissue (**Fig. 2.19**). Softened enamel is vulnerable to mechanical forces that would have no effect on sound enamel, for example, friction from the tongue or toothbrushing.[65] Consequently, the softened tissue can be lost quite soon after the erosive challenge (**Fig. 2.19**), and repeated challenges eventually result in visible loss of tissue.[65] Erosion of dentin creates a superficial layer of demineralized dentin matrix which is vulnerable to the action of bacterial proteases and then to abrasion.[66]

SUMMARY

Dental caries consists of the loss of mineral from dental hard tissues, as a result of the conversion of dietary sugars to acid within a bacterial biofilm (dental plaque) formed in sheltered locations on the tooth surfaces. The loss of mineral can be reversed by crystal growth driven by precipitation of mineral ions derived from the oral fluids (remineralization). Caries lesions progress when demineralization outweighs remineralization and ultimately break down to form cavities, with consequently impaired tooth function. The rate of progress is influenced by the plaque flora, diet, salivary biochemistry, oral hygiene, and numerous behavioral and socioeconomic factors. Fluoride is perhaps the most important factor, because it both reduces demineralization and enhances remineralization. Fluoride reduces solubility of tooth mineral through reactions at the crystal surfaces. It is thus considered that topical application to maintain low but effective fluoride concentrations in the tooth environment is more effective than systematic routes of fluoride delivery. Dental erosion is less localized than caries, is caused by more severe acid challenges, and poses difficult problems of prevention.

REFERENCES

1. Edgar WM, Dawes C, O'Mullane D, eds. Saliva and Oral Health. 3rd ed. London: BDJ Books; 2004

2. Hay DI, Moreno EC. Macromolecular inhibitors of calcium phosphate inhibition in human saliva. Their roles in providing a protective environment for the teeth. In: Kleinberg I, Ellison SA, Mandel ID, eds. Saliva and Dental Caries. New York: IRL Press; 1979:45–58

3. Marsh PD, Martin M. Oral Microbiology. 3rd ed. London: Chapman Hall; 1992

4. Marsh PD, Nyvad B. The oral microflora and biofilms on teeth. In: Fejerskov O, Kidd, EAM, eds. Dental Caries. The Disease and its Clinical Management. Oxford: Blackwell Munksgaard; 2003: 29–48

5. Keyes PH, Jordan HV. Factors influencing the initiation, transmission, and inhibition of dental caries. In: Harris RS, ed. Mechanisms of Hard Tissue Destruction. New York: Academic Press; 1963:261–283

6. Fejerskov O, Kidd EAM, eds. Dental Caries. The Disease and its Clinical Management. Oxford: Blackwell Munksgaard; 2003

7. ten Cate JM, Featherstone JD. Mechanistic aspects of the interactions between fluoride and dental enamel. Crit Rev Oral Biol Med 1991;2(3):283–296

8. Harris R, Nicoll AD, Adair PM, Pine CM. Risk factors for dental caries in young children: a systematic review of the literature. Community Dent Health 2004; 21(1, Suppl):71–85

9. Shellis RP, Duckworth RM. Studies on the cariostatic mechanisms of fluoride. Int Dent J 1994; 44(3, Suppl 1):263–273

10. Lussi A, ed. Dental Erosion. Basel: Karger; 2006. Monographs in Oral Science; vol 20

11. Tanzer JM. Dental caries is a transmissible infectious disease: the Keyes and Fitzgerald revolution. J Dent Res 1995;74(9): 1536–1542

12. Tanzer JM, Livingston J, Thompson AM. The microbiology of primary dental caries in humans. J Dent Educ 2001;65(10):1028–1037

13. Loesche WJ. Role of Streptococcus mutans in human dental decay. Microbiol Rev 1986;50(4):353–380

14. Takahashi N, Nyvad B. Caries ecology revisited: microbial dynamics and the caries process. Caries Res 2008;42(6):409–418

15. Beighton D. The complex oral microflora of high-risk individuals and groups and its role in the caries process. Community Dent Oral Epidemiol 2005;33(4):248–255

16. Marsh PD. Are dental diseases examples of ecological catastrophes? Microbiology 2003;149(Pt 2):279–294

17. Hayes ML, Carter EC, Griffiths SJ. The acidogenic microbial composition of dental plaque from caries-free and caries-prone people. Arch Oral Biol 1983;28(5):381–386

18. Minah GE, Lovekin GB, Finney JP. Sucrose-induced ecological response of experimental dental plaques from caries-free and caries-susceptible human volunteers. Infect Immun 1981;34(3):662–675

19. van Ruyven FOH, Lingström P, van Houte J, Kent R. Relationship among mutans streptococci, "low-pH" bacteria, and lodophilic polysaccharide-producing bacteria in dental plaque and early enamel caries in humans. J Dent Res 2000;79(2):778–784

20. Becker MR, Paster BJ, Leys EJ, et al. Molecular analysis of bacterial species associated with childhood caries. J Clin Microbiol 2002;40(3):1001–1009

21. Corby PM, Lyons-Weiler J, Bretz WA, et al. Microbial risk indicators of early childhood caries. J Clin Microbiol 2005;43(11):5753–5759

22. Russell RRB. How has genomics altered our view of caries microbiology? Caries Res 2008;42(5):319–327

23. Meyer JL, Fleisch H. Calcification inhibitors in rat and human serum and plasma. Biochim Biophys Acta 1984;799(2):115–121

24. Ten Cate JM, Larsen MJ, Pearce EIF, et al. Chemical interactions between the tooth and oral fluids. In: Fejerskov O, Kidd EAM, eds. Dental Caries. The Disease and its Clinical Management. Oxford: Blackwell Munksgaard; 2003:49–70

25. Young RA, Brown WE. Structures of biological minerals. In: Nancollas GH, ed. Biological Mineralization and Demineralization. Berlin: Springer; 1982:101–141

26. Elliott JC. Structure and Chemistry of the Apatites and other Calcium Phosphates. Amsterdam: Elsevier; 1994

27. Shellis RP. A scanning electron-microscopic study of solubility variations in human enamel and dentine. Arch Oral Biol 1996;41(5):473–484

28. Christoffersen MR, Christoffersen J, Arends J. Kinetics of dissolution of calcium hydroxyapatite VII. The effect of fluoride ions. J Cryst Growth 1984;67:107–114

29. Wong L, Cutress TW, Duncan JF. The influence of incorporated and adsorbed fluoride on the dissolution of powdered and pelletized hydroxyapatite in fluoridated and non-fluoridated acid buffers. J Dent Res 1987;66(12):1735–1741

30. de Leeuw N. Resisting the onset of hydroxyapatite dissolution through the incorporation of fluoride. J Phys Chem B 2004;108:1809–1811

31. Arends J, Christoffersen J. Nature and role of loosely bound fluoride in dental caries. J Dent Res 1990;69(Spec No):601–605, discussion 634–636

32. Brown WE, Gregory TM, Chow LC. Effects of fluoride on enamel solubility and cariostasis. Caries Res 1977;11(Suppl 1):118–141

33. Moreno EC, Kresak M, Zahradnik RT. Physicochemical aspects of fluoride-apatite systems relevant to the study of dental caries. Caries Res 1977;11(Suppl 1):142–171

34. Groeneveld A, Van Eck AAMJ, Backer Dirks O. Fluoride in caries prevention: is the effect pre- or post-eruptive? J Dent Res 1990;69(Spec No):751–755, discussion 820–823

35. Marsh PD. Dental plaque as a microbial biofilm. Caries Res 2004;38(3):204–211

36. Schroeder HE, de Boever J. The structure of microbial dental plaque. In: McHugh WD, ed. Dental Plaque. Edinburgh: Livingstone; 1970:49–74

37. Gao XJ, Fan Y, Kent RL Jr, Van Houte J, Margolis HC. Association of caries activity with the composition of dental plaque fluid. J Dent Res 2001;80(9):1834–1839

38. Dibdin GH. Effect on a cariogenic challenge of saliva/plaque exchange via a thin salivary film studied by mathematical modelling. Caries Res 1990;24(4):231–238

39. Paes Leme AF, Koo H, Bellato CM, Bedi G, Cury JA. The role of sucrose in cariogenic dental biofilm formation—new insight. J Dent Res 2006;85(10):878–887

40. Lingström P, van Houte J, Kashket S. Food starches and dental caries. Crit Rev Oral Biol Med 2000;11(3):366–380

41. Rose RK, Dibdin GH, Shellis RP. A quantitative study of calcium binding and aggregation in selected oral bacteria. J Dent Res 1993;72(1):78–84

42. Theuns HM, Driessens FCM, van Dijk JWE, Groeneveld A. Experimental evidence for a gradient in the solubility and in the rate of dissolution of human enamel. Caries Res 1986;20(1):24–31

43. Weatherell JA, Robinson C, Hallsworth AS. Variations in the chemical composition of human enamel. J Dent Res 1974;53(2):180–192

44. Johnson NW. Some aspects of the ultrastructure of early human enamel caries seen with the electron microscope. Arch Oral Biol 1967;12(12):1505–1521

45. Arends J, Christoffersen J. The nature of early caries lesions in enamel. J Dent Res 1986;65(1):2–11

46. Shellis RP. Relationship between human enamel structure and the formation of caries-like lesions in vitro. Arch Oral Biol 1984;29(12):975–981

47. Margolis HC, Moreno EC, Murphy BJ. Effect of low levels of fluoride in solution on enamel demineralization in vitro. J Dent Res 1986;65(1):23–29

48. ten Cate JM, Duijsters PPE. Influence of fluoride in solution on tooth demineralization. I. Chemical data. Caries Res 1983;17(3):193–199, 513–519

49. Aoba T, Moriwaki Y, Doi Y, Okazaki M, Takahashi J, Yagi T. The intact surface layer in natural enamel caries and acid-dissolved hydroxyapatite pellets. An X-ray diffraction study. J Oral Pathol 1981;10(1):32–39

50. Arends J, Schuthof J, Christoffersen J. Inhibition of enamel demineralization by albumin in vitro. Caries Res 1986;20(4):337–340

51. Schüpbach P, Guggenheim B, Lutz F. Histopathology of root surface caries. J Dent Res 1990;69(5):1195–1204

52. Johnson MW, Taylor BR, Berman DS. The response of deciduous dentine to caries studied by correlated light and electron microscopy. Caries Res 1969;3(4):348–368

53. Daculsi G, LeGeros RZ, Jean A, Kerebel B. Possible physico-chemical processes in human dentin caries. J Dent Res 1987;66(8):1356–1359

54. Øgaard B, Rølla G, Arends J. In vivo progress of enamel and root surface lesions under plaque as a function of time. Caries Res 1988;22(5):302–305

55. ten Cate JM, Damen JJM, Buijs MJ. Inhibition of dentin demineralization by fluoride in vitro. Caries Res 1998;32(2):141–147

56. Rose RK, Shellis RP, Lee AR. The role of cation bridging in microbial fluoride binding. Caries Res 1996;30(6):458–464

57. Vogel GL, Carey CM, Ekstrand J. Distribution of fluoride in saliva and plaque fluid after a 0.048 mol/L NaF rinse. J Dent Res 1992;71(9):1553–1557

58. Dijkman AG, Schuthof J, Arends J. In vivo remineralization of plaque-induced initial enamel lesions—a microradiographic investigation. Caries Res 1986;20(3):202–208

59. Teranaka T, Koulourides T, Butler WT. Protein content and amino-acid content of consolidated carious lesions in human enamel and of experimental lesions in bovine enamel exposed to the human mouth. Arch Oral Biol 1986;31(6):405–410

60. Fujikawa H, Matsuyama K, Uchiyama A, Nakashima S, Ujiie T. Influence of salivary macromolecules and fluoride on enamel lesion remineralization in vitro. Caries Res 2008;42(1):37–45

61. Zantner C, Martus P, Kielbassa AM. Clinical monitoring of the effect of fluorides on long-existing white spot lesions. Acta Odontol Scand 2006;64(2):115–122

62. Zero DT, Lussi A. Etiology of erosion: intrinsic and extrinsic factors. In: Addy M, Embery G, Edgar WM, Orchardson R, eds. Tooth Wear and Sensitivity. London: Martin Dunitz; 2000: 121–130

63. Lussi A, Jaeggi T. Chemical Factors. Monogr Oral Sci 2006;20: 77–87

64. Millward A, Shaw L, Harrington E, Smith AJ. Continuous monitoring of salivary flow rate and pH at the surface of the dentition following consumption of acidic beverages. Caries Res 1997; 31(1):44–49

65. Addy M, Shellis RP. Interactions between attrition, abrasion and erosion in tooth wear. Monogr Oral Sci 2006;20:17–31

66. Ganss C, Schlueter N, Hardt M, von Hinckeldey J, Klimek J. Effects of toothbrushing on eroded dentine. Eur J Oral Sci 2007;115(5): 390–396

67. Shellis RP. A synthetic saliva for cultural studies of dental plaque. Arch Oral Biol 1978;23(6):485–489

68. Miller WD. The Microorganism of the Human Mouth [Article in German] Dtsch med Wochenschr 1892;18(45):1016–1018

Histological and Clinical Appearance of Caries

Wolfgang Buchalla

3

The clinical appearance of caries is of great interest to the dental professional, because it tells something of the history of a caries lesion and provides valuable information for adequate noninvasive and invasive treatment. The histology of the caries lesion provides fundamental understanding of the disease process; hence it supports the dental professional with information necessary to make the right treatment decision (Chapters 9 and 20). Much of today's histological knowledge of the caries process was discovered many years ago. Besides advances in oral biology, an understanding of the role of dental biofilm and the invention of the transmitted light microscope, particularly using polarized light, has fostered our knowledge of the caries process. But also other techniques, such as transmission and scanning electron microscopy, fluorescence microscopy, and microradiography have added to our understanding of how caries develops within a tooth.

This chapter will address the following:

- How do enamel and dentin caries appear clinically and histologically?
- How does the caries lesion manifest using different investigative methods—for example, light microscopy, scanning electron microscopy, microradiography (mineral content), hardness testing and fluorescence?
- Caries is a dynamic process—how can caries activity be recognized?
- Where are the bacteria within a caries lesion?
- Can the caries process be stopped and dental hard tissue even be remineralized?
- Dental erosion—not caries, but also destructive to the dentition.

Enamel Caries

Location in the Teeth

Since it is caused by acids produced from a **biofilm** covering the tooth surface, carious dissolution of dental hard tissue (i.e., enamel, dentin, and cementum) always starts on a tooth's surface, which is accessible to the oral environment. Clinically, this may be at the enamel surface, root cementum, or exposed dentin. For simplicity we look first at caries affecting the enamel layer only, and then follow the histological and clinical appearance of the caries process as it penetrates deeper into the tooth. As observed clinically, caries most often develops at typical anatomical sites of the teeth, the **plaque stagnation areas** (**Fig. 3.1**; see also Chapter 1). Caries in pits and fissures is typical for younger people. Caries at interproximal surfaces and at the gingival margin, particularly when root cementum and dentin are exposed, is typical for older patients. These caries predilection sites all facilitate plaque accumulation, because there is some local protection from mechanical cleaning, notably from tongue and cheek movements, and from toothbrushing. Although caries lesions develop predominantly at specific sites, the specific properties of the overlying biofilm (**Figs. 3.1a** and **3.2**) are largely responsible for determining whether or not caries will develop, rather than specific properties of the enamel itself (**Fig. 3.1f**; see also Chapter 2). In principle, the fundamental processes of caries development act the same way, irrespective of the location. Every caries process in

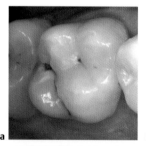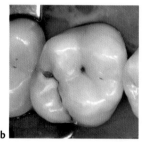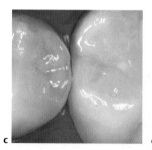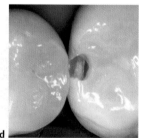

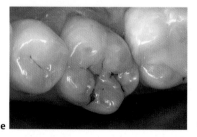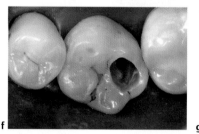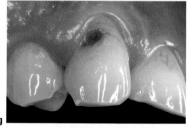

Fig. 3.1a–g Caries lesions start developing at plaque stagnation areas.

a, b Plaque accumulation in the fossae of an upper molar tooth (**a**). After cleaning, this tooth shows a deep (distal) and less developed (central) caries lesion (**b**).

c, d Interproximal (approximal) plaque accumulation has led to caries development below the contact point of a lower molar tooth, which cannot easily be seen by visual examination (**c**) but

extends well into dentin as can be seen during operative treatment (**d**).

e–g It is not the properties of enamel or dentin tissue of the site itself that facilitates caries development, but plaque accumulation, as can be seen at a rotated lower molar tooth (**e**) with deep interproximal caries at an unusual site (**f**). Caries at the cervical region of an upper canine tooth (**g**).

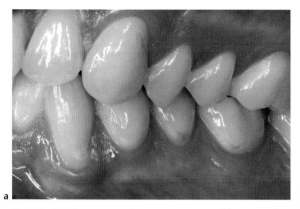

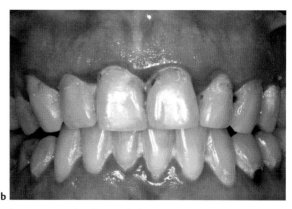

Fig. 3.2a,b Plaque accumulation at interproximal (approximal) and cervical regions, which already has caused cervical caries.
a Small amounts of plaque with cervical caries beginning underneath (young patient).

b Interproximal and cervical plaque deposition with cervical caries at several teeth (older patient suffering from hyposalivation). Note: gingivitis following plaque accumulation at the gingival margin.

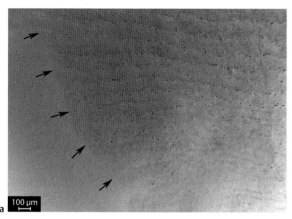

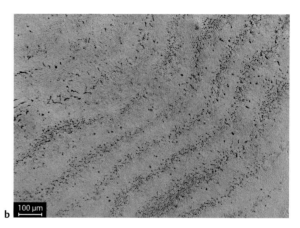

Fig. 3.3a–c SEM images of an interproximal (approximal) site of a molar tooth following extraction and vigorous ultrasonication in NaOCl solution to remove the dental plaque without damaging the surface.
a The border of an early caries lesion (indicated by black arrows) separates sound enamel (left side) from etched, slightly demineralized enamel.
b Surface porosities scattered along the perikymata.
c Quite often a honeycomblike structure is revealed, indicating a preferred dissolution pattern.

enamel starts with slight "etching" of the surface (**Fig. 3.3a**) under a layer of dental plaque.[1] It can be assumed that this process occurs frequently under almost any plaque-covered area and starts as soon as the plaque fluid becomes **undersaturated** with respect to any enamel mineral present (Chapter 2). At a very early stage, the "etching" is reversible. Only under cariogenic circumstances does the dissolution process progress, leaving **micro-**

porosities at the enamel surface (**Fig. 3.3**) that start to extend deeper into the enamel (**Fig. 3.4**). These microporosities are typically located at the prism boundaries and, with further progression, within the prism cores (Chapters 1 and 2).

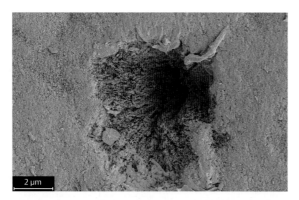

Fig. 3.4 SEM image from a micropore surrounded by enamel of low porosity (intact surface layer). The micropore extends several micrometers into the enamel. Such micropores are often the entrance into channels that extend several hundred micrometers into the enamel.

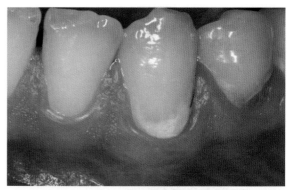

Fig. 3.5 Cervical white spot lesion of a lower canine following removal of the overlying plaque and brief air-drying. Note the dull, matt appearance indicating an active lesion. The cervical caries lesion of the premolar has already developed further including breakdown of the cervical enamel layer. The blood pooling at the gingival margin of the canine is due to tooth cleaning before taking the photograph, indicating gingivitis in this area.

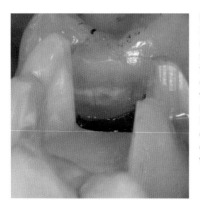

Fig. 3.6 Interproximal (approximal) white spot lesion with central brownish discoloration that became visible during preparation of the neighboring tooth. The oblong shape is typical for interproximal white spot lesions.

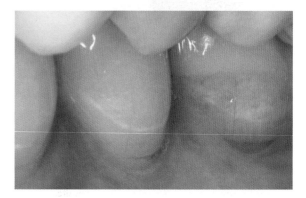

Fig. 3.7 Band-shaped white spot lesions of lower premolars parallel to, but distinctly above the gingival crest. These lesions must have developed at an earlier age when the patient's teeth were not fully erupted.

NOTE

Caries lesions begin to form at specific sites in plaque stagnation areas. To begin with, the caries lesion is no more than a slight, not clinically recognizable etching of the surface underneath a layer of biofilm.

The White Spot Lesion

The first **clinical signs** (visible to the eye of the dental professional) of caries are the so-called **"white spot"** lesions. These lesions can be seen when plaque is removed from the enamel surface and this surface is dried with compressed air for a few seconds (**Fig. 3.5**). At a more advanced stage of disease, white spot lesions are visible also when the enamel surface is still wet. At this stage the caries process may have advanced through the entire enamel layer and into the dentin.[2–4] White spot lesions appear white, because a greater proportion of the incoming light is being backscattered as compared with the

surrounding sound enamel. This is due to an increase in pore volume, which is an increase of porosities in size and number when enamel becomes demineralized, and the difference of the refractive indices of air (or electrolyte) filling those porosities and adjacent enamel.

Activity of White and Brown Spot Lesions

When located interproximally, natural white spot lesions typically appear as oblong shapes below or around the contact point, where they cannot be viewed directly under normal conditions (**Fig. 3.6**). When located at the vestibular or oral aspect of the tooth just above the gingival margin, they are spread out in a line. In some instances, a whitish, sometimes discolored band can be found parallel to, but at some distance from, the gingival margin in teeth of the permanent dentition (**Fig. 3.7**). In this case, most likely, the lesion has developed when the tooth was not fully erupted, which also is a period during which tooth cleaning is often neglected. Following com-

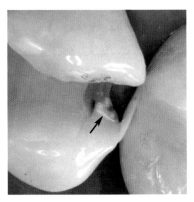

Fig. 3.8 Section through an interproximal (approximal) caries lesion exposed by operative treatment procedures. The enamel caries (arrow) is typically cone-shaped in appearance.

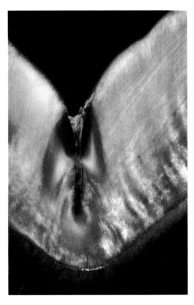

Fig. 3.9 Histological section through the crown of a premolar tooth with fissure caries without cavitation viewed by reflected light microscopy. Lesion development follows the prism orientation, leading to the shape of an inverted cone ("butterfly"). The deepest demineralization of this long fissure occurred at the fissure entrance, most likely due to a better nutritional situation for the plaque bacteria at this site.

nett loss of minerals, they have more porosities at the surface than lesions that are not active. Therefore, an active white spot lesion shows a matt, dull surface, while an inactive lesion presents a shiny surface.[1,8] White spot lesions that are not covered by plaque are clinically almost certainly shiny and inactive, mainly due to incorporation of minerals (remineralization), and abrasion and polishing related to plaque removal.[1]

Lesion progression of white spot lesions within enamel roughly follows the rod/prism direction. The three-dimensional morphology of small white spot lesions on the approximal surface resembles a cone with its base at the enamel surface and its tip toward the enamel–dentin junction (EDJ) (**Fig. 3.8**). The three-dimensional morphology of the occlusal fissure lesion is with the tip at the surface and the base toward the EDJ due to the directions of the prisms in the fissure area (**Fig. 3.9**).

> **NOTE**
>
> The first clinically visible sign of caries-affected enamel is the white spot lesion, which can be as deep as several hundred micrometers. This lesion is composed of a porous body covered by a well-mineralized surface zone. The appearance and porosity of this surface layer is influenced by the lesion activity. Lesion development follows the direction of the enamel prisms.

Transmitted and Polarized Light Microscopy

Many of the findings from histology of the caries lesion were obtained using transmitted and polarized light microscopy. A caries lesion that is well developed within enamel and has not reached the dentin, and thus likely is not cavitated, has typical histological features. These features can also be found in part within lesions in a more advanced state with a cavitated surface.

BACKGROUND

In transmitted light microscopy thin sections of dental hard tissue can be viewed making use mainly of differences in scattering and absorption. Changes within enamel due to carious demineralization lead to a higher degree of scattering and backscattering, whereby these areas appear darker compared to the surrounding, sound areas. Additional incorporation of pigments leads to increased absorption that adds to the effect of backscattering.

Polarized light microscopy makes use of the optical anisotropy of crystals, that is, the ability of a crystal to split incident polarized light into two parts composed of waves that oscillate perpendicularly to each other and travel at different speeds, due to different refraction indices. This property is called birefringence. It occurs in many but not all crystalline materials, and also in regu-

plete eruption, the local ecosystem may have changed due to better cleaning, which is why the demineralized band stabilizes, remaining an inactive white spot lesion, sometimes turning into a brown spot.

When located occlusally, white spot caries lesions develop locally in particular in the fossa areas and grooves (Chapter 1).[5–7] Quite often white spot lesions incorporate exogenous pigments from food, which adds a brownish tint (brown spot lesion). It is believed that exogenous pigments are incorporated with time, indicating that **brown spot lesions** have existed for longer already than white spot lesions. This would mean that brown discoloration is a sign of slow progression or low activity. Certainly, the pigmentation of white spot lesions relies on several factors like nutritional habits, surface porosity, and so on. In some instances, white spot lesions remain white for many years and therefore it cannot be assumed that the absence of brown discoloration in enamel lesions is a sign of high caries activity and fast progression.

A more reliable marker for **lesion activity** is the appearance of the surface of a white spot lesion following removal of the biofilm. While active lesions are in a state of larly constructed organic materials, like some proteins. One of the two refractive indices is called the extraordinary refractive index (n_e) which is defined as parallel to the optical axis of the crystal as opposed to the ordinary refractive index (n_o) which occurs perpendicular to the optical axis of that crystal.[9] The crystal is optically isotropic only for light propagating parallel to the optical axis. For all other directions of incoming light the crystal is anisotropic, meaning that the incoming light wave is split into two waves that travel under the influence of two different refractive indices, n_o and n_e, with their oscillating planes perpendicular to each other. For $n_e > n_o$ a crystal or object is referred to as being positive birefringent, for $n_e < n_o$ it is negative birefringent.

In the presence of porosities alongside such crystals, the matter that fills these porosities (the imbibition medium, e.g., air, Canada balsam, quinoline, or other fluids) adds a third refractive index. The relationship between the three refractive indices and the pore volume in the object determines the maximum amount of light passing through the second polarizer that, within a polarization microscope, sits on the ocular side of the object. By variation of the imbibition media having different refractive indices and turning the object between the two crossed polarizers, information on the nature of the tissue under investigation and on the pore volume within the tissue can be obtained.

Traditional histology performed on thin sections perpendicular to the surface and through the enamel lesion describes four distinct zones within carious enamel that can be visualized using transmitted and polarized light microscopy (**Fig. 3.10**). At the lesion front is a zone that can be seen in about 50% of all samples.[10] It appears brighter than healthy, sound enamel and shows hardly any structural features in transmitted light microscopy using an index matching fluid (a fluid with a refractive index close to enamel, i.e., quinoline with n = 1.625 at 589nm). This **translucent zone** contains porosities larger than the size of quinoline molecules that are mainly located at the prism boundaries.[11] The pore volume in sound enamel is around 0.1%. In the translucent zone the pore volume is increased up to 1%[12] (**Fig. 3.11**). Examined with polarized light microscopy, the translucent zone, like sound enamel, shows negative birefringence. In the translucent zone, crystals of slightly smaller size than in sound enamel (40nm diameter) can be found, indicating initial demineralization.

The next zone after the translucent zone toward the enamel surface is commonly named the **dark zone** and can be found in most sections through enamel lesions.[10] It appears dark-brownish in transmitted light microscopy using quinoline as an index matching fluid. This indicates the presence of porosities smaller than the size of quinoline molecules. Because these small porosities remain filled with air, light scattering is increased in this area

leading to more backscattering, which explains the dark appearance in transmitted light and bright appearance in reflected light microscopy. Presence of small porosities, besides larger porosities that can be filled with quinoline, is also confirmed by polarized light microscopy. Due to the presence of these air-filled small porosities, negative birefringence, typical for sound enamel and the translucent zone, turns into positive birefringence in the dark zone. Using an index matching fluid of smaller molecular size (Thoulet solution, $n = 1.62$), the dark zone becomes bright in transmitted light microscopy and negatively birefringent in polarized light microscopy. The pore volume of the dark zone has been estimated to be 2%–4%. Demineralization in the dark zone was also found to affect prism boundaries, but to a greater extent than in the translucent zone. There is some evidence that the small porosities (that cannot be penetrated by quinoline) are partly remineralized larger porosities.[10] An indication that remineralization is part of the processes taking part within the dark zone is the presence of crystals of larger diameter (50–100nm) as compared with the crystals of sound enamel (40nm).[13] Recently, the presence of exogenous lipids and proteins in the porosities within the dark zone has been reported and it was concluded that they may hamper mineral precipitation and thus remineralization.[14]

The next zone toward the enamel surface is the **body of the lesion**, which shows the highest degree of demineralization within the carious lesion. The body of the lesion is present in all samples prepared from enamel caries lesions. This zone is clearly visible by microradiography (see below) but also with clinical radiography when not superimposed by too high an amount of sound dental hard tissue (see Chapter 6). Using imbibition in quinoline as an index-matching fluid, the body of the lesion appears bright, similar to sound enamel in transmitted light, meaning the presence of porosities with a relative large diameter. In polarized light microscopy the body of the lesion shows positive birefringence (as opposed to negative birefringence of sound enamel). Using water as an imbibition medium that has a refractive index different from enamel mineral ($n_{water} = 1.333$), the body of the lesion stays positive birefringent using polarized light microscopy (sound enamel is negative birefringent under these conditions). In this zone striae of Retzius are clearly visible. Crystals become partly or completely dissolved along the prism boundaries but crystal dissolution can also be observed within the prisms (see TEM below). The pore volume of all zones within enamel is highest in the body of the lesion, being 5%–25% and higher.[15]

The outermost zone of enamel caries is the **surface zone**, sometimes referred to as the intact or pseudo-intact surface layer with a typical thickness of 10–50μm, but it may extend up to 120μm.[16] Its unique property is a relatively high mineral content and a pore volume that can be below 5% due to remineralization processes (see Chapter 2). Therefore, crystal size is somewhat larger (40–80nm) than in sound enamel. The surface zone is clearly visible

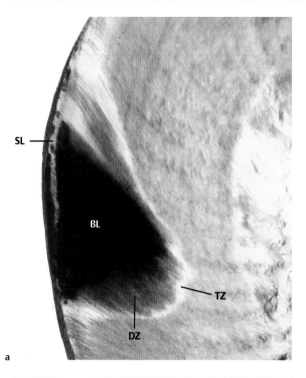

SL

BL

TZ

DZ

a

Fig. 3.10a–c   Light microscopy of a histological section through an enamel caries lesion not reaching the enamel–dentin junction.
a   Transmitted light microscopy shows (starting at the outer surface) an intact surface layer (SL), the body of the lesion (BL), the dark zone (DZ), and the translucent zone (TZ).
b   Polarized light microscopy of the same specimen. The translucent zone and parts of the surface zone show positive birefringence. The body of the lesion is negative birefringent.
c   Polarized light microscopy using a lambda-plate. The translucent zone and parts of the surface zone show positive birefringence. The body of the lesion is negative birefringent.

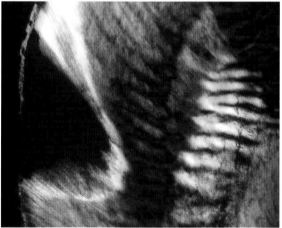

b

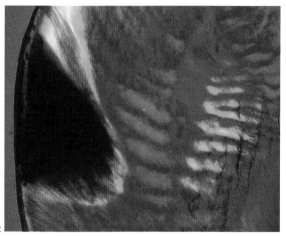

c

using microradiography (see below). Using polarized microscopy, the surface zone is negative birefringent, being the same as sound enamel using water as the imbibition medium ($n = 1.333$) and also (in most cases) using no additional imbibition medium (air with $n = 1.000$).

NOTE

The classical caries zones of enamel caries with an intact surface have been identified on the basis of differences in the amount and size of porosities using transmitted light microscopy (starting at the outer enamel surface):
- Surface zone
- Body of the lesion
- Dark zone
- Translucent zone

Using imbibition media of varying optical refractive indices with transmitted light microscopy or polarized light microscopy, information on the size of the porosities and the pore volume within sound and carious enamel can be obtained.

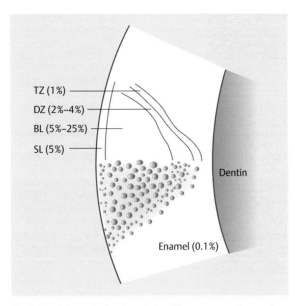

Fig. 3.11 Schematic drawing of the different zones of enamel caries not reaching the enamel–dentin junction, porosities (lower part of the drawing), and pore volume (in parentheses). SL: surface layer; BL: body of the lesion; DZ: dark zone; TZ: translucent zone.

Transverse Microradiography (TMR)

The "beauty" of microradiography is that **mineral content** is measured straightforwardly by the high x-ray absorption of enamel (and dentin) minerals as opposed to the organic and water content present in dental hard tissue. Transverse microradiography (TMR) is considered to be the "gold standard" for determination of the spatial distribution of mineral content across caries lesions from the surface into the deeper layers. Most commonly, 80–100 µm thick sections are prepared perpendicularly to the tooth surface through the caries lesion.[17] These sections are mounted in front of a high-resolution x-ray sensitive film or plate together with an aluminum step wedge for calibration. This set-up is irradiated with Cu K-α x-rays perpendicularly to the film and the cut surface, which is also referred to as transverse or transversal microradiography. The developed film is viewed under a microscope and can be used for qualitative assessment of the carious lesion (**Fig. 3.12**). By using optical densitometry of the film and correlation with gray values from the aluminum calibration step wedge, the mineral content at any given point of the specimen can be calculated, provid-

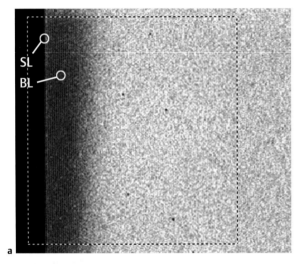

Fig. 3.12a, b

a Microradiograph (detail of a TMR x-ray exposure) of a surface-perpendicular cut through an artificial, early caries lesion of the enamel. The dotted line encloses the area that was analyzed and is represented in (**b**). The dotted square encloses 265 × 277 µm. A thin reasonably well mineralized surface layer and the lesion body are clearly visible.

b Microradiogram of the microradiograph in (**a**). The mineral profile shows a typical artificial enamel caries with the mineral-rich surface layer (SL), the body of the lesion with the lesion body point (BL), the lesion depth (LD) at 73 µm, the sound mineral content at 87 vol%, and the integrated mineral loss (ΔZ) which is the blue area above the mineral profile. Natural caries lesions in their early state show the same features, albeit with a lesion body which is less demineralized, and a wider and higher mineralized surface layer.

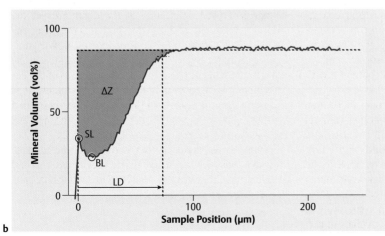

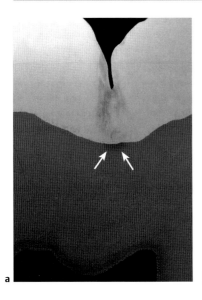 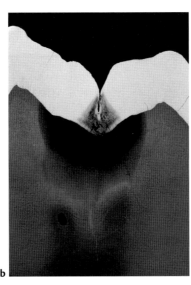

Fig. 3.13a, b Image of a cut through a carious lower molar tooth by backscatter SEM. Lighter gray levels indicate a higher mineral content.
a Early fissure caries with intact enamel surface. Note the unhomogeneous mineral loss within the enamel and the small amount of demineralization within the dentin.
b Deep dentin lesion with the enamel surface still intact. Despite severe demineralization within the enamel, its surface is still intact, most likely due to a lack of mechanical impact in this area. Dentin close to the enamel–dentin junction (EDJ) is severely demineralized. Closer to the pulp, brighter, well-mineralized zones have developed. The circular dark area in the lower third of the image is pulp that was exposed during sample preparation.

ing a quantitative method.[18,19] Using **backscatter-electron imaging** of tooth sections with a scanning electron microscope (**Fig. 3.13**), qualitative information can be gained similarly to microradiography.

The nature of white spot caries lesions can be investigated using **artificially created lesions**. Typically, enamel specimens with a natural or a ground-and-polished surface are exposed to an acidic buffer solution or gel. Depending on the demineralization method used, a carious lesion forms within hours and up to several weeks or months.[1,20, 21] These lesions show most features of natural caries lesions (**Fig. 3.12**). From the outside toward the EDJ the mineral-rich surface layer is clearly visible as is the body of the lesion. From the area of the deepest demineralization on, the mineral content increases continuously toward deeper layers until it reaches the mineral content of sound enamel. The position of the dark and translucent zone visible in transmitted and polarized light microscopy cannot be identified separately in a microradiograph. In other words, the relative clear borders of these zones visible in transmitted and polarized light microscopy do not correspond to abrupt changes in mineral content. Whereas artificially created, carieslike lesions progress almost parallel to the enamel surface, natural enamel lesions develop in a more irregular pattern. This may be caused by the irregular distribution and properties of the cariogenic plaque covering the enamel surface and, in addition, changes of the plaque cariogenic potential with time.

A feature quite often observed with natural enamel caries is the formation of zones with varying mineral content, or bands of higher mineral content that extend through the body of the lesion. These bands run quasi-parallel to the surface, but may be curvy in shape, with the convex aspect toward the EDJ. In an artificial caries model with cyclic de- and remineralization, these bands may also appear. This supports the assumption that the mineral layering within a carious lesion is due to changes in car-

iogenicity of plaque covering the enamel. However, it also was suggested that layers of increased mineral content within the body of the lesion resemble the advancing front of the lesion at an earlier stage.[22]

Scanning Electron Microscopy (SEM)

Scanning electron microscopy of the enamel surface reveals the early stages of caries demineralization. Often, surface porosities can be observed in the imbrication lines of Pickerill along the perikymata (see **Fig. 3.3a, b**). A closer look reveals an enlargement of the interprismatic spaces that may extend from the surface into the depth of the lesion. Beneath areas of dissolution of the interprismatic space, dissolution of the prism core can be found (**Fig. 3.14**). In both cases, at the crystal level, the dissolution process starts from the intercrystal space, enlarging the intercrystal space and reducing crystal diameter and length. Also, dissolution from inside the crystals has been observed (see "TEM" section below). It has been reported that even in the body of the enamel lesion the outer area of the prisms sometimes is less prone to demineralization than the prism core. Reasons suggested for this are a change in crystal orientation at the outer area of the prisms[23,24] as well as the higher organic content of the prism sheath. Also, remineralization (crystal growth) during the caries process[25–27] can be assumed, because in the outer area of prisms of carious enamel, crystals of thicker diameter have been found (120–150nm diameter) as is the case in sound enamel. In this case the newly formed crystals most likely contain more fluoride and are less soluble than native enamel crystals (Chapter 2).

Overall, while caries lesions show an intact surface clinically even when the demineralization has reached the dentin, SEM reveals the presence of small cavitations at earlier stages of the disease.

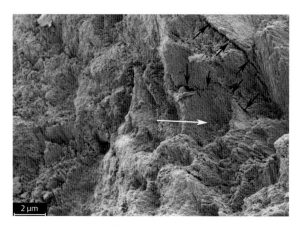

Fig. 3.14 SEM image of a partially cavitated, interproximal white spot lesion. The black arrows indicate an enlarged interprismatic space. The white arrow points at dissolution and wear of a prism core.

Transmission Electron Microscopy (TEM)

Transmission electron microscopy is a technique for investigation of enamel at the ultrastructural level with a theoretical resolution limit of about 0.05 nm. Using TEM it is possible to show specific features of carious enamel, particularly of the crystals. Individual crystals seem to dissolve either from the outside,[28] starting with etching of the crystal surface, or from the inside along the lattice c-axis (longitudinal axis).[28-30] It is not clear so far, under which circumstances either one is the preferred form of crystal dissolution. On the enamel surface of initial caries lesions lacunaelike defects can be found of about 5μm width and depth (see **Fig. 3.4**) that are filled with plaque, including bacteria. Although TEM reveals highly resolved images of ultrathin enamel sections, it shows differences between caries and sound dental enamel only from the body of the lesion, with a pore volume of about 10%–25%. Formation of narrow gaps (30–100 nm width) around prisms of the body of the lesions can be seen in TEM images, but it is still not clear whether this is a sign of demineralization or an artifact from specimen preparation.[28]

> **NOTE**
>
> - A white spot lesion of enamel consists of a surface layer with mineral content lower than sound enamel, but higher than the underlying body of the lesion.
> - Within a white spot lesion, prisms dissolve from the outside, starting with widening of the interprismatic space, but also dissolution of the prism core can be observed.
> - Enamel crystals dissolve either from the outside, getting shorter and smaller in diameter over time, or along the crystal c-axis, leading to hollow tubelike crystals.

Dentin Caries

Whether the caries process that started at the enamel surface will progress into deeper layers depends on the microenvironment at the enamel surface. Under cariogenic conditions the caries process continues and reaches the EDJ and the underlying dentin. As long as the caries is limited to enamel, the carious area located at smooth surfaces and interproximal areas is bigger at the outer enamel and decreases in size toward the EDJ (see **Fig. 3.8**).

As soon as the EDJ is reached, the caries may **spread along the EDJ** to a certain extent and from there into the dentin (**Figs. 3.13, 3.15, 3.16**). The EDJ is known to have higher organic and lower mineral content than enamel and dentin.[31-33] Hence, its higher content of water and organic material may enable lateral spreading of cariogenic acids and assist demineralization of the EDJ area. The same may apply for the proteolytic action of certain bacterial enzymes (see later for more detail). However, the caries process does not extend evenly into underlying dentin from affected areas of the EDJ. The most prominent changes in dentin occur in the center where carious enamel reaches the EDJ. The width of the cariously affected dentin decreases from the EDJ toward the pulp during the advancement of the caries process. The spread of the caries process within dentin follows the direction of the dentinal tubules.

However, lateral spreading of disease along the EDJ is observed more often at a more advanced stage of the caries process with breakdown of the enamel surface rather than with the latter still intact. The reason for this is not fully understood, and some authors have shown results indicating that the mineral content of the EDJ decreases continuously from enamel to dentin,[34,35] which casts doubt on the theory that the EDJ is more vulnerable to acids than the dentin.

It is important to realize that there is a fundamental difference in reaction mechanisms between enamel and dentin. Enamel is a cell-free tissue which does not show any cellular response in the case of caries attack; enamel reaction is based on chemical dissolution and precipitation phenomena. Dentin is different, because it has to be considered as **vital tissue**, since it contains living cellular processes from the odontoblasts lining the pulpo-dentinal wall.[36,37] In dentin, the odontoblasts and the pulp are closely related to one another. Dentin shows reactions that are due to cellular mechanisms of the odontoblasts and therefore it is well justified to consider dentin and the pulp as a physiological unit (Chapter 1). The **dentin–pulp unit** is an organ in itself, consisting also of blood and lymphatic vessels, connective tissue, nerve tissue, stem cells, etc. This allows the dentin–pulp unit to react to stimuli, albeit physiological masticatory forces, traumatic injury (thermal, mechanical or chemical), or caries.[38,39] In that sense, the dentin–pulp unit can be compared with bone, whose inorganic fraction is modulated by osteo-

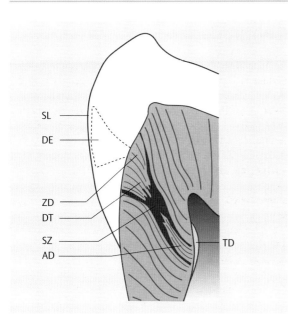

Fig. 3.15a–c Schematic illustration of caries into dentin with the enamel surface intact (**a**), enamel surface cavitated (**b**) and enamel completely broken in (**c**).

a Appearance of dentin caries with an intact enamel surface layer (SL). Demineralized enamel (DE) has reached the enamel–dentin junction. Within dentin, the affected area has a broad base at the enamel–dentin junction, where the zone of demineralization (ZD) is often enclosed from the side by the sclerotic zone (SZ) that converges to a clearly visible zone deeper toward the pulp. Between the zone of demineralization and the sclerotic zone, a zone with "dead tracts" (DT) can be observed. Between the sclerotic zone and the pulp, dentin is hardly distinguishable from "normal" dentin, but it can be considered as affected dentin (AD), because the otherwise reactive or tertiary dentin (TD) would not be formed by the odontoblasts during the carious attack. Note that with the enamel surface intact, single bacteria may penetrate the porosities in enamel, but cannot be found within dentin.

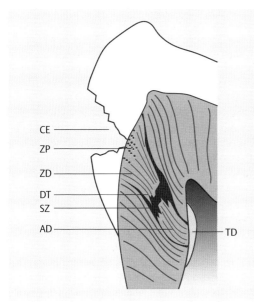

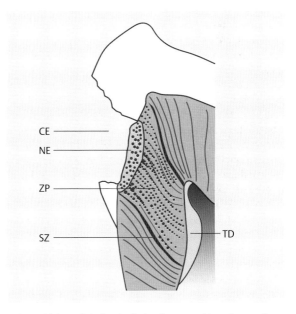

b With cavitated enamel (CE), bacteria (red dots) soon reach dentin and penetrate the dentinal tubules, referred to as the zone of bacterial penetration (ZP). As long as the bacteria are confined to the outer dentin, the characteristic zones within dentin persist: zone of demineralization (ZD), dead tracts (DT), sclerotic zone (SZ), "normal," but affected dentin (AD), and tertiary dentin (TD). During the process of bacterial penetration, the zones spread toward the pulp, the dead tracts disappear, and the sclerotic zone becomes thinner.

c In a widely cavitated caries lesion the enamel layer has partly gone (cavitated enamel, CE) and dentin is readily exposed to plaque accumulation (not shown). The superficial dentin layer, the zone of necrosis (NE), is heavily loaded with bacteria (red dots), is soft, and does not show the tubular structure of dentin any more. Underneath is the zone of bacterial penetration (ZP) that extends more and more toward the pulp. The demineralized zone advances in front of the zone of bacterial penetration at the expense of the sclerotic zone and the "normal" but affected dentin, but is overrun by bacterial penetration with time. Within the zone of bacterial penetration the dentin tubules are heavily loaded with bacteria. During the caries process the zone of bacterial penetration also widens laterally, shifting the sclerotic zone (SZ) sideways. The tertiary dentin (TD) is still present but is also penetrated by bacteria with time.

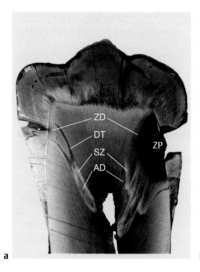
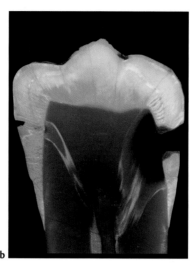

Fig. 3.16a, b Histological mesiodistal section through the crown of a premolar tooth with an interproximal dentin lesion with light (left side of tooth section) and heavy enamel breakdown (right side of tooth section).

a Transmitted light microscopic view. Within dentin the zone of demineralization (ZD, red-brown), the dead tracts (DT, dark), the sclerotic zone (SZ, bright), and "normal," affected dentin (AD) can be seen in both lesions. The zone of bacterial penetration (ZP) is confined to the dark red-brown discolored area of the lesion on the right side, but its borders cannot be identified exactly. Tertiary dentin is hardly visible in this section.

b Reflected light microscopic view of the same section as in (**a**). Other than in transmitted light, the dead tracts appear bright and the sclerotic zone is hardly visible.

cytes and osteoblasts, which also react to physiological or pathological stimuli.[40]

The histology of caries, as it extends into the dentin, reveals a sequence of different zones. While the order of these zones is always the same, the presence or absence of individual zones relates to the progress of the caries as it proceeds toward the pulp (**Fig. 3.15**).

Early Signs of Dentin Reaction

With continuing demineralization of the enamel layer and increasing enamel porosity, acids and toxins of bacterial origin are able to reach and penetrate the underlying dentin. This may be the case well before breakdown of the enamel surface integrity. At this stage, the bacteria are still organized within the plaque covering the enamel surface and do not penetrate the enamel or dentin just yet or only in small numbers.

A first sign of dentin reaction is **tubular sclerosis** (see next paragraph). To avoid confusion, we start by looking at the changes within dentin from the pulpal side toward the EDJ. Usually, after the process of tubular sclerosis has begun, the odontoblasts start building a layer of **reactive dentin**, also referred to as **reparative** or **tertiary dentin** (**Fig. 3.15**; see also an advanced lesion in **Fig. 3.17a**). Since odontoblastic processes and nerve fibers extend well into the dentinal tubules, it is conceivable that the advent of toxins into dentin tubules already triggers the synthesis of reactive dentin by the odontoblasts. Reactive dentin can be found when the caries process reaches deeper into dentin, but it is absent in some cases (**Fig. 3.16**). When the caries process develops slowly over a long time, reactive dentin has a more regular structure with dentinal tubuli, which may be very similar to normal primary or secondary dentin. Under highly cariogenic conditions— that is, rapidly evolving caries which imposes a strong stimulus on the pulp, particularly on the odontoblasts—the expression of reactive dentin is accelerated and its structure may be poorly organized (dysplastic)

with lack of dentinal tubules, and is called osteodentin or fibrodentin. Mature tertiary dentin consists of **type I collagen**, as normal dentin does, while its predentin also comprises **type III collagen**.[41] In the earlier state of dentin affected by the caries process, a layer of normal, unaffected dentin remains below the reactive dentin.

NOTE

Dentin reacts to caries before the demineralization process reaches the enamel–dentin junction (EDJ) and long before the enamel surface breaks down. The first sign of dentin reaction is tubular sclerosis. At this stage no bacteria can be found in the dentin and, as long as the enamel surface is macroscopically intact, hardly any bacteria penetrate the enamel owing to the small size of the enamel porosities at the surface.

Further on, in the direction of the EDJ, a layer of **sclerotic dentin** (earlier referred to as the **translucent zone**) is visible in thin sections using transmitted light microscopy. It is broadest (in the centripetal direction) close to the underlying layer of normal, unaffected dentin, but has "wings" extending almost parallel to the dentinal tubules toward the EDJ. This zone appears bright in transmitted light microscopy, but dark in reflected light microscopy, because the dentin is more translucent due to a better match of the refractive indices of the sclerotic tubules and intertubular dentin. Sclerotic dentin shows occluded tubules with a thick peritubular layer, and a calcified tubular lumen that contains predominantly highly organized apatite crystals and, to a lesser degree, crystals of the Whitlockite type.[42] Keep in mind that these properties are true for a state of caries development where the enamel surface is porous, but still intact, and the dentin itself is hardly demineralized. The properties and shape of the sclerotic zone change with the progression of demineralization.

The next zone toward the outside of the tooth appears relatively dark in transmitted light microscopy. Formation of this zone, referred to as "**dead tracts**," is a consequence of tubular occlusion in the underlying zone consisting of sclerotic dentin. The dead-tract zone is ideally completely enclosed within the sclerotic zone (**Fig. 3.15**). Due to tubular occlusion within the sclerotic zone and retraction of the odontoblastic cellular processes, the dentinal tubules in the dead-tract zone appear empty and cut off from the living odontoblast; that is why it is commonly termed "dead tract." This term comes from experiments in which a dye was placed in the pulp chambers of extracted teeth with dentinal caries and its penetration back into dentin was observed in sections using transmitted light microscopy.[43] It was observed that the dye penetrated into the dentinal tubules of healthy dentin. In areas at the border of carious lesions, dye penetration came to a halt at the sclerotic dentin and could not penetrate further. Dead-tract dentinal tubules easily fill with air in thin sections. They may contain remnants of the odontoblastic processes and are typically more permeable for incoming acids and proteolytic enzymes than tubules within healthy dentin. Therefore, this zone is *less resistant* toward further progression of the caries process. At later stages of the caries process involving enamel cavity formation, bacteria are well able to penetrate the dentinal tubules within the dead-tract zone.

Between the dead tracts and the EDJ the so-called **demineralized zone** can be found, usually when carious enamel demineralization reaches the EDJ. It is caused by the penetration of organic acids of bacterial origin into the dentin. Although this zone is considerably demineralized, it appears rather similar to healthy dentin in transmitted and reflected light microscopy. The zone of demineralization contains less mineral (approximately down to 25% and less) and has lower hardness (approximately down to as low as 10KHN and less) than the sclerotic dentin. As long as the enamel has not collapsed, it is unlikely that bacteria penetrate the underlying dentin. This means that the cariogenic acids, enzymes, and toxins of bacterial origin are synthesized in the dental plaque covering the enamel surface and, consequently, travel deep into the dentin by diffusion as long as the enamel surface has not broken down.

NOTE

With the enamel surface still intact, the caries process reaches the EDJ. With further caries development the following zones can be seen using transmitted light microscopy (from the enamel–dentin junction toward the pulp):
- Zone of demineralization
- Dead tracts
- Sclerotic zone
- Normal, but affected dentin
- Tertiary dentin

Continuing Caries Progression into Dentin

Collapse of the (pseudo-)intact enamel surface means a significant change in caries progression and prognosis. As long as the enamel surface is macroscopically intact, penetration of dental plaque, bacteria, or their components is very much limited. Collapse of the intact enamel surface not only means that the enamel porosities have become so big that they no longer support mechanical stability, it also means that huge numbers of bacteria are able to penetrate the enamel lesion. Consequently, removal of bacteria and dental plaque from the porosities and the enamel crater by mechanical means is not possible any more for most occlusal and interproximal lesions. From this point on, depending on the available nutritional conditions, further lesion development is most likely to occur. With invasion of huge numbers of bacteria into the porous enamel, bacteria soon reach the EDJ and invade the dentin, forming the **zone of penetration**, which takes over the former zone of demineralization. Still at this point, the zone of demineralization precedes the bacterial invasion. This is of some clinical relevance, because it means that demineralized dentin does not necessarily contain bacteria and may be left during excavation (Chapter 18). Also, irreversible pulpal inflammation is typically seen only at later stages, with the bacteria advancing as close to the pulp as around 0.5mm.[44]

With penetration of bacteria deeper into the demineralized zone, the demineralized zone itself moves toward the zone of sclerotic dentin at the expense of the dead-tract zone (**Fig. 3.15c**). While the sclerotic dentin with its mineralized tubules shows some resistance against further demineralization and penetration of bacterial cells, the dead-tract area with its relatively wide tubules shows relatively little resistance against demineralization and bacterial invasion. The diameters of bacterial cells are similar in range to those of dentin tubules. With further progression of the bacterial front, the sclerotic dentin disappears completely, usually before the advancing front of bacteria reaches the pulpal wall. At this stage the enamel layer may have been broken down completely, thus exposing a large area of carious dentin. As long as the dentin surface, now opened up, stays covered by plaque, the complete degradation of dentin continues. While at the earlier stages of dentin involvement, demineralization by **bacterial acids** plays the major role, at the later stages **hydrolytic** and **proteolytic enzymes** successfully degrade the demineralized dentin matrix. The remaining soft material, consisting of remnants of demineralized dentin and dental plaque, is often referred to as the **zone of destruction**. Still, remnants of the sclerotic zone may be present enclosing the cariously affected dentin from the sides (**Figs. 3.15c, 3.16**). With the zone of penetration reaching the dental pulp, **irreversible pulpal inflammation** cannot be avoided.[45,46]

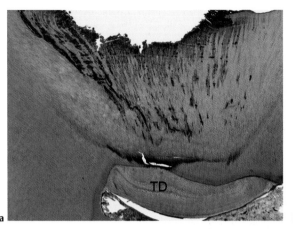
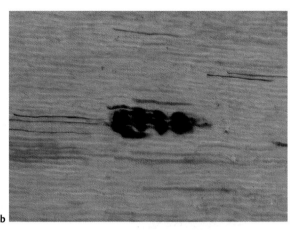

a
b

Fig. 3.17a, b Decalcified section through carious dentin (H&E stain).

a Cross-section through carious dentin with deeply stained bacterially infected dentin tubules and liquefaction foci. A well-developed layer of tertiary dentin (TD) is also visible.

b Conjugated liquefaction foci with accumulation of multiple bacteria show the high elasticity of dentin, giving the impression that the adjacent dentinal tubules were pushed to the side.

NOTE

With breakdown of the intact enamel surface, bacteria can penetrate deeper into enamel and reach the dentin. With further progress of the caries lesion, bacteria finally penetrate and enzymatically dissolve the demineralized dentin, which replaces a part of the zone of demineralization forming the zone of bacterial penetration. The underlying zones travel deeper into the dentin.

Spread of Bacteria within Dentin

With the first bacteria crossing the EDJ, bacteria can be found within the dentinal tubules as single cells, but more often grouping together. Tubule penetration is not a uniform process where tubules fill up with bacteria at the same rate. Longitudinal sections through carious dentin reveal that the depth of infection and also the bacterial density vary markedly from tubule to tubule. However, in the zone of penetration, a high number of dentinal tubules can be found which are completely or in part densely packed with bacterial cells (~10^5 vital bacteria/g).[15] The tubule diameter in these cases is enlarged due to demineralization and proteolytic action. Concomitantly, the intertubular side branches are also filled with bacteria. A specific histomorphological property, associated with caries only, is the local enlargement of densely filled tubules in the form of ampullae, referred to as **liquefaction foci**. Tubules beside a liquefaction focus are pushed to the side, bending around it (**Fig. 3.17**). Parallel with the incremental growth lines, **clefts** can be found that are also heavily infected with bacteria (**Fig. 3.18**). The necrotic zone contains a vast number of bacteria (~10^8 vital bacteria/g).[15]

Bacterial composition inside carious dentin is considerably different to that of dental plaque. Bacteria at the advancing front within carious dentin are acid-producing, aciduric species, predominantly **lactobacilli**. Within the body of the lesion bacterial composition is more complex, but dominated by strict and facultative anaerobes owing to the anaerobic conditions.[47,48] Overall, lactobacilli are the dominant bacteria found in carious dentin.

Hardness of Carious Dentin

BACKGROUND

In vitro, microhardness (after Knoop or Vickers) is used extensively to evaluate the quality and extent of enamel and dentin affected by the caries process. Using microhardness, one should be aware that its use on dentin contains a systematic error. Microhardness of a material is measured by placing a diamond (indenter) of known geometry on a flat and polished surface for a specific time using a specific load. Following removal of the indenter, the size of the impression left behind is measured under a microscope and used for calculation of a hardness number. This method works nicely on material that is plastic rather than elastic, like most metals. It also works on more brittle material like dental enamel, because the impression leaves relatively clear edges with a clearly defined rim of built-up material and its size does not change significantly upon releasing the load and removing the indenter. The problem with dentin is that it has considerable elastic properties. The indent left behind is therefore smaller then as it was during loading, highly influenced by the load and also the delay between unloading and measurement. Also, the area around the indent recedes elastically during

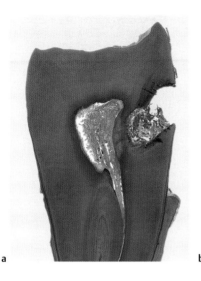

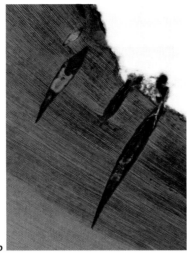

Fig. 3.18a, b Decalcified section through carious dentin (H&E stain).

a Overview of the dentin lesion comprising all histological caries zones, including the zone of necrosis on the outside and the tertiary dentin along the pulpal wall. On the coronal side of the lesion, clefts have developed within an area of well stained, heavily demineralized dentin perpendicular to the dentinal tubules.

b Detail from the same tooth. Transversal clefts filled with bacteria have formed perpendicular to the dentinal tubules, most likely along incremental dentin growth lines.

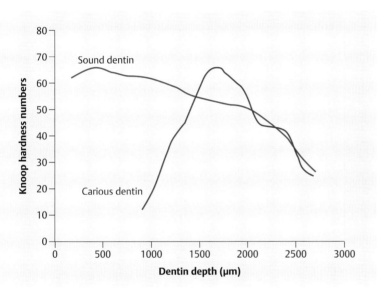

Fig. 3.19 Cross-sectional microhardness (Knoop) profiles from sound and carious dentin. Sound dentin reaches its hardness maximum a few hundred micrometers from the enamel–dentin junction and shows decreasing hardness from there on, toward the pulp. Carious dentin is very soft to start with at the bottom of the cavity. From there on, hardness increases and may reach hardness values at or above those of sound dentin—if a sound dentin layer is still present under the carious dentin lesion. Further toward the pulp within sound dentin, the hardness values decrease again (redrawn after Fusayama et al.[49]).

loading and bounces back after unloading. Therefore, microhardness numbers from dentin should not be compared as absolute values, while comparison of relative values measured under identical conditions may be a valid procedure, assuming that the plastic and elastic properties do not change within the sample.

The hardness of dentin is used clinically to estimate the presence of carious dentin (Chapter 18). When considering the hardness of carious dentin it is important to bear in mind that microhardness of healthy dentin already shows great variation within a single tooth and between teeth. Typically, **microhardness** of sound dentin increases from the EDJ inward due to the low mineral content of the EDJ, but soon (within a few hundred micrometers) reaches its maximum. From there on, microhardness decreases continuously and significantly toward the pulp (**Fig. 3.19**). Knoop hardness numbers

(KHNs) range approximately from up to 70 for outer dentin to 20 close to the pulp.[49] This drop in KHN may partly be attributed to the larger fraction of dentinal tubules per area cross-section and larger tubular diameter close to the pulp, as well as to a lower degree of mineralization of peritubular and intertubular secondary dentin. The overall mineral content is lower close to the pulp as can be seen by microradiography (see **Fig. 3.26**). Carious dentin is even more variable regarding hardness, meaning that the values given here are examples and qualitative in nature and should be used with caution. In a typical situation, in which is dentin caries not fully advanced toward the pulp, it is generally the case that lesion hardness increases from the EDJ toward the sound dentin underlying carious dentin. Within the sound dentin zone underlying the caries, microhardness decreases toward the pulp as described for sound (non-

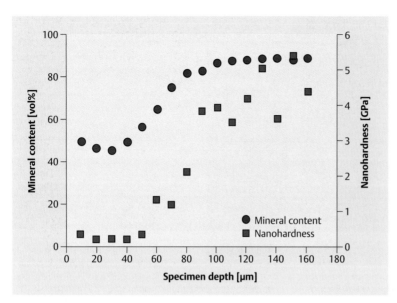

Fig. 3.20 Comparison of nanohardness values (Berkovich, right y-axis) with mineral content (TMR, left y-axis) of an artificially created enamel caries lesion. Both methods show some similarity in the shape of the profiles. The intact surface layer can be seen with both methods, as well as the body of the lesion. Mineral content of 50vol% or less causes severe tissue softening, with nanohardness values below 5GPa. Mineral content increases faster toward the end of the lesion. In this case, the end of the lesion concerning mineral content can be found at ca. 110μm where nanohardness has not yet reached "sound" values. The scattering of the measured values is bigger for nanohardness than for mineral content, which is partly attributed to the small probing diameter of the Berkovich indenter.

carious) dentin. The sclerotic zone between the zone of demineralization and sound dentin may be slightly harder close to the zone of healthy dentin than sound dentin at the same depth.[49] But more likely for a more advanced state of caries development, it has been reported that within the zone of sclerotic dentin the Knoop microhardness decreased from sound values (~40–70 KHN) at the pulpal side of the sclerotic zone to 25–30 KHN at the lesion side of the sclerotic zone.[50] In this case one must assume that mineral deposition by growth of peritubular dentin or within the tubules is not as pronounced toward outer areas of this zone, because additional demineralizing effects interact in this area. Thus, demineralization does not end at the border of the demineralized zone, but may extend well into the sclerotic zone.

The hardness of sound enamel also shows some variability, decreasing toward the pulp. In a typical, artificially created enamel carious lesion, the hardness profile from the surface toward the EDJ shows some correlation with mineral content derived from microradiography. The same could be observed by nanohardness measurements using a Berkovich indenter (**Fig. 3.20**).[51]

NOTE

Within carious enamel, hardness and mineral content show some correlation, but not to an extent that allows calculation of exact values for one method from the other. Within carious dentin, hardness increases from demineralized dentin, which is soft, toward sclerotic dentin, which in some parts is a little harder than sound dentin. Between the sclerotic zone and the pulp, hardness decreases again, in a similar way as if no caries were present.

Fluorescence Properties of Carious and Healthy Dental Hard Tissue

Although fluorescence of human and animal tissue was discovered many years ago,[52] the use of native **autofluorescence** of teeth for diagnostic purposes[53–57] and caries therapy[58] became valued only recently. **Figure 3.21** shows a fluorescence image of a slice (100μm) prepared through differently developed carious areas of two teeth. When excited with violet light, healthy enamel and dentin fluoresce yellow-green, but dentin yellow-green autofluorescence is markedly brighter. The noncavitated interproximal caries (**Fig. 3.21a**) shows a demineralized zone within enamel that does not reach the EDJ. Nevertheless, within the underlying dentin a "darker zone" extends two-thirds of the way toward the pulp, which is identical to the zone of sclerotic dentin found in transmitted light microscopy.[59] On the other hand, *red* autofluorescence is emitted from bacterially infected enamel of the interproximal lesion. Note that the infected, red fluorescing zone is limited to enamel, while the underlying dentin already shows signs of reaction due to diffusion of acids and other metabolites. The occlusal lesion present in this tooth slice shows bacterial activity (red autofluorescence) at the bottom of the fissure, but has not penetrated the dentin. However, the dark-appearing sclerotic dentin zone surrounds a bright yellow-green fluorescing zone. This is the demineralized zone, which is brighter due to dequenching of yellow-green fluorophores.[60] A fluorescence image of a slice through a more advanced occlusal lesion with enamel breakdown (**Fig. 3.21b**) shows penetration of bacteria into the dentin (red autofluorescence), a zone of demineralization (bright yellow-green zone), and a less fluorescent zone (darker appearance) of sclerotic dentin.

The cause of the red autofluorescence is **porphyrin** compounds which are produced by bacteria.[61] These porphyrins, mainly coproporphyrin and protoporphyrin IX,[62] are

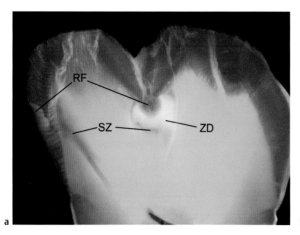
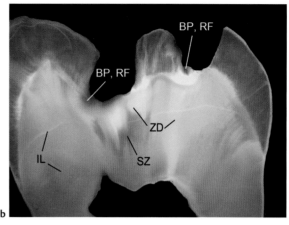

Fig. 3.21 a, b   Fluorescence images from tooth sections using an excitation wavelength of 405 nm viewed though a 530-nm high-pass filter. Generally, healthy dentin fluoresces more strongly than does enamel. Sound enamel and sound dentin fluoresce green. Bacterially contaminated areas fluoresce red due to the presence of bacterially synthesized porphyrin compounds. The cracks through enamel and dentin are artifacts due to the preparation procedure.

a Oral and occlusal carious lesion with macroscopically intact enamel of a bucco-oral cut through a lower molar tooth. The less developed oral lesion shows a bright green fluorescence of the demineralized enamel, and red fluorescence (RF) in the outer demineralized enamel which is contaminated with bacteria. Although the bacteria and enamel demineralization has not reached the inner third of the enamel layer, within the underlying dentin an area fluorescing less than sound dentin can be traced, stretching toward the pulp. This area is identical with the sclerotic zone (SZ). The increased mineral depositions within the dentinal tubules cause a quenching of the fluorophores, which are most likely organic in nature. The occlusal fissure lesion shows bacterial

activity (red fluorescence, RF) in the fissure just starting to penetrate the dentin. The sclerotic zone (SZ) appears less fluorescent (dark) around the demineralized zone (ZD) which fluoresces brighter green than sound dentin. The bright green fluorescence of demineralized dentin is caused by dequenching of the green fluorophores.

b Within the dentin, two thin fluorescent horizontal lines are present, which may resemble two less mineralized incremental lines (IL), although tetracycline intake during the respective growth phase cannot be fully excluded as being the cause. From the occlusal plane two differently severely cavitated lesions have caused histological changes within the dentin. The bigger lesion (left hand side) shows bacterial penetration (BP; red fluorescence, RF) mainly into the enamel and just beginning into the dentin. Within the dentin the brightly green fluorescing zone of demineralization (ZD) and the underlying less fluorescing sclerotic zone (SZ) can be identified. The smaller cavitated lesion on the right hand side shows a narrow zone of demineralization (ZD) all the way through the pulp.

immobilized within the dental hard tissue and constitute an excellent marker for areas with heavy bacterial infection. Single bacteria scattered within dentinal tubules do not produce sufficient amounts of porphyrin compounds. Therefore, it has been suggested to use the contrast between red-fluorescing, heavily infected dentin and yellow-green fluorescing, healthy dentin as a means for caries detection during caries excavation[58,63]

> **NOTE**
>
> Carious enamel and dentin exhibit a strong red autofluorescence which is different from the green autofluorescence emitted from healthy teeth when excited with violet light. This can be differentiated with the naked eye.

Caries of the Exposed Root

Caries of the exposed root has shown increased prevalence over the past few years, particularly among the elderly.[64] Development of root caries relies on the exposure of root areas, mostly due to gingival recession, and the accumulation of plaque (**Fig. 3.22**). With regard to plaque accumulation, the development of root caries is not so much different from caries development at other sites, e.g., interproximal, occlusal, and smooth surfaces. The cementum layer may cover the outer surface of the exposed root. This layer can be removed with time by toothbrushing or dental therapeutic removal of tartar, polishing, or periodontal treatment (scaling and root planing). It is known that dentin is more vulnerable to demineralization than enamel, and the same applies to the cementum layer (see Chapter 2). In most cases root caries spreads across the cementum or dentin surface to a certain extent, while initially its depth is limited. The dentin of the root has fewer dentinal tubules than coronal dentin and it is already in a "mature" state when root caries develops, due to a history of external stimuli following root exposure, or simply age, with a high degree of

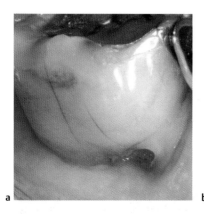 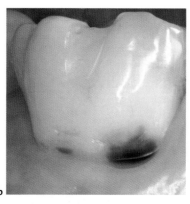

Fig. 3.22a, b Cervical caries lesions of different activity from two different patients.

a Active root caries in a lower molar of an elderly patient. The cavitated caries lesion is partly filled with plaque. The gingiva is inflamed in the area of the lesion and reaches into the cavity.

b Arrested root caries lesion in a lower molar of a middle-aged patient. The lesion was arrested following a change in tooth-brushing habits. The surface is shiny and hard and acquired a pattern of tooth-brushing abrasion. The discoloration of arrested root caries lesions tends to get darker with time.

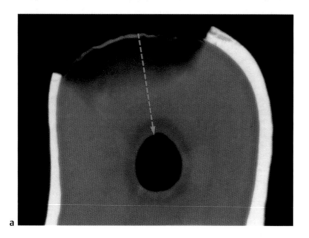

Fig. 3.23a, b Microradiography of a carious cervical lesion of a lower molar cut just above the cemento-enamel junction.

a Due to the severe carious circumstances the enamel layer in the area of the caries lesion has been lost. The exposed dentin shows a remineralized layer at the surface.

b Microradiogram showing the mineral content of the cervical caries lesion along the dashed arrow in (**a**). The high mineral content of the mineralized zone at the surface, the low mineral content at the center of the caries lesion, and a continuous increase in mineral content toward the end of the lesion can be seen. Also, in the sound part of the microradiogram, a decrease in mineral content toward the pulp is visible.

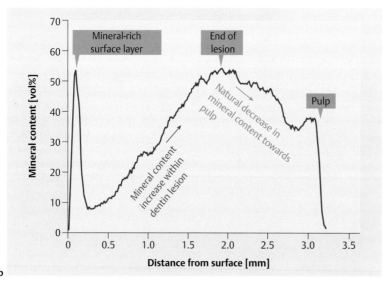

sclerosis.[65] It has been observed that bacteria are already able to penetrate the cementum layer in an early state of root caries development, while bacteria penetrate into the underlying dentin at a later state of lesion development. A **well-mineralized surface zone** forms at the surface of the cementum or dentin (when cementum is absent). The body of the lesion underneath this mineral-rich surface zone is heavily demineralized with about 50% or less of the natural mineral content of sound dentin[66] (see **Fig. 3.23**). The histological layering within root dentin is similar to coronal dentin. However, a cross-section through a root caries lesion shows that root caries lesions are rather shallow, and saucer-shaped in most cases.

For development of root caries the same principles apply as for coronal caries, but there are a few points that facilitate the development of caries within cementum and dentin at the cemento-enamel margin. Two major factors contribute to root caries: the exposure of the cervical region in conjunction with the fact that cementum and dentin are more vulnerable to demineralization than enamel; and patient age, which is associated not only with root exposure, but also with lower salivary flow and reduced tooth-cleaning capabilities.

Caries Arrest and Remineralization

The caries process is driven by carbohydrate-consuming, acid-producing bacteria, organized in a biofilm, that is, the dental plaque (Chapters 1 and 2). The caries process will continue as long as the **microenvironment** at the tooth surface does not change its cariogenicity. In other words, caries arrest is possible only when the surface conditions change, owing to sufficient **plaque removal**. If a patient is able to significantly improve the microenvironment at the tooth surface of a formerly progressing caries lesion, there is a good chance that the caries process may be halted. As soon as the improvements to the microenvironment wear off, the caries process most likely will continue.

Daily dental practice provides many examples of **caries arrest**. A prime example is the band-shaped enamel white spot lesion at the buccal side of molars and other teeth that developed during tooth eruption along the gingival margin due to lack of plaque removal in this area. Quite often, with further eruption of these teeth, lesion progression stops. What remains is a "scar," a shiny band-shaped white spot parallel to, but clearly above, the gingival margin (see **Fig. 3.7**).

Another example is cervical caries lesions in dentin or cementum, which do not necessarily need operative treatment and filling therapy. In an active state these lesions are covered by plaque. Following plaque removal, in most cases a (light-) brownish, soft ("leathery") surface appears. As to the degree of discoloration, a wide range of brownish hues is possible. If the patient is able to avoid plaque accumulation by daily cleaning of the respective area, such lesions will arrest (**Fig. 3.22**); the surface becomes harder and, in most cases, the lesion becomes darker in color. This process usually takes months.

It is widely accepted that primary caries lesions, as soon as the overlying plaque is removed, do not progress further. The situation is not that simple in case of secondary caries (caries adjacent to restorations). In some cases of secondary caries there is a gap between the restoration and the enamel or dentin wall. Most likely, this gap is filled with plaque, but daily removal of dental plaque from this gap is not practically possible. To avoid complete removal of the restoration, sealing of this gap is an option (Chapter 19). By sealing the marginal gap, progression of a secondary caries lesion can be avoided and the lesion becomes arrested.

So far we have seen that lesion arrest is possible under clinical conditions. However, beyond lesion arrest, complete lesion remineralization would be desirable. Complete **remineralization** seems possible only for very shallow (a few micrometers deep only), artificially created, carious enamel lesions. Natural caries lesions limited to enamel show mineral accumulation in the outer layers, but deeper areas of the lesion seem not to remineralize properly. The reasons for this are not exactly known, but the presence of incorporated protein within the lesion as well as reduced diffusion due to blocked diffusion channels within the remineralized surface layer may play a role. Under the respective clinical conditions (e.g., regular plaque removal, provision of fluoride) the surface zone (pseudo intact surface layer) that is less mineralized than sound enamel, but more mineralized than the body of the lesion, gains mineral and widens (**Fig. 3.24**). Under ideal circumstances it can contain almost as much mineral as sound enamel. The body of the lesion may accumulate mineral but always stays less mineralized than sound enamel. Particularly under the influence of fluoride, a layering (intermittent zones of more-mineralized enamel) within the body of the lesion forms. In in-vitro experiments using artificially created carieslike enamel lesions, the lesions gained mineral, but the depth of the lesion increased further, albeit to a small extent.

Caries lesions extending into dentin with macroscopically intact enamel have a chance to remineralize, limited to the enamel as described above. In those lesions it is highly unlikely that the dentin will undergo significant remineralization. However, caries lesions very **deep into dentin** show a tendency toward remineralization if they are cut off from caries attack from outside of the tooth. This can be seen during a **stepwise excavation procedure**, where bulk caries is removed, but close to the pulp carious, soft dentin is left behind to avoid pulp exposure. Upon re-entry after typically 6 or 12 months following temporary restoration with a sub-base of $Ca(OH)_2$, clinically it can be observed that the former soft dentin close to the pulp becomes harder due to remineralization in most cases. To date there is no clear proof where the minerals come from, but most likely both the calcium reservoir from $Ca(OH)_2$ and pulpal tubular fluid (calcium and phosphate) are involved.

Cervical caries lesions with dentin (or cementum) at the surface show a significant potential for remineralization. However, remineralization of dentin is mostly attributed to mineral deposition in the dentinal tubules. In-vitro experiments of remineralization of dentin with artificially created carieslike lesions showed hypermineralization (**Fig. 3.25**). In this case the mineral content of the remin-

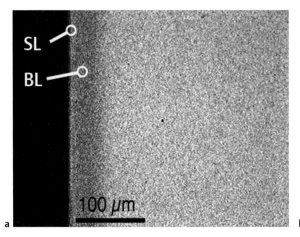

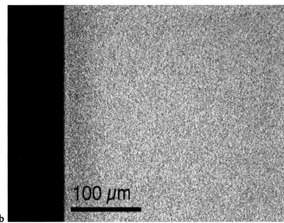

Fig. 3.24a–c TMR from artificial enamel caries following demineralization and remineralization.

a Microradiograph (detail of a TMR x-ray exposure) of a surface-perpendicular cut through an artificial early enamel caries lesion directly after the demineralization regimen. Surface layer (SL) and lesion body (BL) are clearly visible.

b Microradiograph of the same specimen as in (**a**), but after 14 days remineralization in situ. The lesion body is less pronounced than in (**a**), indicating remineralization.

c Microradiogram of the microradiographs of (**a**) and (**b**) shows a mineral uptake throughout the entire lesion body of this shallow carious lesion of the enamel.

eralized dentin at the dentin surface showed a higher mineral content than sound dentin. The body of the lesion within the dentin, however, remained hypomineralized.

In addition to successful plaque removal, **presence of fluoride** facilitates remineralization of caries lesions by shifting the chemical balance from net-demineralization to net-remineralization.

NOTE

Caries arrest can be observed clinically quite often. To turn the caries process round from net-demineralization to net-remineralization the local conditions at the tooth surface must change. Specifically, the overlying biofilm needs to be completely removed or at least significantly reduced. Arrestment influences in particular the surface zone and the dark zone in enamel caries lesions. Even deep parts of dentin caries can remineralize when the overlying caries process is interrupted, a mechanism that is used during stepwise excavation.

Correlation of Histology with Radiography and Clinical Appearance of Caries

The correlation between histology, and clinical and radiographic appearance of caries much depends on the circumstances. These include the development of the actual caries lesion, lesion site, and how well radiography and clinical observation can be performed. However, there is some correlation between histology, clinical appearance and radiography.[67] In **Table 3.1** the typical correlation between histology, clinical radiography, and clinical appearance is provided, but it is important to recognize that some variation is possible.

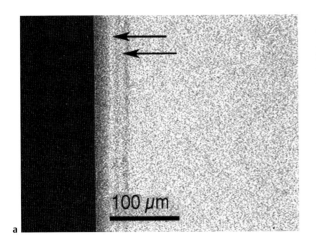

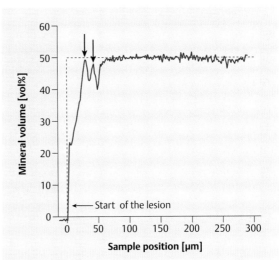

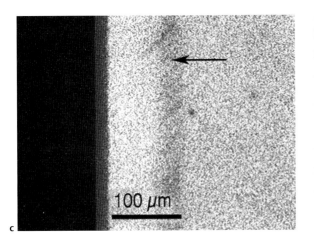

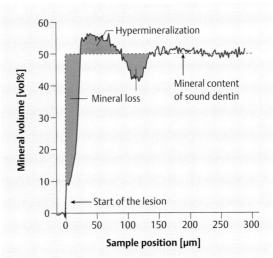

Fig. 3.25 a–d TMR from artificial dentin caries following remineralization with intermittent fluoride exposure.

a Microradiograph (detail of a TMR x-ray exposure) from a former 60 μm deep dentin lesion after 1 day of remineralization with three exposures by a 1500 ppm fluoride solution for 5 min every 8 h. Within the lesion body two distinct layers of mineral accumulation can be seen (arrows).

b Microradiogram of the microradiograph in (**a**) shows the same two mineral-rich layers (black arrows) with almost the mineral content of sound dentin (50 vol%).

c Microradiograph (detail of a TMR x-ray exposure) from a former 60 μm deep dentin lesion after 5 days of remineralization with exposure to 1500 ppm fluoride solution for 5 min every 8 h (experiment from **3.24a** continued). Within the lesion body a wide hypermineralized layer has formed that is delineated toward sound dentin by a demineralized layer (black arrow). Note that the lesion (demineralized layer) has shifted deeper into the dentin.

d Microradiogram of the microradiograph in (**a**) shows the same wide hypermineralized layer and the demineralized layer that has travelled deeper into the dentin.

Erosion—a Noncarious Defect

Noncarious defects, if not caused by direct traumatic injury, are due either to wear (attrition, abrasion, abfraction, and erosion) or defects that were established during tooth development (molar-incisor-hypomineralization, trauma, fluorosis). In particular, erosive defects have come under scrutiny in the last decade.

The etiology of **dental erosion** is different from caries (Chapter 2), and so is the histology. Erosion, however, is not caused by bacteria, but by the direct dissolution of enamel and dentin due to acids.[68] Those acids may originate from the nutrition (acidic food and drinks) or stomach (by reflux or vomiting). In some cases, environmental reasons (e.g., poorly maintained swimming pools or frequent exposure to acidic vapors in industry) or individual habits may account for dental erosion. Under erosive conditions calcium and phosphate dissolved from enamel or dentin are immediately detached from the enamel or dentin surface and not "parked" in a reservoir like dental

Table 3.1   Correlation between histological, radiographical, and clinical appearance of developing caries. For radiography and clinical appearance ideal conditions are assumed (approximal caries for radiography but directly accessible to the naked eye regarding its clinical appearance)

Histology	Radiography	Clinical appearance
–	–	Sound
Surface etching	–	–
Shallow (approx. <100 μm) enamel subsurface lesion with intact surface layer	–	White (brown) spot, visible only under dry conditions
Enamel subsurface lesion extending halfway to the EDJ with intact surface layer	Hardly visible, maybe slightly in outer enamel	White (brown) spot, visible only under dry conditions (no cavitation)
Caries lesion extending to the EDJ with enamel surface still intact. Dentin reactions comprising development of different zones and tertiary dentin	Translucency in enamel	White (brown) spot, visible under dry conditions, but often also visible under wet conditions (no cavitation)
Dentin reactions comprising different zones and build-up of tertiary dentin. Within localized areas of enamel breakdown, bacteria penetrating the enamel can be found	Translucency in outer third of dentin	White (brown) spot, visible under dry and wet conditions. Small, localized breakdown of the enamel surface may be visible
Following enamel breakdown, bacteria can be found within dentin tubules. Dentin reactions comprising different zones and tertiary dentin	Translucency in middle third of dentin	Well developed macroscopic cavitation, usually within a white (brown) spot. Possibility of discomfort or pain
Dentin is exposed further. The exposed dentin surface starts to disintegrate (necrotic zone) and the zone of penetration reaches deeper into dentin. In an advanced state bacteria can have penetrated up to the pulp	Translucency in inner third of dentin	Well developed cavity with increased likelihood for discomfort or pain

plaque for some time, and for this reason they become immediately and irreversibly lost.

With respect to erosive **mineral dissolution** of enamel, two different types of dissolution occur that are relevant to the further destiny of the damaged enamel. Consider a single exposure to an acidic solution under laboratory conditions: a certain amount of material, a layer of ca. 0–1 μm, is completely lost and cannot be remineralized in any way. (Under harsh laboratory conditions—not comparable to the clinical situation—this can exceed 1 μm.) The newly exposed surface is softened and porous up to about 10 μm, showing some similarity to the acid-etch pattern after exposure to 35%–40% phosphoric acid that is used prior to placing an adhesive restoration (**Fig. 3.26**). The softened surface zone is not homogeneously soft, but shows a gradient of increasing hardness from a more softened surface to the sound enamel underneath. This gradient extends to a depth of up to 10 μm, but usually is less than that. For this reason, surface microhardness measurements (such as Vickers and Knoop) may not work reliably, because the tip of the indenter rests on harder material, probably sound enamel already, indicating microhardness values harder than the actual hardness of the outermost layer.[69]

The **softened layer** is highly vulnerable to mechanical forces, such as attrition, abrasion or toothbrushing.[70,71] While erosion leads to irreversible tooth substance loss

of the outermost layer of enamel, the softened layer may be remineralized, at least to a certain extent and hereby regain its mechanical resistance toward toothbrushing and other mechanical forces. It has been shown in situ that saliva takes much longer than one hour to remineralize softened eroded enamel to restore its original mechanical resistance.[71] In an effort to combat enamel erosion, timing of toothbrushing (i.e., before or after erosive meals) may be crucial (Chapter 10), but also fluoride has been found to be effective, to a limited degree.[72,73]

In the clinical situation, the **acquired pellicle** seems to have an important protective effect against erosion, particularly when the erosive attack is not too severe. Most studies on enamel erosion to date have been performed under laboratory conditions without enamel protected by an acquired pellicle. Due to the protective effect of the pellicle, the loss from erosive substance in the mouth is far less than that predicted from experiments on polished yet unprotected enamel surfaces. This may explain why people of older age with "normal" eating habits still have their own teeth in function, despite regular consumption of acidic fruit, vegetables, and beverages.

An erosive attack on **dentin** leaves collagen fibers at the surface, a phenomenon that is also known from acid etching in adhesive dentistry. It is known that the *exposed collagen* network on the surface of dentin acts protectively toward further erosion of the surface, but may be damaged by proteolytic enzymes, such as pepsin in the case of esophageal reflux or vomiting as the cause of erosion.[74] Newer strategies against dentin erosion consider particularly the collagen matrix of dentin. The role of metallo-matrix proteinases (MMPs) present in dentin seem to play a role in dentin degradation due to caries and erosion,[75] and hence ways of reducing the MMP-activity are currently under investigation.[76]

NOTE

Erosion is loss of dental hard tissue due to direct dissolution by acids from the nutrition, the stomach, or the environment that are not of bacterial origin. During an erosive attack, calcium and phosphate are lost irreversibly and the remaining enamel or dentin surface is demineralized up to a few micrometers. Areas covered by plaque are protected from erosion. The acquired pellicle seems to play an important role in prevention of erosive substance loss.

SUMMARY

The cause of caries lesion development—the accumulation of dental plaque—is facilitated at specific, mechanically protected areas. Caries lesions typically initiate at these so-called predilection sites / plaque stagnation areas. The development of a caries lesion starting at the enamel surface and spreading toward dentin and further toward the pulp follows the same mechanisms, independently of the site of such a lesion. Histology reveals different zones within a caries lesion, depending on the depth of the lesion, but also on whether and to what extent the enamel surface has broken down. With a caries lesion that is limited to enamel, the outer layer of the enamel is less mineralized than sound enamel, but more mineralized than the subsurface lesion. As long as the enamel surface is macroscopically intact, only a few bacteria can be found within the enamel. With breakdown of the intact enamel surface, lesion development is accelerated and bacteria can spread deeper and in large numbers into both enamel and dentin. Usually, the demineralized areas within a well-developed dentin caries lesion precede the bacterially infected areas. Among the histological techniques used to investigate enamel and dentin caries lesions, light microscopy can be used to reveal different zones within enamel and dentin caries that correspond to different pore volumes and size distribution of such porosities. Microradiographic techniques are able to analyze exactly the mineral content as a function of lesion depth. Scanning electron microscopy shows changes at the enamel surface at early lesion states and within a lesion at the enamel prism level, while transmission electron microscopy provides insight into changes at the crystal

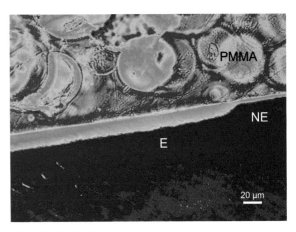

Fig. 3.26 Section through enamel after 1 min of erosion in citric acid (false colors). The enamel specimen was embedded in acrylic (PMMA) following erosion and sectioned perpendicularly to the surface through eroded (E) and noneroded (NE) enamel. The green band on top of the enamel surface in the eroded area represents a layer of demineralized, but at this stage not completely lost, enamel of 10 μm thickness.

level. Even when a caries lesion progresses, demineralization is interrupted by phases of remineralization. Net remineralization can be achieved only when the biological and chemical conditions at the surface of such a lesion change toward a less cariogenic environment. Clinically, this means successful regular plaque removal and administration of fluoride. Under these conditions, the caries process can come to halt and remineralization of the outer layers of enamel or exposed dentin is possible. However, the result of lesion remineralization can be considered to be a "scar," because complete remineralization in the sense of a "restitutio ad integrum" does not occur. Remineralization of deeper lesions most likely leaves behind a less mineralized area.

Both caries and erosion cause loss of mineral from a tooth, but the etiology and the histology are considerably different. Erosion is not caused by bacteria, but by the direct dissolution of enamel and dentin due to acids that originate from the nutrition, the stomach, or other environmental sources. Erosion leads to immediate irreversible loss of calcium and phosphate from the enamel or dentin surface and creates only a shallow softening of the surface. This softened surface is prone to abrasive loss, but may be remineralized when left mechanically undisturbed for some time.

Acknowledgments. The author would like to thank Prof. Dr. Hans Ulrich Luder, University of Zurich, Center for Dentistry, Institute for Oral Biology for kindly providing **Figs. 3.9, 3.10, 3.13, 3.16, 3.17**, and **3.18** and for numerous valuable discussions. I also would like to thank Dr. Hao Yu for preparation and imaging of **Figs. 3.3, 3.4**, and **3.14** and PD Dr. Áine M. Lennon for providing **Fig. 3.21.**

REFERENCES

1. Thylstrup A, Bruun C, Holmen L. In vivo caries models—mechanisms for caries initiation and arrestment. Adv Dent Res 1994; 8(2):144–157

2. Ekstrand KR, Kuzmina I, Bjørndal L, Thylstrup A. Relationship between external and histologic features of progressive stages of caries in the occlusal fossa. Caries Res 1995;29(4):243–250

3. Ekstrand KR, Martignon S, Ricketts DJ, Qvist V. Detection and activity assessment of primary coronal caries lesions: a methodologic study. Oper Dent 2007;32(3):225–235

4. Ekstrand KR, Ricketts DN, Kidd EAM, Qvist V, Schou S. Detection, diagnosing, monitoring and logical treatment of occlusal caries in relation to lesion activity and severity: an in vivo examination with histological validation. Caries Res 1998;32(4):247–254

5. Carvalho JC, Ekstrand KR, Thylstrup A. Dental plaque and caries on occlusal surfaces of first permanent molars in relation to stage of eruption. J Dent Res 1989;68(5):773–779

6. Carvalho JC, Ekstrand KR, Thylstrup A. Results after 1 year of non-operative occlusal caries treatment of erupting permanent first molars. Community Dent Oral Epidemiol 1991;19(1):23–28

7. Carvalho JC, Thylstrup A, Ekstrand KR. Results after 3 years of non-operative occlusal caries treatment of erupting permanent first molars. Community Dent Oral Epidemiol 1992;20(4):187–192

8. Nyvad B, Machiulskiene V, Baelum V. Reliability of a new caries diagnostic system differentiating between active and inactive caries lesions. Caries Res 1999;33(4):252–260

9. Hecht E. Optics. 3rd ed. Reading: Addison-Wesley; 1998

10. Silverstone L. Structure of carious enamel, including the early lesion. Oral Sci Rev 1973;3:100–160

11. Silverstone LM, Johnson NW, Hardie JM, Williams RAD. Enamel caries. In: Silverstone LM, Johnson NW, Hardie JM, Williams RAD, eds. Dental Caries: Aetiology, Pathology and Prevention. London: Macmillan; 1981:133–161

12. Darling A. Studies of the early lesion of enamel caries. Br Dent J 1958;105:119–135

13. Silverstone LM. Remineralization and enamel caries: significance of fluoride and effect on crystal diameter. In: Leach SA, Edgar WM, eds. Demineralization and Remineralization of Teeth. Oxford: IRL Press: 1983:185–205

14. Shellis RP, Hallsworth AS, Kirkham J, Robinson C. Organic material and the optical properties of the dark zone in caries lesions of enamel. Eur J Oral Sci 2002;110(5):392–395

15. Schroeder HE. Karies und Erosion. Pathobio Oral Struktur 1997; 3:95

16. Meyer-Lueckel H, Paris S, Kielbassa AM. Surface layer erosion of natural caries lesions with phosphoric and hydrochloric acid gels in preparation for resin infiltration. Caries Res 2007;41(3):223–230

17. Buchalla W, Attin T, Schulte-Mönting J, Hellwig E. Fluoride uptake, retention, and remineralization efficacy of a highly concentrated fluoride solution on enamel lesions in situ. J Dent Res 2002;81(5):329–333

18. Angmar B, Carlström D, Glas JE. Studies on the ultrastructure of dental enamel. IV. The mineralization of normal human enamel. J Ultrastruct Res 1963;8:12–23

19. de Josselin de Jong E, ten Bosch JJ, Noordmans J. Optimised microcomputer-guided quantitative microradiography on dental mineralised tissue slices. Phys Med Biol 1987;32(7):887–899

20. Arends J, Christoffersen J. The nature of early caries lesions in enamel. J Dent Res 1986;65(1):2–11

21. Magalhães AC, Moron BM, Comar LP, Wiegand A, Buchalla W, Buzalaf MA. Comparison of cross-sectional hardness and transverse microradiography of artificial carious enamel lesions induced by different demineralising solutions and gels. Caries Res 2009;43(6):474–483

22. Weatherell JA, Robinson C, Hallsworth AS. Microanalytical studies on single sections of enamel. In: Stack MV, Fearnhead RW, eds. Tooth Enamel II: Its Composition, Properties, and Fundamental Structure. Report of the Proceedings of a Second International Symposium on the Composition, Properties, and Fundamental Structure of Tooth Enamel, held at the London Hospital Medical College, 16/17 June 1969. Bristol: Wright and Sons; 1971:31–38

23. Boyde A. The structure of developing mammalian dental enamel. In: Stack MV, Fearnhead RW, eds. Tooth Enamel: Its Composition, Properties, and Fundamental Structure: Bristol: Wright and Sons; 1965:163–167

24. Meckel AH, Griebstein WJ, Neal RJ. Structure of mature human dental enamel as observed by electron microscopy. Arch Oral Biol 1965;10(5):775–783

25. Johansen E. The nature of the carious lesion. Dent Clin North Am 1962;6:305–320

26. Johnson NW. Some aspects of the ultrastructure of early human enamel caries seen with the electron microscope. Arch Oral Biol 1967;12(12):1505–1521

27. Silverstone LM, Poole DF. Histologic and ultrastructural features of remineralized carious enamel. J Dent Res 1969;48(5):766–770

28. Johnson NW. Transmission electron microscopy of early carious enamel. Caries Res 1967;1(4):356–369

29. Johansen E. Comparison of the ultrastructure and chemical composition of sound and carious enamel from human teeth. In: Stack MV, Fearnhead RW, eds. Tooth Enamel: Its Composition, Properties, and Fundamental Structure. Bristol: Wright and Sons; 1965:177–181

30. Johnson NW. Differences in the shape of human enamel crystallites after partial destruction by caries, EDTA and various acids. Arch Oral Biol 1966;11(12):1421–1424

31. Almer JD, Stock SR. High energy X-ray scattering quantification of in situ-loading-related strain gradients spanning the dentino-enamel junction (DEJ) in bovine tooth specimens. J Biomech 2010;43(12):2294–2300

32. Stock SR, Vieira AE, Delbem AC, Cannon ML, Xiao X, Carlo FD. Synchrotron microComputed Tomography of the mature bovine dentinoenamel junction. J Struct Biol 2008;161(2):162–171

33. Tesch W, Eidelman N, Roschger P, Goldenberg F, Klaushofer K, Fratzl P. Graded microstructure and mechanical properties of human crown dentin. Calcif Tissue Int 2001;69(3):147–157

34. Schulze KA, Balooch M, Balooch G, Marshall GW, Marshall SJ. Micro-Raman spectroscopic investigation of dental calcified tissues. J Biomed Mater Res A 2004;69(2):286–293

35. Xu C, Yao X, Walker MP, Wang Y. Chemical/molecular structure of the dentin-enamel junction is dependent on the intratooth location. Calcif Tissue Int 2009;84(3):221–228

36. Kamal AM, Okiji T, Kawashima N, Suda H. Defense responses of dentin/pulp complex to experimentally induced caries in rat molars: an immunohistochemical study on kinetics of pulpal Ia antigen-expressing cells and macrophages. J Endod 1997;23(2):115–120

37. Steinman RR. Physiologic activity of the pulp-dentin complex. Quintessence Int 1985;16(10):723–726

38. Cooper PR, Takahashi Y, Graham LW, Simon S, Imazato S, Smith AJ. Inflammation-regeneration interplay in the dentine-pulp complex. J Dent 2010;38(9):687–697

39. Lee YL, Liu J, Clarkson BH, Lin CP, Godovikova V, Ritchie HH. Dentin-pulp complex responses to carious lesions. Caries Res 2006;4(3):254–264

40. Larmas M, Kortelainen S, Bäckman T, Hietala EL, Pajari U. Odontoblast-mediated regulation of the progression of dentinal caries. Proc Finn Dent Soc 1992;88(Suppl 1):313–320

41. Karjalainen S, Söderling E, Pelliniemi L, Foidart JM. Immunohistochemical localization of types I and III collagen and fibronectin in the dentine of carious human teeth. Arch Oral Biol 1986; 31(12):801–806

42. Zavgorodniy AV, Rohanizadeh R, Bulcock S, Swain MV. Ultrastructural observations and growth of occluding crystals in carious dentine. Acta Biomater 2008;4(5):1427–1439

43. Fish EW. Surgical pathology of the mouth. London: Pitman and Sons; 1948

44. Shovelton DS. The maintenance of pulp vitality. Br Dent J 1972;133(3):95–101

45. Langeland K. Tissue response to dental caries. Endod Dent Traumatol 1987;3(4):149–171

46. Reeves R, Stanley HR. The relationship of bacterial penetration and pulpal pathosis in carious teeth. Oral Surg Oral Med Oral Pathol 1966;22(1):59–65

47. Hoshino E. Predominant obligate anaerobes in human carious dentin. J Dent Res 1985;64(10):1195–1198

48. Martin FE, Nadkarni MA, Jacques NA, Hunter N. Quantitative microbiological study of human carious dentine by culture and real-time PCR: association of anaerobes with histopathological changes in chronic pulpitis. J Clin Microbiol 2002;40(5): 1698–1704

49. Fusayama T, Okuse K, Hosoda H. Relationship between hardness, discoloration, and microbial invasion in carious dentin. J Dent Res 1966;45(4):1033–1046

50. Ogawa K, Yamashita Y, Ichijo T, Fusayama T. The ultrastructure and hardness of the transparent layer of human carious dentin. J Dent Res 1983;62(1):7–10

51. Buchalla W, Imfeld T, Attin T, Swain MV, Schmidlin PR. Relationship between nanohardness and mineral content of artificial carious enamel lesions. Caries Res 2008;42(3):157–163

52. Stübel H. Die Fluoreszenz tierischer Gewebe in ultraviolettem Licht. Arch Ges Physiol 1911;142:1–14

53. Alfano RR, Yao SS. Human teeth with and without dental caries studied by visible luminescent spectroscopy. J Dent Res 1981; 60(2):120–122

54. Buchalla W. Comparative fluorescence spectroscopy shows differences in noncavitated enamel lesions. Caries Res 2005;39(2): 150–156

55. Buchalla W, Lennon ÁM, Attin T. Comparative fluorescence spectroscopy of root caries lesions. Eur J Oral Sci 2004;112(6): 490–496

56. de Josselin de Jong E, Sundström F, Westerling H, Tranaeus S, ten Bosch JJ, Angmar-Månsson B. A new method for in vivo quantification of changes in initial enamel caries with laser fluorescence. Caries Res 1995;29(1):2–7

57. Hibst R, Paulus R. New approach on fluorescence spectroscopy for caries detection. In: Featherstone JDB, Rechman P, Fried D, eds. Lasers in Dentistry V. Proc SPIE 1999;3593:41–147

58. Lennon ÁM. Fluorescence-aided caries excavation (FACE) compared to conventional method. Oper Dent 2003;28(4):341–345

59. Lennon ÁM, Buchalla W, Stookey GK. A new fluorescence method to detect residual caries. Caries Res 2001;35:265 (Abstract)

60. van der Veen MH, ten Bosch JJ. The influence of mineral loss on the auto-fluorescent behaviour of in vitro demineralised dentine. Caries Res 1996;30(1):93–99

61. Lennon AM, Buchalla W, Brune L, Zimmermann O, Gross U, Attin T. The ability of selected oral microorganisms to emit red fluorescence. Caries Res 2006;40(1):2–5

62. Buchalla W, Attin T, Niedmann Y, Lennon ÁM. Porphyrins are the cause of red fluorescence of carious dentin: Verified by gradient reversed-phase HPLC. Caries Res 2008;42:223 (Abstract)

63. Lennon AM, Buchalla W, Rassner B, Becker K, Attin T. Efficiency of 4 caries excavation methods compared. Oper Dent 2006;31(5): 551–555

64. Micheelis W, Schiffner U. Vierte Deutsche Mundgesundheitsstudie – (DMS IV): neue Ergebnisse zu oralen Erkrankungsprävalenzen, Risikogruppen und zum zahnärztlichen Vorsorgungsgrad in Deutschland 2005. Institut der Deutschen Zahnärzte (IDZ). IDZ Materialreihe Band 31. Köln: Deutscher Ärzte-Verlag; 2006

65. Schüpbach P, Guggenheim B, Lutz F. Human root caries: histopathology of initial lesions in cementum and dentin. J Oral Pathol Med 1989;18(3):146–156

66. Schüpbach P, Guggenheim B, Lutz F. Human root caries: histopathology of advanced lesions. Caries Res 1990;24(3):145–158

67. Ekstrand KR, Ricketts DN, Kidd EAM. Reproducibility and accuracy of three methods for assessment of demineralization depth of the occlusal surface: an in vitro examination. Caries Res 1997;31(3):224–231

68. Lussi A, Jaeggi T. Erosion—diagnosis and risk factors. Clin Oral Investig 2008;12(Suppl 1):S5–S13

69. Attin T. Methods for assessment of dental erosion. Monogr Oral Sci 2006;20:152–172

70. Addy M, Shellis RP. Interaction between attrition, abrasion and erosion in tooth wear. Monogr Oral Sci 2006;20:17–31

71. Attin T, Knöfel S, Buchalla W, Tütüncü R. In situ evaluation of different remineralization periods to decrease brushing abrasion of demineralized enamel. Caries Res 2001;35(3):216–222

72. Lagerweij MD, Buchalla W, Kohnke S, Becker K, Lennon AM, Attin T. Prevention of erosion and abrasion by a high fluoride concentration gel applied at high frequencies. Caries Res 2006; 40(2):148–153

73. Wiegand A, Attin T. Influence of fluoride on the prevention of erosive lesions—a review. Oral Health Prev Dent 2003;1(4): 245–253

74. Schlueter N, Ganss C, Hardt M, Schegietz D, Klimek J. Effect of pepsin on erosive tissue loss and the efficacy of fluoridation measures in dentine in vitro. Acta Odontol Scand 2007;65(5): 298–305

75. van Strijp AJ, Jansen DC, DeGroot J, ten Cate JM, Everts V. Host-derived proteinases and degradation of dentine collagen in situ. Caries Res 2003;37(1):58–65

76. Magalhães AC, Wiegand A, Rios D, Hannas A, Attin T, Buzalaf MA. Chlorhexidine and green tea extract reduce dentin erosion and abrasion in situ. J Dent 2009;37(12):994–998

Paradigm Shift in Cariology

Sebastian Paris, Hendrik Meyer-Lueckel

4

The previous chapters have addressed the etiology, pathogenesis, and clinical appearance of caries. This brief chapter will discuss the effects of scientific caries models and paradigms as well as approaches to treat the disease. Furthermore, pathogenesis will be illustrated in a model that will allow us to categorize the various options for intervention in Chapter 9. This chapter addresses the following topics:

- The influence of scientific paradigms on dentists' approaches to treat caries
- The specific and ecological plaque hypotheses
- A current model of the pathogenesis of caries

Scientific Paradigms

Paradigms are understood to be the generally accepted scientific concepts and the worldview in a particular era. Paradigms are based on theories and models and form the scientific framework in which the scientists work. Abstract, idealized, and simplified models are frequently used to make the complex phenomena and interrelationships of nature comprehensible, explicable, and predictable. Of course, simplifications, idealizations, and abstractions can be problematic. Paradigms as well as the models and theories that underlie them come up against limits in certain situations. A paradigm, with its associated theories and models, is always accepted by the scientific community within a particular field as long as it is capable of satisfactorily explaining the relationships in nature and making reliable predictions. Once a paradigm meets its limits, it needs to be modified or replaced by a competing paradigm with its own theories and models. The new paradigm is then gradually accepted by more and more members of the scientific community, and the old one is finally abandoned. This process is termed a "scientific revolution."[1,2]

Dentistry and medicine are also influenced by scientific paradigms. For example, the dentistry that is practiced in many countries, and which is represented in this book, is based on what is generally termed "Western academic medicine." Contrastingly, "traditional Chinese medicine" avails itself of different paradigms which are mostly incompatible with Western academic medicine. The various medical paradigms naturally influence the ways in which we treat illnesses. Consequently, the therapeutic approaches in "Western academic medicine" are completely different from those in traditional Chinese medicine.

Paradigms and theories also reflect the scientific and social experiences of the scientists who created them. For example, the specific plaque hypothesis and the forms of therapy that are derived from it (see below), which were created during the beginning of the second half of the last century, reflect the widespread concept of human domination, scientifically and technologically, of a specific (hostile) environment. The ecological plaque hypothesis that was developed in recent decades arose during a period in which people, particularly in industrialized nations, became aware that fighting the environment has negative consequences. Hence protecting the environment and species is recommendable from both ethical and pragmatic points of view. In medicine, it was revealed that microorganisms are not harmful per se, and that they have irreplaceable, positive functions in our body.[3] Consequently, the ecological plaque hypothesis does not point to the environment (infection with certain bacteria) as the primary cause of caries, but rather to our own behavior.

The present abandonment of the specific plaque hypothesis and embracing of the ecological plaque hypothesis is a classic paradigm shift that is bringing about a sustainable change in treatment concepts in dentistry.[4]

How Paradigms Influence Our Clinical Approach

The Specific Plaque Hypothesis

The chemo-parasitic theory that was founded by Miller in the beginning of the last century[5] described the metabolic activity of bacteria as the main cause of caries. Later experiments with gnotobiotic (germ-free) rodents identified certain specific types of bacteria such as mutans streptococci and lactobacilli as essential factors in the etiology of caries.[6–8] It was revealed that gnotobiotic hamsters did not develop caries even when they consumed sugar-containing food, whereas hamsters infected with *Steptococcus mutans* developed caries when they consumed cariogenic food. The resulting **specific plaque hypothesis** describes the infection of a host with specific pathogenic germs (e.g., *S. mutans* or *Lactobacillus* spp.). Consequently, caries was, and is, described frequently as a "transmittable infectious disease."[9] This view has influenced dentistry for many years.

If caries is considered an infectious disease, the most attractive preventive measure, as is the case with other classic infectious diseases, is to **avoid contact with the pathogen.** This consequentially led to preventive methods for avoiding the transfer of germs, for example, from the mother to the child. It was frequently recommended that the mother and child avoid the exchange of saliva.[10] This led to recommendations that young mothers not put pacifiers or their children's spoons in their mouth.[11] Parents however, found that it was almost impossible to prevent the transfer of colds between the parent and child and vice versa. How was this to be prevented with mutans streptococci? Where else should children acquire their physiological oral flora if not from their closest contact person? Whether it is in fact possible or even desirable to consistently avoid the transmission of bacteria from parents to children is hence questionable. After an individual acquires a classic infectious disease, the therapy focuses on **fighting the pathogen** (if possible) with, for example, antimicrobial substances. In caries therapy, this means mechanically or chemically removing the pathogen, or at least decimating the bacterial plaque. Attempts were even made to regularly deliver antibiotics in toothpaste.[12] The **complete excavation of caries** in the dentin is based on the belief that the disease can only be stopped by completely eradicating the pathogen. Also immunological approaches such as the development of vaccines against *S. mutans* are an extension of the specific plaque hypothesis.[13]

NOTE

The specific plaque hypothesis views caries as primarily originating from an infection with specific bacteria and leads to therapeutic approaches that seek to completely eradicate the pathogenic germs.

The Ecological Plaque Hypothesis

Critics of the specific plaque hypothesis argue that mutans streptococci are also found in individuals who are clinically free of caries.[4,14] Contrastingly, *S. mutans* sometimes cannot be found in patients suffering from caries. Since the varied bacterial flora of the digestive system are essential to our body which continuously interacts with the environment, it is inappropriate to view a modification of the bacterial composition within our body as an infection. It is known that other factors are necessary to produce caries such as the regular supply of fermentable carbohydrates which promote the growth and metabolism of cariogenic bacteria. The presence of cariogenic microorganisms such as *S. mutans* therefore appears to be a necessary but not a sufficient factor for generating caries. These considerations have led the paradigm of the specific plaque hypothesis to be increasingly questioned.[4]

In contrast to the specific plaque hypothesis, the **ecological plaque hypothesis** in favor today does not focus on infection with pathogenic microorganisms, but rather explains caries as a disturbance in the homeostasis of the oral microflora.[15] This is caused by the selective favoring of (potentially) pathogenic microorganisms (such as *S. mutans*) by a sugar-rich diet. It is assumed that it is not an exogenous infection with pathogenic species that is responsible for caries. Rather, these species are a part of the physiological (endogenous) flora in healthy humans, and only the qualitative and quantitative changes are pathological.[4] The increased consumption of fermentable carbohydrates favors microorganisms that efficiently metabolize these sugars into organic acids (acidogenic) and also tolerate the resultant low pH (aciduric).

This ecological approach also influences therapy. Proceeding from the ecological plaque hypothesis, prevention no longer focuses on avoiding the transmission of germs. It is even probable that the transmission of a healthy bacterial oral flora from mother to child is preferable. Instead of avoiding the transmission of pathogens which is probably impossible, the development of a physiological bacterial oral flora in the mother is supported by

appropriate interventions and recommendations. More recent approaches even seek to specifically reinforce a physiological bacterial flora through probiotic products.[16] **Avoiding** the mother-to-child transmission of **disease-promoting behaviors** (sugar consumption) appears to be a more useful way to prevent caries. If caries and hence a pathogenic flora exist, the therapeutic goal is not to eradicate or decimate all bacteria, in contrast to earlier approaches, since this would harm the physiological flora. In addition, the decimation of a cariogenic species would probably enable another potentially pathogenic species to fill the ecological niche, which would lead to similar problems. Instead, the primary goal of therapy is to **restore the physiological equilibrium** (Chapters 9–12). If caries is not an infection, the necessity of complete excavation of infected dentin has to be put in question. The **incomplete excavation** of caries and creation of local conditions unfavorable to cariogenic bacteria (no room for the formation of a biofilm, cut off the source of nutrition with a sealant) can be sufficient to control the disease (Chapters 15–18).

NOTE

Based on our present knowledge, the ecological plaque hypothesis appears to be the most attractive and widely accepted theory on the etiology and pathogenesis of caries. The ecological plaque hypothesis focuses on the ecological equilibrium in the oral cavity as the source of caries which leads to therapeutic approaches that seek to control the different physiological factors of the process.

A Current Model of Caries

The **etiology** of caries has been described in various models and ways.[17–20] The famous Venn diagram by Keyes (see **Fig. 2.1**, p. 22) shows the three essential etiological factors for caries: "bacteria," "tooth," and "sugar."[17] Later, König suggested including "time" as a fourth essential factor.[18] Both models are based on the specific plaque hypothesis and—for reasons of simplicity—ignore other influencing factors. The model introduced by Fejerskov and Manji (see **Fig. 21.1**, p. 307) in contrast, shows caries as a multifactorial disease.

Figure 4.1 shows a **pathogenesis** model of caries based on the ecological plaque hypothesis: According to our present understanding, a sugar-rich diet plays a primary role in the etiology and pathogenesis of caries.[21] A greater role has been assigned to sugar because caries is a disease of civilizations that consume a greater amount (or excess?) of sugar, which was not the case throughout most of human history.[22] The excessive consumption of fermentable carbohydrates appears to be less physiologically normal than the regular existence of small numbers of

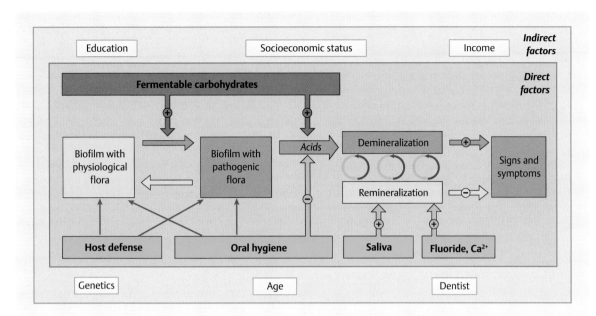

Fig. 4.1 The pathogenesis of caries. The primary causal pathogenic factor (dark red) for caries is the frequent consumption of fermentable carbohydrates (sugars). This causes an ecological shift in the oral biofilm favoring acidogenic and aciduric species (pathogenic flora). The increased metabolic activity of the biofilm, which is also triggered by sugar consumption, causes the formation of organic acids. This leads to demineralization of dental hard tissues, which consequently results in the characteristic signs and symptoms of caries. On the contrary there are several protective factors (dark green): the host defense (immune system) and the oral

hygiene limit the number of microorganisms. By oral hygiene the biofilm can be completely removed at least locally, and thus acid formation can be avoided. In addition, the components of saliva as well as locally applied fluorides and calcium enhance the remineralization of dental hard tissues, which may alleviate the signs and symptoms of caries. Besides these (local) direct factors there are several indirect (distant) factors, which only indirectly influence the caries process but may be strongly associated with caries. For simplicity, not all associations are marked.

potentially cariogenic bacteria in the physiological flora. The frequent consumption of fermentable carbohydrates causes a pathological shift in the oral microflora and promotes acidogenic and aciduric species.[15] Consuming fermentable carbohydrates also causes potentially cariogenic bacteria such as *S. mutans* to produce organic acids that demineralize the enamel and dentin. This finally causes the characteristic signs and symptoms of caries. Protective factors also influence the development of caries. Both the host's defenses and the patient's oral hygiene limit the growth and metabolism of the oral biofilm and hence the production of acids. With its buffering properties and minerals, saliva promotes the remineralization of the enamel. The remineralizing effect of saliva can be supported by the application of fluorides and calcium compounds.[23] In addition to these local, direct factors, other behavioral and socioeconomic factors are associated with caries as revealed by epidemiological investigations.[24] However, these only indirectly influence the caries process through the local factors.[4]

With the exception of the consumption of fermentable carbohydrates that is shown in **Fig. 4.1** as a **pathogenic**

factor (dark red), all of the other factors that locally influence the caries process are shown as **protective factors** (dark green). However, the minimization or elimination of protective factors can have a significant influence on the caries process. For example, the elimination of saliva's protective function in patients with hyposalivation frequently causes caries to progress extremely fast, even though other factors are scarcely modified.[25] The **risk factors** for caries are accordingly increasing the pathogenic factor of fermentable carbohydrates as well as eliminating or reducing protective factors.

According to our present understanding, caries is a **multifactorial disease**. If and how fast caries develops depends on the complex interrelationships between the various pathogenic and protective factors. If the protective factors predominate, caries does not develop, or existing caries is arrested or healed. However, if the pathogenic factors predominate, the disease progresses.[20] This dynamic character of the caries process enables the disease to be influenced in every stage. Approaches for preventing caries therefore seek to minimize the pathogenic factors and support the protective factors.

SUMMARY

Scientific paradigms guide our understanding of diseases and therefore also influence our preventive/therapeutic approaches. The paradigm of the specific plaque hypothesis leads to preventive approaches for avoiding infection with cariogenic microorganisms and forms of therapy to eliminate all cariogenic microorganisms. Contrastingly, the ecological plaque hypothesis is based on environmental and behavioral influences and consequently leads to interventions for reducing pathogenic factors and/or promoting protective factors.

REFERENCES

1. Kuhn TS. Die Struktur wissenschaftlicher Revolutionen. Frankfurt: Suhrkamp; 1979
2. Chalmers AF. Wege der Wissenschaft. Berlin: Springer; 2007
3. Hooper LV, Wong MH, Thelin A, Hansson L, Falk PG, Gordon JI. Molecular analysis of commensal host-microbial relationships in the intestine. Science 2001;291(5505):881–884
4. Fejerskov O. Changing paradigms in concepts on dental caries: consequences for oral health care. Caries Res 2004;38(3):182–191
5. Miller WD. Textbook of conservative dentistry. [Lehrbuch der Conservirenden Zahnheilkunde]. 2nd ed. Leipzig: Thieme; 1898
6. Orland FJ, Blayney JR, Harrison RW, et al. Use of the germfree animal technic in the study of experimental dental caries. I. Basic observations on rats reared free of all microorganisms. J Dent Res 1954;33(2):147–174
7. Fitzgerald RJ, Jordan HV, Stanley HR. Experimental caries and gingival pathologic changes in the gnotobiotic rat. J Dent Res 1960;39:923–935
8. Keyes PH. The infectious and transmissible nature of experimental dental caries. Findings and implications. Arch Oral Biol 1960;1:304–320
9. Tanzer JM. Dental caries is a transmissible infectious disease: the Keyes and Fitzgerald revolution. J Dent Res 1995;74(9):1536–1542
10. Caufield PW, Cutter GR, Dasanayake AP. Initial acquisition of mutans streptococci by infants: evidence for a discrete window of infectivity. J Dent Res 1993;72(1):37–45
11. Suhonen J. Mutans streptococci and their specific oral target. New implications to prevent dental caries? Schweiz Monatsschr Zahnmed 1992;102(3):286–291
12. Hill TJ, Sims J, Newman M. The effect of penicillin dentifrice on the control of dental caries. J Dent Res 1953;32(4):448–452
13. Taubman MA, Nash DA. The scientific and public-health imperative for a vaccine against dental caries. Nat Rev Immunol 2006;6(7):555–563
14. Marsh PD, Martin M. Oral Microbiology. 3rd ed. London: Chapman and Hall; 1992
15. Marsh PD. Microbial ecology of dental plaque and its significance in health and disease. Adv Dent Res 1994;8(2):263–271
16. He X, Lux R, Kuramitsu HK, Anderson MH, Shi W. Achieving probiotic effects via modulating oral microbial ecology. Adv Dent Res 2009;21(1):53–56
17. Keyes PH. Recent advances in dental caries research. Bacteriology. Bacteriological findings and biological implications. Int Dent J 1962;12:443–464
18. König KG. Karies und Kariesprophylaxe. München: Goldmann; 1971
19. Fejerskov O, Manji F. Risk assessment in dental caries. In: Bader JD, ed. Risk Assessment in Dentistry. Chapel Hill: University of North Carolina Dental Ecology; 1990:215–217
20. Featherstone JD. Prevention and reversal of dental caries: role of low level fluoride. Community Dent Oral Epidemiol 1999;27(1):31–40
21. Zero DT. Sugars—the arch criminal? Caries Res 2004;38(3):277–285
22. Moore WJ. The role of sugar in the aetiology of dental caries. 1. Sugar and the antiquity of dental caries. J Dent 1983;11(3):189–190
23. ten Cate JM, Featherstone JD. Mechanistic aspects of the interactions between fluoride and dental enamel. Crit Rev Oral Biol Med 1991;2(3):283–296
24. Harris R, Nicoll AD, Adair PM, Pine CM. Risk factors for dental caries in young children: a systematic review of the literature. Community Dent Health 2004; 21(1, Suppl):71–85
25. Fox PC. Salivary enhancement therapies. Caries Res 2004;38(3):241–246

Visual–Tactile Detection and Assessment

Kim R. Ekstrand, Stefania Martignon

5

The terms **detection** and **assessment** with respect to caries lesions have not been widely adopted so far. Instead the term **diagnosis** is used to describe the result of the clinical and radiographic examination. The current international glossary of key terms states that[1]:

- **Lesion detection** implies a process involving the recognition (and/or recording), traditionally by optical or physical means, of changes in enamel and/or dentin, and/or cementum, which are consistent with having been caused by the carious process.
- **Lesion assessment** is the assessment of the characteristics of a carious lesion, once it has been detected. These characteristics may include optical, physical, chemical, or bio-chemical parameters, such as color, size, or surface integrity and its activity status.
- **Caries diagnosis** should imply the human professional summation of all the signs and symptoms of disease to arrive at an identification of the past or present occurrence of the disease, caries (see Chapter 9).

Looking up the word diagnosis in the dictionary, one will find that it originates from the two Greek words: *"dia"* which corresponds to "through," and *"gnosis"* which corresponds to "knowledge." Consequently, it is only through knowledge about diseases that the professional summation or the correct diagnosis can be established.[2] Hence Chapters 1–4 have informed about the structure of the teeth, the etiology, and pathogenesis of caries on histological and clinical levels as well as the caries process depicted as a theoretical model.

It follows from the above, then, that diagnosis is a process.[3] Here, several signs and symptoms of a disease (as caries) are detected and assessed by means of different qualitative or quantitative methods or tools. Basically, for caries the diagnostic process either leads to the assumption that the **lesion is likely to progress** or not. In the first case, further loss of mineral is expected, if relevant factors of the disease are not changed[4], and either a non-, micro-, or minimal-invasive treatment should then be performed. The therapy that offers the best **prognosis** to prevent lesion progression without damaging too much sound and diseased hard tissue should be advocated. If the diagnostic process leads to the assumption that the lesion is **arrested**, no further mineral loss would be expected under the current oral conditions. In consequence, no cariologic treatment is currently necessary (Chapters 9 and 20)[4].

> **NOTE**
>
> Detection and assessment of various signs and symptoms of a disease are summarized together with other parameters to reach a diagnosis.

In this chapter we will begin by introducing the visual–tactile method, the main tool for the **clinical part** of the diagnostic process. The next chapter will deal with radiographs and other caries detection methods. The visual–tactile method comprises the use of the eye and a thin explorer, the latter is said to "lengthen the eye of the examiner." Hereby a caries lesion can be:

1. Detected, which implies a subjective method of determining whether or not a caries lesion is present
2. Assessed according to severity status (depth)
3. Assessed according to activity status

> **NOTE**
>
> Visual–tactile examination of the teeth is just one of several detection and assessment methods for caries, but still the most important.

In detail, this chapter will cover:

- Requirements for visual–tactile examination of the teeth
- Visual–tactile indices to record or score caries lesions
- Relationships between visual signs of caries and the histological depth
- How to assess activity status of caries lesions
- Differences between caries and other diseases of the tooth hard substance

General Remarks

Caries develops where a cariogenic biofilm accumulates. In consequence, caries most often develops next to gingival margins, cervical to approximal contact areas, and in the grooves and fossae of the occlusal surfaces. Caries is very seldom seen on the incisal edge or at the cusps of teeth. In elderly people root caries can frequently be observed where the gingiva is recessed.

Basically, **primary caries,** which is caries on unrestored surfaces and **caries adjacent to a restoration** (old terminology: secondary caries or recurrent caries), can be observed both on crowns and roots. **Residual caries** means that demineralized tissue, often dentin, was left behind for some reason before a restoration has been placed.

Good light as well as clean and dry teeth are required when examining for caries and other dental hard tissue defects.[4–5] These are particularly important to identify early stages of caries[3–6] (**Fig. 5.1**). **Professional tooth cleaning** can be performed by means of rotating brushes or simply by manual toothbrushing. Approximal surfaces are most easily cleaned by flossing. Cotton rolls are placed in the maxillary sulci to control saliva from the parotid glands. Suction and/or cotton rolls might be used lingually as supplement. Each tooth is then examined, starting for example in the maxilla in the right side of the mouth on the most posterior tooth (tooth 18). Distal, occlusal, oral, buccal, and finally the mesial/distal interproximal surfaces are examined separately under clean and dry conditions. The examination proceeds in the anterior direction, completing first the upper and then the lower arch. A **thin**

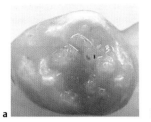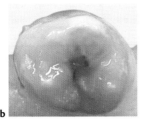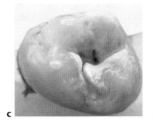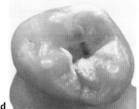

a   b   c   d

Fig. 5.1a–d Occlusal aspect of an extracted tooth with biofilm covering the surface (**a**). After professional cleaning it is possible to detect caries on the occlusal surface (**b**). Caries becomes more visible after air-drying (**c**). Hard probing has created breakdowns in the surface integrity (**d**).

probe and a **dental mirror** are needed. **Visually,** color changes compared with the appearance of structurally sound teeth are noticed; **tactilely,** irregularities in the morphology of the tooth surface are sensed.

Thus, changes in color compared with the appearance of structurally sound teeth can be **seen**, while irregularities in the morphology of the tooth surface can be **felt**.

During recent years it has been increasingly popular for dental professionals to use **magnifying glasses**. It has been be assumed that magnification increases the accuracy of detection and assessment of caries lesions, in particular of initial ones. However, studies show inconclusive results with respect to improvement in caries examination by using magnification compared to the naked eye.[8,9]

Histological and Clinical Features of Caries

Coronal Caries Lesions

Caries on the crowns mainly develops in the groove–fossa system (fissure system), on the approximal and the smooth surfaces near the gingival margins. Early stages of caries on approximal surfaces are hidden from visual inspection due to the adjacent tooth. Caries in the groove–fossa system develops most often at the entrance to the fissure parts and in the bottom part of the grooves. However, after cleaning and drying, initial and also more mature stages of occlusal caries lesions can be visually identified.[3,10,11]

Wherever a cariogenic biofilm is established, signs and subsequently symptoms (tenderness or pain) of caries may become evident. The **first changes** recognized visually are changes in color from yellowish white to chalky white. If the carious challenge continues, the white area becomes more obvious in time. In the next stage small **breakdowns** (discontinuations/microcavities) occur in the enamel and/or a dark shadow due to underlying carious dentin is observed. This stage is followed by different sizes of breakdown of enamel and also parts of the dentin. Eventually the surface/tooth is completely destroyed due to the demineralization process (**Fig. 5.2**, **Fig. 5.11**). If progression stops at an early stage, very often the whitish appearance, in particular on the occlusal surfaces, discolors (brownish) and stays like that as a scar (**Fig. 5.2**).

The change in color from yellowish white to chalky white can be explained by dissolution of mineral. Consequently, the intercrystalline spaces will be bigger and the pore volume increases. Hereby light will be scattered, which is recognized visually as an opaque area that is different from the surrounding translucent sound enamel. This phenomenon can be explained physically by the different **refractive indices** of various media/structures. Air has a refractive index (RI) of 1.0, water/saliva of 1.33, and enamel of 1.62.[12,13] If, in the laboratory, a liquid (e.g., quinoline) with a refractive index of 1.62, being similar to that of the surrounding sound enamel, is applied onto a white spot caries lesion, the lesion will disappear (see Chapter 3). Clinically, we can only dry the lesions and re-wet them with water to identify small lesions with a very low increase in pore volume. After drying, a caries lesion that is normally 'bathed in saliva' will be more distinctively visible, since the RI in the most demineralized parts is now changed to 1.0. After applying water the RI in these pores will again (similarly to saliva) increase to 1.33; the lesion is no longer visible, or at least less. If whitish, these initial caries lesions on enamel are called **white spots**. Stains arising from nutrition or smoking might change these into **brown spots** over time.

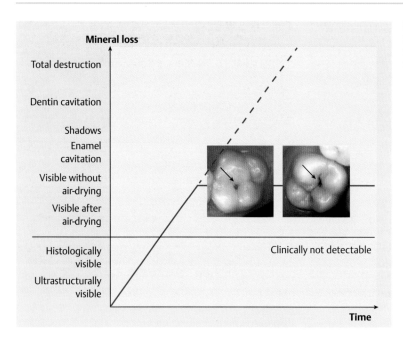

Fig. 5.2 Relevant stages of caries within a certain period of time. Brown-spot lesions are visible without prior air drying and often do not progress.

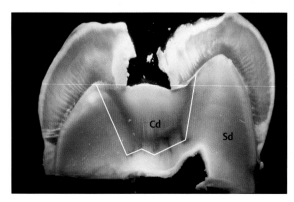

Fig. 5.3 Section of the coronal part of the tooth showing color changes in the demineralized dentin (Cd; marked with lines) compared with surrounding normal dentin (Sd).

When acids reach the dentin they will dissolve the mineral in the dentin. Demineralized dentin varies in color from that of sound dentin—it appears more yellowish or brownish (**Fig. 5.3**). Sometimes the change in color can be

seen through the overlying enamel as a shadow (**Fig. 5.4**). Thus, if a shadow from the underlying dentin can be identified, demineralization of the dentin has taken place. It is important to emphasize that **demineralized dentin** is not the same as dentin harboring **microorganisms**, or even **biofilms**. As long as the caries lesion is not cavitated, occasionally single microorganisms, but not established biofilms, will be present within the lesion. If the lesion is **cavitated**, larger numbers of microorganisms enter into the enamel and may build up cariogenic biofilms there as well.[14,15] Microcavities are cavities in outer parts of the demineralized enamel that covers the demineralized dentin. If all the enamel is gone, this is called a dentin cavitation.[16]

CLINICAL PEARL

Breakdown of tooth structure due to caries can clinically be verified by gently drawing a probe across the area (*feeling*).

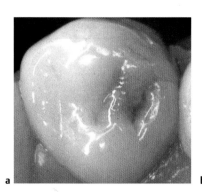
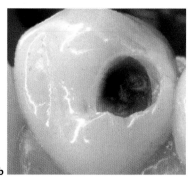

Fig. 5.4a, b Shadowed lesion on the occlusal/distal aspects of tooth 34 (**a**). After removal of some enamel parts demineralized and dark dentin appears (**b**).

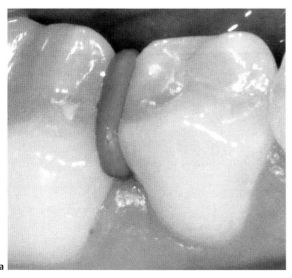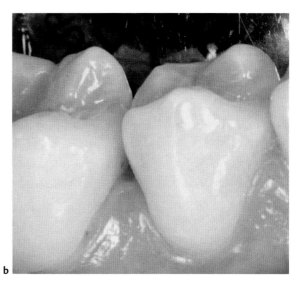

Fig. 5.5a, b Steps in tooth separation for visual–tactile caries detection and assessment on approximal surfaces.

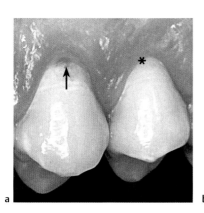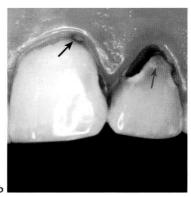

Fig. 5.6a, b Different stages of root caries in one patient: Slight gingival recession on tooth 25, but no caries lesion (✱). A noncavitated caries lesion visible on tooth 24 (**a**, arrow). Cavitated root caries lesions (depth < 0.5 mm) on tooth 21 (black arrow) and more pronounced on tooth 22 (depth > 0.5 mm; red arrow) (**b**).

Caries lesions on approximal surfaces are often obscured by the adjacent tooth surface, which hinders adequate visual examination. Placement of an orthodontic elastic band (0.8 mm) for two days **(Fig. 5.5)** creates some space, large enough to examine both approximal surfaces visually and tactilely. High interrater-reproducibility when assessing cavitation status has been reported for this technique.[17] Few patients seem to experience discomfort when using separators.[18] Nevertheless, in dental practice this method does not seem to be adopted on a large scale owing to two patient visits being needed. The use of a thin probe without prior separation or a floss (a floss will crack if it is run over a cavity) might be of help at least to distinguish between cavitated and noncavitated approximal lesions.

Root Caries Lesions

Caries on the roots will only develop when the gingiva is recessed due to either inflammation or trauma (e.g., following incorrect toothbrushing). Even normal brushing will then abrade the cementum covering the root dentin.

If a cariogenic biofilm is frequently established in these areas, apatite crystals will be dissolved and the dentin will change in color and texture. Root caries pathogenesis differs slightly from that of enamel, since caries in dentin follows the tubules. Microorganisms will quite easily penetrate into these, already in the very early stages of root caries formation. Preformed sclerotic dentin as well as access to saliva and gingival fluid may slow down the progression rate. Nonetheless, root caries also tends to circle around the neck of the tooth rather than to penetrate very deeply into the tissue. As for enamel, root caries lesions will first be noncavitated **(Fig. 5.6)**.

CLINICAL PEARL

When sound dentin is probed, the texture feels hard. Demineralized dentin is softer than sound dentin, which can be sensed with the probe. Often the dentin feels sticky, which means that the dental professional has to pull back the probe.

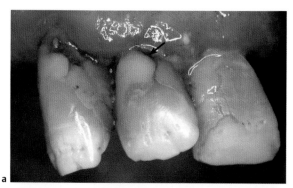

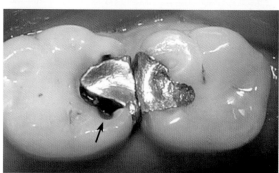

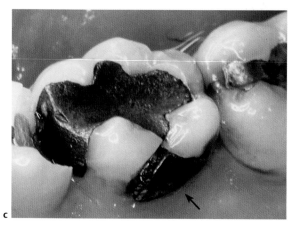

Fig. 5.7a–c Examples of an early caries lesion adjacent to a restoration (CAR) (**a**), a more severe CAR lesion (**b**), and an amalgam restoration that is loose (**c**).

Caries Adjacent to Restorations

Caries adjacent to or at the margin of restorations (**Fig. 5.7a, b**) has many designations, for example, **secondary caries** to distinguish it from primary caries and **recurrent caries** to reflect the results of lack of plaque control. The preference in this chapter is **caries adjacent to restorations** (CAR), which relates to the supposition that CAR in principle follows the pathogenesis delineated for primary caries, whether coronal or in root dentin.[19–21] From histological examination it has been suggested to describe the CAR enamel lesion in two parts: an outer primary lesion next to the restoration, and a wall lesion between the restoration and the cavity. Initially in enamel

and dentin lesions, the wall lesion is narrow, but when the lesion reaches the enamel–dentin junction (EDJ) there may be some lateral spread. The outer primary enamel lesion is a subsurface lesion, which spreads further into the enamel following the directions of the prisms. When the lesion reaches the EDJ, dentin demineralization occurs mainly along the affected dentinal tubules. The initial root CAR lesion also follows the shape of the dentinal tubules.

In addition, a restoration can be imperfect, possibly loose (**Fig. 5.7c**), and then traps plaque, which can lead very quickly to development of caries.

Indices for Clinical Recording of Caries Lesions

Numerous indices for visual/tactile recording of various stages of caries lesions, restorations, and sealants have been described. The reliability in terms of intra- and interrater-reproducibility of the individual indices is often expressed in kappa values. To ease readability of this paragraph the reliability of the individual indices will be graduated according to the three following levels (modified from Landis and Koch[22]) Thus, if a recording system has the following "scores," ☺☺☺, ●●●, this means that both intra- and interrater-reproducibility are almost perfect (**Table 5.1**).

Historical Perspective

Numerous classification systems to record caries have been developed over the years.[23] Each system fulfilled a particular aim, such as to be used in epidemiological investigations, clinical studies, or for daily use in clinical practice.

In the past 50 years a system for epidemiological investigations advocated by the World Health Organization ☺☺☺, ●●● has been widely adopted.[24] Here, only caries at the cavity level—a quite late stage of the disease (**Fig. 5.8**)—is reported. This is understandable, as the system was primarily developed to record caries under **field conditions**, without cleaning and drying of the teeth, and using nonprofessional light sources. As caries is recorded at the cavity level, there are no good reasons to have codes for either active or arrested caries lesions, as all cavitated lesions in this system are regarded as being active. Another system (Radike [X,●●])[25] also only scores caries at the cavity level or for those caries lesions where the probe is **caught**.

The modern approach is to prevent caries before it requires restorations, and therefore it is necessary to record initial, noncavitated stages as well as cavitated stages.[26][X,X, 27] ☺☺☺, ●●●, [28]☺☺☺, ●●●, [29]☺☺☺, ●●●. Such indices may also be used in **clinical trials** where small changes within short periods from baseline to final examination need to be recorded. **Table 5.2** shows the scoring system used by Kuzmina et al.[28] where primary caries

Table 5.1 Scoring of Indices at three levels

Score	Symbol
Intrarater-reproducibility	
Poor	☺
Moderate/substantial	☺☺
Almost perfect	☺☺☺
Not evaluated	x
Interrater-reproducibility	
Poor	●
Moderate/substantial	●●
Almost perfect	●●●
Not evaluated	x

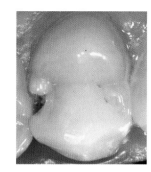

Fig. 5.8 Example of a cavitated caries lesion, which is registered as caries in the WHO classification system (see text).

caries on children in the Public Child Dental Health Service in Denmark.[30–31] This system, ☺☺☺, ●●●, has been used since the 1970s on a daily basis by both dentists and dental hygienists. This recording system was amongst the first where scores for a whole child population could be transferred to a computer, where mean dmfs/t-DMFS/T and percentages of children with dmft-DMFT = 0 could be expressed at the individual level, and at the municipality, county, and national levels.

There are several other recording systems worth mentioning, also covering root caries; however, they are linked to the depth of the lesions evaluated histologically and/or the activity state of the lesions. These will be discussed in the following paragraphs.

is divided into four scores: 1 = initial, noncavitated caries; 2 = caries with microcavitation; 3 = caries with dentin cavitation; and 4 = deep dentin caries.

Figure 5.9 shows a formula used for recording primary caries and CAR, root treatments, and extractions due to

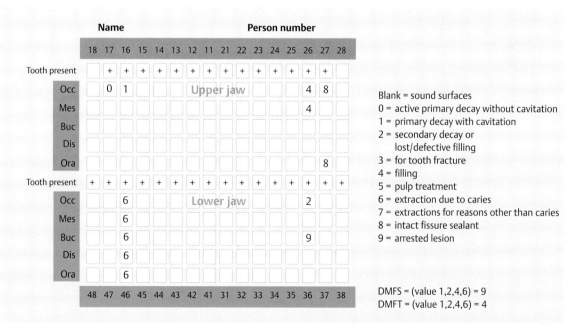

Name **Person number**

	18	17	16	15	14	13	12	11	21	22	23	24	25	26	27	28
Tooth present		+	+	+	+	+	+	+	+	+	+	+	+	+	+	
Occ		0	1				Upper jaw							4	8	
Mes														4		
Buc																
Dis																
Ora															8	
Tooth present	+	+	+	+	+	+	+	+	+	+	+	+	+	+	+	+
Occ			6				Lower jaw							2		
Mes			6													
Buc			6												9	
Dis			6													
Ora			6													
	48	47	46	45	44	43	42	41	31	32	33	34	35	36	37	38

Blank = sound surfaces
0 = active primary decay without cavitation
1 = primary decay with cavitation
2 = secondary decay or lost/defective filling
3 = for tooth fracture
4 = filling
5 = pulp treatment
6 = extraction due to caries
7 = extractions for reasons other than caries
8 = intact fissure sealant
9 = arrested lesion

DMFS = (value 1,2,4,6) = 9
DMFT = (value 1,2,4,6) = 4

Fig. 5.9 Form and scores used in the Danish Public Child Dental Health system for recording caries. The scores and descriptions are seen to the right. All permanent teeth are present (+) apart from 18 and 28. Occlusally, on 17 there is an active noncavitated lesion (score 0). Occlusally, on 16 there is a primary cavitated lesion (score 1). Occlusally/mesially, on 26 there is a restoration (score 4). Oc- clusally and orally, on 27 sealants are placed. Occlusally, on 36 there is a cavitated lesion (secondary, score 2) seen next to a restoration, and buccally, there is an arrested lesion (score 9). Tooth 46 has been extracted due to caries (score 6). The figure also gives the DMFS and the DMFT values.

Table 5.2 Classification of different stages of caries expressed by the Kuzmina system [28]

Classification of caries	Scores
Normal enamel translucency (sound)	0
Opaque enamel with a dull-whitish surface (active caries without cavitation)	1
Dull-whitish enamel with localized surface destruction in enamel, but not reaching the dentin (cavitation in enamel)	2
Initial dentin cavitation	3
Deep dentin caries	4
Active caries with cavitation on filled surface	5
Secondary caries	6
Filled surface	7
Shiny appearance of the surface of the opaque area with different degrees of brownish discoloration (arrested lesion)	8
Sealed surfaces	9

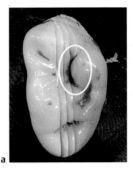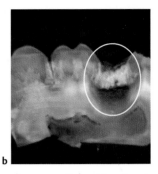

a   b

Fig. 5.10a, b A dark shadow can be seen on the serial sectioned occlusal surface (**a**), caries is seen in the enamel and rather deep into the dentin (**b**).

NOTE

Traditional caries indices have focused on lesions at the cavitation (into dentin) level. More recent ones include the recording of noncavitated caries lesions. The majority of indices have not been adequately evaluated scientifically, although reproducibility seems to be quite good for most of them.

Correlation between Histology and Clinical Severity: the ICDAS System

Traditionally, the relationship between clinical signs of caries and the corresponding histological changes has been examined on extracted teeth, which were serially sectioned or hemisectioned through the selected areas of the tooth (**Fig. 5.10**).[6,16,32] To express the relationship between the clinical sign, often expressed as scores (e.g., score 0–4), and the depth of the lesions, also expressed as scores (e.g., score 0–4), either the correlation coefficient was used and/or terms such as sensitivity and specificity to describe the accuracy (validity) of the recording system. Irrespective of the method, certain **thresholds** of the caries disease had to be defined.

Coronal Caries Lesions

For occlusal caries lesions, a visually ranked scoring system using five visual severity grades (**Table 5.3**) has been related to lesion depth, which is also separated into five severity grades scientifically☺☺☺,●●●.[16] The accuracy of this recording system is substantial to excellent, meaning that a score of 1 visually corresponded well to a score of 1 histologically, and so forth. This system was the forerunner of the most recent classification system: the **International Caries Detection and Assessment System (ICDAS)** ☺☺,●●, which has been developed by a group of cariologists and epidemiologists (**Fig. 5.11**).[33–35] For primary caries there are seven visual severity stages (codes) starting from sound surfaces, to first visible changes after air-drying, distinct changes being visible without air-drying, microcavitated surfaces, shadowed lesion, dentin cavitation, and ending up with defects where more than half of the surface has been lost due to caries. ICDAS is closely related to the histological findings occlusally (**Table 5.4**)[35] but also on approximal surfaces.[36] The intention of the ICDAS system is that it can be used for any type of investigation—**field, longitudinal, or interventional studies**. A guideline for using ICDAS for coronal primary caries has been developed[37] (www.icdas.org). Moreover, in this book a way of implementing ICDAS in daily dental practice will be proposed (Chapters 9 and 24–26).

With respect to **bacterial colonization** a significant correlation between lesion depth and number of microorganisms at the enamel–dentin junction (EDJ) has been observed for primary coronal caries lesions.[15] At most, a few microorganisms were seen at the EDJ in noncavitated lesions. Substantial numbers of microorganisms were observed at the EDJ in micro cavitated and shadowed lesions.

Based on these findings, it seems clinically relevant to describe three severity stages when expressing the relationship between visual sign of caries on the surface and the corresponding depth of the coronal caries lesions: these are **superficial, medium, and profound lesions**[4] (**Table 5.5**).

Table 5.3 The classification system devised by Ekstrand et al.[16] for occlusal caries detection and estimation of depth

Score	Visual appearance	Histological depth
0	No, or slight, change in enamel translucency after prolonged air-drying (>5 s)	No enamel demineralization or a narrow surface zone of opacity (edge phenomenon)
1	Opacity (white or brown) hardly visible on the wet surface but distinctly visible after air-drying	Enamel demineralization limited to the outer 50% of the enamel layer
2	Opacity (white or brown) distinctly visible without air-drying	Demineralization involving 50% of the enamel and up to one-third of the dentin
3	Localized enamel breakdown in opaque or discolored enamel and/or grayish discoloration from the underlying dentin	Demineralization involving the middle third of the dentin
4	Cavitation in opaque or discolored enamel exposing the dentin	Demineralization involving the inner third of the dentin

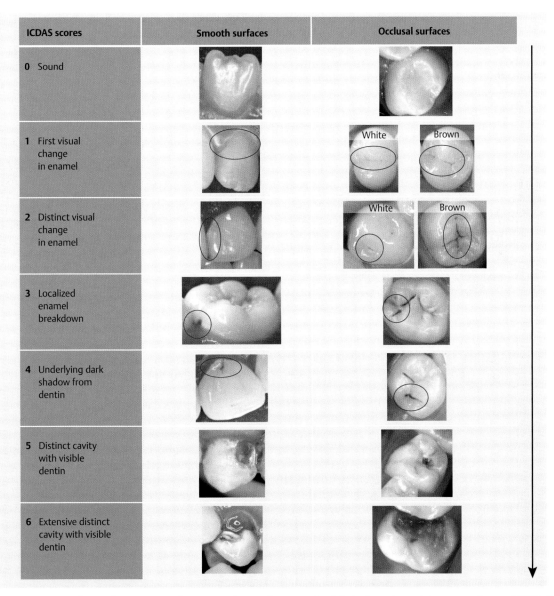

Fig. 5.11 Scoring of coronal primary caries lesions according to the International Caries Detection and Assessment System (ICDAS). The arrow indicates increasing severity of caries lesions from first signs (ICDAS 1) to extensive cavitation (ICDAS 6)

Table 5.4 Relation between ICDAS scores and depth of the caries lesions (according to Ekstrand et al. 2007[35])

Histology ICDAS Score	Sound	Outer half enamel	Inner half enamel, outer third dentin	Middle third dentin	Inner third dentin	Total
0 Sound	35	2				37
1 W/B dry	3	16	1			20
2 W/B wet		3	21	5		29
3 Microcav.			4	7	2	13
4 Shadow			1	7	1	9
5 D-cavit		5		5	13	18
6 D-cavit					13	13
Total	38	21	27	24	29	139

[a]Surfaces that are visually scored as sound are also histologically sound in most cases (35 out of 37). Surfaces showing a white (W) spot lesion, which are only identified after air-drying, or a small brown (B) spot (ICDAS 1) are in most cases limited to the outer half of the enamel. White spot lesions identified without air-drying or more mature brown spot lesions (ICDAS 2) are histologically extended into the inner half of the enamel to outer third of the dentin. Microcavitated or shadowed lesions (ICDAS 3 and 4) are depthwise generally restricted to the middle third of the dentin, whereas lesions showing cavitations into the dentin (ICDAS 5 and 6) are histologically confined to the inner third of the dentin or have even progressed into the pulp.

Table 5.5 Relationship between visual classification of sign of caries and the histological changes and designated term

Visual classification	Histological findings	Term
White or brown spot lesions, no visible breakdown	Enamel caries and if caries in the dentin it is limited at max. to the outer third	Superficial
Microcavitation and/or shadow	Dentin caries in the middle third	Medium
Dentin cavitation	Dentin caries in the inner third	Profound

Root Caries Lesions

The ICDAS group also developed a classification system for primary root caries lesions. ☺☺☺,X [33,37] The codes are:
- 0: sound root surface (see **Fig. 5.6a***)
- 1: a demarcated area on the root surface or at the EDJ that is discolored (light/dark brown, black). Still, no cavitation deeper than 0.5 mm is present (see **Fig. 5.6a, b** arrows).
- 2: a demarcated area on the root surface or at the EDJ that is discolored (light/dark brown, black). A cavitation ≥ 0.5 mm is present (see **Fig. 5.6b** red arrow).

No studies have related the visual appearance of root caries lesions to the histological depth of the corresponding lesions. However, clinical experience indicates that noncavitated root caries lesions are less deeply demineralized than microcavitated ones (cavitation depth < 0.5 mm), which again are less deeply demineralized than more severely cavitated lesions (> 0.5 mm). This seems also to be true for root caries lesions adjacent to restorations.

Tooth anatomy tells us that the distance from the surface of the roots to the pulp tissue is within a range of 1–4 mm. Therefore, as with coronal caries, it is convenient to differentiate between superficial (non cavitated), medium (cavitated < 0.5 mm), and profound (cavitated > 0.5 mm) caries lesions (see **Fig. 5.6a, b**).

Caries Adjacent to Restorations

To the best knowledge of the authors there are no studies which have related the visual appearances of CAR to the corresponding histological changes. As CAR act as primary caries[19–21] it is assumed that the histological changes related to CAR are the same as in primary caries lesions. Therefore, ICDAS operates with the same codes for CAR lesions as for both primary coronal as well as primary root caries lesions. No reliability and validity data for these scoring systems are currently available.

Caries Activity Assessment

In combination with lesion severity recording (e.g., by the ICDAS system) caries activity assessment should also be performed. This means that the dental professional needs to distinguish active caries lesions from inactive ones. **Caries activity assessment** should be semantically differentiated from **caries risk assessment of the person/patient** (individual level). Caries activity describes the probability of a caries lesion to progress, taking into account information mainly from the visual–tactile examination of the caries lesion and its surroundings. Caries risk assessment takes into account several other individual signs (e.g., caries experience, nutrition, or general plaque status).

Coronal Caries Lesions

There seems to be no single variable (predictor) that accurately predicts whether a lesion is active or arrested.[4,38,39] It has been suggested that the most important clinical predictors are the presence of **plaque, location** of the lesion, **the visual appearance** of the lesion including luster/shine and the **tactile feeling** when a probe is drawn gently across the lesion.[4,39–41] In addition, the **status of gingiva** in terms of bleeding after gentle probing also seems to be a good predictor when the lesion is close to the gingival margin.[42]

Demineralized surface enamel which is frequently affected by a cariogenic biofilm may **feel** rougher compared with the surrounding sound enamel, when a probe is gently passed along the surface.[43] If this area is now kept clean by brushing, the brush may polish the former rough area, which then becomes smooth again. Hence, some abrasion of the softened demineralized enamel may occur (**Fig. 5.12**). Thus, roughness and smoothness of the lesion can indicate the activity stage of the lesion.

The visual appearances of the lesions seem also to be of value in this sense. Ekstrand et al.[39] ☺☺☺,●●● described noncavitated white spot lesions in plaque stagnation areas which were judged as active, whereas noncavitated brown spot lesions were mainly arrested. In addition, shadowed or cavitated lesions were also considered as active in this system. In the "**Nyvad criteria**" (**Table 5.6**)[41,44] ☺☺☺,●●●, activity is related to the plaque occurrence and characteristics like **color** of the lesion, **luster** or **opacity,** as well as **roughness** of the caries lesion. According to the authors "A typical, active noncavitated lesion is whitish/yellowish opaque surface with loss of luster, exhibiting a chalky or neo-white appearance. The surface feels rough when the tip of a sharp probe is moved gently across it." In contrast, "the inactive enamel caries lesions are generally shiny and feel smooth on gentle probing." Both systems showed substantial to excellent accuracy, meaning they were both good at finding active and arrested lesions.[35,39,41]

An add-on activity system to the ICDAS has been devised,[4,35] allocating points to each of the four clinical

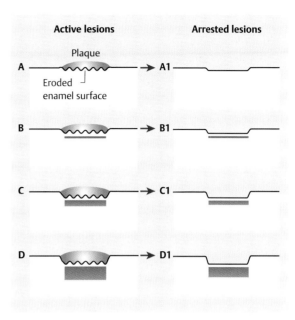

Fig. 5.12 Illustrations showing the principle appearances of the outermost enamel surface as well as the subsurface enamel for active lesions (A–D) and when these are arrested (A1–D1). Active lesions tend to be rough when a probe is run over them, whereas the same lesions if arrested tend to be more smooth. A "scar" will stay in the tooth when a lesion is arrested.
A Plaque-covered enamel. Eroded very initial surface lesion but without subsurface lesion.
B–D Plaque-covered enamel. Eroded initial surface lesion now with subsurface lesion.
A1–D1 Corresponding stages of lesion formation as A–D; however, arrested due to constant plaque control. The eroded surface enamel is partly or fully removed due to wear (abrasion), but the subsurface lesion remains almost the same as when the lesion was active (modified from Thylstrup et al. 1994[43]).

predictors named above (**Fig. 5.13**). Accordingly, a total score of more than 7 points is a strong indicator for the lesion being **active**, while a total score of 7 points or less indicates that the lesion has **arrested (inactive)**. Accuracy of the scoring system seems to be acceptable.[4,35]

It appears that current plaque levels are not a part of the ICDAS activity add-on system, which is related to the fact that ICDAS coding is performed on clean and dry teeth to minimize the risk of being unable to detect, in particular, initial caries lesions.[5] Thus, as a surrogate for occurrence of plaque, **plaque stagnation area** is used, since caries will most likely develop in these areas[45] (see Chapter 1).

Root Caries Lesions

Figure 5.14 shows one of the most detailed recording systems[46] devised to record caries on the roots and caries adjacent to restorations on the roots☺☺☺,X, and to distinguish lesions which are active from inactive lesions. The accuracy of the recording system has not been evaluated.

A similar add-on activity system for coronal caries (ICDAS) has been devised for assessing the activity of

Table 5.6 Details of Nyvad's[41] diagnostic criteria

Score	Category	Criteria
0	Sound	Normal enamel translucency and texture (slight staining allowed in otherwise sound fissure)
1	Active caries	Surface of enamel is whitish/yellowish opaque with loss of luster; (intact surface) feels rough when the tip of the probe is moved gently across the surface; generally covered with plaque No clinically detectable loss of substance Smooth surface: Caries lesion typically located close to gingival margin Fissure/pit: Intact fissure morphology; lesion extending along the walls of the fissure
2	Active caries	Same criteria as score 1 Localized surface defect (microcavity) in enamel only (surface discontinuity) No undermined enamel or softened floor detectable with the explorer (probe)
3	Active caries	Enamel/dentin cavity easily visible with the naked eye Surface of cavity feels soft (cavity) or leathery on gentle probing There may or may not be pulpal involvement
4	Inactive caries	Surface of enamel is whitish, brownish, or black. Enamel may be shiny and feels (intact surface) hard and smooth when the tip of the probe is moved gently across the surface No clinically detectable loss of substance Smooth surface: Caries lesion typically located at some distance from gingival margin Fissure/pit: Intact fissure morphology; lesion extending along the walls of the fissure
5	Inactive caries	Same criteria as score 4. Localized surface defect (microcavity) in enamel only (surface discontinuity) No undermined enamel or softened floor detectable with the explorer
6	Inactive caries	Enamel/dentin cavity easily visible with the naked eye Surface of cavity may be shiny and feels hard on probing with gentle pressure No pulpal involvement
7	Filling	(no adjacent caries)
8	Filling + active caries	Caries lesion may be cavitated or noncavitated
9	Filling + inactive caries	Caries lesion may be cavitated or noncavitated

root caries lesions.[47] **Table 5.7** presents the four predictors, the characteristics, and the related points. A total score between 3 and 5 points indicates that the lesion is arrested; a higher score than 5 indicates that the root caries lesion is active. The accuracy in terms of predicting active lesions versus arrested lesions was substantial.[47]

Caries Adjacent to Restorations

While there is some evidence of reliability (reproducibility) and validity (accuracy) for activity assessment of primary caries lesions,[35,41,47] whether coronal or in roots, there is very limited evidence of activity assessment of caries lesions adjacent to restorations (CAR). As we assume that CAR acts as do primary caries,[19–21] the above considerations about primary caries should also be used for CAR. The following variables *do not* reliably predict active caries adjacent to a filling[19,48]:

• Ditching around an amalgam restoration
• Staining around an amalgam restoration
• Staining around a tooth-colored restoration

Thus, replacement of a restoration showing these characteristics and no other, more severe, defects does not seem to be indicated at all. A loose restoration and/or marginal defects > 400 μm[21] adjacent to a restoration result in plaque stagnation with cariogenic potential. Here, either repair or renewal of the restoration is indicated.

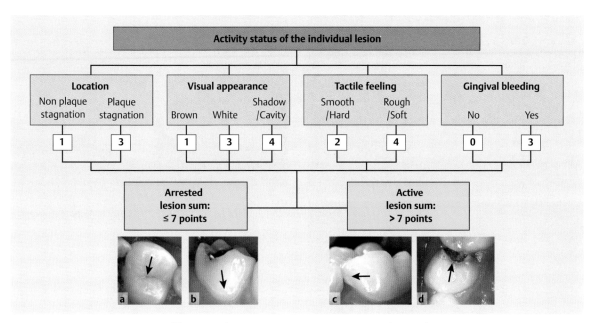

Fig. 5.13 Caries activity assessment of four coronal primary caries lesions. The gingival status is only used when the lesion is near to the gingiva, thus not in case A.

a Location: 3; visual: 1; tactile: 2   6
b Location: 1; visual: 3; tactile: 2; Gingiva: 0 =   6
c Location: 3; visual: 3; tactile: 4; Gingiva: 3 = 13
d Location: 3; visual: 4; tactile: 4; Gingiva: 3 = 14

- Inactive lesion without surface destruction
- Inactive lesion with cavity formation
- Active lesion without definitive surface destruction
- Active lesion with surface destruction (cavitation), but cavitation is estimated not to exceed 1 mm in depth (visually)
- Active lesion with a cavity, exceeding 1 mm, but not involving the pulp
- Lesion expected to penetrate into the pulp
- Filling confined to the root surface or extending from a coronal surface onto the root surface
- Filling with an active (secondary) lesion along the margin
- Filling with an inactive (secondary) lesion confined to the margin

Fig. 5.14 Criteria for root surface caries according to Fejerskov et al. 1991.[46]

Table 5.7 Predictors for caries activity of root surface lesions and weighted scores according to Ekstrand et al.[47]

Predictors	Characteristics	Score
Location of the lesion	>1 mm away from the gingiva	0
	along the gingiva (≤ 1mm)	1
Appearance of the lesion	Brownish	0
	Yellowish	1
Texture	Hard	0
	Leathery	1
	Soft	3
Contour	No cavitation or the border of the cavitation is smooth	0
	Cavitation/border is irregular	1

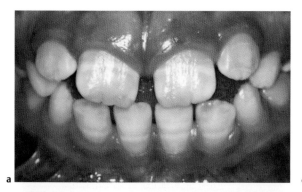

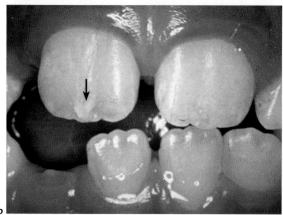

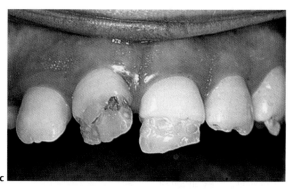

Fig. 5.15a–c Dental fluorosis appears rather homogenous on contralateral teeth (**a**), whereas hypomineralization (arrow), e.g., due to trauma of the pulp of deciduous teeth, is mostly observed on a single tooth (**b**). Example of a tooth with enamel hypoplasia (**c**).

The Visual Difference between Caries and other Dental Hard Tissue Defects

The initial stages of **dental fluorosis** (**Fig. 5.15a**) and enamel opacities/hypomineralization (**Fig. 5.15b**) appear white, like early caries lesions, because they all lack mineral. **Table 5.8** presents among other things the views of Russel[49] and coworkers in describing mild forms of dental fluorosis and opacities not related to dental fluorosis (hypomineralization) and how they differ in particular from caries and erosions, but also from **molar-incisor hypomineralization** and **erosions**. As caries is a localized disease, which develops in plaque stagnation areas, the location and shape of the lesion can be used to differentiate caries from dental fluorosis or enamel opacities. In addition, dental fluorosis occurs on contralateral teeth, which is seldom the case for caries and very seldom opacities. Finally, while very early stages of caries lesions become more obvious with air-drying and diminish when re-wetted with water/saliva, opacities do not change color or size with water or air-drying.

The different fluorosis indices (e.g., Dean and Thylstrup/ Fejerskov index) are discussed in Chapter 12. Hypomineralization is often separated into opacities alone (**Fig. 5.15b**) (no hypoplasia) and cases with hypoplasia (**Fig. 5.15c**).

The last decade has seen a lot of focus on another developmental disturbance in the enamel, namely the **molar-incisor hypomineralization** (**MIH**, cheesy teeth)[50] (**Fig. 5.16**). MIH affects between 1 and 4 permanent first molar teeth often in combination with hypomineralization of incisors. However, other teeth can also be affected. In contrast to the diffuse appearance of opacities seen in dental fluorosis, MIH is characterized by demarcated lesions, where the hypomineralized enamel can chip off easily and a fast caries progression rate can be observed. Prevalence varies in different countries. In Sweden[51] 20% of young children showed MIH (see also Chapter 8). One-third was minimally affected, one-third moderately, and one-third severely. Several etiological factors such as respiratory diseases, environmental changes, breast feeding[50] and most recently infections treated with amoxicillin (e.g., otitis media) have been related to MIH.[52]

The appearance of dental erosion is different from other diseases of the dental hard tissues.[53,54] The explanation is that caries, dental fluorosis, and hypomineralization are characterized by an increasing pore volume between the apatite crystals. Erosive defects are also very superficially demineralized, but the disease is mainly characterized by a tooth substance loss starting at the surface (see Chapters 2 and 3). **Figure 5.17a** is an example of a permanent dentition of a 20-year-old male with no or very superficial stages of erosion while **Fig. 5.17b–d** shows examples of erosion of increasing severity.

Table 5.8 Characteristics of caries as well as milder forms of dental fluorosis, nonfluoride opacities of enamel (hypomineralization), molar-incisor hypomineralization, and erosions (modified from Russel 1961[49])

Characteristics	Caries	Mild forms of fluorosis[48]	Nonfluoride opacities[48]	Molar incisor hypomineralization	Erosion
Affected areas	Plaque stagnation areas	On or near tips of cusps or incisal edges; usually centered in smooth surface	Centered on smooth surfaces; may affect the entire crown	On tips of cusps on one or more first molars and incisors	May affect most of the crown; approximal areas are less affected and areas close to the gingiva mainly unaffected
Shape of the lesion	Follow the extension of plaque	Follow incremental lines	Often round or oval	From very localized to involving most of the surface	Related to the exposition to acid
Demarcation	Clearly differentiated from adjacent normal enamel	Shades of hypomineralized enamel into sound enamel	Clearly differentiated from adjacent normal enamel	Shades of hypomineralized enamel into sound enamel	Clearly differentiated from adjacent normal enamel
Color	More opaque than sound enamel (chalky/dull), if not colored secondarily	Slightly more opaque than sound enamel (frosted appearance)	Creamy yellow to dark reddish orange. Can be pigmented at time of eruption	Creamy yellow to brownish	Initial stages: Normal color. More mature stages: color of the dentin
Teeth affected	Any tooth	Any tooth, but in homologous pairs of teeth	Any tooth	Most frequently first molars and incisors	All tooth types
Gross hypoplasia	Breakdown/cavitation occurs in late stage of the disease	Pitting occurs in more severe stages	Absent to severe	Pitting occurs in more severe stages	None, but the surfaces become smooth and shiny, in later stages surface characteristics disappear

SUMMARY

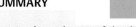

The visual–tactile part of the diagnostic process for caries involves the following:
1. Detect a lesion and decide that it is caries and nothing else
2. Assess its depth/severity
3. Assess its activity status

To find all stages of caries the clinical examination has to be performed on cleaned and air-dried teeth using a proper light source.

There are numerous indices and recording systems for caries lesions. The reliability of the majority of the caries indices is moderate to excellent. There is a moderate to strong relationship between visual appearance of caries and the depth (histology) of the lesion for both primary and permanent teeth. However, it is rather difficult to assess approximal caries lesions by visual–tactile techniques, although tooth separation might help. Based on the visual appearance of the caries lesion it is possible to predict the depth of the caries lesion: noncavitated

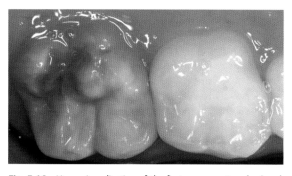

Fig. 5.16 Hypomineralization of the first permanent molar (moderate form of MIH). In this 7-year-old, all first molars were moderately affected (courtesy of H. Meyer-Lueckel).

lesions are mainly restricted to the enamel or just entering the dentin (a superficial lesion); microcavitated lesions or shadowed caries lesions; depthwise, are most often in the enamel and reaching into the middle third of the dentin (a medium lesion); while dentin cavitated lesions, depthwise, are in the enamel and in the inner

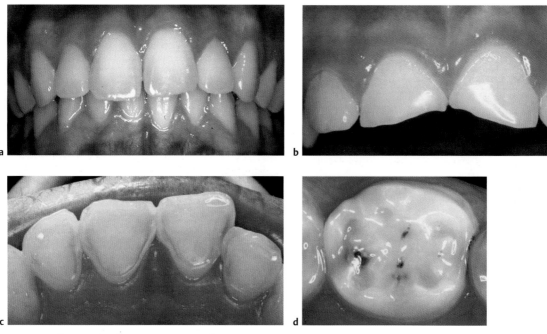

Fig. 5.17a–d Examples of no or minor stages of erosions (**a**), erosions limited to the enamel (**b**), and erosions where the dentin is involved (**c, d**)

third of the dentin, thus close to the pulp (a profound lesion).

No single clinical variable can reliably and accurately assess activity status of a caries lesion; a combination of current plaque accumulation, location of the lesion on the surface, its visual appearance, its tactile feel and gingival status seem to result in the best prediction. The detection and assessment methods described in this chapter should eventually lead to a reliable statements as to whether a lesion is due to caries, whether the caries lesion is a superficial, medium, or a profound lesion, and whether the lesion is active or arrested. There are several diseases/conditions which show a similar visual appearance to caries; these are dental fluorosis and enamel hypomineralization, including molar-incisor hypomineralization. In particular, the location of the "lesion" can be used in a differential diagnostic process. Erosions do not have the same visual appearance as other "lack of mineral" diseases in the dental hard tissues.

REFERENCES

1. Longbottom CL, Huysmans MC, Pitts NB, Fontana M. Glossary of key terms. In: Pitts N. Detection, Assessment, Diagnosis and Monitoring of Caries. Monogr Oral Sci 2009;21:209–216

2. Thylstrup A, Fejersjov O. Textbook of Cariology. Copenhagen: Munksgaard; 1986

3. Ekstrand KR, Ricketts DN, Kidd EAM. Occlusal caries: pathology, diagnosis and logical management. Dent Update 2001;28(8): 380–387

4. Ekstrand KR, Zero DT, Martignon S, Pitts NB. Lesion activity assessment. Monogr Oral Sci 2009;21:63–90

5. Möller IJ, Poulsen S. A standardized system for diagnosing, recording and analyzing dental caries data. Scand J Dent Res 1973;81(1):1–11

6. Ekstrand KR, Kuzmina I, Bjørndal L, Thylstrup A. Relationship between external and histologic features of progressive stages of caries in the occlusal fossa. Caries Res 1995;29(4):243–250

7. Ekstrand K, Qvist V, Thylstrup A. Light microscope study of the effect of probing in occlusal surfaces. Caries Res 1987;21(4): 368–374

8. Forgie AH, Pine CM, Pitts NB. The use of magnification in a preventive approach to caries detection. Quintessence Int 2002;33(1):13–16

9. Haak R, Wicht MJ, Hellmich M, Gossmann A, Noack MJ. The validity of proximal caries detection using magnifying visual aids. Caries Res 2002;36(4):249–255

10. Ekstrand KR, Bjørndal L. Structural analyses of plaque and caries in relation to the morphology of the groove-fossa system on erupting mandibular third molars. Caries Res 1997;31(5): 336–348

11. Carvalho JC, Ekstrand KR, Thylstrup A. Dental plaque and caries on occlusal surfaces of first permanent molars in relation to stage of eruption. J Dent Res 1989;68(5):773–779

12. Silverstone LM. The Histopathology of Enamel Lesions Produced in Vitro and their Relation to Enamel Caries [PhD Thesis]. Bristol: University of Bristol; 1967

13. Silverstone LM. Structure of carious enamel, including the early lesion. Oral Sci Rev 1973;3:100–160

14. Thylstrup A, Qvist V. Principal enamel and dentine reactions during caries progression. In: Thylstrup A, Leach SA, Qvist V, eds. Dentine and Dentine Reactions in the Oral Cavity. Oxford: IRL Press; 1987

15. Ricketts DN, Ekstrand KR, Kidd EAM, Larsen T. Relating visual and radiographic ranked scoring systems for occlusal caries detection to histological and microbiological evidence. Oper Dent 2002; 27(3):231–237

16. Ekstrand KR, Ricketts DNJ, Kidd EAM. Reproducibility and accuracy of three methods for assessment of demineralization depth of the occlusal surface: an in vitro examination. Caries Res 1997;31(3):224–231

17. Hintze H, Wenzel A, Danielsen B, Nyvad B. Reliability of visual examination, fibre-optic transillumination, and bite-wing radiography, and reproducibility of direct visual examination following tooth separation for the identification of cavitated carious lesions in contacting approximal surfaces. Caries Res 1998; 32(3):204–209

18. Rimmer PA, Pitts NB. Temporary elective tooth separation as a diagnostic aid in general dental practice. Br Dent J 1990;169 (3-4):87–92

19. Kidd EAM. Diagnosis of secondary caries. In: Stookey GK, ed. Early Detection of Dental Caries. Proceedings of the 1st Annual Indiana Conference. Indianapolis: Indiana University School of Dentistry; 1996:157–162

20. Kidd EAM, Joyston-Bechal S. Essentials of Dental Caries. The Disease and its Management. Bristol: Wright; 1987:158–170

21. Özer L, Thylstrup A. What is known about caries in relation to restorations as a reason for replacement? A review. Adv Dent Res 1995;9:394–402

22. Landis JR, Koch GG. The measurement of observer agreement for categorical data. Biometrics 1977;33(1):159–174

23. Ismail AI. Visual and visuo-tactile detection of dental caries. J Dent Res 2004;83 Spec No C(Spec.):C56–C66

24. World Health Organization (WHO). Oral Health Surveys: Basic Methods. 4th ed. Geneva: World Health Organization; 1997

25. Radike AW. Criteria for diagnosing dental caries. In: American Dental Association. Proceedings of the Conference on the Clinical Testing of Cariostatic Agents; October 14–16, 1968; Chicago: American Dental Association; 1972:87–88

26. Marthaler TM. A standardized system of recording dental conditions. Helv Odontol Acta 1966;10(1):1–18

27. Ekstrand KR, Kuzmina IN, Kuzmina E, Christiansen ME. Two and a half-year outcome of caries-preventive programs offered to groups of children in the Solntsevsky district of Moscow. Caries Res 2000;34(1):8–19

28. Kuzmina IN, Kuzmina E, Ekstrand KR. Dental caries among children from Solntsevsky—a district in Moscow, 1993. Community Dent Oral Epidemiol 1995;23(5):266–270

29. Kuzmina I. A Caries Preventive Program Among Children in a District of Moscow [PhD Thesis]. Copenhagen: University of Copenhagen; 1997

30. Friis-Hasché E. Child Oral Health Care in Denmark. Copenhagen: Copenhagen University Press; 1994

31. Friis-Hasché E. Skolebørns sundhedstilstand. Copenhagen: Odontologisk Boghandels; 1981

32. Downer MC. Concurrent validity of an epidemiological diagnostic system for caries with the histological appearance of extracted teeth as validating criterion. Caries Res 1975;9(3): 231–246

33. Pitts N. "ICDAS"—an international system for caries detection and assessment being developed to facilitate caries epidemiology, research and appropriate clinical management. Community Dent Health 2004;21(3):193–198

34. Ismail AI, Sohn W, Tellez M, et al. The International Caries Detection and Assessment System (ICDAS): an integrated system for measuring dental caries. Community Dent Oral Epidemiol 2007;35(3):170–178

35. Ekstrand KR, Martignon S, Ricketts DJ, Qvist V. Detection and activity assessment of primary coronal caries lesions: a methodologic study. Oper Dent 2007;32(3):225–235

36. Ekstrand KR, Luna LE, Promisiero L, et al. The reliability and accuracy of two methods for proximal caries detection and depth on directly visible proximal surfaces: an in vitro study. Caries Res 2011;45(2):93–99

37. ICDAS Foundation. International Caries Assessment and Detection System (ICDAS) Web site. http://www.icdas.org

38. Pitts NB, ed. Detection, Assessment, Diagnosis and Monitoring of Caries. Basel: Karger; 2009. Monographs in Oral Science; vol 21

39. Ekstrand KR, Ricketts DNJ, Kidd EAM, Qvist V, Schou S. Detection, diagnosing, monitoring and logical treatment of occlusal caries in relation to lesion activity and severity: an in vivo examination with histological validation. Caries Res 1998;32(4):247–254

40. Ekstrand KR, Ricketts DNJ, Longbottom C, Pitts NB. Visual and tactile assessment of arrested initial enamel carious lesions: an in vivo pilot study. Caries Res 2005;39(3):173–177

41. Nyvad B, Machiulskiene V, Baelum V. Reliability of a new caries diagnostic system differentiating between active and inactive caries lesions. Caries Res 1999;33(4):252–260

42. Ekstrand KR, Bruun G, Bruun M. Plaque and gingival status as indicators for caries progression on approximal surfaces. Caries Res 1998;32(1):41–45

43. Thylstrup A, Bruun C, Holmen L. In vivo caries models—mechanisms for caries initiation and arrestment. Adv Dent Res 1994; 8(2):144–157

44. Nyvad B, Machiulskiene V, Baelum V. Construct and predictive validity of clinical caries diagnostic criteria assessing lesion activity. J Dent Res 2003;82(2):117–122

45. Thylstrup A, Birkeland JM. Prognosis of Caries. In: Thylstrup A, Fejerskov O, eds. Textbook of Cariology. Copenhagen: Munksgaard; 1986:358–367

46. Fejerskov O, Luan WM, Nyvad B, Budtz-Jørgensen E, Holm-Pedersen P. Active and inactive root surface caries lesions in a selected group of 60- to 80-year-old Danes. Caries Res 1991; 25(5):385–391

47. Ekstrand KR, Martignon S, Holm-Pedersen P. Development and evaluation of two root caries controlling programmes for home-based frail people older than 75 years. Gerodontology 2008; 25(2):67–75

48. Kidd EAM, Joyston-Bechal S, Beighton D. Marginal ditching and staining as a predictor of secondary caries around amalgam restorations: a clinical and microbiological study. J Dent Res 1995;74(5):1206–1211

49. Russell AL. The differential diagnosis of fluoride and nonfluoride enamel opacities. J Public Health Dent 1961;21:143–146

50. Weerheijm KL, Jälevik B, Alaluusua S. Molar-incisor hypomineralisation. Caries Res 2001;35(5):390–391

51. Jälevik B, Klingberg G, Barregård L, Norén JG. The prevalence of demarcated opacities in permanent first molars in a group of Swedish children. Acta Odontol Scand 2001;59(5):255–260

52. Laisi S, Ess A, Sahlberg C, Arvio P, Lukinmaa PL, Alaluusua S. Amoxicillin may cause molar incisor hypomineralization. J Dent Res 2009;88(2):132–136

53. Ganss C, Lussi A. Diagnosis of erosive tooth wear. Monogr Oral Sci 2006;20:32–43

54. Lussi A. Dental erosion clinical diagnosis and case history taking. Eur J Oral Sci 1996;104(2 (Pt 2)):191–198

Radiographic and Other Additional Diagnostic Methods

Rainer Haak, Michael J. Wicht

6

Many sites that have a predilection for caries naturally lie in regions of the dentition that are difficult to view. Consequently, for diagnostic purposes, a visual–tactile examination of the approximal regions, deep fissures and grooves, and the margins of restorations is frequently insufficient to detect and evaluate early caries lesions. Other methods can be used to provide additional, valuable diagnostic information.

The most widely used additional diagnostic aid is bitewing radiographs. Caries lesions are visualized by means of the increased radiotranslucency of the dental hard substance associated with mineral loss. Bitewing radiographs provide useful additional diagnostic information on approximal and occlusal lesions or enable them to be detected for the first time.

Other diagnostic methods are based on the transillumination of teeth using visible light (fiber-optic transillumination), the fluorescence of healthy or carious dentin and enamel (DIAGNOdent, camera systems), or the electrical conductivity of caries (measurement of electrical resistance, impedance spectroscopy). This chapter addresses the various additional diagnostic methods and describes their clinical use as well as their advantages and disadvantages.

In particular, the following will be discussed:
- How to use bitewing x-ray radiography
- Analogue and digital radiographic systems
- Evaluation and relevance of radiographic findings
- Bitewing radiograph diagnostics and follow-up intervals
- Diagnostic methods based on visible light
- Caries diagnostics using electrical current

Radiographic Caries Diagnostics

Context of Radiographic Caries Detection

Primary caries lesions arise with greater frequency in children and adolescents.[1] The time window for the elevated risk of developing occlusal caries lesions in the permanent dentition starts with the eruption of the teeth, whereas approximal defects arise at a greater rate beginning at 13 years of age. Today, the number of initial caries lesions that have not penetrated the surface is substantially greater than the number of established defects or filled tooth surfaces,[2] and this makes it significantly more difficult to identify and evaluate caries lesions.[3]

Whereas the discovery of a carious lesion used to be an indication for restorative therapy, the present goal of therapy is to stop the progress of caries by attacking the underlying cause, such as by controlling the bacterial biofilm or providing nutritional education, etc. Only when the biofilm directly contacts the dentin there is a sufficiently potent bacterial invasion to cause demineralization and destruction of the organic dentin components.

Consequently, at this stage restorative measures are generally indicated. However, reactive changes in the dentin to a carious process in the tooth surface are an unsuitable indication for invasive therapy.[4]

NOTE

The primary goal of the causal therapy of caries is to stop or at least slow the progress of the lesion by controlling the biofilm.

The quality of the surface is currently held to be the decisive criterion for restorative treatment, since it can be directly influenced by hygiene; that is, it is the primary factor in the ability of the cariogenic biofilm to be removed through hygiene. When a cavity exists, the entire metabolism of the biofilm changes.[5]

NOTE

When there is surface cavitation, the options for non-invasive preventive measures are generally exhausted, and restorative treatment is indicated.

The primary goal of radiographic diagnostic methods is to detect and evaluate caries lesions in areas that are clinically inaccessible, or are only accessible with difficulty. This holds true particularly for **approximal surfaces** but also for **occlusal surfaces** and caries in restorations. Radiographic methods therefore enhance diagnostic sensitivity (detection). Furthermore, radiographic findings can also refine clinical findings through additional details on the extent of caries (assessment). Series of radiographs taken over an extended period also provide a longitudinal view of caries lesions and provide information about their progression (**Fig. 6.1**).

NOTE

Radiographic diagnostic methods primarily focus on the detection and assessment of caries lesions in approximal surfaces that cannot be clinically visualized as well as occlusal surfaces and existing restorations.

Radiographic images visualize caries lesions due to a decreased radiopacity of demineralized dentin and enamel (**Fig. 6.2**). When x-rays are used to detect caries, intraoral images should be used in the bitewing projection.[6,7] Bitewings were introduced in 1925 and have only been modified slightly since that time.[8] They have a film holder and bite tab that reduces proximal overlap and projection errors.[9]

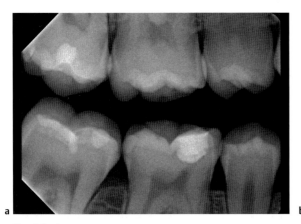

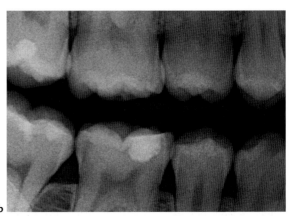

Fig. 6.1a, b

a Bitewing radiograph of the right jaw of a 21-year-old patient with an average caries risk. The distal lesion at tooth 46 has just penetrated the enamel–dentin junction. At this time, the therapy consisted of closely monitoring aggressive prophylactic measures.

b The follow-up radiograph after 6 months revealed a marked progression of the lesion with a radiologic propagation into the 2nd third of the dentin (D2).

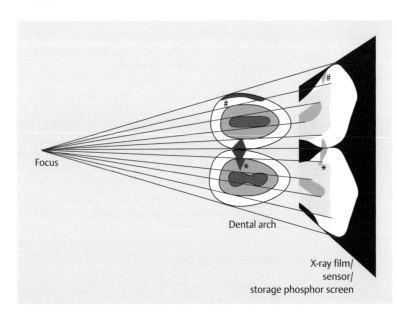

Fig. 6.2 Diagram of the bitewing x-ray technique. The x-ray beam passes from the focus of the x-ray tube, through the object (dental arch), and contacts the x-ray film or sensor or storage phosphor screen. The beam is attenuated, depending on the radiopacity and thickness of the transirradiated tissue. A two-dimensional image of overlapping three-dimensional anatomical structures is created. The (histological) extent of the caries tends to be underestimated due to this overlapping effect (*). However, the depth of the caries can be overestimated if the caries is long and runs parallel to the beam path (#).

Validity and Reliability of Radiographic Caries Detection

Which Gold Standard?

The radiographic detection of caries is only an additional tool in the overall effort to diagnose caries. It does not enable the dentist to determine whether surface cavitation exists. This clinically relevant criterion for therapy can only be estimated from the demineralization revealed in the bitewing radiographs. Consequently, when considering how scientific reports on the quality of radiographic caries diagnoses relate to the choice of therapy, one always needs to consider which validation method or "gold standard" was employed in the study. In most investiga-

tions of the radiographic detection of caries, the **depth of lesion penetration** is used as the reference criterion, which is determined histologically or clinically.[10] These may or may not be relevant to practice, however (see Chapter 9).[11] Rather, the gold standard is relative to the specific questions posed in the study.[12] When assessing the informational quality of the radiographic detection as it relates to potential restorative treatment, the (indirect) evaluation of potential **surface cavitation** is the primary determinant of validity. It is true that data from in-vitro studies reveal a moderate correlation between the clinical appearance and the radiographic extension of approximal and occlusal lesions.[13] However, the radiographic extension of caries only allows one to indirectly predict the probability of surface cavitation.

Sensitivity and Specificity

With in-vitro investigations, the sensitivity (fraction of correctly detected carious teeth) of dental lesion detection ranges from 50% to 70%, whereas specificity (fraction of correctly detected sound teeth) fluctuates from 70% to 97%.[14] In contrast, it is much more difficult to detect caries lesions in the enamel.[15,16] There is unanimous agreement that more caries lesions can be identified by combining radiographic information with clinical findings than by visual inspection alone.[17–19] When bitewing x-ray images are used, it has been demonstrated that the number of identified caries lesions can be increased 827% over visually detected caries lesions.[20] In other words, this means that only 10.8% of carious defects are discovered through visual inspection in comparison to combined visual and radiographic findings.

NOTE

The additional information provided by a radiographic image in combination with the clinical examination significantly increases the number of correctly detected caries lesions.

Reproducibility

The reproducibility of detections from bitewing radiographs assumes a moderate-to-good inter observer agreement.[20,21] This means, however, that the subjective element involved in analyzing radiographs influences the conclusion just as much as the basic ability to identify visual information in an x-ray photo.

Conventional and Digital Bitewing X-ray Imaging

Systems

Over the years, numerous digital systems have become available in addition to conventional x-ray equipment that use intraoral film.[22,23] In addition to digitizing conventional radiographs, both direct and indirect **semiconductor sensors** or **luminescence films** are used to create digital intraoral images. At the beginning of the digital era, the analog/digital conversion of intraoral x-ray films was extensively investigated to determine digital processing options.[24–26] Over time, only direct techniques gained currency in digital intraoral radiology.[27–29] Semiconductor sensors on CCDs (charge coupled devices) or CMOS (complementary metal oxide semiconductors) use a luminescent film to convert the x-rays into visible light that is detected by the back-illuminated CCD chips, or the x-ray is converted directly into an electrical signal in the silicon circuits without an intermediate carrier. In comparison to a CCD sensor, a CMOS sensor has a somewhat higher sensitivity with a slightly greater level of noise, and re-

quires less space and power. At the moment, however, both systems are apparently considered equivalent. Imaging plates first need to be read by a scanner, but they are easier to position than sensors.[30]

Advantages of Digital Technologies

In comparison to conventional techniques, digital intraoral radiographs possess numerous advantages. Due to the higher exposure tolerance, fewer imaging errors arise, and technical and environmental problems associated with wet chemistry no longer exist. In addition, the exposure time and dose can be reduced, and digital images can be processed electronically.[6] However, each new system that appears on the market must demonstrate that the images possess a level of validity and reproducibility at least similar to conventional techniques for the depiction of caries.[14,19] This has been demonstrated for numerous available digital systems and dental films,[31–34] so it can therefore be assumed that **digital and analog imaging** systems are at least **equivalent**. In addition, digital systems allow computer-supported image processing.[35] The goal of digital image manipulation is to more clearly depict information relevant to the detection of caries and suppress irrelevant details.[24] Software programs with their own image processing features are available for all digital systems.[36] Although these types of manipulation can be described with the specific terminology used in the field, generally individual descriptions or buttons with icons are employed which makes the programs difficult to compare. It is unclear, however, whether programs that offer the same types of modifications and filters produce the same results, or whether the options can be freely combined with each other.[36] Consequently, further investigations are required to determine the effectiveness of image modifications relative to various diagnostic issues and especially the detection of caries.

NOTE

Digital radiography possesses advantages over conventional radiography with regard to clarity, exposure tolerance, environmental compatibility, the required time, and radiation dose.

Tuned-Aperture Computed Radiography and Digital Volume Tomography

Since there is no perfect correlation between the detectable demineralization front and surface quality,[37] the search continues for a way to obtain this essential diagnostic information for visually inaccessible tooth surfaces. **Three-dimensional (3-D) radiographic techniques** could be particularly suitable, since the summation effect of classic intraoral x-ray photos is eliminated by the relevant information obtained from the structures in the beam path. Furthermore, the position of the slice from the 3-D volu-

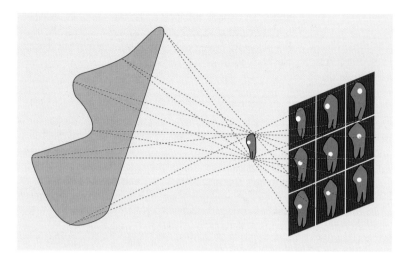

Fig. 6.3 Principle of tuned aperture volume tomography (TACT). The object is recorded from several different projections that are not predetermined. A three-dimensional representation of the object is constructed by a computer program from the two-dimensional images and a metal sphere on the object, which is used as a reference.

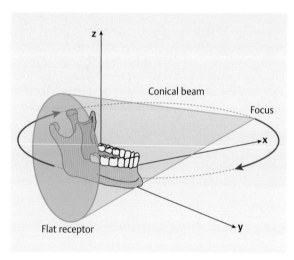

Fig. 6.4 Principle of digital volume tomography (DVT) / cone beam tomography. A conical beam together with a flat sensor travels 360° around the object. Complex algorithms are used to calculate a three-dimensional image of the object from this data.

metric record is freely determinable, which frees one from the bucco-oral projection and the associated image obtained from conventional intraoral radiographs. The conventional form of radiographic imaging, also termed transmission radiography, is characterized by a dot-shaped beam source and a flat beam receptor. The radiograph accordingly results from the attenuation of the transmission beam in the tissue. Two-dimensional reproductions of a 3-D configuration of tissues with overlapping anatomical structures can produce false negatives or false positives when (for example) buccal or oral caries lesions appear as a single lesion on the approximal surfaces in the radiograph.[38]

One approach for accommodating radiographic data in a 3-D matrix is **tuned-aperture computed tomography (TACT)**.[39] At least three different projected digital radiographs are overlapped using a reference point, and a 3-D record is generated that can be portrayed in the form of slices or a 3-D animation[40] (**Fig. 6.3**).

Whereas artificial lesions are more discernible in comparison with conventional x-ray film and CCD sensors,[41] there was no discernible improvement on the detection of occlusal and approximal caries.[42,43]

Another approach is **cone-beam computer tomography** or **digital volume tomography (DVT)**. Similar to conventional computed tomography, an x-ray beam executes a maximum 360° orbit as it scans the object. Different than conventional computer tomography, in which the object is scanned using a fan-shaped x-ray beam and a ring-shaped detector, a conical x-ray beam and flat detector are employed (**Fig. 6.4**).

Current publications have demonstrated experimentally that the detection of caries can be improved using local slice images.[44] The question therefore arises of whether cavitation from approximal caries can be detected better with cone-beam computer tomograms than with conventional intraoral x-rays. It was revealed that 80% sensitivity was achievable with a specificity of 96% in cone beam images, whereas only 29% of caries lesions with cavitation were correctly identified in bitewing x-ray images.[45]

These results indicate that cone-beam technology can be helpful in differentiating between intact and cavitated tooth surfaces in the approximal region. It was also demonstrated in isolated cases that occlusal lesions extending into the dentin are easier to identify by this method than in classic radiographs (**Fig. 6.5**). One problem that needs to be overcome before the method can be used in practice is the formation of artifacts in radiopaque materials, which always arise in tomographic imaging and can mask defects. It remains to be demonstrated whether the substantial investment that this technique requires will actually allow it to be employed in the evaluation of caries.

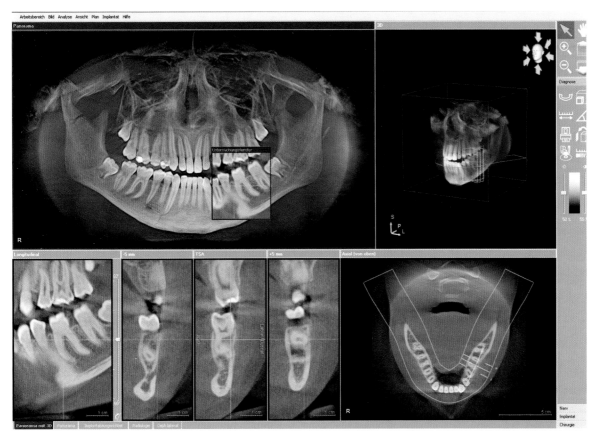

Fig. 6.5 In the slices of the digital volume tomograph, occlusal lesions are clearly identifiable in teeth 26 and 36. In addition to the more precise identification of interruptions in continuity, the more precise discernment of dentin participation in the occlusal defects is considered an advantage of digital volume tomography.

> **NOTE**
>
> In comparison with two-dimensional bitewing x-ray images, the use of three-dimensional tomographic imaging yields a higher detection rate of approximal cavitation, although it is not yet ready for widespread use.

Bitewings

Traditionally, it is recommended to image a region extending from the distal surface of the canine to the distal surface of the terminal molar,[19] so that generally two size 2 films are required on each side of the mouth. If a long bitewing film (size 3) is used instead, the radiation exposure can be reduced, but this yields increased overlapping, projection errors and undisplayed approximal surfaces.[46] Since the probability of developing caries lesions in canines and first premolars is rather low in most patients today, it can be assumed that lesions will be rarely overlooked when only one x-ray is taken per side.[47] In addition, the approximal surfaces between the canine and premolar can frequently be visually evaluated.

Preparations

There are a few basic rules regarding patient positioning, the positioning of the film or sensor, and the alignment of the central beam when creating bitewing images. Beforehand, the patient should be asked about any previous medical exposure to ionizing radiation. Pregnancy should be excluded in women of childbearing age, radioprotective shielding should be draped over the patient, and removable dentures should be removed as well as jewelry, glasses, etc.

Taking Bitewing X-ray Photos

As mentioned above, digital radiography offers distinct advantages, especially in regard to radiation exposure, environmental considerations, and the avoidance of imaging errors. Consequently, the following clinical images were exclusively generated by a digital system (Xios, Sirona, Bensheim), but other systems can be used as well. Special bitewing holders are provided with a tab for technical reasons to which the sensor is mechanically anchored (**Fig. 6.6**). Attached to the centering rod extending out of the mouth is an aiming ring as a positioning tool for the tube that allows the orthoradial alignment of the

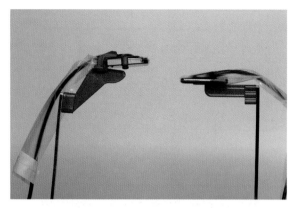

Fig. 6.6 With bitewing holders for digital radiography, the sensor in a plastic sleeve is either pushed onto the tab (left, XCP Dentsply Rinn bitewing holder) or adhered (right, Xios, Sidexis). In the version where the sensor is pushed on, mishandling and wear can cause the sensor to lose its perpendicular alignment with the tube more quickly, thus distorting the images.

central beam. The patient's head should be stabilized with a headrest, and the bipupillary line as well as the occlusal plane should be aligned approximately parallel to the floor. This is followed by the intraoral positioning of the sensor. The bite plate of the holder is fixed between the occlusal surfaces of the upper and lower posterior teeth, and the sensor is placed as close as possible to the oral surfaces of the relevant teeth (**Fig. 6.7**). Due to the aforementioned epidemiological situation, it is frequently suf-

ficient to create one bitewing per jaw half. If two x-ray images are indicated for anatomical reasons, however, it is recommended to start with the anterior projection since it is more difficult due to the bulkiness of the sensor. Errors in imaging generally impair quality and decrease the available information in the radiographs or render them useless in case of doubt.

> **NOTE**
>
> Using special bitewing holders, including an aiming ring and centering rod, and correct patient positioning enable an orthoradial and hence overlap-free projection of the approximal areas.

Reproducible Adjustment

If the radiographic progression or arrest of a caries lesion is to be assessed in longitudinal monitoring, the imaging parameters should ideally be the same each time. The projection can only be reproducible if the intraoral position of the tab, the position of the film (sensor), and path of the central beam remain the same. Special film holders (**Fig. 6.8**) enable the projections to be reproducible and also allow special x-ray software to be used for digital subtraction radiography. By subtracting the pixels of two images recorded under identical conditions, a new image is generated that visualizes the differences between the radiographs.

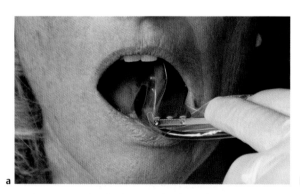

a

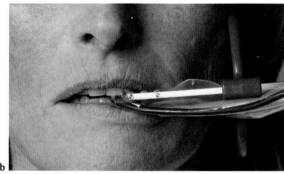

b

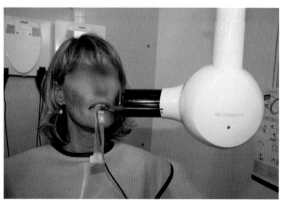

c

Fig. 6.7a–c A slight rotation is used to position the sensor in the mouth by first horizontally inserting the holder and then turning it toward the alveolar process (**a**). The patient is asked to close her mouth slowly until the bite plate is held firmly (**b**). The aiming ring is then pushed toward the cheek as far as it will go, and the tube is aligned in two planes parallel to the centering rod (**c**). This aligns the central beam parallel with the bitewing which runs tangentially through the contact point between the second premolar and first molar when a single bitewing radiograph is taken per side.

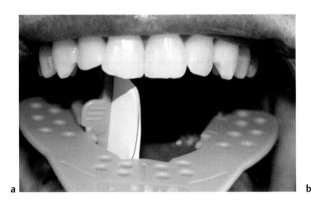

a

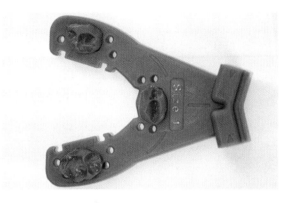

b

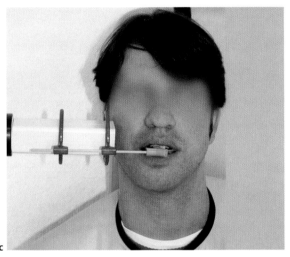

c

Fig. 6.8a–c The bitewing holder (TenoLux, DMG) (**a**) with a bite registration (**b**) and double aiming ring (Rinn, Dentsply) (**c**) enables the film to be consistently placed in the same position, which in turn enables reliable comparison of images during longitudinal monitoring of lesions.

Documenting the Findings of Bitewing Images

Radiographic Extension and Clinical Findings of Approximal Superficial Lesions

The radiologic findings need to be documented to make well-founded therapeutic choices and for the longitudinal monitoring of caries lesions (**Figs. 6.9, 6.10**).

> **NOTE**
>
> When assessing therapies, the detailed documentation of radiologic findings is essential so that changes in lesions can be tracked over a long period.

For the choice of therapy, it is particularly important to identify a possible surface break down (cavitation) since, due to the difficulties in cleaning, this generally represents the threshold for invasive therapy. In a comparison of the penetration depth of lesions determined in radiographs with the corresponding surface findings (**Table 6.1**), it was found that the surface of initial enamel lesions (E1) was almost always intact. Lesions that reached the

inner half of the enamel (E2) in the radiograph manifested clinical cavitation in only 10.5% of cases. Given a radiologic extension into the outer half of the dentin, 59% of surfaces remained intact. Only when radiolucency was observed within the second half of the dentin, surface cavitation should be assumed in almost 100% of cases.[37] A comparable clinical investigation revealed that, on average, 32% of radiologic lesions that extended into the first third of the dentin manifested cavitation; this was true for 72% of lesions extending into the middle third of the dentin.[48] The radiologic penetration depth at which one can assume that the surface is cavitated is accordingly the middle third of the dentin. The classification presented in **Table 6.2** identifies five degrees of caries or penetration depths that take into account this important observation.[49,50]

With grade E1 and D3 lesions, the radiologic findings are a relatively true reflection of the clinical surface findings (whether or not there is cavitation) and hence can be relied on when discussing a therapy, since invasive procedures are generally only indicated when there is cavitation. With lesions of categories E2, D1, and D2, this inference is somewhat less probable.

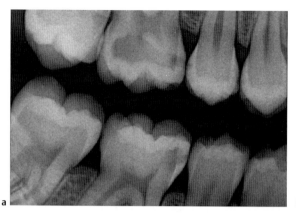 a

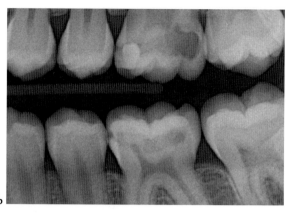 b

Fig. 6.9a, b   Bitewing images of a 13-year-old female with occlusal and approximal primary lesions of different severity. At teeth 16, 26, and 36, we clearly see occlusal lesions extending into the middle third of the dentin (tooth 36; D2) and inner third of the dentin (teeth 16, 26; D3). Buccal demineralization of the two upper six-year molars also overlap this clear finding. Teeth 16, 36, and 46 also manifest mesial dentin lesions that have reached the inner third of the dentin in tooth 46 (D3) and the middle third of the dentin in teeth 16 and 36 (D2). The mesio-occlusal fossa of tooth 26 was restored at an earlier time and manifests mesial translucency like the other first molars, which indicates an approximal primary lesion extending to the restoration. In the distal contact area, tooth 15 reveals initial demineralization of the enamel (outer half of the enamel; E1). Since the patient is young, we must assume a very high caries risk and progression rate, especially since the premolars reveal clinical and radiologic signs of demineralization. A radiologic follow-up in 6 months is recommendable, even after restoration of the advanced lesions.

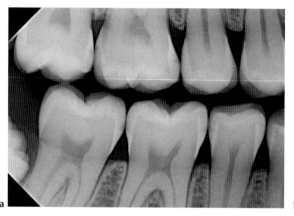 a

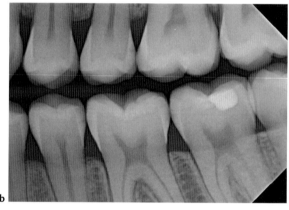 b

Fig. 6.10a, b   Bitewing x-ray images of an 18-year-old female patient with a moderate caries risk. No clinical signs of carious lesions were identified. The patient stated that tooth 37 was restored when she was 13 years old. The bitewing radiographs reveal that all premolars and molars have initial lesions limited to the enamel (E1, E2) indicative of insufficient hygiene of the approximal region. These findings stabilized over four years through appropriate training in oral hygiene and the consistent use of dental floss. The initial radiological follow-up interval of 6 months was extended to one year.

NOTE

The propability of approximal caries being cavitated only exeeds 50% when the lesion radiographically has reached the middle or inner third of the dentin (D2, D3).

Evaluating Occlusal Surfaces

With certain restrictions, this classification can also be transferred to occlusal caries. Examining bitewing radiographs to determine occlusal lesions enhances the sensitivity of the visual detection. This is particularly true in the case of obvious dentin lesions, whereas initial lesions are more difficult to detect due to overlaps. Compared with histological sections as an external validation criterion, about 50% of occlusal lesions are overlooked in the radiograph.[51]

Table 6.1 Categorization of radiological findings to describe the lesion depth of approximal caries (modified after Tveit et al.[49] and Hinze et al.[50])

Degree	Description
E 1	Radiolucency in the outer half of the enamel
E2	Radiolucency in the inner half of the enamel
D1	Radiolucency in the outer third of the dentin
D2	Radiolucency with obvious propagation within the middle third of the dentin
D3	Radiolucency in the inner third of the dentin

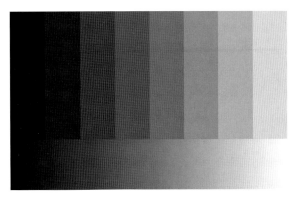

Fig. 6.11 The Mach band effect describes the enhancement of contrasts between two levels of gray due to the particular functioning of the light receptors in the retina. The strips on the right appear darker than the ones on the left. In actuality, the grayscale of each strip on the right and left is identical. The same effect can cause a false-positive assessment of dentin caries.

Estimating the Probability of Caries Progression

A single x-ray photo does not provide the dentist with any clues as to whether caries is likely to progress or not. A comparison of several sequential bitewing x-rays taken over an appropriate period can be useful. If only an individual radiograph is available, however, the estimation of progression can be supported using clinical parameters if necessary. In addition to existence of plaque and the width of the contact point, the inflammation of the neighboring papilla can provide indications of the probable progression of approximal caries.[54] Lesions that cause the neighboring papilla to bleed in response to careful probing are more likely to progress than those with uninflamed neighboring papilla. To prevent misinterpretation, it should be determined beforehand that the patient does not suffer from generalized gingivitis, and the patient should undergo professional cleaning in the approximal region (see Chapter 5).

Determining the Radiologic Follow-up Interval

Relevant Factors

The available literature does not provide a clear guideline for determining the frequency and intervals of bitewing x-rays.[55–57] The existing guidelines allow a degree of freedom for individual decisions and considerations.[58–60] There is only unanimity about one thing: there is no such thing as a fixed interval that universally applies to all patients. Dentists need to base their judgment on the individual situation and weigh the risk of an incorrect decision. The recommendations are presented from the European guidelines on protection against radiation in dental radiology[59] (**Table 6.2**) and the American Dental Association[60] (**Table 6.3**).

The Mach Band Effect

One should be particularly aware of the Mach band effect. This perceptual phenomenon artificially enhances the perception of contrast next to a boundary due to lateral inhibition within the eye.[29,52] At the border between light and dark surfaces (the enamel–dentin border), a narrow, brighter strip is perceived on the bright side of the boundary (**Fig. 6.11**). Correspondingly, a narrow, particularly dark strip appears on the dark side of the boundary, which can incorrectly be interpreted as dentin caries.[53]

Table 6.2 Recommendations of the European Commission for follow-up intervals in radiological caries diagnosis[59]

Age	High caries risk	Moderate caries risk	Low caries risk
Children	6 months	1 year	Primary teeth: 18–24 months[a]
			Second dentition: 2 years[a]
Adults	6 months	1 year	2 years[a]

[a]Longer intervals are possible when there is a low caries risk over the long term.

NOTE

There are no fixed guidelines for setting the follow-up interval. The frequency should be primarily based on the patient's risk of caries and age. The patient needs to perceive the benefit of each x-ray photo session.

When establishing a patient-oriented framework for the radiological diagnostics of caries that focuses on prevention, one primary consideration is **radiation exposure**. In addition to the unambiguous legal requirement of minimizing radiation exposure, unnecessary radiographs should be avoided for ethical reasons.[59] In addition, the **caries risk** should be considered when setting the correct interval between bitewing x-ray examinations.[55,56] This calculation needs to be made more than once; the risk needs to be regularly re-evaluated so that changes can be taken into consideration.[55] Various parameters need to be considered when assessing the caries risk such as the caries incidence, the quantity of saliva, nutrition, etc., and any existing lesions of the enamel and dentin in the radiograph as well as the age of the patient (see Chapters 7 and 24).

A radiographic baseline examination during the initial visit may be useful and is generally recommended.[55,56,59,60] During this first visit, the caries risk is assessed to determine the interval for the first radiological

follow-up. It needs to be remembered that the intervals for the clinical and radiological follow-up visits do not have to be the same.[55,56] In addition, the radiological caries diagnostic is only a supplement to, and not a substitute for the clinical examination.[57] One reference point for determining the length of time between two follow-up x-ray sessions is the average time it takes an enamel lesion to penetrate into the dentin. For age groups with a low caries risk, a minimum of four years can be assumed[61,62]; in Scandinavia, 6–8 years is cited in the literature.[63] This period is reflected in the recommendations from 1992[55] for age groups above 25 years. The time should be shorter for age groups with an elevated risk such as children with mixed dentition and adolescents. Since the progression and establishment of caries lesions can vary from individual to individual, the follow-up interval should be recalculated after each radiologic examination.[56] If no new lesions arise after a long period and no progression of existing lesions is observable, the interval to the next radiologic examination can be extended. The longer the retrospective period, the longer the follow-up interval.[55]

Special Considerations for Children and Adolescents

Frequent follow-ups every 6–12 months are recommendable for children and adolescents with a high caries risk.[55–57] This recommendation is reflected in current guidelines.[59,60,64] Children and adolescents in particular are at an elevated risk of developing approximal lesions.[57] Consequently, radiological examinations are held to be useful for these age groups. An initial examination of 5-year-olds is recommendable since 30%–50% of children at this age already have approximal caries lesions. A second radiological examination is recommended for children of age 8–9 years to detect and assess lesions in the mesial approximal surfaces of the first permanent molars. Additional radiologic examinations should occur at ages 12–13 and 15–16 years. The follow-up interval can be significantly extended for children and adolescents who do not manifest any caries in the radiographs to reduce radiation exposure. In any case, it is useful to perform a radiologic examination of children aged 15–16 who have a

Table 6.3 Radiological examination schedule recommended by the American Dental Association[60]

	Child with primary teeth	Child with mixed dentition	Adolescent with second dentition	Adult full/partial dentition
New patient	First bitewing radiographs[a]			
Follow-up patient with visible caries or high caries risk	6–12 months[a]			6–18 months
Follow-up patient without visible caries and low caries risk	12–24 months[a]		18–36 months[a]	24–36 months[a]

[a]If the approximal tooth surface cannot be clinically evaluated.

low caries risk, since this age is considered a high risk phase for approximal lesions after the eruption and establishment of approximal contacts.[56]

NOTE

Bitewing radiographs are indicated for deciduous teeth as well, since children and adolescents are at an elevated risk of developing approximal lesions.

In the past decades the importance of radiographic caries diagnostics has increased for two main reasons. First, due to the altered appearance and incidence of caries, lesions which are inaccessible to visual inspection are found relatively more often. Secondly, the comparison of consecutive radiographic images allows the monitoring of lesion progression (or stagnation) over time, which is particularly important to evaluate the progression of lesions as well as the treatment success of non- and microinvasive measures.

Other Caries Diagnostic Methods

Fiber-optic Transillumination

Fiber-optic transillumination (FOTI) is a method based on **visible light** for detecting and evaluating approximal and occlusal caries lesions. The light is directed from a strong light source through an optical fiber and fine tip (0.3–0.5 mm) onto the tooth surface. The light shines through the dentin and enamel and is scattered and absorbed differently, depending on the translucence of the tissues. Sound enamel is relatively translucent to visible light. When the pore volume within the dentin and enamel is increased due to demineralization and there is brownish discoloration in the dentin, the light within the caries is scattered and absorbed to a greater extent, which causes shading.

To detect approximal caries, the light probe is placed on a buccal or lingual contact point, and the transillumination of the light is determined either at the opposite side, or from an occlusal direction at the marginal ridge (**Fig. 6.12**). To detect occlusal demineralization, the probe is moved back and forth in a buccal or lingual direction, and the transillumination is determined from the occlusal side. It is recommendable to turn off the operating light and dim other sources of light as well.

Shadows that do not proceed beyond the marginal ridge with a diameter less than 2 mm at the occlusal surface frequently only extend into the enamel or outer dentin. Contrastingly, caries that generates more shade, generally extends deeper into the dentin.[65–67]

Most available studies of FOTI evaluate the sensitivity and specificity of the method for detecting lesions in the

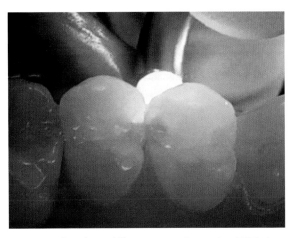

Fig. 6.12 Clinical use of fiber-optic transillumination (FOTI). Approximal caries, mesial 25 and distal 23, is identifiable as a dark shade.

enamel and dentin.[65,68–70] The use of FOTI can nearly double the number of approximal lesions that are detected in comparison to visual-tactile detection alone. However, bitewing radiographs are more sensitive than the two other techniques combined: only about one-fifth of radiographically detected enamel lesions and one-half of lesions radiographically extending into the dentin were identified using a combination of visual-tactile detection and FOTI.[70]

The primary advantage of FOTI in comparison to bitewing radiographs is the lack of radiation exposure and comparative harmlessness of the method, which is why FOTI can be used without restriction, especially to diagnose caries in children. The primary disadvantage is the reduced sensitivity of the method, particularly in detecting enamel lesions.

NOTE

By means of fiber-optic transillumination (FOTI), a greater number of early lesions can be detected than with visual-tactile diagnostics. However, the sensitivity of FOTI in detecting these lesions is significantly less than that of bitewing radiographs.

Methods Based on Fluorescence

Several fluorescence-based methods for caries diagnostics have been investigated in scientific studies.[71,72] However, many have not gained wide acceptance among dentists. The most widespread clinical method is the DIAGNOdent device (KaVo, Biberach, Germany). This method is based on the measurement of fluorescence of certain chromophores that occur in caries lesions.

The DIAGNOdent generates a red laser light (655 nm) that is conducted through an optical fiber into a fine tip. The tip is guided over the tooth surface and the laser light is absorbed by the organic components, especially in the

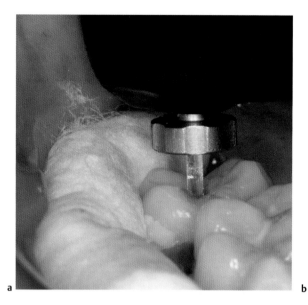

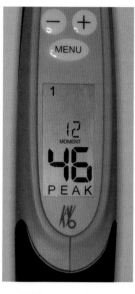

Fig. 6.13a, b
a Evaluation of occlusal caries with DIAGNOdent.
b The device shows the current measured fluorescence and maximum in the form of relative values (0–99).

dentin, and thereby excites the electrons in these components. The electrons briefly jump to a higher energy level and then return to their original state. During this process, they release energy in the form of light at a longer wavelength. This release is termed fluorescence. Fluorescent light is conducted through optical fibers into the handpiece, filtered, and quantified (**Fig. 6.13**). The intensity of the fluorescence correlates to the extension of the lesion and is indicated over a range of 0 to 99. The fluorescence of caries lesions is probably caused by porphyrins, which are metabolic products of microorganisms.

In the case of occlusal lesions, the DIAGNOdent pen is able to distinguish fairly reliably between lesions restricted to the enamel and those extending into the dentin (sensitivity + specificity ~1.6).[73,74] A threshold of 30 is proposed at which dentin caries is assumed. One problem of this method is the large proportion of measurements that are frequently too high, especially when a low threshold is chosen. In addition, tooth surfaces that have not been cleaned influence the measurements owing to the fluorescence of impurities such as plaque and calculus.[74]

The newest version of DIAGNOdent contains optical systems for use on occlusal and approximal surfaces. However, its use for approximal surfaces is relatively new and has not been extensively validated.[75] A few problems such as the relatively thick and fragile approximal optical system as well as the overly high measurements generated by plaque and calculus reduce the practicality of this method in the approximal region.

Over the years, various intraoral camera systems have been marketed that have different light filters and allow fluorescence images to be taken. Frequently, various filters are used together, which enable the autofluorescence of healthy dentin and enamel to be visualized in addition to the aforementioned fluorescence of carious dental hard substance (**Fig. 6.14**). However, only a handful of studies of these systems have been performed, and therefore nothing definitive can be said about their diagnostic quality.[76,77]

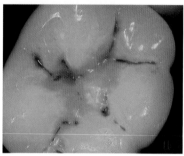

Fig. 6.14   Occlusal surface of a molar taken with a fluorescence camera (Sopro-Life by Aceton). The healthy hard substance is green, and the caries is red. As with DIAGNOdent, plaque and calculus fluoresce similarly to caries and therefore appear red.

Electrical Conductivity

The evaluation of caries by means of electric current is based on the greater conductivity or reduced electrical resistance of demineralized, porous in comparison to sound enamel. Similarly to the electrometric determination of length in endodontology, weak AC or DC current is applied to a tooth surface using an electrode (**Fig. 6.15**). A second electrode is either applied to the patient's mouth, or the patient holds it in his or her hand. The current flows from the electrode through the caries lesion, the dental hard substance (especially dentin), and through the pulp and soft tissue to the second electrode. The level of the current is measured, and a relative value for the depth of the caries is calculated and shown on a display. At present, the method is restricted to occlusal surfaces, while moisture is carefully controlled, since any moisture on the tooth surface causes the circuit to flow through the gingiva and yield incorrect results. For occlusal surfaces the sensitivity of electrical conductance measurement is higher in comparison with visual-tactile assessment but sensitivity is lower[78–81].

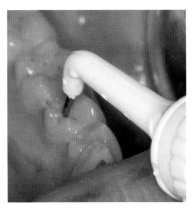

Fig. 6.15 Detection and assessment of caries using electrical conductivity (CariesScan).

SUMMARY

Beyond visual inspection, the radiographic imaging of caries lesions in bitewing radiographs is an essential tool in the overall diagnosis of caries, and it provides the dentist with clinically relevant information about the status of approximal areas, which are inaccessible to the eye. In addition, occlusal lesions and caries in restorations are detectable by bitewing x-rays with certain restrictions. In comparison to conventional intraoral x-ray imaging, digital x-ray systems offer significant advantages such as less exposure to radiation, less pollution, and less time, and the images can be processed digitally. In addition, the quality of digital images is at least comparable with that of conventional systems. Under laboratory conditions, three-dimensional methods (TACT, DVT) yield promising results in regard to the detection of cavitated approximal surfaces; however, they have not become widely used, especially because of the high investment costs.

When creating intraoral radiographs, the patient should be correctly positioned, and the position of the film/sensor and tube also influence quality. Similar to clinical, visual examinations, it is recommendable to include as much pertinent detail and documentation as possible when evaluating the x-ray photos for a general diagnosis of caries. Various approaches have been described in the literature for categorizing the radiographic extension of caries. It is particularly important to document strategically relevant transitions, for example, from the inner half of the enamel to the dentin, or from the first to the middle third of the dentin. Depending on the individual caries risk, the follow-up interval is determined together with the patient. This can be 6 months with children and adolescents who have a high risk of caries, and 4 years or longer with adult patients who have a documented low risk of caries.

With fiber-optic transillumination (FOTI), visible light shines through the dentin and enamel, and caries appears as a dark shade. The advantage of this method in comparison to radiographic methods is that ionizing radiation is not used. However, the sensitivity of FOTI is much less than bitewing radiographs, particularly in the early stages of the lesions. Different diagnostic methods, such as the DIAGNOdent approach or camera systems, use the fluorescence of certain organic components of caries lesions. The diagnosis of caries using electrical conductivity exploits the fact that the porosity of caries lesions conducts electrical impulses better than healthy dentin and enamel. The last-mentioned principles can only be used on surfaces that are easily accessible (smooth occlusal surfaces), and more scientific research is required.

REFERENCES

1. Mejàre I, Stenlund H, Zelezny-Holmlund C. Caries incidence and lesion progression from adolescence to young adulthood: a prospective 15-year cohort study in Sweden. Caries Res 2004;38(2):130–141

2. Hannigan A, O'Mullane DM, Barry D, Schäfer F, Roberts AJ. A caries susceptibility classification of tooth surfaces by survival time. Caries Res 2000;34(2):103–108

3. Weerheijm KL, Gruythuysen RJ, van Amerongen WE. Prevalence of hidden caries. ASDC J Dent Child 1992;59(6):408–412

4. Thylstrup A, Fejerskov O. Clinical and pathological features of dental caries. In: Thylstrup A, Fejerskov O, eds. Textbook of Clinical Cariology. Copenhagen: Munksgaard; 1996:111–148

5. Fejerskov O, Scheie AA, Manji F. The effect of sucrose on plaque pH in the primary and permanent dentition of caries-inactive and -active Kenyan children. J Dent Res 1992;71(1):25–31

6. Kidd EA, Mejare I, Nyvad B. Clinical and radiographic caries diagnosis. In: Fejerskov O, Kidd EA, eds. Dental Caries: The Disease and its Clinical Management. Oxford: Blackwell Munksgaard; 2003:111–128

7. Akarslan ZZ, Akdevelioğlu M, Güngör K, Erten H. A comparison of the diagnostic accuracy of bitewing, periapical, unfiltered and filtered digital panoramic images for approximal caries detection in posterior teeth. Dentomaxillofac Radiol 2008;37(8):458–463

8. Raper HR. Practical clinical preventive dentistry based upon periodic roentgen-ray examinations. J Am Dent Assoc 1925;12:1084–1100

9. Pitts NB. Film-holding, beam-aiming and collimating devices as an aid to standardization in intra-oral radiography: a review. J Dent 1984;12(1):36–46

10. Hintze H, Wenzel A. Diagnostic outcome of methods frequently used for caries validation. A comparison of clinical examination, radiography and histology following hemisectioning and serial tooth sectioning. Caries Res 2003;37(2):115–124

11. Nyvad B. Diagnosis versus detection of caries. Caries Res 2004;38(3):192–198

12. ten Bosch JJ, Angmar-Månsson B. Characterization and validation of diagnostic methods. Monogr Oral Sci 2000;17:174–189

13. Ratledge DK. A clinical and laboratory investigation of the tunnel restoration. [PhD thesis]. London: University of London; 1999

14. Wenzel A. Current trends in radiographic caries imaging. Oral Surg Oral Med Oral Pathol Oral Radiol Endod 1995;80(5):527–539

15. Hintze H, Wenzel A, Jones C. In vitro comparison of D- and E-speed film radiography, RVG, and visualix digital radiography for the detection of enamel approximal and dentinal occlusal caries lesions. Caries Res 1994;28(5):363–367

16. White SC, Yoon DC. Comparative performance of digital and conventional images for detecting proximal surface caries. Dentomaxillofac Radiol 1997;26(1):32–38

17. Kidd EA, Pitts NB. A reappraisal of the value of the bitewing radiograph in the diagnosis of posterior approximal caries. Br Dent J 1990;169(7):195–200

18. Pitts NB, Kidd EA. Some of the factors to be considered in the prescription and timing of bitewing radiography in the diagnosis and management of dental caries. J Dent 1992;20(2):74–84

19. Wenzel A. Bitewing and digital bitewing radiography for detection of caries lesions. J Dent Res 2004;83 Spec No C:C72–C75

20. Poorterman JH, Aartman IH, Kalsbeek H. Underestimation of the prevalence of approximal caries and inadequate restorations in a clinical epidemiological study. Community Dent Oral Epidemiol 1999;27(5):331–337

21. Hintze H, Wenze A. Clinical and laboratory radiographic caries diagnosis. A study of the same teeth. Dentomaxillofac Radiol 1996;25(3):115–118

22. Kaeppler G. Digitale Röntgentechniken im Zahn- und Kieferbereich – eine Übersicht. Dtsch Zahnarztl Z 1996;51:194–205

23. Wenzel A. Digital imaging for dental caries. Dent Clin North Am 2000;44(2):319–338, vi

24. Versteeg CH, Sanderink GC, van der Stelt PF. Efficacy of digital intra-oral radiography in clinical dentistry. J Dent 1997;25 (3-4):215–224

25. Attaelmanan A, Borg E, Gröndahl HG. Digitisation and display of intra-oral films. Dentomaxillofac Radiol 2000;29(2):97–102

26. Janhom A, van Ginkel FC, van Amerongen JP, van der Stelt PF. Scanning resolution and the detection of approximal caries. Dentomaxillofac Radiol 2001;30(3):166–171

27. Wenzel A, Gröndahl HG. Direct digital radiography in the dental office. Int Dent J 1995;45(1):27–34

28. Miles DA. The deal on digital: the status of radiographic imaging. Compend Contin Educ Dent 2001;22(12):1057–1062, quiz 1064

29. Williams CP. Digital radiography sensors: CCD, CMOS, and PSP. Pract Proced Aesthet Dent 2001;13(5):395–396

30. Bahrami G, Hagstrøm C, Wenzel A. Bitewing examination with four digital receptors. Dentomaxillofac Radiol 2003;32(5):317–321

31. Wenzel A. Digital radiography and caries diagnosis. Dentomaxillofac Radiol 1998;27(1):3–11

32. Syriopoulos K, Sanderink GC, Velders XL, van der Stelt PF. Radiographic detection of approximal caries: a comparison of dental films and digital imaging systems. Dentomaxillofac Radiol 2000;29(5):312–318

33. Uprichard KK, Potter BJ, Russell CM, Schafer TE, Adair S, Weller RN. Comparison of direct digital and conventional radiography for the detection of proximal surface caries in the mixed dentition. Pediatr Dent 2000;22(1):9–15

34. Haak R, Wicht MJ, Noack MJ. Conventional, digital and contrast-enhanced bitewing radiographs in the decision to restore approximal carious lesions. Caries Res 2001;35(3):193–199

35. Williams CP. Digital radiography sensors: contemporary software. Pract Proced Aesthet Dent 2001;13(8):644–646

36. Lehmann TM, Troeltsch E, Spitzer K. Image processing and enhancement provided by commercial dental software programs. Dentomaxillofac Radiol 2002;31(4):264–272

37. Pitts NB, Rimmer PA. An in vivo comparison of radiographic and directly assessed clinical caries status of posterior approximal surfaces in primary and permanent teeth. Caries Res 1992;26(2):146–152

38. Wenzel A, Hintze H. Perception of image quality in direct digital radiography after application of various image treatment filters for detectability of dental disease. Dentomaxillofac Radiol 1993;22(3):131–134

39. Webber RL, Horton RA, Tyndall DA, Ludlow JB. Tuned-aperture computed tomography (TACT). Theory and application for three-dimensional dento-alveolar imaging. Dentomaxillofac Radiol 1997;26(1):53–62

40. Webber RL, Webber SE, Moore J. Hand-held three-dimensional dental X-ray system: technical description and preliminary results. Dentomaxillofac Radiol 2002;31(4):240–248

41. Nair MK, Tyndall DA, Ludlow JB, May K, Ye F. The effects of restorative material and location on the detection of simulated recurrent caries. A comparison of dental film, direct digital radiography and tuned aperture computed tomography. Dentomaxillofac Radiol 1998;27(2):80–84

42. Abreu M Jr, Tyndall DA, Ludlow JB. Detection of caries with conventional digital imaging and tuned aperture computed tomography using CRT monitor and laptop displays. Oral Surg Oral Med Oral Pathol Oral Radiol Endod 1999;88(2):234–238

43. Shi XQ, Han P, Welander U, Angmar-Månsson B. Tuned-aperture computed tomography for detection of occlusal caries. Dentomaxillofac Radiol 2001;30(1):45–49

44. van Daatselaar AN, Tyndall DA, van der Stelt PF. Detection of caries with local CT. Dentomaxillofac Radiol 2003;32(4):235–241

45. Haak R, Wicht MJ, Ritter L, et al. Cone beam tomography for the detection of approximal carious cavitations. Caries Res 2006;40:346

46. Kaffe I, Gordon M, Laufer B, Littner MM. Detection of proximal carious lesions: two-film versus four-film bitewing radiography. Oral Surg Oral Med Oral Pathol 1984;57(5):567–571

47. Hintze H, Wenzel A. A two-film versus a four-film bite-wing examination for caries diagnosis in adults. Caries Res 1999;33(5):380–386

48. Hintze H, Wenzel A, Danielsen B, Nyvad B. Reliability of visual examination, fibre-optic transillumination, and bite-wing radiography, and reproducibility of direct visual examination following tooth separation for the identification of cavitated carious lesions in contacting approximal surfaces. Caries Res 1998;32(3):204–209

49. Tveit AB, Espelid I, Skodje F. Restorative treatment decisions on approximal caries in Norway. Int Dent J 1999;49(3):165–172

50. Hintze H, Wenzel A, Danielsen B. Behaviour of approximal carious lesions assessed by clinical examination after tooth separation and radiography: a 2.5-year longitudinal study in young adults. Caries Res 1999;33(6):415–422

51. Wenzel A, Fejerskov O. Validity of diagnosis of questionable caries lesions in occlusal surfaces of extracted third molars. Caries Res 1992;26(3):188–194

52. Mach E. Über die Wirkung der räumlichen Vertheilung des Lichtreizes auf die Netzhaut. Sitzungsberichte der Kaiserlichen Akademie der Wissenschaften, Wien. Mathematisch-naturwissenschaftliche Classe, Zweite Abteilung. 1865;52:303–322

53. Moereau JL. [The dangers of the supposed "Mach band" effect in dental radiography. Apropos of 3 cases]. Chir Dent Fr 1985;55(309):37–39

54. Ratledge DK, Kidd EA, Beighton D. A clinical and microbiological study of approximal carious lesions. Part 1: the relationship between cavitation, radiographic lesion depth, the site-specific gingival index and the level of infection of the dentine. Caries Res 2001;35(1):3–7

55. Pitts NB, Kidd EA. The prescription and timing of bitewing radiography in the diagnosis and management of dental caries: contemporary recommendations. Br Dent J 1992;172(6):225–227

56. Stodt T, Attin T. Bitewing examinations as a part of preventive dentistry—a review. [Article in German] Schweiz Monatsschr Zahnmed 2004;114(9):882–889

57. Mejàre I. Bitewing examination to detect caries in children and adolescents—when and how often? Dent Update 2005;32(10): 588–590, 593–594, 596–597

58. Pitts NB, Kidd EA. 'Selection criteria for dental radiography'. Br Dent J 1992;173(7):227

59. European Commission. Radiation Protection 136. European Guidelines on Radiation Protection in Dental Radiology. The Safe Use of Radiographs in Dental Radiology. Luxembourg: Office for Official Publications of the European Communities; 2004

60. American Dental Association (ADA). Council on Dental Benefit Programs; Council on Scientific Affairs; US Department of Health and Human Services; Public Health Service; Food and Drug Administration (FDA). The selection of patients for dental radiographic examinations. Food and Drug Administration (FDA); 2004. http://www.fda.gov/Radiation-EmittingProducts/RadiationEmittingProductsandProcedures/MedicalImaging/MedicalX-Rays/ucm116504.htm (accessed 23rd July 2012)

61. Darvell BW, Pitts NB. A mathematical model for the progression of approximal carious lesions through enamel. Aust Dent J 1984; 29(2):111–115

62. Mejàre I, Källest l C, Stenlund H. Incidence and progression of approximal caries from 11 to 22 years of age in Sweden: A prospective radiographic study. Caries Res 1999;33(2):93–100

63. Mejàre I, Stenlund H. Caries rates for the mesial surface of the first permanent molar and the distal surface of the second primary molar from 6 to 12 years of age in Sweden. Caries Res 2000; 34(6):454–461

64. Espelid I, Mejàre I, Weerheijm K; EAPD. EAPD guidelines for use of radiographs in children. Eur J Paediatr Dent 2003;4(1):40–48

65. Friedman J, Marcus MI. Transillumination of the oral cavity with use of fiber optics. J Am Dent Assoc 1970;80(4):801–809

66. Côrtes DF, Ekstrand KR, Elias-Boneta AR, Ellwood RP. An in vitro comparison of the ability of fibre-optic transillumination, visual inspection and radiographs to detect occlusal caries and evaluate lesion depth. Caries Res 2000;34(6):443–447

67. Côrtes DF, Ellwood RP, Ekstrand KR. An in vitro comparison of a combined FOTI/visual examination of occlusal caries with other caries diagnostic methods and the effect of stain on their diagnostic performance. Caries Res 2003;37(1):8–16

68. Stephen KW, Russell JI, Creanor SL, Burchell CK. Comparison of fibre optic transillumination with clinical and radiographic caries diagnosis. Community Dent Oral Epidemiol 1987;15(2): 90–94

69. Verdonschot EH, Bronkhorst EM, Wenzel A. Approximal caries diagnosis using fiber-optic transillumination: a mathematical adjustment to improve validity. Community Dent Oral Epidemiol 1991;19(6):329–332

70. Peers A, Hill FJ, Mitropoulos CM, Holloway PJ. Validity and reproducibility of clinical examination, fibre-optic transillumination, and bite-wing radiology for the diagnosis of small approximal carious lesions: an in vitro study. Caries Res 1993;27(4): 307–311

71. de Josselin de Jong E, Sundström F, Westerling H, Tranaeus S, ten Bosch JJ, Angmar-Månsson B. A new method for in vivo quantification of changes in initial enamel caries with laser fluorescence. Caries Res 1995;29(1):2–7

72. Neuhaus KW, Longbottom C, Ellwood R, Lussi A. Novel lesion detection aids. Monogr Oral Sci 2009;21:52–62

73. Lussi A, Imwinkelried S, Pitts N, Longbottom C, Reich E. Performance and reproducibility of a laser fluorescence system for detection of occlusal caries in vitro. Caries Res 1999;33(4): 261–266

74. Ricketts D. The eyes have it. How good is DIAGNOdent at detecting caries? Evid Based Dent 2005;6(3):64–65

75. Lussi A, Hack A, Hug I, Heckenberger H, Megert B, Stich H. Detection of approximal caries with a new laser fluorescence device. Caries Res 2006;40(2):97–103

76. Jablonski-Momeni A, Schipper HM, Rosen SM, et al. Performance of a fluorescence camera for detection of occlusal caries in vitro. Odontology 2011;99(1):55–61

77. Matos R, Novaes TF, Braga MM, Siqueira WL, Duarte DA, Mendes FM. Clinical performance of two fluorescence-based methods in detecting occlusal caries lesions in primary teeth. Caries Res 2011;45(3):294–302

78. Lussi A, Firestone A, Schoenberg V, Hotz P, Stich H. In vivo diagnosis of fissure caries using a new electrical resistance monitor. Caries Res 1995;29(2):81–87

79. Ricketts DN, Kidd EA, Liepins PJ, Wilson RF. Histological validation of electrical resistance measurements in the diagnosis of occlusal caries. Caries Res 1996;30(2):148–155

80. Ekstrand KR, Ricketts DN, Kidd EA. Reproducibility and accuracy of three methods for assessment of demineralization depth of the occlusal surface: an in-vitro examination. Caries Res 1997; 31(3):224–231

81. Longbottom C, Huysmans MC. Electrical measurements for use in caries in clinical trials. J Dent Res 2004;83 Spec NoC: C76–79

Caries Risk Assessment and Prediction

Cor van Loveren

7

The terminology associated with assessing or predicting future development of caries can easily lead to confusion. Throughout this chapter we will define and use only very few terms and show their practical utility in dental clinics. **Caries risk** can be defined as the probability of an individual developing at least a certain number of carious lesions reaching a given stage of disease progression during a specified period, conditional on the exposure status remaining stable during the period at issue.[1–3] Caries risk assessment or caries prediction can be based on several predictors, namely risk factors, risk indicators, and risk markers: the first is involved in the caries process, the second and third are only associated with the process itself. We will use the terms predictor and risk factors in this chapter and both terms can mean environmental, behavioral, or biological factors.

This chapter will cover:

- the following concepts in caries prediction: prevalence, sensitivity, specificity, crude hit rate, expected utility, and receiver operating characteristics (ROC) curves;
- the usefulness of various predictors such as past signs of caries experience;
- the Cariogram computer program for caries prediction;
- the value of early caries diagnosis for the preventive treatment planning for individual occlusal surfaces; and
- the Nexø program.

The Dentist's Clinical Judgment

For the benefit of the patients and a responsible use of resources, dentistry should avoid both overtreatment and undertreatment as much as possible. For caries preventive measures this means that the dental professional should try to differentiate between those people who will develop caries, including new lesions in addition to existing ones (high risk: high focus on prevention), and those who will not develop new caries (low risk: no or minor focus on prevention). In daily practice this prediction is frequently based on the **clinical judgment of the dental professional**. What is this prediction worth?

> **NOTE**
>
> Caries risk is the probability of an individual developing new caries lesions during a specified period.

In a study where 15 dentists were asked to predict whether children would develop dentinal caries lesions needing restoration within the next year, it turned out that dentists recognized 35%–79% of the children who developed dentinal caries and 75%–97% of the children who remained free of new caries into the dentin.[4,5] The terminology for this is that dentists showed a **sensitivity**, meaning the ability to recognize those who would develop dentin caries (the disease) varying from 35% to

79%, and a **specificity**, meaning the ability to recognize those who will not develop dentin caries (no disease) of 75%–94% (**Table 7.1**). When looking at the individual dentists, the one (dentist A) with the lowest sensitivity (35%: the dentist recognized 35% of those who later developed dentinal caries) recognized 92% of those who remained free of caries into the dentin (specificity 92%) and the one (dentist B) with the highest sensitivity (79%) showed a specificity of 75%. It was interesting to note that the prediction tended to be only slightly better if the dentist had treated the same children for several years as compared with when the prediction was done at first examination; the average sensitivity of the dentists increased from 40% to 50%, but the average specificity remained at about 90%.[4] When the children were without cavities or restorations at baseline (DMF = 0, see Chapter 8) the mean sensitivity decreased to 23%, indicating a high number of false negative predictions (dentin caries is present but the clinical judgment failed to predict it) suggesting that the dentists were misled by the caries-free status.

Based on the above, several questions arise:

- Should (these) dentists follow their clinical judgment when selecting caries-active children for preventive measures?
- What do the differences between these dentists A and B mean for their patients? Would you rather be a patient of dentist A or of dentist B?
- Which type of dentist are you, yourself?
- Are there any tests using risk factors systematically that perform better than the clinical judgment of these two dentists?

In spite of the mass of literature on caries prediction, the last question is difficult to answer because the outcome measures of the studies differ in the amount of caries to predict and the periods over which the predictions are made. In discussing the differences between dentists A and B, this chapter will introduce **crude hit rate** and **expected utility,** two methods to evaluate the performance of clinical judgment, and frequently suggested tests to predict caries and compare their performances against using no test at all.

Crude Hit Rate of a Predictor

There are different methods to express the accuracy of the prediction—for example, the sensitivity, specificity, and the crude hit rate. All of them require that data are dichotomized, meaning that data are structured in a two-by-two table where, for example, the prediction is divided into "caries increment expected" or "no caries increment expected" and the actual caries increment at a certain threshold level (the truth observed during the study) is yes or no (**Table 7.1**). The crude hit rate is the number of true positive predictions plus the number of true negative predictions divided by the total number of predictions

Table 7.1   A 2x2 table for evaluating the accuracy of a dichotomous predictor and formulae for some selected measures of accuracy

		Actual caries increment		
		Yes (1 or more dentinal lesions)	No (no dentinal lesions)	Total
Predic-tor	Increment	**True positive (TP) correct treatment**	**False positive (FP) overtreatment**	TP + FP
	No increment	**False negative (FN) undertreatment**	**True negative (TN) correct (no) treatment**	FN + TN
Total		TP + FN	FP + TN	n =TP + FP + FN + TN
Prevalence		(TP + FN)/n		
Sensitivity (Se)		TP/(TP + FN)		
Specificity (Sp)		TN/(TN + FP)		
1 – Prevalence		(FP + TN)/n		
Crude hit rate		(TP+TN)/n Or: (prevalence × Se) + (1 – prevalence) × Sp/n (Correct treatment + correct no-treatment)/no. of persons Can be expressed in % by multiplying by 100%		
Utility		Numerical value for a health outcome, e.g., correct treatment (TP), correct no-treatment (TN), undertreatment (FN) or overtreatment (FP)		
Expected utility		Prevalence × [Se × utility$_{(TP)}$+ (1 – Se) × utility$_{(FN)}$] + (1 – prevalence) × [Sp × utility$_{(TN)}$+ (1 – Sp) × utility$_{(FP)}$] If utility$_{(TP)}$ = utility$_{(TN)}$ =1 and utility$_{(FP)}$ = utility$_{(FN)}$ =0, then expected utility = crude hit rate		

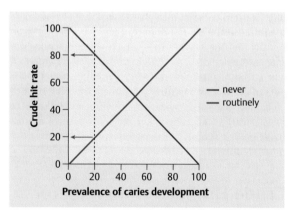

Fig. 7.1   Crude hit rate (% true positive + % true negative allocations of treatment) in relation to the percentage of children showing caries development (prevalence) when preventive measures are never or routinely applied. The vertical line indicates the corresponding crude hit rate for a prevalence of dentin caries of 20% in case of routinely (crude hit rate: 20) or never performed (crude hit rate: 80) preventive measures.

(**Table 7.1**). The crude hit rate can be expressed as a percentage by multiplying the fraction by 100%.

Figure 7.1 shows the crude hit rates (in this case the percentage of true allocations of preventive measures) in relation to the prevalence of caries development when preventive measures are either routinely or never applied. If, for example, 20 out of 100 persons who all routinely are given preventive measures developed dentin caries (prevalence of caries development: 20%), the crude hit rate of this strategy is 20. So in case of routine preventive measures the crude hit rate equals the prevalence of caries development. On the other hand, if none of the persons received preventive measures and 20 out of 100 were to develop caries, the crude hit rate is 80%: thus 80% (1 – prevalence of caries development) of the persons correctly receive no treatment.

BACKGROUND

In this chapter we use the term "prevalence of caries development" instead of "caries incidence" to correspond better to the 2×2-table presented in **Table 7.1**.

When only the number of good decisions counts and they count equally, strategies with high crude hit rates are better than strategies with lower crude hit rates. It is clear that when the prevalence of caries development is above 50% it is better to apply preventive measures routinely rather than never, but when the prevalence is below 50%, it is better never to apply a preventive measure than to do it routinely.

The crude hit rate can also be estimated for dentist A and dentist B; however, it requires calculations, as we initially only know the sensitivity and specificity of the dentists and the prevalence of caries development. The number of true positive predictions (TP) equals the prevalence × sensitivity (**Table 7.1**), and the number of true negative predictions (TN) equals (1 − prevalence) × specificity. Thus, the number of true positive and true negative predictions can be calculated for dentist A, remembering that his sensitivity was 35% and specificity was 92%, and for dentist B for whom the sensitivity was 79% and the specificity 75%. The crude hit rates for dentists A and B are calculated in **Table 7.2** for increasing prevalence of caries development. For example, if the prevalence of developing dentin caries is 50%, the number of true positive predictions of dentist A is 50 × 0.35 = 17.5 and his number of true negative predictions is 50 × 0.92 = 46 and added together the crude hit rate is 63.5. In **Fig. 7.2a, b** the crude hit rates of dentists A and B are added to the crude hit rates when preventive measures are given to all or to none of the patients as depicted in **Fig. 7.1**. Again, when strategies with high crude hit rates are better than strategies with lower crude hit rates, it is clear that dentist A should not use his clinical judgment when caries prevalence is less than 18% (crude hit rate < 83 against the crude hit rate for never doing prevention at > 84), and dentist B should not when caries prevalence is below 25%. Under those conditions, in practices with these low prevalences of caries development, the dentists should follow the strategy of never applying the preventive strategy. At higher prevalences, > 18% and > 25% respectively, dentists A and B should use their clinical judgment. However, when prevalences of caries development increase above 60% or 78%, dentists A and B, respectively, should no longer use their clinical judgment but always apply the preventive strategy. When superimposing **Fig. 7.2a, b**, it can be noted that with prevalences < 28%, the crude hit rate of dentist A is higher than that of dentist B (**Fig. 7.2c**). So dentist A, then, would be the more accurate dentist. With prevalences > 28%, the crude hit rate of dentist B is higher than that of dentist A, thus making dentist B the "better" dentist.

NOTE

When only the number of good decisions counts and they count equally, strategies with high crude hit rates are better than strategies with lower crude hit rates.

Utilities of Predictors

The above outcome, viz. that dentist A is better than dentist B when caries development prevalence is below 28%, relates not to the fact that dentist A has more true positive predictions, but to the fact that dentist A has more true negative predictions (see columns in **Table 7.2**). One can argue that true positive predictions (patients who will develop new caries are identified) are more important than true negative predictions (patients who will not develop new caries are identified). Then, in the formula of the crude hit rate a higher value can be given to the true positive prediction compared with the true negative prediction. This will change the comparison between dentist A and dentist B. A numerical value given to a (health) outcome is called a **utility**. Utilities can also be given to false positive and false negative predictions. Those predictions are wrong and that should be reflected in the utility assessment.

NOTE

A numerical value given to a (health) outcome is called a utility. Utilities can be given to true and false positive and true and false negative outcomes (TP, TN, FN, FP predictions). Unfortunately, there are no generally accepted values for utilities that should be assigned to the outcomes of a predictor.

Unfortunately, there are no generally accepted values for utilities that should be assigned to the outcomes of a predictor (TP, TN, FN, FP calls). It may be clear that dental professionals, patients, and finance officials may disagree on the utilities that should be given. In **Table 7.3** suggestions are made for utilities, and these values are used in the calculations in this chapter. If readers do not agree with these values and want to change the ratio between the values, they have to redo the calculations in this chapter with their own values. By doing so, such a reader may reach other conclusions than those of the author.

When utilities are assigned, the expected utility (EU) of a prediction or predictor can be calculated (see **Table 7.1**). In **Table 7.4** the expected utilities of dentist A are calculated (using the formula presented in **Table 7.1**), where the values for true positives are multiplied by the numerical value 2, true negatives by 1, false positives by −1 and false negatives by −2. The justification of these multipliers is addressed in **Table 7.3**.

The same calculations can be made for the strategies "treat never" and "treat routinely" for dentist B. The outcomes of these calculations are depicted in **Fig. 7.3**, which shows that up to a prevalence of 10% and 15% for dentists A and B, respectively, both dentists should go for the "no preventive treatment" strategy. From a prevalence of above 10% and 15% to, respectively, 42% (dentist A) and 65% (dentist B), they should follow their own judgment

Table 7.2 Calculation of the crude hit rate for dentists A and B in relation to the prevalence of children developing caries lesions

Population characteristics		Dentist A (sensitivity: 35%; specificity: 92%)			Dentist B (sensitivity: 79%; specificity: 75%)		
Prevalence	(1 – prevalence)	True positives +	True negatives =	Crude hit rate	True positives +	True negatives =	Crude hit rate
% of children developing dentinal lesion	% of children not developing dentinal lesion	Prevalence × sensitivity	(1 – prevalence) × specificity	True positives + true negatives	Prevalence × sensitivity	(1 – prevalence) × specificity	True positives + true negatives
0	100	0.0	92.0	92.0	0.0	75.0	75.0
10	90	3.5	82.8	86.3	7.9	67.5	75.4
20	80	7.0	73.6	80.6	15.8	60.0	75.8
30	70	10.5	64.4	74.9	23.7	52.5	76.2
40	60	14.0	55.2	69.2	31.6	45.0	76.6
50	50	17.5	46.0	63.5	39.5	37.5	77.0
60	40	21.0	36.8	57.8	47.4	30.0	77.4
70	30	24.5	27.6	52.1	55.3	22.5	77.8
80	20	28.0	18.4	46.4	63.2	15.0	78.2
90	10	31.5	9.2	40.7	71.1	7.5	78.6
100	0	35.0	0.0	35.0	79.0	0.0	79.0

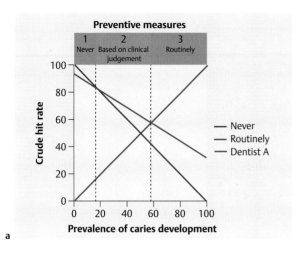

a

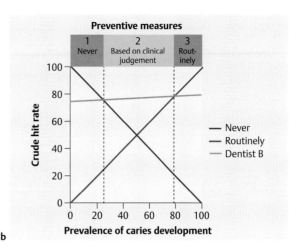

b

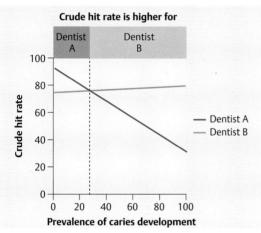

c

Fig. 7.2 a–c

a, b Crude hit rate in relation to the percentage of children showing caries development when preventive measures are never or routinely applied and when applied based on the clinical judgment prediction of dentist A (**a**) and dentist B (**b**). Region 1: no clinical judgment should be used nor preventive strategy be applied; region 2: clinical judgment should decide whether or not to apply preventive strategy; region 3: always apply preventive strategy.

c Crude hit rate in relation to the percentage of children showing caries development when preventive measures are applied based on the clinical judgment prediction of dentist A or dentist B. Below 28%, dentist A is the better dentist; above 28%, dentist B is the better.

Table 7.3 Suggestions for utilities for outcomes of a predictor

	Utility	Factors affecting the utility value
True positive prediction	2	Treatment is assigned to those who are in need Effectiveness of the treatment Costs of the treatment
True negative prediction	1	Prevents overtreatment
False positive prediction	−1	Causes overtreatment: • Costs without effect • Treatment time is wasted for those who are in need of treatment • Harms of the treatment
False negative prediction	−2	Causes undertreatment • Treatment is not given to those who are in need • Effectiveness of the treatment • Costs of the treatment

and above those prevalences they should follow the "treat all" strategy. When superimposing the expected utilities of dentist A and dentist B, it can be seen (**Fig. 7.3 c**) that with a prevalence <18% dentist A is the more accurate dentist, and with a higher prevalence of caries development dentist B is the more accurate.

NOTE

When utilities are assigned, the expected utility (EU) of a prediction or predictor is the sum of the products of the percentages TP, FN, TN and FP and their assigned utilities.

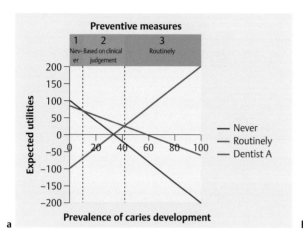

a

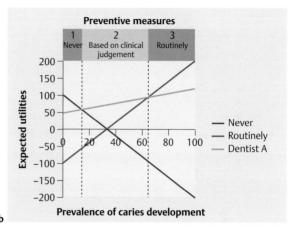

b

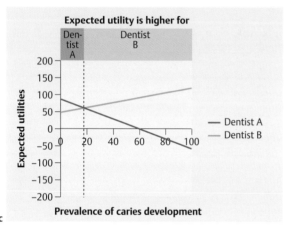

c

Fig. 7.3a–c

a, b Expected utilities in relation to the percentage of children showing caries development when preventive measures are never or routinely applied and when applied based on the clinical judgment prediction of dentist A (a) and dentist B (b). Region 1: no clinical judgment should be used nor preventive measures be applied; region 2: clinical judgment should decide whether or not to apply preventive measures; region 3: always apply preventive measures.

c Expected utilities in relation to the percentage of children showing caries development when preventive measures are applied based on the clinical judgment prediction of dentist A or dentist B. Below 18% dentist A is the better dentist, above 18% dentist B is the better.

Objective Predictors

A disadvantage of the clinical judgment strategy as discussed above is that no dentist or patient knows how good the dentist is. Therefore, there is a need for more **objective prediction models.** The following predictors/ risk factors are most often included in the models: signs of past caries experience; amount of dental plaque; dietary tests; microbiologic salivary tests; and salivary tests such as flow rate and buffering capacity. It has been shown that the usefulness of tests depends on the age of the individuals to whom they are applied, and that past **caries experience**, especially, is the most significant risk indicator of future caries development.[6] The status of the most recently erupted/exposed surface was the most appropriate measure of past caries experience. When **bacterial levels** were included in prediction models, they did not improve or only moderately improved the fit of the models.[7,8] Although salivary lactobacilli and *Streptococcus mutans* counts had some predictive value on their own, they did not add to the prediction when the counts were combined with DMFS score (see Chapter 8) including initial lesions. The caries predictive power of **salivary flow rate** in healthy people is very modest and that of **buffering capacity** is very low, so neither can be used.[1] True hyposalivation,

however, is a serious threat to oral health and patients with compromised salivary flow are in need of intensified preventive programs. Yet, salivary flow rate tests should only be used to confirm hyposalivation when there is a firm suspicion.

Although a high sucrose diet and bad oral hygiene contribute importantly to caries etiology (see Chapter 2), the predictive power of these parameters is very low in populations where the use of fluoride is widespread.[7,9] When fluoride is not adequately used these factors could have predicted value, but in these populations there might be little variation in the sucrose intake or in the level of oral hygiene. This compromises the predictive power of these tests.

NOTE

Past caries experience is the most significant risk indicator of future caries development. The status of the most recently erupted/exposed surface was the most appropriate measure of past caries experience. When bacterial levels were included in prediction models, they did not improve or only moderately improved the fit of the models.

Table 7.4 Calculation of the expected utility (EU) of the prediction by dentist A in relation to the prevalence of children developing caries lesions

Population characteristics		Dentist A (sensitivity: 35%; specificity: 92%)									
Prevalence	(1 – prevalence)	EU true positives	+	EU false negatives	+	EU true negatives	+	EU false positives	=	Total EU	
% of children developing dentinal lesion	% of children not developing dentinal lesion	Prevalence × sensitivity × utility(TP)	+	Prevalence × (1 – sensitivity) × utility(FN)	+	(1 – prevalence) × specificity × utility(TN)	+	1 – prevalence × (1 – specificity) × utility(FP)	=	Total EU	
0	100	$0 \times 0.35 \times 2 = 0$	+	$0 \times 0.65 \times -2 = 0$	+	$100 \times 0.92 \times 1 = 92.0$	+	$100 \times 0.08 \times -1 = -8.0$	=	84.0	
10	90	$10 \times 0.35 \times 2 = 7$	+	$10 \times 0.65 \times -2 = -13$	+	$90 \times 0.92 \times 1 = 82.8$	+	$90 \times 0.08 \times -1 = -7.2$	=	69.6	
20	80	$20 \times 0.35 \times 2 = 14$	+	$20 \times 0.65 \times -2 = -26$	+	$80 \times 0.92 \times 1 = 73.6$	+	$80 \times 0.08 \times -1 = -6.4$	=	55.2	
30	70	$30 \times 0.35 \times 2 = 21$	+	$30 \times 0.65 \times -2 = -39$	+	$70 \times 0.92 \times 1 = 64.4$	+	$70 \times 0.08 \times -1 = -5.6$	=	40.8	
40	60	$40 \times 0.35 \times 2 = 28$	+	$40 \times 0.65 \times -2 = -52$	+	$60 \times 0.92 \times 1 = 55.2$	+	$60 \times 0.08 \times -1 = -4.8$	=	26.4	
50	50	$50 \times 0.35 \times 2 = 35$	+	$50 \times 0.65 \times -2 = -65$	+	$50 \times 0.92 \times 1 = 46.0$	+	$50 \times 0.08 \times -1 = -4.0$	=	12.0	
60	40	$60 \times 0.35 \times 2 = 42$	+	$60 \times 0.65 \times -2 = -78$	+	$40 \times 0.92 \times 1 = 36.8$	+	$40 \times 0.08 \times -1 = -3.2$	=	-2.4	
70	30	$70 \times 0.35 \times 2 = 49$	+	$70 \times 0.65 \times -2 = -91$	+	$30 \times 0.92 \times 1 = 27.6$	+	$30 \times 0.08 \times -1 = -2.4$	=	-16.8	
80	20	$80 \times 0.35 \times 2 = 56$	+	$80 \times 0.65 \times -2 = -104$	+	$20 \times 0.92 \times 1 = 18.4$	+	$20 \times 0.08 \times -1 = -1.6$	=	-31.2	
90	10	$90 \times 0.35 \times 2 = 63$	+	$90 \times 0.65 \times -2 = -117$	+	$10 \times 0.92 \times 1 = 9.2$	+	$10 \times 0.08 \times -1 = -0.8$	=	-45.6	
100	0	$100 \times 0.35 \times 2 = 70$	+	$100 \times 0.65 \times -2 = -130$	+	$0 \times 0.92 \times 1 = 0$	+	$0 \times 0.08 \times -1 = 0$	=	-60.0	

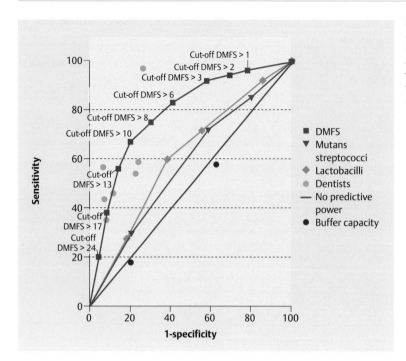

Fig. 7.4   ROC curves of various predictors (data taken from refs. 7,10). Persons with lower values than the cut-off values are predicted not to develop caries, while persons with the cut-off or higher values are predicted to do so (data for the dentist are taken from refs. 4,5).

ROC curve

The ROC (receiver operating characteristics) curve is a graphic presentation of the sensitivity and 1–specificity of the various possible cut-off values of a predictor. In **Fig. 7.4** ROC curves of various predictors discussed above are depicted (data taken from refs. 4, 5, 7, and 10). The more the line moves to the left upper corner of the plot area (high sensitivity and high specificity), the better the predictor. The diagonal in the plot area from the left lower to the right upper corner represents the values of no predictive power. It should be seen that **DMFS is the most powerful predictor** with the most cut-off values. Lactobacilli counts perform worse and have four cut-off points. Mutans streptococci counts perform about equally to lactobacilli counts but have 3 cut-off points and buffering capacity (2 cut-off points) has no predictive power. The individual studies perform better or equal to the tests.[4,5]

> **NOTE**
>
> A receiver operating characteristics (ROC) curve depicts the sensitivity against (1–specificity) for each possible cut-off value of the predictor.

Cariogram

An interactive program for the PC called **Cariogram** has been developed, which combines information on the following risk factors and indicators: past caries experience; caries related diseases; diet in terms of content and frequency of sugar intake; oral hygiene; use of fluoride; and saliva analyses including mutans streptococci, buffering capacity, and secretion rate. The Cariogram program operates basically in such a way that information collected about the patient is transferred to "scores" which are then entered into the program. According to its built-in algorithm, the program evaluates the data and presents the summarized result expressed as a pie-diagram illustrating the "chance of avoiding cavities" in the future (**Fig. 7.5**).[11]

In a two-year prospective study, 446 schoolchildren, 10–11 years old, were divided into 5 groups according to the assessed caries risk at baseline. Where the Cariogram predicted a 0%–20% (high risk), 21%–40%, 41%–60%, 61%–80%, and 81%–100% (low risk) chance of avoiding new lesions, 8, 35, 42, 73, and 83% of the children, respectively, had no new dentinal lesions after two years.[12] Thus, the predictive power of the program in this test seemed acceptable.

The question remains of how the choice for preventive measures relates to the various subgroups. The answer to the latter question can be found when the categories of chance of the Cariogram outcomes are laid over **Fig. 7.3** (**Fig. 7.6**):

- In the three subgroups with less than 60% chance to remain free of dentinal caries (high-to-moderate risk), all children should receive preventive treatment (the expected utility values of "routinely" treatment are higher than those of "never" treatment).
- In the subgroup with 61%–80% chance to remain free of dentinal caries, the strategy is unclear (because the expected utility lines of "never" and "routinely" treatment

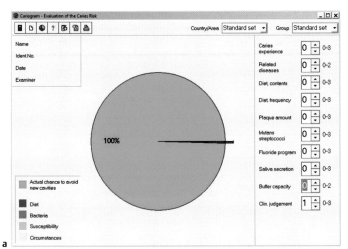

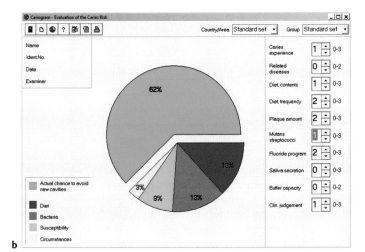

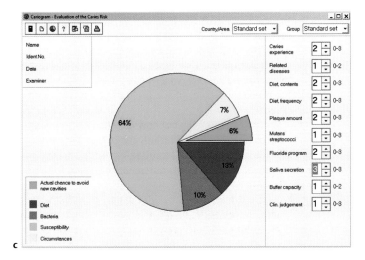

Fig. 7.5a–c Examples of cariograms showing different risks.
a No risk, as all risk factors are adequate.
b Moderate risk, as a few of the risk factors are inadequate.
c High risk, as several risk factors (e.g., hyposalivation) are inadequate.

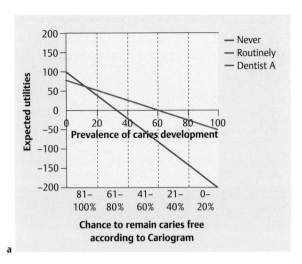

a

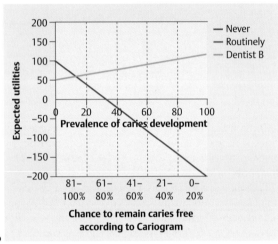

b

Fig. 7.6a, b   The outcome categories of the Cariogram prediction laid over the expected utilities in relation to the percentage of children showing caries development when preventive measures are never or routinely applied and when applied based on the clinical judgment prediction of dentist A (**a**) and dentist B (**b**). For each Cariogram category it can been seen which preventive strategy gives the highest expected utility.

cross) and in the group with >80% chance to remain free of dentinal caries (low caries risk) no preventive treatment should be applied (the expected utility values of "never" treatment are higher than those of "routinely" treatment).

- In the two subgroups with 41%–60% and 61%–80% chance to remain free of dentinal caries, the clinical judgment of the dentist may overrule the outcome of the Cariogram as the expected utilities of these judgments could be higher.

A Swedish study compared the caries risk profiles of children (10–11 years at baseline) and senior adults (age groups 55, 65, and 75 at baseline) with the Cariogram program, and after two and five years the incidence of caries was re-evaluated and compared to the predictions.[13] Of the senior adults, 26% belonged to the highest caries risk group versus 3% of the children (**Table 7.5**). The mean DFS increment per year for the total group of children was 0.4±0.8 (SD) and 1.2±1.9 for the senior adults. (DFS: sum of decayed and filled surfaces, see Chapter 8). Individual factors contributing significantly to the higher risk profiles for the adults were higher plaque scores, higher counts of mutans streptococci, and lower buffering capacity. Overall, the risk for caries, as assessed by the Cariogram, was twice as high for the adults. This study emphasized the need for preventive programs for senior citizens but also the need of simple prediction models for older people.

Inclusion of salivary and microbial measurements makes the Cariogram very laborious and expensive, which contributes negatively to the utility score (see the comments in the last column of **Table 7.3**). The costs may even be higher than the treatment itself and then the question is justified: why not go for a treat-all strategy? Alternatively, the Cariogram can be run by only 7 scores of the included 10 risk factors, for example by **leaving out the expensive mutans and buffering capacity tests.**

The Cariogram identifies individuals' individual risk factors. Knowing all the caries etiology-related dietary, salivary and oral hygiene risk factors of an individual may prove of value in directing the individual strategies for the prevention of future caries. Moreover, this knowledge

Table 7.5   Caries risk expressed as % chance of avoiding caries and percentage of senior adults and children in the different groups according to the predictions made by the Cariogram[13]

% chance of avoiding caries requiring operative dentistry according to Cariogram evaluations	0%–20% (high risk)	21%–40%	41%–60%	61%–80%	81%–100% (low risk)
% of senior adults	26	17	36	19	2
% of children	3	7	14	26	50

could be used to **motivate patients** to continue their efforts and re-assessments to allow for evaluation of the effectiveness of the preventive measures.

The results of the Cariogram prediction have been compared with clinicians' ability to range patients according to the caries risk. This exercise provoked discussions among the clinicians about the relative impact of etiological factors of caries. This suggests that the Cariogram may also serve as a tool to sharpen clinicians' ability to predict caries.[11]

NOTE

The Cariogram is an interactive PC-based program combining information on the following risk factors and indicators: past caries experience; caries related diseases; diet in terms of content and frequency of sugar intake; oral hygiene; use of fluoride; and saliva analyses including mutans streptococci, buffering capacity, and secretion rate.

CLINICAL PEARL

The Cariogram software can be downloaded at: http://www.mah.se/fakulteter-och-omraden/Odontologiska-fakulteten/Avdelning-och-kansli/Cariologi/Cariogram/

Signs of Past Caries Experience

The signs of past caries experience, both initial stages of visible caries as well as restorations and extractions, are definitely part of the clinical judgment. Past caries summarizes the cumulative effect of all risk factors to which an individual has been exposed. The use of past caries experience as a predictor for future caries increment has been criticized by the argument that the aim should be to detect high-risk, susceptible individuals before there are any signs of caries experience. But since past caries experience is a powerful predictor it means that children with (early signs of) caries continue to develop caries and there is still the need to prevent caries.

When using past caries experience as predictor, there are many possible cut-off values to regard people as being at risk, or at more risk than others. In a study from Finland, the sensitivity and specificity was calculated of various DMFS cut-offs to predict 3-year caries increment (≥4 surfaces) in 13-year-old children (**Table 7.6**).[7] Using at baseline the cut-off value between 0 (not having caries) and ≥1 DMFS (having any caries) in a population where in reality only 27% of the children will develop ≥4 surface caries in the 3-year period:

70% of the children were predicted to develop caries: TP + FP = (TP = prevalence × sensitivity) + (FP = [1 − prevalence] × [1 − specificity]) = (TP = 0.27 × 0.92) + (FP = 0.73 × 0.62) = 0.70 (see **Table 7.6**)

Table 7.6 Prediction of 3-year caries increment (≥5) by base line D_3MFS score in a cohort of initially 13-year-old children[7]

Baseline DMFS score	Se (%)	Sp (%)
≥1	92	38
≥2	83	54
≥3	74	65
≥4	63	74
≥5	55	80
≥6	44	85
≥7	38	90
≥8	32	92
≥9	24	95
≥14	10	100

Thus, 45% of the studied population were erroneously marked as being at caries risk and would erroneously receive preventive therapy: FP = (1 − prevalence) × (1 − specificity) = 0.73 × 0.62 = 0.45 (see **Table 7.6**).

The study stated that this number was an unacceptable outcome for a prediction model (too much FP) and suggested a cut-off value of between DMFS <4 and ≥ 4. With that cut-off value: 35% of the population was classified as being at risk (TP + FP = (TP = prevalence × sensitivity) + (FP = [1 − prevalence] × [1 − specificity]) = (TP = 0.27 × 0.6) + (FP = 0.73 × 0.26) = (TP = 0.16) + (FP = 0.19) = 0.35 (see **Table 7.6**), while the FP fraction was 19%, which was thought to be acceptable. What the study implies is that at a prevalence of 27%, the negative expected utilities of the false predictions outweigh the positive expected utilities of the true predictions when using a cut-off DMFS between 0 and ≥1, but not when a cut-off DMFS between <4 and ≥4 is used. Nothing is stated in the study to tell us which values were assigned to the various utilities.

In **Fig. 7.7** the expected utilities of both cut-off values are given and compared with treating either never or routinely. It is again clear that the best strategy depends on the prevalence of the development of caries (or individually on the chance to develop caries):

- Up to a prevalence of ca. 16%, the "never treat" strategy would be the best one to follow.
- Until a prevalence of ca. 38%, the best strategy would be to treat the patients with baseline DMFS ≥4.
- At a prevalence between 38% and 75%, the best strategy would be to treat all children with caries (cut-off DMFS ≥1).
- Above a prevalence of 75%, all children should be treated, irrespective of whether they have caries or not.

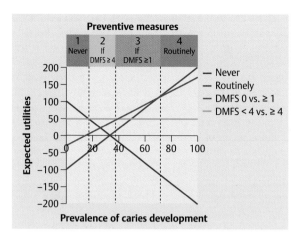

Fig. 7.7 Expected utilities in relation to the percentage of children showing caries development when preventive measures are based on "never treat" or "treat routinely" strategy, or when DMFS is used as sole predictor with the cut-off values of 0 vs. ≥1 and <4 vs. ≥4. Region 1: no clinical judgment should be used nor preventive measures be applied; region 2: preventive measures for those with DMFS ≥4; region 3: preventive measures for those with DMFS ≥1; region 4: always apply preventive measures.

Unfortunately, we cannot make a comparison between dentists A and B, because they were not asked to predict which children would develop ≥4 cavities within the next 3 years.

Caries experience in the primary dentition has been used to predict caries development in the permanent dentition. One study demonstrated that the sensitivity and specificity of caries in primary teeth (at 6 years old) were 57% and 85%, respectively, to select the 25% of children with the highest caries experience at the age of 13 years.[14] For caries experience of the permanent dentition, the sensitivity to select this upper quartile was only 28% at the age of 6 years, reached 68% at the age of 9 years, and remained at that level until age 12 years. Specificity decreased from 92% (6 years) to 85% (9 years) and then steadily increased to 93% (12 years).

When screening for high caries increment in young children below the age of 9 years, caries in the primary dentition seems to be a better screening criterion than caries in permanent first molars. When the aim is to identify those patients who will get high caries increment later on, screening at age 9 years seems to be as accurate as that done at a later age.

A method of caries prediction by using past caries experience as predictor for children with a mixed dentition has been developed in Switzerland.[15,16] Low numbers of sound primary molars and high numbers of pre-cavitated lesions in permanent first molars (discolored pit and fissures in the 7/8-year-olds and white spots on lingual and buccal smooth surfaces in 10/11-year-olds) proved to be the best variables in identifying high risk of future caries in the children. Inclusion of radiographic variables did not

substantially increase the quality of the prediction. The Swiss method of caries prediction was validated on a population of Dutch children and proved to be robust despite slight differences in the ages of the Dutch population and small differences in the method of caries diagnosis.[8] While the Swiss model included the presence of slightly brown discolored fissures, which may be difficult to detect, the Dutch model showed the prediction was at least as good when more advanced incipient and cavitated lesions were regarded. This would make the prediction easier in general dental practice.

Both the Swiss and Dutch systems calculate an individual risk value for each person using a regression formula. In principle, the higher the value, the more likely that an individual will develop caries; therefore, individuals can be ranked in order of caries risk. The percentage of individuals declared at-risk can then be decided upon, considering the available resources. Depending on the age of the children, the prediction periods, and the amount of caries to predict (≥2, ≥4 or ≥6 new lesions within 4 years), the sensitivities of the models varied from 65% to >80% and the specificities between 70% and 80%.[16,17] An advantage of these models is that the individual risk values can readily be calculated on any personal computer or programmed pocket calculator.

The predictive value of DMF may be reduced in older people, since DMF is a cumulative measure. This means that when high-risk persons change their behavior, the DMF will remain high. Nevertheless, an association between coronal DMF and the risk of developing root caries has been found.[18,19]

NOTE

When screening for high caries increment in young children below the age of 9 years, caries in the primary dentition seems a better screening criterion than caries in permanent first molars. When the aim is to identify those patients who will get high caries increment later on, screening at age 9 years seems as accurate as that done at a later age.

Too Young to Have Past Caries Experience

Patients may be too young to have past caries experience. For them, **scoring the presence of visible plaque** may be a good alternative. One study assessed four variables for their ability to identify 19-month-old children who would experience caries during the subsequent 1.5-year period.[20] The variables were (i) visible plaque on the labial surfaces of the maxillary incisors, (ii) the use of a nursing bottle, (iii) mother's caries prevalence, and (iv) mother's salivary level of mutans streptococci. Visible plaque and the use of a nursing bottle were strongly associated with the caries development, while the other two variables had weak or no statistically significant associations. The best indicator of risk was visible plaque showing a sensitivity of 83% and specificity of 92%. Overall, 91% of the children were correctly classified with this variable.

> **NOTE**
>
> Patients may be too young to have past caries experience. For them, scoring the presence of visible plaque is a good alternative to estimate caries risk.

Active versus Nonactive Lesions

For preventive measures that are aimed at individual teeth it is necessary to predict caries risk at the individual tooth level. This question is most urgent for placing pit and fissure sealants. One study presented a visual–tactile scoring system for activity on intact lesions[21] (see Chapter 6). Intact, active lesions were described as having a whitish/yellowish opaque surface with loss of luster, feeling rough when the tip of a probe was moved gently across the surface, and generally covered with plaque. Inactive caries was described as caries with a whitish, brownish, or black shiny, intact surface. The enamel would feel hard and smooth on gentle probing. In a later publication the authors presented a clinical validation of this method, describing the transitions of the surfaces after a 3-year period.[22]

This study was done with two populations of children, of which one group brushed their teeth with fluoride toothpaste under daily supervision at school, while the fluoride toothpaste use of the other group was sparse and not controlled. From the data presented it can be calculated that in the group using fluoride toothpaste at school, the predictor "active noncavitated versus inactive noncavitated lesions in pits and fissures" had a sensitivity and specificity of 38% and 71%, respectively, for the outcome active noncavitated caries, cavity, or filling (**Table 7.7**). For the cut-off point between sound fissures versus fissures with either inactive or active noncavitated lesions, the sensitivity was 80% and the specificity 70% (**Table 7.7**).

Figure 7.8a shows the expected utilities of this predictor for the implementation of a preventive treatment. For the children using fluoride toothpaste only for a small prevalence interval (30%–35%), it might be useful to make a discrimination between active and nonactive lesions, but in most populations this discrimination would not contribute to a higher expected utility. However, to discriminate between sound fissures and fissures with either inactive or active noncavitated lesions would be a good strategy when the prevalence of caries development in fissures varies between around 18% and 65% (**Fig. 7.8b**). Below a prevalence of 18% the no-treatment option has the highest expected utility, and above 65% the treat-all strategy has the highest expected utility.

Table 7.7 Upper part is original data (fluor dated group) from the article of Nyvad et al. (2003).[21] The lower part explains how the sensitivity (Se) and specificity (Sp) can be calculated from these data

Total N	Recording at baseline	Status after 3 years			
		Sound (%)	Inactive noncavitated (%)	Active noncavitated (%)	Cavity or filling (%)
1112	Sound	80	14	0	5
463	Inactive noncavitated	9	61	3	27
219	Active noncavitated	27	35	5	34

Calculation of Se and Sp of the cut-off of inactive noncavitated (n = 463) versus active noncavitated lesions (n = 219) with the caries outcome of active noncavitated lesions, cavity, or filling.

TP = 39% × 219 = 85.4	FN = 30% × 463 = 138.9	Se = TP/(TP + FN) = 85.4/(85.4 + 138.9) = 0.38
TN = 70% × 463 = 324.1	FP = 61% × 219 = 133.6	Sp = TN/(TN + FP) = 324.1/(324.1 + 133.6) = 0.71

Calculation of Se and Sp of the cut-off of sound (n = 1112) versus inactive noncavitated + active noncavitated lesions (n = 463 + 219) with the caries outcome of active noncavitated lesions, cavity, or filling

TP = 39% × 219 + 30% × 463 = 224.3	FN = 5% × 1112 = 55.6	Se = TP/(TP + FN) = 224.3/(224.3 + 55.6) = 0.80
TN = 94% × 1112 = 1045.3	FP = 61% × 219 + 70% × 463 = 457.3	Sp = TN/(TN+FP) = 1045.3/(1045.3 + 457.3) = 0.70

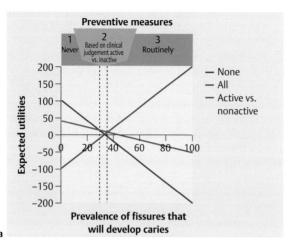

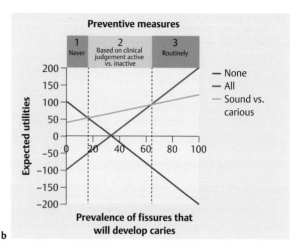

Fig. 7.8a, b Expected utilities for preventive treatment of fissures in relation to the percentage of fissures with initial caries in which the caries may be active or progress when the initial caries is diagnosed as either active or nonactive (**a**); and in fissures diagnosed as either sound or having initial inactive or active noncavi- tated lesions (**b**). Region 1: no clinical judgment should be used nor preventive measures be applied; region 2: clinical judgment should decide whether or not to apply preventive measures; region 3: always apply preventive measures.

NOTE

For preventive measures that are aimed at individual teeth it is necessary to predict caries risk at an individual tooth level. A cut-off point between sound fissures versus fissures with any signs of noncavitated caries seems to be better than a cut-off between active versus nonactive, noncavitated lesions.

The Nexø Model

Can we offer our patients the right preventive programs? The indications are that it is difficult and that even intensified preventive programs may not sufficiently reduce the caries risk.[23–26] One reason may be that most programs are not individualized and do not encourage an individual's own responsibility and resources to prevent oral disease.[27] One program that uses both the dentist's skills to select risk children and a child's (parent's) own responsibility and resources for prevention is known as the Nexø program. This program differs from all other programs, because in addition to all the mentioned risk factors it also includes the eruption period of molar teeth as a special risk factor.[28–29]

A more in-depth description of the program will be given in Chapter 21.

SUMMARY

The possibilities of predicting future caries are discussed and various predictors and risk factors are compared. These comparisons are compromised among other things by differences in study design, by the cut-off levels used, by the amount of caries to be predicted, and by variations in the population studied. None of the available studies reported confidence intervals of the outcomes. For these reasons comparisons can only give a superficial view. Nevertheless, it is clear that clinical predictors may be the best predictors and that dentists have the ability to summarize these clinical predictors and make use of them in their clinical judgment; they are probably as good as any test to select the most caries-prone individuals. Dentists should train themselves in caries prediction, and computer programs such as Cariogram may be helpful in this. The Nexø program is a good example, where the clinical judgment of dentists is successfully used to offer an effective preventive program to the individual child which is related to his or her risk.

REFERENCES

1. Hausen H, Seppä L, Fejerskov O. Can caries be predicted? In: Thylstrup A, Fejerskov O, eds. Textbook of Clinical Cariology. Copenhagen: Munksgaard; 1994:393–410

2. Bratthall D, Ramanathan Stjernswärd J, Hänsel Pettersson G. Assessment of caries risk in the clinic – a modern approach. In: Wilson NHF, Roulet JF, Fuzzi M, eds. Advances in Operative Dentistry. Chicago: Quintessence; 2001:61–72

3. Fontana M, Zero DT. Assessing patients' caries risk. J Am Dent Assoc 2006;137(9):1231–1239

4. Alanen P, Hurskainen K, Isokangas P, et al. Clinician's ability to identify caries risk subjects. Community Dent Oral Epidemiol 1994;22(2):86–89

5. Isokangas P, Alanen P, Tiekso J. The clinician's ability to identify caries risk subjects without saliva tests—a pilot study. Community Dent Oral Epidemiol 1993;21(1):8–10

6. Powell LV. Caries prediction: a review of the literature. Community Dent Oral Epidemiol 1998;26(6):361–371

7. Hausen H. Caries prediction. In: Fejerskov O, Kidd EAN, eds. Dental Caries: the Disease and its Clinical Management. 2nd ed. Oxford: Blackwell Munksgaard; 2008:527–542

8. van Palenstein Helderman WH, Mikx FH, Van't Hof MA, Truin G, Kalsbeek H. The value of salivary bacterial counts as a supplement to past caries experience as caries predictor in children. Eur J Oral Sci 2001;109(5):312–315

9. Burt BA, Pai S. Sugar consumption and caries risk: a systematic review. J Dent Educ 2001;65(10):1017–1023

10. Hausen H. Caries prediction. In: Fejerskov O, Kidd EAM, eds. Dental Caries: the Disease and its Clinical Management. Oxford: Blackwell Munksgaard; 2003:327–339

11. Petersson GH, Bratthall D. Caries risk assessment: a comparison between the computer program 'Cariogram', dental hygienists and dentists. Swed Dent J 2000;24(4):129–137

12. Hänsel Petersson GH, Twetman S, Bratthall D. Evaluation of a computer program for caries risk assessment in schoolchildren. Caries Res 2002;36(5):327–340

13. Petersson GH, Fure S, Twetman S, Bratthall D. Comparing caries risk factors and risk profiles between children and elderly. Swed Dent J 2004;28(3):119–128

14. Seppä L, Hausen H, Pöllänen L, Helasharju K, Kärkkäinen S. Past caries recordings made in Public Dental Clinics as predictors of caries prevalence in early adolescence. Community Dent Oral Epidemiol 1989;17(6):277–281

15. Helfenstein U, Steiner M, Marthaler TM. Caries prediction on the basis of past caries including precavity lesions. Caries Res 1991;25(5):372–376

16. Steiner M, Helfenstein U, Marthaler TM. Dental predictors of high caries increment in children. J Dent Res 1992;71(12):1926–1933

17. van Palenstein Helderman WH, Van't Hof MA, van Loveren C, Bronkhorst E. Utility technology in the assessment of the cut-off between a negative and a positive test in a caries prediction model. Caries Res 2007;41(3):165–169

18. Ravald N, Hamp SE, Birkhed D. Long-term evaluation of root surface caries in periodontally treated patients. J Clin Periodontol 1986;13(8):758–767

19. Vehkalahti MM. Relationship between root caries and coronal decay. J Dent Res 1987;66(10):1608–1610

20. Alaluusua S, Malmivirta R. Early plaque accumulation—a sign for caries risk in young children. Community Dent Oral Epidemiol 1994;22(5 Pt 1):273–276

21. Nyvad B, Machiulskiene V, Baelum V. Reliability of a new caries diagnostic system differentiating between active and inactive caries lesions. Caries Res 1999;33(4):252–260

22. Nyvad B, Machiulskiene V, Baelum V. Construct and predictive validity of clinical caries diagnostic criteria assessing lesion activity. J Dent Res 2003;82(2):117–122

23. Seppä L, Hausen H, Pöllänen L, Kärkkäinen S, Helasharju K. Effect of intensified caries prevention on approximal caries in adolescents with high caries risk. Caries Res 1991;25(5):392–395

24. Hausen H, Kärkkäinen S, Seppä L. Application of the high-risk strategy to control dental caries. Community Dent Oral Epidemiol 2000;28(1):26–34

25. Källestål C. The effect of five years' implementation of caries-preventive methods in Swedish high-risk adolescents. Caries Res 2005;39(1):20–26

26. Heyduck C, Meller C, Schwahn C, Splieth CH. Effectiveness of sealants in adolescents with high and low caries experience. Caries Res 2006;40(5):375–381

27. Hausen H, Seppä L, Poutanen R, et al. Noninvasive control of dental caries in children with active initial lesions. A randomized clinical trial. Caries Res 2007;41(5):384–391

28. Ekstrand KR, Kuzmina IN, Kuzmina E, Christiansen ME. Two and a half-year outcome of caries-preventive programs offered to groups of children in the Solntsevsky district of Moscow. Caries Res 2000;34(1):8–19

29. Ekstrand KR, Christiansen ME. Outcomes of a non-operative caries treatment programme for children and adolescents. Caries Res 2005;39(6):455–467

Epidemiology of Caries and Noncarious Defects

U. Schiffner

8

The early chapters of this book (Chapters 1–3) dealt with the fundamental ecology of the oral cavity with particular reference to teeth. Factors were presented that could trigger an imbalanced equilibrium between teeth and biofilm, resulting in caries. The origin of noncarious defects of enamel and dentin was also considered. In the subsequent chapters, a caries model (Chapter 4) as well as clinical aspects of caries and noncarious defects were introduced (Chapters 5–7). From all of this it becomes clear that the caries process is also influenced by a series of more indirect factors that do not directly affect the surface of the tooth. For example, a parent's lack of education can affect a child's knowledge as well as his or her attitude and behavior towards toothbrushing, which in turn directly affects the rate of caries. If only for this reason, the knowledge and assessment of indirect (population-based) factors affecting the development of caries and other defects of the tooth's hard substances are crucial for the dental professional. The evaluation of these indirect factors is part of **epidemiology**.

Beyond the observations and findings regarding the patient and his or her teeth as well as an awareness of indirect factors, a specific treatment decision also depends on the frequency and severity of caries that the dentist observes and will then expect again in the patient population. To prevent the injection of subjectivity when assessing the prevalence, incidence, and distribution of a disease, knowledge of the empirical data is essential to more accurately evaluate the disease load. The treatment decision for the individual (tooth surface) should be based on an awareness of the relevant data in the respective population. These data are provided by epidemiology.

The term "epidemiology" refers to a scientific method that describes the spread, distribution, and severity of a disease in the overall population or individual groups of the population, along with the factors that influence the disease. The descriptive field of epidemiology answers the questions of "how many" and "which" persons are affected, and "the degree of severity" of the disease. These purely **descriptive epidemiological investigations** are primarily observational.[1] In addition, information can be gained about the etiology of the disease by using epidemiological methods to investigate the factors that may play a role for disease pathogenesis (**analytical epidemiology**). Analytical epidemiology also promotes an awareness of the cofactors and options for controlling diseases. Furthermore, the methods of epidemiology are used in scientific studies to determine the effects of specific measures for controlling or preventing diseases. One example of the latter is to investigate the influence of fluoridation on the caries incidence (**experimental or interventional epidemiology**).

In detail, this chapter covers the following topics:
- The importance, fundamentals, and methods of epidemiology
- The validity and limits of conventional indices for describing caries and noncarious defects

- Current developments in the prevalence and occurence of caries
- The prevalence of noncarious defects of the dental hard tissues.

> **NOTE**
>
> - **Descriptive epidemiology:** Provides statistics about disease conditions (spread, severity, and alterations).
> - **Analytical epidemiology:** Statistical analysis of factors related to disease, recovery, and prevention that provide information on the etiology of diseases and options for controlling them.
> - **Experimental epidemiology:** Analyzes the influence of factors being related to prevention or recovery from a disease under controlled conditions.

General Relevance of Epidemiology

From the statistics on the prevalence of diseases, specific conclusions can be drawn about medical treatments and/or the need for medical care. Oral epidemiology allows to evaluate preventive and therapeutic interventions and can be used as a basis for cost-benefit analyses. Epidemiology is an established, essential resource for planning and evaluating strategies in dental care, and for answering questions in medical research. Beyond its descriptive power, epidemiology provides the necessary information for political and health policy decisions that go far beyond a numerical understanding of disease conditions and can have significant medical and social consequences.[2]

Since epidemiology is playing an increasingly greater role in the fundamental research of health and health care, the planning, implementation, evaluation, and interpretation of epidemiological studies have to fullfil a series of requirements.[1,2] In addition to the relevant quality assurance measures required in research (calibration of the investigator, e.g., by repeated examinations to identify reliability within and between rates), the principles of medical ethics and data protection[3] must also be considered. Furthermore, the authors of a study are expected to interpret the results of their epidemiological research and to communicate their findings through scientific and public media.[4]

Study Types

Epidemiology uses different types of study. In **cross-sectional studies,** the prevalence of a disease and its potential causative or at least associated factors can be determined.[5] In cross-sectional studies, caution is required when offering interpretations that go beyond mere

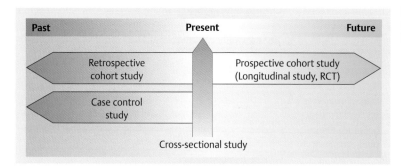

Fig. 8.1 Types of study in epidemiology (see also Note box). RCT: randomized controlled trial.

descriptions, since distorting influences (termed confounders) are frequently large because the factors are determined retrospectively.

Longitudinal studies require at least two examinations of the same study population, using the same investigative methodology. The collected data provide information on the incidence of diseases, and the conclusions regarding the etiological disease parameters are generally more accurate than those derived from cross-sectional studies. Furthermore, longitudinal studies are divided into retrospective and prospective cohort studies. In retrospective studies, current findings are collected and evaluated using historical information. In prospective studies, a study hypothesis is postulated and tested by comparing existing data with data collected in the future (**Fig. 8.1**).

Important parameters used to characterize the investigated cohort population are gender, age, geographic location, and **social status** of the investigated individuals. Social strata are assigned using the variables "education," "occupation," or "income." Sociological parameters also generally cover the opinions and behavior of the specific study population. In considering the sociological parameters, medical and dental information is weighed and sociological relationships are identified which can be used to help in describing or clarifying the phenomena of oral morbidity.[2]

NOTE

Types of **epidemiological study:**

- **Cross-sectional study:** Collection of disease data, possibly including the determination of potential associated factors at a single point in time. Offers fast results and is economical, but subject to the danger of misinterpretation. Example: Caries and plaque status on 5-, 12- and 15-year-olds in a certain period.
- **Retrospective cohort study:** Longitudinal studies extending into the past. A survey of present data is evaluated with reference to influences from the past. Fast results and economical, but no proof of a causal relationship. Provides plausible hypotheses. Example: Caries status of children from various regions related to the level of fluoride in the drinking water back in time.

- **Prospective cohort study:** Longitudinal study extending into the future. Data are collected in the future to test a hypothesis. Takes a long time, is expensive, and confirms causal relationships. Example: Caries status as well as urinary fluoride concentration of children is followed from ages 2 to 6 and their relation evaluated.

Descriptive Epidemiology of Caries and Noncarious Defects

Epidemiological Identification of Caries

Caries can be identified either clinically or radiologically (Chapters 5 and 6). Caries is identified much more sensitively by radiologic means.[6] However, in addition to organizational reasons that may preclude the taking of x-ray images, in many countries x-rays for purely epidemiological purposes are not permitted. Consequently, most epidemiological data regarding caries are derived from clinical investigations under **field conditions** (under non-optimal conditions). Frequently, caries lesions are only identified under difficult conditions in accessible tooth surfaces (little light, no dry surfaces, no tooth cleaning before the examination). This limits the detection of caries lesions in epidemiological studies and must be taken into consideration when interpreting the results.

Frequently, the epidemiological description of caries is in terms of prevalence. **Prevalence** means the **occurrence of a disease within a group at a specific point in time.** The percentage of individuals suffering from the disease is given in relation to the entire investigated population. Occasionally, however, "prevalence" is misinterpreted as the investigation of individuals and subsequent averaging of the extent of caries and its consequences for the group. This type of calculation yields the DMF number that is correctly identified as the **caries experience** (see below).

Instead of the prevalence of caries expressed as a percentage of the individuals affected by caries, sometimes the percentage of individuals who do not have the disease is used (**caries-free persons**). Various aspects need to be taken into consideration when using this term. In the

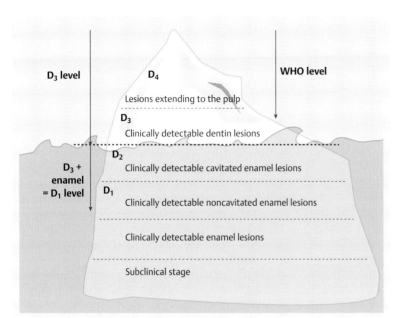

Fig. 8.2 Describing caries as an iceberg[4] illustrates the fact that mainly advanced stages of caries (D_3 level) are detected with visual–tactile methods; these caries lesions "extend out of the water", so to speak. Initial lesions lie "below the surface of the water" and are difficult to identify. This is true especially when the field conditions are suboptimal (such as insufficient light and moisture control) in a series of investigations.[63]

epidemiology of caries, "diseased" persons are to be understood both as those with untreated carious defects and those with treated caries. In addition, the underlying categorization of caries as a disease also needs to be considered. Frequently, only lesions involving dentin are defined as carious defects in epidemiological terms.[7]

This perspective negates the view of caries as a dynamic process at the tooth surface that proceeds from initial demineralization over long periods and results in macroscopically identifiable caries. Generally, only the advanced stages of the disease are considered. Restricting the epidemiological identification of caries to this late stage—which is also characterized as the identifiable tip of the **"caries iceberg"**[8]—does not consider the long developmental process leading to this stage. Thus, the choice of threshold for when to record the tooth or surface as carious is an important issue in epidemiological studies. Frequently caries is recorded only when it is cavitated or at least clearly extended into dentin. This way, only the top of the caries iceberg is considered. However, if caries is recorded also in noncavitated stages (e.g., a white spot lesion), then the caries prevalence or experience will be higher (**Fig. 8.2**).

Earlier, the frequency of individuals *without* caries in a population was also defined as the percentage of people with **"naturally healthy dentition."** Today, this term is not used, since it suggests the complete absence of any oral disease. The term **caries-free** which was preferred for a long time is now also deprecated, since it can be misinterpreted as referring to an absence of untreated carious lesions, and this overlooks fillings which are in fact treated caries lesions.[5]

For both *caries experience* and *caries prevalence*, a definition of the threshold is required at which a tooth surface can be considered diseased, to allow the reported data to be properly interpreted. Individuals *without caries experience* do not reveal any untreated caries lesions at the specified caries level, and they also do not show any consequences of caries (fillings or extractions). A group of people in which all the members exhibit this finding at a specific time has a caries prevalence of 0%.

Indices for Coronal Caries

Data on the caries prevalence of a population, especially in age groups with a generally high caries experience, do not sufficiently describe the disease since the average extent of the disease in individuals is not identified. More precise survey instruments are required such as the **DMF index**.[9]

The DMF index, suggested in the late 1930s (Klein et al. 1938), includes carious changes and their therapies such as fillings or extractions:[9]

- **"D"** stands for decayed teeth or tooth surfaces that have been "destroyed" by caries,
- **"M"** stands for missing teeth that were removed due to carious decay, and
- **"F"** stands for filled teeth or tooth surfaces due to caries.

The DMFT index ("T" = teeth) can be calculated from these data from the combined findings for a tooth. If either a D, M, or F component applies to a tooth, the tooth is included in the index. The DMFT value equals the sum of corresponding teeth for an individual; in cohort studies, the DMFT values of the individual members of the cohort are averaged. If wisdom teeth are not included, the DMFT can range from 0 to 28 (**Table 8.1**).

If at least one tooth surface is carious or filled, the entire tooth is identified as a DMF tooth. The DMFT index pro-

Table 8.1   Indices for documentation of caries experience

Variations of the DMF (decayed, missing, filled) index[a]	
DMFT	Sum of carious, extracted and filled permanent teeth due to caries
D$_3$MFT or D$_{3-4}$ MFT	The sum of carious, filled and extracted permanent teeth due to caries with the explicit understanding that D teeth show carious lesions that clinically extend into the dentin (= 3; 4 = pulp involvement)
D$_1$MFT or D$_{1-4}$ MFT	The sum of carious, filled and extracted permanent teeth due to caries with the explicit understanding that D teeth can have carious lesions of every severity (including the clinically visible initial stages)
dmft	Sum of carious, extracted and filled deciduous teeth due to caries
DMFT+ dmft	The grand total of all carious, filled and extracted teeth due to caries of mixed dentition
deft	Sum of carious, filled and extracted deciduous teeth due to caries. The "e" explicitly refers to the teeth that are missing from extraction (in contrast to exfoliated teeth). This is rarely used today
dft	Sum of deciduous carious and filled teeth due to caries. The occasionally difficult assignment of missing teeth in mixed dentition due to caries is thereby circumvented
DMFT/S = 0 deft/s = 0	No decayed (D$_3$ or D$_4$ level), missed, and filled surfaces due to caries. Often expressed as % of a group/population ("caries-free")

[a]The different indices can also refer to tooth surfaces (S instead of T).

vides a more precise description of dental health than just the prevalence. Nevertheless, equating (for example) a tooth which has one surface with a filling to an extracted tooth does not precisely reflect the level of the disease. Consequently, **surveys at the tooth surface level taking into account decayed, filled, or missing components separately** are customary for detailed investigations, especially in analytical or experimental oral epidemiology.

The sum of tooth surfaces affected by caries is the **DMFS value** (S = surfaces). Although the DMFS is the more reasonable survey instrument, the World Health Organization (WHO) prefers the DMFT index, since it is easier to standardize under a range of investigative conditions and is therefore easier to compare.[7,10] Worldwide more investigations are performed with the DMFT, and this index is therefore generally used in comparisons.

By definition, the **DMF index** refers to **caries and its consequences.** It therefore should only include teeth or tooth surfaces that are filled or missing due to caries. This means that teeth missing due to tooth agenesis or other causes, or teeth that are provided with restorations for other reasons than caries, are not included in the index. If permanent teeth are missing, it is generally assumed that they were extracted due to caries unless stated otherwise by the investigated individual, or unless typical configurations (such as the absence of all first premolars) render this scenario implausible. Due to the uncertainty associated with this assumption regarding the actual reason for tooth loss, the DMF index can only approximate the caries incidence in adults and seniors.

Permanent teeth are counted in the DMF index. If the index is to reflect the caries of **deciduous teeth,** the index is in lower case as the **dmf index.** If not otherwise indicated, only permanent teeth are included in mixed dentition; deciduous teeth are not included even if they are carious. However, it may be appropriate to indicate the overall incidence of caries (dmft + DMFT or dmfs + DMFS) in certain investigations/age groups. For epidemiological surveys of caries during the transitional dentition phase, different indices are used such as the **def index** (e = extracted), or the index is restricted to d and f (df index) to differentiate between teeth that are missing from caries or physiological reasons, or to circumvent this differentiation.

For epidemiological purposes, caries in the crown is generally only identified visually and not by using a sharp probe. This procedure corresponds to the WHO recommendations for epidemiological field studies[7] in which a standardized **blunt periodontal probe** is preferred over a dental probe. This takes into consideration the fact that the aggressive use of a sharp probe would not improve the detection and evaluation of occlusal caries, for example. As noted in Chapter 5, the improper use of a sharp-tipped probe to detect and evaluate caries can damage the surface enamel and thereby promote the progression of formerly noncavitated caries lesions.[11,12] A thin probe of course has certain advantages over a thicker, blunt probe when applied without pressure to detect and evaluate changes to approximal caries. Since, however, the time to examine a large number of persons is frequently restricted in epidemiological studies, sharp probes are not used, in order to spare the investigated surface of the crowns from the aggressive use of the sharp instrument.

Restricting the epidemiological investigation of caries to lesions that involve the dentin (D$_3$ lesions) has increasingly been considered inappropriate.[4] Such defects represent an advanced stage of caries. Limiting the noted caries to such defects overlooks developing caries since initial lesions or those limited to the enamel are not included. When only D$_3$MFT changes are considered, it remains unclear whether a reduction of caries includes a reduction of **early stages of caries,** or whether the disease has merely reverted to earlier stages of caries without cavitation. In addition, a problem with this procedure is that a greater percentage of the actual caries experience remains unrecorded as the prevalence of severe forms of caries decreases. For this reason, the occurrence of noncavitated caries lesions is also noted in current surveys (D_1 level[4]) (**Fig. 8.3**). In addition, the lesions can be divided into active and nonactive lesions.

In Health Services Research, it is meaningful to consider the individual components of the DMF index (D, M, or F components). This can yield important information on the Unmet Restorative Treatment (UNT) index. The UNT is the percentage of untreated carious teeth in relation to the overall caries[4]; in children, this is preferably in relation to the sum of untreated and filled teeth (DT * 100/[DT+FT]).

In children and adolescents, caries is not normally distributed[4,5,14] (**Fig. 8.4**). Consequently, the calculations of the DMF average and standard deviation are helpful for comparative purposes, but do not provide a sufficiently precise picture of the disease. In the case of skewed distributions, the distribution frequency of individual levels of findings is useful. Another proposed instrument for describing the epidemiological prevalence of caries in risk groups is the **significant caries index (SiC)**, the DMFT value for the one-third of children with the highest caries incidence.[15] It is not a separate survey instrument and is based on the DMF distribution.[5]

One result of the attempt to identify lesions as early as possible by epidemiological means is to use the **ICDAS criteria** (International Caries Detection and Assessment System, see Chapter 5) for epidemiology.[16] Initial efforts have revealed that this is possible in principle.[17] It remains to be seen whether this detection and assessment system for caries that was validated for identifying caries in occlusal surfaces[18] will gain acceptance, despite the fact that it is more time-consuming,[18] under epidemiological field conditions.

Indices for Root Caries

In addition to coronal caries, the identification of root caries is a field of epidemiological research that is gaining many importance in view of the demographic shift in countries with established market economies. For root caries to occur, the roots have to be exposed. A general assessment is the percentage of individuals who have at least one root with presence of caries (root caries prevalence). A more precise assessment is the number of root surfaces affected by root caries or filled due to caries. Since this total depends on the number of exposed root surfaces, the **root caries index (RCI)** has been established as a method of measuring the severity of the disease. The RCI describes the percentage of carious teeth or root surfaces in relation to exposed surfaces.[19]

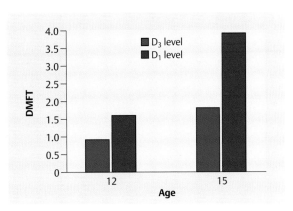

Fig. 8.3 The caries experience in 12- and 15-year-olds in Germany, both not including (D_3 level) and including (D_1 level) initial caries (according to ref. 13).

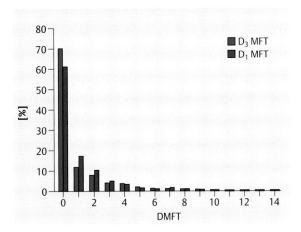

Fig. 8.4 Distribution frequency of the caries experience (DMFT) in 12-year-old children including and excluding D_1 lesions (data from ref. 13).

NOTE

- The prevalence of root caries is equivalent to the percentage of individuals with at least one tooth with root caries (treated or untreated).
- The root caries index (number of tooth surfaces with treated or untreated root caries) generally refers to the number of teeth (tooth surfaces) with exposed roots expressed as a percentage.

With root caries as well, a distinction can be drawn between active and inactive lesions.[20]

Other Indices for Public Health Needs

Additional indices for caries have been proposed for special public health needs. To plan and implement dental treatment systems in nonindustrialized countries, the DMF index is unsuitable, since without further differentiation the D component does not provide any information about more severe decay.[2] A survey instrument that was recently proposed, the **PUFA index,** was developed not only to detect caries, but also to evaluate the clinical consequences of advanced stages of untreated caries and estimate the necessary scope of treatment.[21] The letters of the acronym have the following meanings: **(P)** = pulp involvement, **(U)** = ulceration, **(F)** = fistula, and **(A)** = abscess. The index is particularly suitable for regions without any dental infrastructure.

An additional index, the **FST index,** describes the functionality of the dentition.[22] This index is used to identify the number of filled (F) and healthy (S = sound) teeth (T). Epidemiological data on the mean number of existing original teeth or the prevalence of edentulous individuals are important for public health purposes.[2]

> **NOTE**
>
> Description of dental health for public health needs including caries-related restrictions:
> - PUFA index: The number of decayed teeth with pulp involvement, ulceration, fistulas, and abscess
> - FST index: Number of filled and healthy teeth
> - Information on the mean number of existing original teeth
> - Prevalence of edentulous individuals

Indices for Noncarious Defects

In addition to caries, teeth can show acquired or developmental defects of the enamel or dentin. Indices have been suggested for many of these defects. It should be remembered that 'caries-free' dentition is not synonymous with healthy teeth. In a differential diagnosis, caries lesions can be distinguished from noncarious defects generally by their location (some locations show a predilection for caries), their extent (caries is almost never found in incisal surfaces and rarely affects the entire enamel of the tooth crown), their margins (defects that are developmentally related, frequently have distinct margins), and their distribution in the oral cavity (a number of noncarious defects is symmetrical) (see also Chapters 3 and 5).

Given the continued reduction of the level of caries in children and adolescents, there has been increasing scientific and therapeutic interest in noncarious defects. It is not certain whether this is due to an increase in prevalence (i.e., defects are more easily recognizable in a contest of decreasing caries prevalence) or whether there is a growing awareness of noncarious pathological defects of the dental hard tissues. Examples of dental health indices

for other conditions than caries are the **fluorosis index** (Chapter 12) as well as indices for detecting the loss of tooth substance from **abrasion** (wear) or **erosion.**[23,24]

> **NOTE**
>
> **Note**
> Examples of indices for noncarious defects in the dentin and enamel:
> - Developmental defects (hypoplasia, fluorosis):
>   - Developmental defects of dental enamel (DDE) index
>   - Tooth surface index of fluorosis (TSIF)
>   - Thylstrup–Fejerskov index (TFI) for fluorosis
> - Acquired defects (abrasion, attrition, erosion):
>   - Tooth wear index (TWI)
>   - Basic erosive wear examination (BEWE)

Developmental Defects of the Dental Hard Tissues

Hypoplasia and **Hypomineralization** of enamel and dentin arise while teeth are developing. A distinction is drawn between two types of developmental defects affecting the enamel with and without altering the tooth shape.[25] The latter variant is characterized by discoloration (opacity). Circumscribed time windows in childhood can be identified during which enamel hypoplasia and hypomineralization originate, but it is frequently difficult to ascribe an etiology. In addition to conventional illnesses and malnutrition which can cause hypoplasia and hypomineralization in several (homologous) teeth or all the teeth, impairment of the ameloblasts by fluoride (**fluorosis,** see Chapter 12) or medications can potentially alter the enamel. Single permanent teeth can be altered by local infections of the peri-apex of preceding deciduous teeth, or by trauma to the deciduous teeth that directly affects the permanent tooth underneath a primary tooth.

For epidemiological purposes, the prevalence of enamel hypoplasia and hypomineralization is recorded, and the **DDE index** is used as well (index of developmental defects of dental enamel[26,27]). This index classifies structural anomalies according to the kind, number, location, extent or **demensations** of the defects, and it does not refer to their etiology.

In recent years, there has been an increased incidence of highly hypomineralized or hypoplastic changes in six-year molars and incisors which has been termed **molar-incisor hypomineralization (MIH).** The etiology of these generally sharply delimited changes has not been satisfactorily clarified, although the influence of common illnesses and antibiotic therapy is suspected.[28]

In view of the different and sometimes ambiguous origins as well as the different locations and types of hypoplasia, the prevalence of MIH is generally noted. The extent or severity of the defects is noted less frequently, since the DDE index is held to be insufficient for this purpose.[29] There is, however, a consensus regarding which symptoms should be used to indicate the MIH prevalence for epidemiological purposes (including circumscribed opacities, posteruptive enamel breakdown, and atypically placed restorations). Various indices have been suggested for indicating the severity of MIH, which have yet to be uniformly applied.

> **NOTE**
>
> Criteria for the epidemiological recording of molar-incisor hypomineralization (MIH)[30]:
> - Circumscribed opacity
> - Posteruptive enamel breakdown
> - Atypically placed restorations
> - Extractions due to hypomineralization
> - Non-eruption of molars and incisors

Acquired Defects of the Dental Hard Tissues

Among the acquired noncarious defects, **erosion** from the effects of acids and **attrition** and **abrasion** due to mechanical forces are the most significant. A series of indices has been proposed to identify them for clinical and epidemiological purposes.[31] A distinction is drawn between indices that define changes to the enamel and dentin apart from their etiology (such as the tooth wear index)[24] and indices that identify changes with specific etiologies such as **erosion** (e.g., the **basic erosive wear examination; BEWE**).[32] Of the etiology-independent indices, the **tooth wear index** (TWI) has gained wide acceptance. This includes the occurrence, average number of abraded teeth, and severity of the change in which each tooth surface is subject to a defect evaluation with five gradations.[24] These gradations, which estimate the depth of the defects, render the index unsuitable for large epidemiological studies. A simplified version (the simplified TWI[33]) assesses the presence of exposed dentin using four levels.

Erosion is defined as acid-related damage to the tooth surface without bacteria being involved. A series of erosion indices have been proposed in response to the increasing clinical and scientific interest in erosive tooth damage. In this case as well, the range of index definitions extends from the more complex in which separate tooth surfaces are evaluated using different criteria (such as the erosion index according to Lussi[34]) to simple scoring systems that can be used in epidemiology (e.g., the BEWE).[23] The BEWE uses a four-level scale to identify the most significant erosion in each sextant, and the total score is used for clinical recommendations.

> **NOTE**
>
> Basic erosive wear examination; BEWE[23]:
> - **Score of 0:** No enamel loss
> - **Score of 1:** Initial loss of surface structure
> - **Score of 2:** Significant damage with loss of enamel comprising less than 50% of the tooth surface
> - **Score of 3:** Significant damage with loss of enamel comprising more than 50% of the tooth surface
>
> The highest value is recorded for each sextant.
> The sum of the scores equals the cumulative BEWE score.

The use of erosion indices (e.g. BEWE) presumes that erosive defects are identified according to recognized definitions. The indices reach their limits where combined defects from erosive and mechanical origins overlap.

Occurrence and Distribution of Caries

The epidemiology of caries can be investigated far into the past by examining **skulls.** These investigations have revealed that caries has always existed, but its prevalence was much less than today.[5,35,36] Industrialization was associated with an epidemic spread of caries (**Fig. 8.6**). Since scientific recording of caries experience started after the implementation of the DMF index, an increasing caries rate has been documented in industrialized countries, interrupted only by food shortages, for example, during World War II.[5,35] This trend has reversed in industrialized countries since the 1970s. In parallel, the prevalence of caries in nonindustrialized countries has rapidly increased. In the early 1980s, less caries was recorded in industrialized countries than in nonindustrialized countries for the first time[35,37] (**Fig. 8.5**).

The development of caries lesions is not evenly distributed over the entire lifespan; the risk of caries is elevated within certain **age groups.** This especially relates to the phases during the eruption of the primary teeth and permanent molars in the oral cavity.[38] There is a particular interest in collecting epidemiological data on these age groups. During the phases with an elevated risk of new caries, distinct locations on the tooth (caries predilection sites) are in particular danger in regard to caries development. Of the permanent teeth, the occlusal surfaces of the six-year molar are particularly affected by caries, followed by the approximal surfaces are subject to an elevated risk starting in adolescence.[39] In adults and seniors, the root surface is primarily where new caries originates (**Fig. 8.6**).

In consideration of this risk distribution, the WHO recommends collecting epidemiological caries data for 5-year-olds, 12-year-olds, and 15-year-olds. The WHO also recommends investigating the prevalence of caries

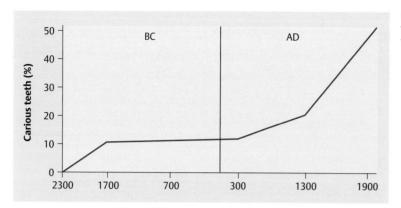

Fig. 8.5 Percentage of carious teeth as revealed by investigated skulls in Greece (data from ref. 36).

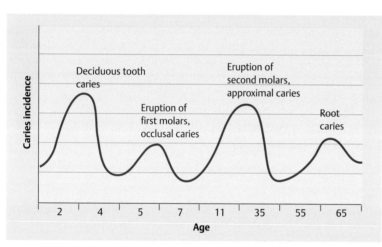

Fig. 8.6 Phases of different caries incidence (after ref. 38 with the addition of root caries).

in the additional age groups of 35–45-year-old adults and 65–74-year-old seniors.

Trends in Caries Epidemiology

Global Considerations

The most comprehensive international collection of data on the prevalence of caries exists for **12-year-olds**.[40] According to the WHO,[7] this group is best suited for international comparisons since 12-year-olds can be easily accessed through the school systems in most countries. This makes epidemiological surveys easier to organize. However, the second molars have not yet erupted in the oral cavity of many 12-year-old children, and the premolars and canines have only existed in the oral milieu for a short while, which can contribute to a lower prevalence of caries in this age group. When **15-year-old** adolescents are included in epidemiological field studies of caries, these teeth have been present in the mouth for longer.[7]

Today, the prevalence of caries in children and adolescents is very low in most industrialized countries. The current figures on the prevalence and incidence of caries

for specific age groups are accessible in a database maintained by the WHO[40] (**Fig. 8.7**).

Children and Adolescents

A series of recent epidemiological field studies in countries with established market economies, where individual and group prophylactic measures have been pursued for a long time on a broad basis, reveal a significant reduction of the mean caries experience in the permanent teeth of children and adolescents over recent decades[7,41–45] (**Fig. 8.8**).

The trend of caries experience in children and adolescents is revealed by representative national studies, for example, in Germany (**German oral health studies I–IV**[13,14]). The most recent study, in 2005, was a repetition of the survey conducted in 1997 using the same methodology and sampling approach, which allows the comparison of the changes in the epidemiological findings regarding caries. Initial representative studies on the caries experience in Germany were conducted in 1989 and 1992. The 2005 survey revealed a very low DMFT value of 0.7 for 12-year-olds (**Fig. 8.9**). A comparatively low DMFT value of 1.8 was also found for 15-year-olds.

It can be assumed that the use of fissure sealants was an important factor in the significant reduction of caries in

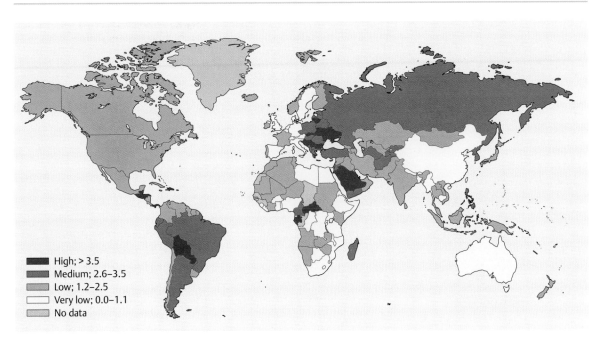

Fig. 8.7 Average number of carious teeth either decayed, missing, or filled (DMFT) in 12-year-old children (2008). Worldwide average: 2.0; highest value: Croatia 6.7; lowest values: Ruanda, Tanzania, Togo 0.3 (after ref. 64).

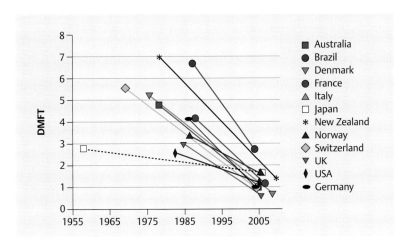

Fig. 8.8 Reduction of caries experience (DMFT) in 12-year-old children in various countries over recent decades (after ref. 40).

12-year-olds in Germany. At least one tooth was sealed in about 75% of 12- and 15-year-olds. These children and adolescents manifested significantly less caries than their contemporaries.[14]

With an average of 0.9 teeth with demineralized or initially carious enamel, there were more teeth that revealed an initial stage of caries compared with the D_3MFT (0.7) which only reflects deeper caries lesions plus the treatment due to caries.[13] This underscores the necessity of ongoing preventive care, even when the caries experience is decreasing. It should not be assumed from the data revealing a reduction of the caries experience that the importance of primary and secondary preventive care has decreased in any way. In addition, positive changes of the caries experience in children and adolescents

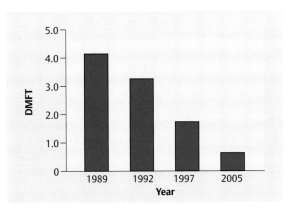

Fig. 8.9 Significant reduction of the D_3MFT (~85%) in 12-year-olds in Germany from 1989 to 2005 (data from refs. 13, 14).

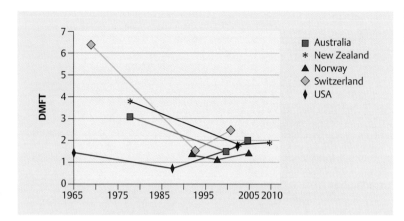

Fig. 8.10 Reduction and rise of caries experience in five- and six-year-old children in different countries (data from ref. 40)

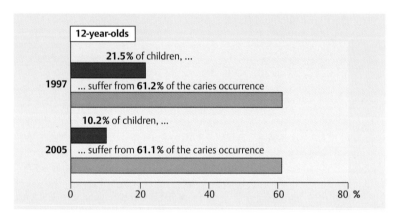

Fig. 8.11 Increasing polarization has occurred in recent years with the preponderance of caries being not prevalent in a small group of people in Germany. Whereas around 20% of 12-year-olds experienced ca. 60% of the total caries in 1997 for that age group, the number of children fell to ca. 10% in 2005. (Data from ref. 13).

should not keep us from recognizing that the situation regarding **deciduous teeth** is unsatisfactory. Many countries report a halt in the reduction or even a rise of the caries experience in primary teeth (**Fig. 8.10**).[8,45–47,]

Association of Caries and Social Status

The reduction of caries experience is not evenly distributed among all individuals in industrialized countries. In contrast, caries prevalence and experience are significantly polarized among children and adolescents[5,8]: the majority of caries lesions in their age group occurs in the mouths of comparatively few individuals (**Fig. 8.11**). Members of the lower social classes experience more caries and have more extracted teeth.[5,13,48,49]

NOTE

The reduction of the caries experience in the permanent teeth of children and adolescents in industrialized countries is subject to significant social stratification.

Adults and Seniors

A general reduction of caries prevalence is also not noticed among adults and seniors, even though the number of extracted teeth has decreased.[50,51] However, the epidemiological data for adults is incomplete.[48] Whereas studies are frequently performed for adolescents, there are only a few studies on 20–35-year-olds and 35–44-year-olds. At present, there is little information on certainary groups, teeth, and conditions being associated with increased caries experience (**Fig. 8.12**). Prospective studies suggest that the caries process in young adults advances slowly but continuously, especially in approximal surfaces.[39,40]

A hypothesis has been aired that the success of caries prevention in children and adolescents will have significant positive consequences on the "caries burden" in adults.[5] This has already been confirmed in adults up to 45 years old in the United States[50] and also to some extent for adults and senior citizens in Germany in 2005 (**Fig. 8.13**). This effect was especially due to the reduced number of caries-related tooth extractions, which was also significantly associated with affiliation to a higher social stratum.[14] From a long-term perspective, a rise in quality of life associated with oral health can be anticipated in industrialized countries due to the **reduced level of edentulism.**

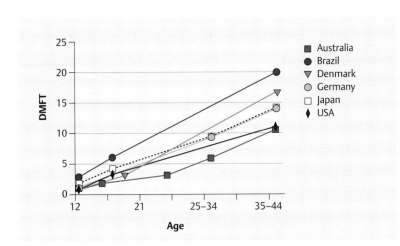

Fig. 8.12 Continuous linear rise of the caries experience in young adults (data from ref. 40).

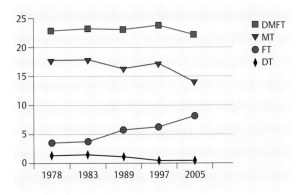

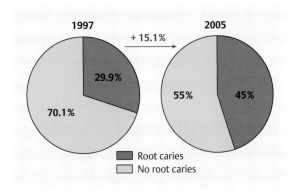

Fig. 8.13 DMFT index and its individual components for 65–74-year-old seniors in western Germany from 1978 to 2005 (data from ref. 13).

Fig. 8.14 Increase in the prevalence of root caries in seniors over recent years in Germany (data from ref. 13).

Root Caries

The increased retention of one's own teeth is also associated with a significant rise in the prevalence of root surface caries. For example, in 2005 in Germany, 21.5% of adults and 45% of seniors had at least one carious or filled root surface (**Fig. 8.14**). The root caries index (RCI) that refers to the number of exposed root surfaces was 9% in adults and 17% in seniors.[13] For the senior cohort, the prevalence found in Germany corresponds to the prevalence of about 50% reported in the United States in the NHANES III (National Health and Nutrition Examination) survey.[52] In Great Britain, 45% of over-65-year-olds have at least one tooth with a restored root surface.[51] In all these countries, root caries is also associated with significant social stratification. These figures reveal a strong need for preventive intervention to avoid the need for invasive treatment of root surface caries.

> **NOTE**
>
> The success of preventive and restorative dentistry (keeping more teeth until a higher age) is associated with a rise in root caries.

Occurrence and Distribution of Noncarious Defects

Developmental Defects

Widely varying numbers have been reported on the prevalence of hypoplasia and hypomineralization. This may be associated with the different indices used for collecting data; nonetheless, actually deviating frequencies of developmental or acquired hypoplasia are discernible. It should be considered that numerous publications analyze the relationship between various factors/diseases and developmental changes, which might lead to the misinterpretation that the prevalence of these is high in general.

The prevalence of **developmental enamel defects** in the general population is indicated as being 4%–60% for deciduous teeth[53] and about 50% for the permanent dentention.[25] Defects in the shape of the enamel are much rarer; these have been observed in 4%–9% of children. Chapter 12 addresses the etiology and prevalence of dental fluorosis.

Clinical and scientific interest in **molar-incisor hypomineralization** (MIH) has increased significantly in recent years. A parallel increase in prevalence rates has been simultaneously reported. A series of systematic reviews[54] has reported a prevalence of 10%–19% in children. Other studies[55,56] describe a greater spread (2%–40%). The underlying reasons for the rise in prevalence remain unclear and are presently being researched.

> **NOTE**
>
> - The prevalence of noncarious defects in the enamel and dentin varies widely across the globe.
> - The prevalence of MIH is apparently rising.

Acquired Defects of Enamel and Dentin

The data on the prevalence of acquired mechanical and chemically-related defects in enamel and dentin vary widely. Since abrasion and erosion are physiological changes that occur while chewing food over the course of life, it is difficult to identify pathological stages, which should always be done by relating the findings to the age of the investigated individual.[32]

The relationship between age and the prevalence of **abrasion** also applies to the deciduous dentition. The prevalence ranges between 0% and 82%.[57] For permanent teeth in children and adolescents, prevalence rates from 0% to 54% have been reported with no discernible relationship to age. In contrast, increasing levels of abrasion are found in older age groups. The prevalence of pathological abrasion ranges from 3% in 20-year-olds to 17% in 70-year-olds.[30]

With regard to **erosion,** prevalence rates of 6%–50% have been reported for preschool children, while rates of 11%–100% have been reported for adolescents and 18%–82% for adults[58]. Another systematic review found an erosion prevalence of 10%–80% for children and adolescents.[59] The BEWE has only been used in a few reports to date. In a cohort of 14–16-year-old adolescents with an erosion prevalence of 58%, the use of the BEWE was shown to be suitable under both scientific and practical aspects.[60]

The prevalence of erosive defects in enamel and dentin apparently differs in different populations. The use of different indices and the examination of different age groups, dentitions, and tooth surfaces need to be considered as additional reasons for widely deviating observations. Representative epidemiological studies on the occurrence of dental erosion are rare. A prevalence of 46% has been reported for 13–19-year-old adolescents in the United States[61]; in Iceland, erosion was found in 16% of 12-year-olds and in 31% of 15-year-olds.[62]

Many investigations reveal a trend toward an increase in the prevalence of erosions.[58] This trend may arise from changes in diet or oral hygiene as well as the increased retention of teeth and decrease in caries therapy. From the submitted data, no conclusions can be drawn regarding public health needs, treatment requirements, or effects on the quality of life of the affected individuals.

> **NOTE**
>
> - The data on the prevalence of erosion show high variations.
> - From the available data on the prevalence of erosive tooth defects, it is difficult to discern the clinical relevance of these changes for the individual or treatment needs.

SUMMARY

Caries epidemiology provides information about the prevalence, distribution and severity of caries in populations or individual subgroups. Although epidemiological investigations are primarily observational in nature and provide descriptive information, suitable study designs are capable of providing information on the status of dental care and treatment needs, on cost-benefit ratios, and public health needs. By applying sociological survey instruments, caries epidemiology can also provide additional insight.

Information on caries is expressed as the prevalence in terms of percentage in the group or population studied with one or more caries lesions (treated and decayed) as well as by the mean number of carious teeth or surfaces (caries experience) in the group or population studied. Data on caries experience are presented by using the long established **DMF index** which is generally used for specific **reference age groups** (5- and 12-year-old children, 15-year-old adolescents, 35–44-year-old adults, and 65–74-year-old seniors). This index identifies carious changes in tooth crowns and their therapeutic consequences such as fillings or extractions. The D component may involve only decayed surfaces which are cavitated or noncavitated lesions as well.

The prevalence of caries in children and adolescents is much lower at present in most industrialized countries than it was 40 years ago. The initial stages of caries comprise the majority of the caries load. However, the reduction of caries has been associated with a significant **polarization of the caries experience.** In the deciduous dentition, the **reduction of caries** has stagnated. Some studies reveal an initial caries reduction in adults. The decreased percentage of extracted teeth is associated with an increased number of teeth with root caries. For this reason and in consideration of initial caries, preventive treatment strategies remain necessary.

Recent years have seen a growing interest in the clinical and epidemiological aspects of **noncarious defects of enamel and dentin.** A series of indices have been proposed to assess such changes for epidemiological purposes. The prevalence of noncarious defects vary widely in the available data. The DDE index is useful for precisely identifying developmental defects, and the tooth wear index is helpful for scoring acquired defects; the BEWE index can be used to document erosion. Of the numerous indices, no single one has become generally accepted which successfully accommodates the competing goal for complexity, precision, and practicality.

REFERENCES

1. Arbeitsgruppe Epidemiologische Methoden der Deutschen Arbeitsgemeinschaft für Epidemiologie (DAE). Leitlinien und Empfehlungen zur Sicherung von Guter Epidemiologischer Praxis (GEP) (April 2004). http://www.gesundheitsforschung-bmbf.de/_media/Empfehlungen_GEP.pdf. Accessed July 17, 2011

2. Schiffner U, Jordan RA, Michaelis W. Clinical Practice Guideline: Aims and methods of the epidemiological recording of oral diseases. [In German] Dtsch Zahnarztl Z 2010;65:496–502

3. Deutsche Arbeitsgemeinschaft für Epidemiologie (DAE), Arbeitskreis Wissenschaft der Konferenz der Datenschutzbeauftragen des Bundes und der Länder. Epidemiologie und Datenschutz (1998). http://www.dgepi.de. Accessed July 14, 2011

4. Pitts NB. Diagnostic tools and measurements – impact on appropriate care. Community Dent Health 1992;10:1–9

5. Burt BA, Eklund SA. Dentistry, Dental Practice and the Community. 6th ed. St. Louis: Elsevier Saunders; 2005

6. Bloemendal E, de Vet HC, Bouter LM. The value of bitewing radiographs in epidemiological caries research: a systematic review of the literature. J Dent 2004;32(4):255–264

7. World Health Organization (WHO). Oral Health Surveys. Basic methods. 4th ed. Geneva: World Health Organization; 1997

8. Pitts NB, Boyles J, Nugent ZJ, Thomas N, Pine CM. The dental caries experience of 5-year-old children in Great Britain (2005/6). Surveys co-ordinated by the British Association for the study of community dentistry. Community Dent Health 2007;24(1):59–63

9. Klein H, Palmer CE, Knutson JW. Studies on dental caries. I. Dental status and dental needs of elementary school children. Public Health Rep 1938;53:751–765

10. World Health Organization (WHO). Oral health global indicators for 2000. Geneva: World Health Organization; 1984

11. Ekstrand K, Qvist V, Thylstrup A. Light microscope study of the effect of probing in occlusal surfaces. Caries Res 1987;21(4):368–374

12. Lussi A. Impact of including or excluding cavitated lesions when evaluating methods for the diagnosis of occlusal caries. Caries Res 1996;30(6):389–393

13. Institut der Deutschen Zahnärzte I (IDZ). Vierte Deutsche Mundgesundheitsstudie (DMS IV). Köln: Deutscher Ärzteverlag; 2006

14. Schiffner U, Hoffmann T, Kerschbaum T, Micheelis W. Oral health in German children, adolescents, adults and senior citizens in 2005. Community Dent Health 2009;26(1):18–22

15. Bratthall D. Introducing the Significant Caries Index together with a proposal for a new global oral health goal for 12-year-olds. Int Dent J 2000;50(6):378–384

16. Ismail AI. Visual and visuo-tactile detection of dental caries. J Dent Res 2004;83 (Spec. C):C56–C66

17. Kühnisch J, Berger S, Goddon I, Senkel H, Pitts N, Heinrich-Weltzien R. Occlusal caries detection in permanent molars according to WHO basic methods, ICDAS II and laser fluorescence measurements. Community Dent Oral Epidemiol 2008;36(6):475–484

18. Braga MM, Oliveira LB, Bonini GA, Bönecker M, Mendes FM. Feasibility of the International Caries Detection and Assessment System (ICDAS-II) in epidemiological surveys and comparability with standard World Health Organization criteria. Caries Res 2009;43(4):245–249

19. Katz RV, Hazen SP, Chilton NW, Mumma RD Jr. Prevalence and intraoral distribution of root caries in an adult population. Caries Res 1982;16(3):265–271

20. Ravald N, Birkhed D. Factors associated with active and inactive root caries in patients with periodontal disease. Caries Res 1991;25(5):377–384

21. Monse B, Heinrich-Weltzien R, Benzian H, Holmgren C, van Palenstein Helderman W. PUFA—an index of clinical consequences of untreated dental caries. Community Dent Oral Epidemiol 2010;38(1):77–82

22. Sheiham A, Maizels J, Maizels A. New composite indicators of dental health. Community Dent Health 1987;4(4):407–414

23. Bartlett D, Ganss C, Lussi A. Basic Erosive Wear Examination (BEWE): a new scoring system for scientific and clinical needs. Clin Oral Investig 2008;12(Suppl 1):S65–S68

24. Smith BGN, Knight JK. An index for measuring the wear of teeth. Br Dent J 1984;156(12):435–438

25. Pieper K. Zahnanomalien und ihre Versorgung. In: Einwag J, Pieper K, Hrsg. Kinderzahnheilkunde. München: Elsevier; 2008: 297–312

26. FDI Commission on Oral Health Research and Epidemiology. An epidemiological index of developmental defects of dental enamel (DDE Index). Commission on Oral Health, Research and Epidemiology. Int Dent J 1982;32(2):159–167

27. FDI Commission on Oral Health Research and Epidemiology. A review of the developmental defects of enamel index (DDE Index). Int Dent J 1992;42(6):411–426

28. Alaluusua S. Aetiology of Molar-Incisor-Hypomineralisation (MIH): A systematic review. Eur Arch Paediatr Dent 2010; 11(2):53–58

29. Weerheijm KL, Duggal M, Mejàre I, et al. Judgement criteria for molar incisor hypomineralisation (MIH) in epidemiologic studies: a summary of the European meeting on MIH held in Athens, 2003. Eur J Pediatr Dent 2003;4:110–113

30. Van't Spijker A, Rodriguez JM, Kreulen CM, Bronkhorst EM, Bartlett DW, Creugers NH. Prevalence of tooth wear in adults. Int J Prosthodont 2009;22(1):35–42

31. Bardsley PF. The evolution of tooth wear indices. Clin Oral Investig 2008;12(Suppl 1):S15–S19

32. Bartlett D, Dugmore C. Pathological or physiological erosion—is there a relationship to age? Clin Oral Investig 2008;12(Suppl 1):S27–S31

33. Bardsley PF, Taylor S, Milosevic A. Epidemiological studies of tooth wear and dental erosion in 14-year-old children in North West England. Part 1: The relationship with water fluoridation

and social deprivation. Br Dent J 2004;197(7):413–416, discussion 399

34. Lussi A. Dental erosion clinical diagnosis and case history taking. Eur J Oral Sci 1996;104(2(Pt 2)):191–198

35. Sheiham A. Changing trends in dental caries. Int J Epidemiol 1984;13(2):142–147

36. Sognnaes RF. A survey of dental caries in Greece. N Y State Dent J 1949;15(1):15–21

37. Downer MC. Changing patterns of disease in the Western world. In: Guggenheim B, ed. Cariology Today. Basel: Karger; 1984:1–12

38. Axelsson P. The effect of a needs-related caries preventive program in children and young adults – results after 20 years. BMC Oral Health 2006;6(Suppl 1):S7

39. Mejàre I, Källestål C, Stenlund H, Johansson H. Caries development from 11 to 22 years of age: a prospective radiographic study. Prevalence and distribution. Caries Res 1998;32(1):10–16

40. World Health Organization (WHO) Collaborating Centre for Education, Training and Research in Oral Health. WHO Oral Health Country/Area Profile Project (CAPP). Country Oral Health Profiles. http://www.whocollab.od.mah.se. Accessed July 14, 2011

41. Brown LJ, Wall TP, Lazar V. Trends in total caries experience: permanent and primary teeth. J Am Dent Assoc 2000;131(2):223–231

42. Hugoson A, Koch G, Göthberg C, et al. Oral health of individuals aged 3–80 years in Jönköping, Sweden during 30 years (1973–2003). I. Review of findings on dental care habits and knowledge of oral health. Swed Dent J 2005;29(4):125–138

43. Pitts NB, Boyles J, Nugent ZJ, Thomas N, Pine CM. The dental caries experience of 11-year-old children in Great Britain. Surveys coordinated by the British Association for the Study of Community Dentistry in 2004 / 2005. Community Dent Health 2006;23(1):44–57

44. Pitts NB, Chestnutt IG, Evans D, White D, Chadwick B, Steele JG. The dentinal caries experience of children in the United Kingdom, 2003. Br Dent J 2006;200(6):313–320

45. Truin GJ, van Rijkom HM, Mulder J, van't Hof MA. Caries trends 1996–2002 among 6- and 12-year-old children and erosive wear prevalence among 12-year-old children in The Hague. Caries Res 2005;39(1):2–8

46. Dye BA, Arevalo O, Vargas CM. Trends in paediatric dental caries by poverty status in the United States, 1988–1994 and 1999–2004. Int J Paediatr Dent 2010;20(2):132–143

47. Haugejorden O, Birkeland JM. Evidence for reversal of the caries decline among Norwegian children. Int J Paediatr Dent 2002;12(5):306–315

48. Pitts NB, Fejerskov O, von der Fehr FR. Caries epidemiology, with special emphasis on diagnostic standards. In: Fejerskov O, Kidd EAM, eds. Dental Caries: The Disease and its Clinical Management. Oxford: Blackwell Munksgaard; 2003:141–163

49. Truin GJ, König KG, Bronkhorst EM, Frankenmolen F, Mulder J, van't Hof MA. Time trends in caries experience of 6- and 12-year-old children of different socioeconomic status in The Hague. Caries Res 1998;32(1):1–4

50. Brown LJ, Wall TP, Lazar V. Trends in caries among adults 18 to 45 years old. J Am Dent Assoc 2002;133(7):827–834

51. Kelly M, Steele J, Nuttall N, et al. Adult Dental Health Survey. Oral Health in the United Kingdom 1998. London: Stationery Office; 2000

52. Winn DM, Brunelle JA, Selwitz RH, et al. Coronal and root caries in the dentition of adults in the United States, 1988–1991. J Dent Res 1996; 75(Spec No)642–651

53. Seow WK. Enamel hypoplasia in the primary dentition: a review. ASDC J Dent Child 1991;58(6):441–452

54. Kellerhoff NM, Lussi A. "Molar-incisor hypomineralization". [Article in French, German] Schweiz Monatsschr Zahnmed 2004;114(3):243–253

55. Jälevik B. Prevalence and diagnosis of Molar-Incisor-Hypomineralisation (MIH): A systematic review. Eur Arch Paediatr Dent 2010;11(2):59–64

56. Willmott NS, Bryan RA, Duggal MS. Molar-incisor-hypomineralisation: a literature review. Eur Arch Paediatr Dent 2008;9(4):172–179

57. Kreulen CM, Van't Spijker A, Rodriguez JM, Bronkhorst EM, Creugers NH, Bartlett DW. Systematic review of the prevalence of tooth wear in children and adolescents. Caries Res 2010;44(2):151–159

58. Jaeggi T, Lussi A. Prevalence, incidence and distribution of erosion. Monogr Oral Sci 2006;20:44–65

59. Taji S, Seow WK. A literature review of dental erosion in children. Aust Dent J 2010;55(4):358–367, quiz 475

60. Margaritis V, Mamai-Homata E, Koletsi-Kounari H, Polychronopoulou A. Evaluation of three different scoring systems for dental erosion: a comparative study in adolescents. J Dent 2011;39(1):88–93

61. McGuire J, Szabo A, Jackson S, Bradley TG, Okunseri C. Erosive tooth wear among children in the United States: relationship to race/ethnicity and obesity. Int J Paediatr Dent 2009;19(2):91–98

62. Arnadottir IB, Holbrook WP, Eggertsson H, et al. Prevalence of dental erosion in children: a national survey. Community Dent Oral Epidemiol 2010;38(6):521–526

From Diagnostics to Therapy

Sebastian Paris, Hendrik Meyer-Lueckel, Kim R. Ekstrand

9

The dental profession remains strongly influenced by a "drill and fill" mentality, that is, the restorative reconstruction of teeth decayed from caries. In recent decades, great progress has been made owing to the development of effective dental materials and techniques that allow tooth-colored minimally invasive restorations of teeth with advanced caries stages. Although this progress represents a significant accomplishment, it should not be forgotten that the restoration of carious defects using dental materials is palliative in nature and not curative.[1] If caries therapy is restricted to the **alleviation of symptoms** without **healing** the disease by addressing etiological factors, new carious defects will occur. As noted in Chapter 4, the process of caries depends on a complex interaction of pathogenic and protective etiological factors. To address the origin of caries, one or more (risk) factors needs to be permanently influenced. Our profession is in the process of change in which the focus of dentistry is slowly shifting from classic surgical restoration toward controling the causes of caries.[2]

A proper diagnosis is a precondition for the right treatment. Therefore, this chapter will discuss the diagnostic basics for an early and cause-related treatment of caries. In addition, this chapter provides an overview of the different approaches and measures for the control of caries, which will be discussed in greater detail in subsequent chapters. The various procedures will be presented along with the associated indications for the different stages and types of caries. In particular, the following topics will be addressed:

- Special aspects of dental diagnostics
- Dealing with diagnostic errors
- Different therapeutic approaches
- Therapeutic options for different predilection sites
- Specific measures that are indicated for specific stages of disease

From Diagnostics...

A proper diagnosis is a prerequisite for the selection of an appropriate therapy. When treating caries, one is frequently tempted to restrict the diagnosis and therapy to individual teeth since they manifest the most acute signs and related symptoms. However, as indicated in the previous chapters, caries is a disease that is not primarily restricted to single teeth; it originates from the patient's behavior (nutrition, oral hygiene, etc.) and the protective influential factors in the oral cavity (such as saliva). For this reason, caries is rarely restricted to single teeth and is typically found in several teeth. The diagnosis should therefore take into consideration the entire patient and not be limited to individual teeth.

Diagnostics at the Individual Level

The aim of patient-level diagnostics is to assess the patient's **caries risk** (i.e., the probability that the patient will develop new caries lesions in the future). This is especially useful when determining the individual need for therapy and diagnostic follow-up interval. In addition, the goal of assessing the risk of caries is to **identify and assess the patient's relevant individual risk factors**. Caries is a disease with several causes, and the weight given to the pathogenic and various protective factors differs from patient to patient, and at different times for individual patients. To arrive at an appropriate caries therapy that addresses the main underlying causes, the patient's relevant risk factors must be identified, and the protective factors must be analyzed. Then a risk-related treatment can be established.

Diagnostics at the Tooth Level

How is Caries Diagnosed?

In medicine, a diagnosis is defined as "the art or act of identifying a disease from its signs and symptoms."[3] In this classic form of diagnosis, the challenge is to ascribe a pattern of certain signs (objective) and symptoms (subjective) that the patient manifests to an underlying disease and exclude other potential diseases in a differential diagnosis.[4] For caries, this form of diagnosis is still found in many countries without a highly developed health care system, and is often used for dental emergency care. The patient appears with complaints (signs and symptoms), and the suspected cause (such as caries, pulpitis) is identified and delimited from all other causes (such as acute periodontitis) in a differential diagnosis. If caries is identified as the cause of the symptoms, it is frequently in an advanced stage and requires emergency treatment.

In many countries with a highly developed health care system, the diagnosis of caries uses a different approach that does not precisely fit the above definition.[5,6] Caries is diagnosed primarily in regular dental health care visits, and the goal is the early detection of the disease. The patient generally does not voice any complaints. In this context, diagnosis takes on the character of a screening. That is, the dentist looks initially for the specific patterns or signs of a known disease (caries in this case), and the number of differential diagnoses for these patterns of signs is very limited.[6] The challenge in this form of diagnosis is detection, including early stages (using appropriate methods), the correct assessment of the lesion, and the subsequent choice of an appropriate therapy. Although this form of diagnosis is very different from classic medical diagnosis,[6] it is not restricted to dentistry and is becoming increasingly relevant in other disciplines of general medicine in which secondary, preventive strategies are pursued in the early diagnosis and therapy of diseases (such as colon cancer or coronary heart disease). Screening examinations enable early detection and consequently non-, micro-, or minimally invasive therapies.

One risk associated with screening examinations is false positive findings that can lead to overtreatment (see below).[7] The intervals between dental check-ups primarily depend on the patient's individual caries risk (see Chapter 7 and 24). Beyond the screening for caries, other oral diseases such as periodontitis and diseases of the mucosa are screened in these check-ups, and the individual's risk of these diseases is also considered.

NOTE

In many countries with a highly developed health care system, the diagnosis of caries has a screening character. This allows an early diagnosis (and therapy) of the disease, but there is a higher risk of false positive findings.

The Truth About Caries

From the aforementioned, we could conclude that it is recommendable to detect the signs of caries as early as possible, so that the disease can be identified and treated promptly. Such an approach is based on an **essentialistic perspective**. That is, it is assumed that a (hidden) process or disease called "caries" exists, which converts the causes of caries into the typical signs and symptoms of the disease (**Fig. 9.1**).[8] Consequently, the aim of diagnostics is to reveal the underlying hidden disease by highly precise methods to find out the "truth", whether caries is there or not. But where does caries actually start? The most characteristic sign of caries is a mineral loss of dental hard tissues. However, the physiological fluctuations of pH in the oral cavity constantly cause mineral losses and subsequent mineral gains. On the one hand, beginning mineral losses (incipient lesions), which might only be detectable with special diagnostic tools, often have no pathological value and may remineralize without intervention. On the other hand, these lesions might also represent early stages of later cavities. According to the essentialistic concept, which assumes the existence of a disease independent of its signs and symptoms, one would say that caries is the underlying cause of these lesions.[8] Thus, many people will be classified as "caries diseased." This might be unjustified, since not every individual will develop cavities from early lesions, possibly causing symptoms and functional problems. From the above said it becomes clear that it is not possible to define a commonly accepted start/beginning of caries.

The **nominalistic approach**, therefore, assumes that there is no disease called "caries" which is independent of the signs and symptoms; rather, we have assigned the name "caries" to the pathological process as well as to its signs and symptoms (**Fig. 9.1**). The logical result is that only the signs and symptoms and not the hidden disease are problematic and hence relevant to the patient. This also means that there is no "truth" about caries: whether a tooth or somebody has caries or not depends on our definition.

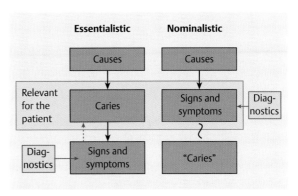

Fig. 9.1 Essentialistic and nominalistic approaches (modified from ref. 8).

The nominalistic approach has consequences for caries diagnostics. Because here, in contrast to the essentialistic concept, no disease is searched for behind the symptoms—it does not make sense to search for early abstract signs of the disease with more and more precise diagnostic tests. In the nominalistic approach, the only the diagnostic information that is relevant is that which yields therapies which will result in a **health benefit for the patient**.[1,8] Strictly speaking, all other diagnoses are then superfluous. This yields a problem, since the quality of diagnostic methods used in scientific examinations is generally measured against their ability in determining signs and symptoms compared with a "gold standard." Often microscopic or laboratory methods are employed in such investigations as gold standards which can detect abstract signs of the disease with high accuracy. The relevance of these signs detected by the gold standards in the prognosis of a disease or the success of the related therapy is generally not investigated, since then such investigations are very time-consuming and expensive. For example, essentialistic thinking resulted in the common practice that in scientific studies diagnostic tools were tested for their ability to detect "dentin caries," that is, the histological effect on dentin, which could be easily proven with microscopic techniques in vitro. Consequently, in the clinic the discovery of discolored dentin during cavity preparation was interpreted as a confirmation of the diagnosis "dentin caries," meaning "this tooth requires a restoration." Today, it is assumed that the histological effect on dentin per se is only of subordinate importance for the prognosis, and consequently in the diagnosis of caries. Rather, cavitation in the surface of the lesion appears to be relevant to the prognosis, and hence diagnosis, in the majority of cases.

NOTE

The aim of caries diagnosis is to record and describe the signs and symptoms of the disease, caries. Diagnostic information is only relevant when it is relevant to therapy.

Table 9.1   Cross table for a diagnostic testing of healthy patients (healthy) versus unhealthy patients (unhealthy)[a]

		Disease		
		Yes	**No**	
Test	**Positive**	True positive	False positive	**Positive predictive value:** $\dfrac{\text{No. true positive}}{\text{No. all positive tested}}$
	Negative	False negative	True negative	**Negative predictive value:** $\dfrac{\text{No. true negative}}{\text{No. all negative tested}}$
		Sensitivity: $\dfrac{\text{No. of true positive}}{\text{No. all unhealthy}}$	**Specificity:** $\dfrac{\text{No. true negative}}{\text{No. all healthy}}$	

[a]In an ideal case, all unhealthy are tested positive (true positive), and all healthy are tested negative (true negative). In reality, the test also gives negative results for healthy (false negative) and positive results for healthy (false positive). The sensitivity expresses the proportion of unhealthy who were correctly tested as unhealthy. The specificity indicates the proportion of the healthy who were correctly identified as being healthy. The positive predictive value expresses the proportion of those who were tested positive who are actually unhealthy. The negative predictive value expresses the proportion of those who were tested negative who are actually healthy. These values can be expressed as a percentage by multiplying the fraction with 100%.

Diagnostic Errors and Their Consequences

As described in the above paragraphs, each diagnostic test is subject to errors. That is, a positive test does not always mean that caries is present, and a negative test does not always guarantee the absence of caries. Frequently, both false positive and false negative test results are produced (**Table 9.1**). As a result, the patient is either overtreated (in the case of false positive findings) or undertreated (in the case of false negative findings).

To better illustrate the problems of diagnostic errors, let us consider an example from the field of jurisprudence: Legal judgments, like medical tests, are also subject to error. A judgment (or "test" in our case) always seeks to condemn only the guilty (true positive) and exonerate the innocent (true negative). However, every judge or jury will make mistakes from time to time and incorrectly exonerate the guilty (false negative) and incorrectly condemn the innocent (false positive).

The sensitivity and specificity of different diagnostic methods has been described in the previous chapters. The better the test, the lower its error rate will be (high level of sensitivity and high level of specificity). Frequently, however, increasing the sensitivity will reduce the specificity. A strict judge (high level of sensitivity) will exonerate fewer of the guilty, but he or she will probably unjustly condemn more of the innocent (low specificity). In contrast, a judge who primarily tries not to condemn the innocent (high level of specificity) will probably tend to exonerate more of the guilty (low level of sensitivity). Similarly, the search for early stages of caries (such as discolored fissures) with the aim of correctly identifying more caries (increased sensitivity) will automatically increase the number of false positive findings and hence reduce the level of specificity.

NOTE

The sensitivity and specificity of a diagnostic method (test) are always closely related. If the sensitivity is increased, the specificity automatically decreases.

Various diagnostic procedures and categorization methods were presented in the previous chapters. Even though dental diagnoses are still based on clinical examinations, additional diagnostic methods can be used to help detect and assess caries, particularly in tooth surfaces that are impossible or difficult to inspect visually. By using additional diagnostic methods, a greater number of caries lesions can frequently be identified to reduce the number of false negative findings (increase of sensitivity). However, in addition to increasing the number of true positive findings (and hence the sensitivity), the number of false positive findings is also increased by merely adding up the positive findings from different methods.[6]

To illustrate this problem, let us again use an analogous example from the legal profession: The fallibility of court judgments is a familiar problem. If every suspect who was exonerated by a court were to therefore undergo a second trial with a different judge and witnesses (additional diagnostic measure), the number of correctly condemned criminals (true positive findings) might be increased, and fewer perpetrators would mistakenly be let free. However, the number of the unjustly condemned would necessarily increase (false positive findings), since more of these errors would also occur. For this reason, not every positive finding should be considered a definite sign of caries, and the positive findings from several methods should not be simply added up. Instead, the **fallibility of each diagnostic method** should be considered, and contradictory results should be carefully evaluated, eventually using additional methods.[8]

NOTE

When several diagnostic methods are used, the number of false positive findings increases. Contradictory results therefore need to be carefully reviewed.

For similar reasons, it is not recommendable to use every method for screening. As explained above, dental examinations frequently take on the character of a **screening**. The sensitivity and specificity of a test always depend on the prevalence of the disease. In a screening, the prevalence of the disease is, however, frequently low (many healthy teeth were examined to find a few diseased teeth). When the prevalence is low, the number of false positive findings increases, and the predictive value of the test decreases.

Once more, we will take an example from the legal profession to provide an illustration: If every citizen were to undergo a trial for any crime without any justifiable suspicion, it is highly probable that more criminals would be justifiably imprisoned. However, the number of innocent prisoners condemned due to a miscarriage of justice would be substantially higher. For similar reasons, it does not make sense to investigate all the occlusal surfaces of a patient using a moderately specificity diagnostic method (such as laser fluorescence). This method would yield an unnecessary number of false positive readings. Instead, such methods should be restricted to tooth surfaces where based on previous clinical or radiological examinations potential caries is assumed.[6]

NOTE

The frequency and probability of a disease in screenings or check-ups is relatively low. For this reason, the number of false positive findings increases, and the predictive value of the test decreases. Additional diagnostic methods should therefore only be used for clinically 'suspect' tooth surfaces and not for screening.

The Diagnostic Process

The diagnostic process in dental check-ups involves several steps. First, the signs and symptoms characteristic of caries need to be identified (**detection**). This is followed by a precise description of the (severity) stage and activity status of the lesion (**assessment**).[9,10] Several methods can be used to detect and describe caries, which will produce both confirmatory as well as contradictory information. The findings are then combined to form a **diagnosis** which is used to select a therapy (**Fig. 9.2**).[2,11] The **therapeutic decision** involves two elements: 1) whether or not the disease needs to be treated; 2) which therapy is appropriate.[5]

During the dental examination, the individual steps of the diagnostic process are frequently performed unconsciously. Unfortunately, diagnostic steps are often combined with therapeutic planning where the dentist only determines which tooth surface needs to be filled with which material.[4,12,13] The reason for this is probably a historical one and linked to the reimbursement system, which in many countries only gives money for operative treatment, not for prevention. Since in earlier times caries was treated almost exclusively with restorations—owing to the few therapeutic alternatives and high prevalence and activity of caries—it was not necessary to identify early stages of caries. Diagnosis primarily consisted of the detection of cavitated lesions (a cavity did or did not exist), and the presence of caries automatically led to restorative therapy.[14]

Today, caries is progressing relatively slowly in many countries and population groups, and there are numerous therapeutic options (see below). To select the right therapy for the specific **stage of caries**, a more precise description of the disease is required. In addition to describing the stage of caries, identifying the **activity of caries** is now considered just as important. Since the goal of many therapies is to arrest the progress of caries, active stages that require treatment need to be distinguished from inactive stages that do not require (any more) therapy. In therapeutic approaches that seek to arrest caries, observing lesions over a longer period is frequently the only way to **monitor the success of therapy**. If the dental findings are restricted to simply documenting the presence or absence of caries, a great deal of information is lost, and the appropriate therapy for the specific stage or cause cannot be selected.

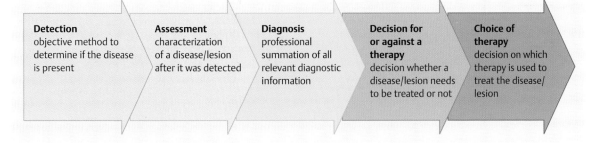

Fig. 9.2 The diagnostic process and choice of therapy.

The stage and activity of caries must be assessed so that an appropriate therapy can be selected. In addition to determining the need for therapy, the diagnosis is also used to assess the success of therapy.

The visual–tactile examination remains the core of caries diagnostics. This examination is supported by other diagnostic methods such as bitewing radiography, fiberoptic transillumination, and laser fluorescence. These methods give the dentist a highly differentiated picture of caries. To properly evaluate the various findings, it is useful to document them in a clearly laid out patient chart (see Chapter 24).

The art of diagnosing consists of **combining the various findings into a diagnosis** on which to base the ideal therapy for the patient and his or her disease. The different bits of information that have been collected (findings) are weighted, interpreted, evaluated and then assembled into a coherent picture for a diagnosis. It is particularly important to consider what is actually measured with the different methods. For example, the visual and tactical findings in the dental office are primarily for evaluating the surface of the lesion and only allow the depth of the caries to be indirectly estimated, based on the knowledge between the visual signs of caries and the histological extent of the lesion[9,10,15](see Chapter 5), whereas bitewing radiographs, fiberoptic transillumination, or laser fluorescence primarily allow one to estimate the depth of caries but cannot provide direct information about the surface.[8] There is, in principle, a certain correlation between the caries depth, activity, and probability of cavitation; nevertheless, these findings can sometimes be contradictory or misleading. As pointed out above, each investigative method can also yield incorrect values, and the error rate can vary depending on the method, tooth surface, and extent of the caries.

In addition to these theoretical considerations, the dentist's decision-making process largely depends on his or her individual experience. In addition, considerations about the consequences of the therapy to the patient and dentist also influence the decision-making process.

Categories and Thresholds

The findings must be categorized to document and weight the signs of caries observed using various methods. This means that the clinical situation, which is frequently highly complex, needs to be simplified and expressed using a reasonable number of categories. Thresholds need to be defined for the individual categories that delimit the categories from each other. As noted in previous chapters, a variety of systems has been developed over time for categorizing clinical and radiographic findings.[16] The question then arises: Which system is the most suitable for clinical practice? According to the nominalistic approach, only those categories are useful that relate to available therapeutic options.

It is useful to draw a distinction between **active and inactive** lesions, since only the former require therapy.[17] In addition, a distinction is frequently made between noncavitated and cavitated lesions, since the former can frequently be treated with noninvasive or microinvasive measures (see below), whereas the latter require restorative therapy, at least in tooth surfaces that are not directly accessible such as approximal surfaces.[18] However, such a dichotomous distinction frequently leaves it unclear whether microcavitation, breakdown of the enamel (ICDAS 3), or dentin caries (ICDAS 5) (see **Table 5.11**, Chapter 5) should be considered "cavitation." The individual distinction depends on the efficacy of the subsequent therapy for the transitional areas (nominalistic approach).[6] The following factors are involved in the categorization of diagnoses:

- The activity of the lesion
- The extent of the lesion
- The location of the lesion

Table 9.2 Therapeutically relevant diagnoses of primary caries

Diagnosis / Findings	Inactive caries (caries non-progressiva)	Sound, but at increased risk (sanus majoris periculi)	Active Caries (caries progressiva) Early (... superficialis)	Active Caries (caries progressiva) Medium (... media)	Active Caries (caries progressiva) Late (... profunda)
Visual-tactile findings	All ICDAS stages, but inactive	0	ICDAS 1–2 (active)	ICDAS 3–4 (active)	ICDAS 5–6 (active)
Radiographic extension	Mainly E0, E1, E2, D1	0	E0, E1, E2, D1	(D1), D2	(D2), D3
DIAGNOdent values	Mainly <50	< 15	0–40	40–99	n/a
Most likely therapy	None	Noninvasive or microinvasive		Minimally invasive	Invasive + pulp preservation or endodontics

Individual cut-offs for different diagnoses are arbitrary and may be individually adapted.

- The available therapeutic options
- Patient-related factors
- The dentist's opinion

Table 9.2 offers a related categorization of **three color-coded diagnoses** that will be used subsequently when determining various therapeutic options and findings relating to caries. It should be noted that transitional stages in particular (such as ICADAS 3, 4) cannot be strictly assigned to the various categories. Several parameters should be considered when diagnosing (and determining a therapy for) caries. Furthermore in the late stages, it can be helpful to distinguish caries lesions that only require restorative intervention (media) from those that also require pulp preserving (e.g., stepwise excavation) or endodontic treatment, or even extraction (profunda).

...to Therapy

Aim of Treatment

In the field of medicine, therapy is defined as "measures for healing a disease. Etiotropic or causal therapy seeks to eliminate the causes, and symptomatic therapy only seeks to alleviate the manifestations of the disease ..."[19] In this regard, caries does not fundamentally differ from other diseases: in the therapy of caries, our goal is to **induce healing**, **alleviate symptoms**, and **restore the functions of the teeth.** In this book we will define the term "therapy" a little more broadly and include, besides measures to treat the disease, also measures that aim to prevent caries. The dichotomous differentiation between "prevention" or "prophylaxis" on the one hand and "therapy" on the other hand is problematic for diseases like caries because, as described above, no generally accepted start of the disease can be defined. Moreover, interventions aiming at the causes of caries may not only prevent the disease, but also may lead to an arrest (healing) of lesions (see below). Therefore, we will use the term "therapy" for all interventions that aim to prevent or heal caries, as well as those interventions that aim to alleviate the signs and symptoms of caries and restore the functions of the teeth. In the past, the focus of dental treatment was only to **alleviate symptoms** and **re-establish function** with restorative measures. Dental therapy only became increasingly focused on **healing the disease** (restoration of the ecological equilibrium in the oral cavity, stopping the progress of lesions) during recent decades.

> **NOTE**
>
> Throughout this book we will use the term "therapy" for all interventions to treat caries, but also to prevent the disease.

Different types of healing are described in general pathology—complete recovery, regeneration, or "restitutio ad integrum" is the ideal form of healing. A complete regeneration of the associated tissue is sought in which the signs and symptoms are no longer detectable (**Table 9.3**). This form of healing is only observed when caries is in its very early stages. In the middle stages, rather, a repair with scarring of the diseased tissue is expected. This type of healing occurs when caries lesions are arrested and the caries process has stopped, but the signs of caries such as discoloration and increased porosity in the lesion body frequently persist (white and brown spots).

One major difference between caries and diseases of other tissues and organs is that the dental hard tissues can not (enamel), or only to a very limited extent (dentin), be actively regenerated by cells. In these tissues healing occurs primarily through mineralization processes in which cells do not directly participate. Remineralization can only occur where there are crystal nuclei. Otherwise, mineral deposits would collect in the oral cavity without restraint. Accordingly, caries lesions that already manifest cavitation cannot be completely repaired in the sense of restoring the original contours of the tooth. If the dentin and enamel have been destroyed to the extent of cavitation, the caries process can only be arrested at best. The primary aim of therapy in this case is to restore the tooth's shape and function through restorative measures and thereby allow the patient to regularly remove plaque.[20]

Table 9.3 Potential therapeutic goals of caries treatment

Aim of treatment	Definition	Disease stage	Invasiveness
Regeneration	"Restitutio ad integrum": Complete restoration of the healthy condition	Very early lesions	Noninvasive
Repair	Improvement of the status without complete restoration of the healthy condition (scarring)	Noncavitated lesions	Noninvasive, microinvasive
Restoration	Artificial restoration of the tooth's shape and function	Cavitated lesions	(minimally) Invasive
Prosthetic rehabilitation	Complete artificial replacement of the tooth	Complete destruction	Invasive

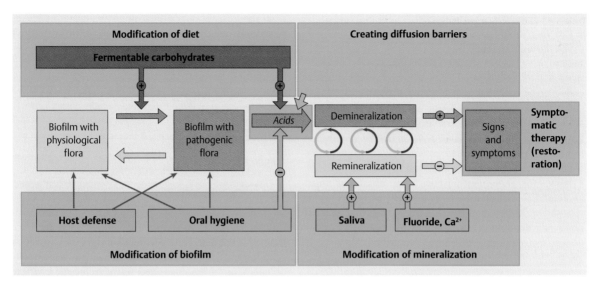

Fig. 9.3 Preventive strategies address the etiological factors of the caries process. By modification of the diet, the biofilm, and mineralization, or by creating a diffusion barrier, the caries process is altered to reduce demineralization and promote remineralization. By contrast, symptomatic (restorative) therapy is restricted to alleviating the clinical signs and symptoms.

NOTE

Caries can "heal" through remineralization processes. Most arrested lesions will remain as a scar in the tooth. If cavitation exists, however, the defect cannot be eliminated through remineralization and needs to be filled in many cases to restore the tooth contour and hence its ability to be cleaned.

Treatment Approaches

The model of caries presented in Chapter 4 describes the various etiological factors influencing the caries process and hence the potential risk factors for caries (see Chapter 8). In principle, all of the etiological factors for caries should be considered when looking for potential targets of preventive strategies and therapies. However, direct factors are particularly suitable for altering the caries process by modifying **diet**, the **biofilm** or **mineralization** (**Fig. 9.3**). In addition, caries prevention can be promoted through indirect factors such as "knowledge" or "health insurance." These indirect factors are often addressed in population or group-based strategies (see Chapter 13). However, in this chapter we will restrict ourselves to the modification of local factors on the tooth and to the individual.

The common element of all causal strategies is that they do not require invasive treatment of the enamel and dentin and are purely **noninvasive**. Some therapeutic options such as sealants or infiltration only slightly modify the enamel and dentin and are therefore considered **microinvasive**. Contrastingly, restorative measures are almost always associated with the loss of dentin and enamel and are **minimally invasive** at best. The term "minimal" expresses the fact that, in contrast to the classic rules of preparation defined by G.V. Black ("extension for prevention"), the restoration of carious defects with adhesive materials today is defect orientated (**Table 9.4**).

Noninvasive Measures

Noninvasive measures include all therapies that do not destroy the enamel and dentin and directly address causal factors. This includes measures for influencing the **biofilm**, **diet**, and **mineralization**. Since caries is frequently a long-lasting, chronic disease and these measures directly affect the caries process, they generally need to be pursued over the long term as well, in order to be effective. It is therefore usually necessary for patients to perform these therapies themselves and preferably integrate them into their lifestyle.

Influencing the Biofilm

The oral biofilm plays a key role in caries; its metabolic activity is the driving force in the caries process.[21] Consequently, regularly and completely removing the biofilm prevents or arrests caries. In addition to purely mechanical methods of **oral hygiene** such as toothbrushing, there are chemical and biological approaches to remove dental plaque or modify it to specifically suppress potentially pathogenic species or promote commensal, nonpathogenic bacteria. The various methods for influencing the biofilm are discussed in Chapter 10.

Influencing Diet

Diet is a primary factor in the etiology of caries. Changing one's diet so that it contains few fermentable carbohydrates can prevent, slow, or arrest caries.[22] Patients are frequently unaware of which foods contain sugar and how frequently they consume them. Diet counseling is therefore a fixed element in caries therapy, particularly for

Table 9.4 Etiological targets for various therapeutic strategies

Target	Intervention	Chapter	Invasiveness
Biofilm	Mechanical: oral hygiene	10	Noninvasive
	Chemical: antimicrobials		
	Biological: probiotics		
Diet	Diet modification	11	
	Sugar substitution		
Mineralization	Provide substances that promote mineralization: fluoride, calcium compounds	12	
	Stimulate salivation: chewing gum		
Diffusion	Sealants	15, 16	Microinvasive
	Infiltration	17	
Signs and symptoms	Restoration	18, 19	Minimally invasive

people at a high caries risk.[23] Unfortunately, the goal of sugar-free nutrition is difficult to achieve owing to the lack of patient adherence, since people probably have an evolutionarily caused predilection for sweet foods. In addition, this tendency, which only becomes pathogenic in times of overabundant nutrition, is reinforced by the advertising of the food and snack industries. Since it is generally impossible to completely avoid sugar, it is often more practical to substitute cariogenic sugars with **sugar alcohols** or **intense sweeteners**. These are not or only slightly cariogenic. Frequently, the mere substitution of cariogenic sugars has an anti-cariogenic effect.[24] In addition some of these substances possess antibacterial properties and stimulate salivation. The various methods for influencing nutrition are discussed in Chapter 11.

Influencing Mineralization

Caries is characterized by the loss of mineral in the enamel and dentin. The healing of caries lesions is caused by remineralization processes in which **fluorides** play an important role. As discussed in Chapter 2, fluorides reduce demineralization and promote the remineralization of the enamel and dentin.[25] Fluoride has a strong caries-inhibiting effect, particularly when small amounts are regularly applied. One significant advantage is that fluoride can be applied relatively easily in the diet (such as in water and table salt) or in toothpaste. The reduced prevalence of caries observed in recent decades in many locations has been ascribed to the widespread use of fluoride toothpaste.[26] However, the use of fluoride is restricted by toxicological considerations. **Calcium and phosphate compounds** are also involved in the complex processes of demineralization and remineralization, and a high concentration of these mineral compounds in the saliva can in principle favorably shift the balance toward remineralization. However, their use as remineralizing substances is

limited by the fact that solutions of calcium and phosphate precipitate at high concentrations. Given the complex functions of saliva in the remineralization of enamel and dentin, **stimulating saliva secretion,** for example by chewing gum, has an anticariogenic effect.[27] The various methods for influencing mineralization are discussed in Chapter 12.

Microinvasive Measures

These are understood to be therapeutic measures that only slightly influence the enamel and dentin (e.g., by etching). This includes **sealing** fissures and smooth surfaces and the **infiltration of caries.**

Sealants

Sealing fissures and pits was originally used for the primary prevention of caries in healthy occlusal surfaces (preventive sealing). This method is based on the idea that deep fissures which are difficult to clean can be rendered easy to clean by filling them with resin or cements. In addition, the sealant creates a diffusion barrier between the potential biofilm and enamel which further limits the demineralization of the enamel. In recent years, also the sealing of caries lesions has been increasingly recommended.[28,29] In addition to fissures, the method is also used to prevent the progression of caries in buccal and approximal smooth surfaces. Sealing is discussed in Chapters 15 and 16.

Infiltration

Whereas sealants create a superficial diffusion barrier, the goal of caries infiltration is to arrest noncavitated caries lesions by infiltrating the pores in the lesion body using special low-viscosity, light-curing resins. In contrast to sealing, the diffusion barrier is not created on the lesion surface but rather inside the lesion which results in a stabilization and arrest of caries progression.[30,31] Caries infiltration is discussed in Chapter 17.

(Minimally) Invasive Measures

These are restorative measures primarily aimed at halting the progression and aggravation of the disease (symptomatic therapy, tertiary prevention) and require the removal and restoration of enamel and dentin that has been destroyed by caries.

Restoration

With the cavitation of a caries lesion, a stage of disease has generally been reached that is almost impossible to heal by remineralization. Advanced forms of caries with cavitation usually do not respond to noninvasive or microinvasive therapies due to the limited potential of the enamel and dentin to regenerate. In these stages of the disease, restorative measures are indicated to restore the tooth's ability to be cleaned as well as the aesthetic and masticatomy function by means of **plastic reconstruction**.[18] Various materials such as amalgams, cements, and composites are used. Generally, the enamel and dentin altered by caries are removed by excavating the caries, primarily to ensure the mechanical stability and seal of the restoration. Caries excavation and restorative therapy are described in Chapters 18 and 19.

Additional Measures

If the carious defects are extensive, restorations using resin materials are frequently too time-consuming or impractical, and therefore restorations fabricated in the laboratory or using CAD/CAM (inlays, onlays, partial crowns) are employed. Furthermore, endodontic treatment is often required in this stage due to the effects on the pulp organ. For a detailed discussion of these topics, refer to the appropriate reference works on restorative dentistry, endodontology, and prosthetics.

Which Measures are Indicated at What Time?

Just as a comprehensive diagnosis of caries includes both the patient (the patient's caries risk) and individual teeth (the stage and activity of a caries lesion), there are different therapeutic measures that address either the patient (individual level) or specific tooth surfaces or teeth (tooth level).

Table 9.5 Systemic therapeutic measures depending on the individual risk factors

Risk factor/ protective factor	Therapeutic measures
Oral hygiene	Biofilm modification: oral hygiene instruction, professional tooth cleaning, supervised toothbrushing
Diet	Diet modification: diet counseling, sugar substitutes and intense sweeteners
Exposure to fluoride	Fluoridation
Amount of saliva	Saliva stimulation, saliva substitutes
General diseases, medication	Consider switching medication in consultation with the treating specialists

Individual Level

The majority of the etiological factors for caries affect the entire oral cavity and not just single teeth. Correspondingly, caries therapy should include both a local therapy of individual teeth (where signs and symptoms become manifest) and a therapy that addresses the patient. **Systemic caries therapy** should therefore address the etiological risk factors for the individual patient, which were identified when determining the caries risk (risk-related intervention) (**Table 9.5**). Another consideration when choosing a therapy is patient compliance. Many noninvasive therapeutic options need to be regularly used or require a change of the patient's habits. Therapeutic approaches need to be chosen that are most likely to be adopted by the patient.

> **NOTE**
>
> At the level of the individual, the primary consideration when choosing an appropriate therapy is the patient's individual risk factor.

Tooth Level

The location, severity, and activity of caries are the primary considerations in choosing the intervention for individual teeth. For healthy teeth, tooth surfaces or groups of teeth with an increased caries risk (such as erupting molars), risk-oriented, noninvasive measures such as local fluoridation and oral hygiene instructions, or microinvasive measures such as fissure sealing are used to prevent caries from occurring (**primary prevention**). Active caries in the early stages should be arrested using the same noninvasive and microinvasive measures as **secondary prevention**. If the caries is already in advanced stages, generally restorative measures as **tertiary prevention** are necessary to prevent the disease from worsening.

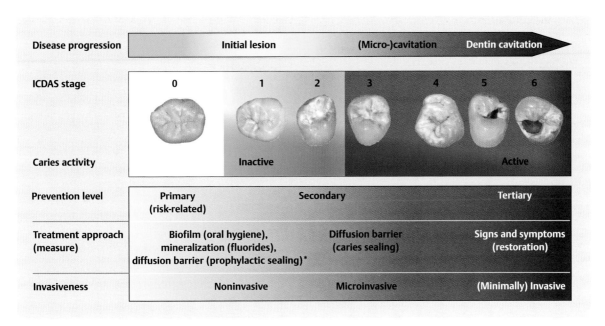

Fig. 9.4 Therapeutic options for various stages in the caries process in occlusal surfaces.
* Prophylactic sealing belongs to microinvasive measures.

At the tooth level, the location, severity, and activity of caries are the primary considerations when choosing a therapy.

Therapeutic Options for Occlusal Caries

Whereas it is frequently difficult to diagnose caries in fissures and grooves, the therapy of caries in these locations is relatively easy since the occlusal surface is generally readily accessible (**Fig. 9.4**). Noninvasive methods such as biofilm control (by mechanical or chemical means) or local fluoridation are used for healthy fissures with an increased caries risk (e.g., during tooth eruption), and for fissures with early-stage caries. In addition, fissure sealing is a very effective microinvasive procedure that can be used for healthy fissures (primary prevention) and noncavitated stages of caries (secondary prevention) to arrest the caries process. In later stages of cavitated caries, generally restorative methods are indicated (caries excavation, restoring the defect).

Therapeutic Options for Approximal Caries

Given its location below the contact point, approximal caries represents both a diagnostic and therapeutic challenge. Noninvasive methods such as plaque control or local fluoridation are appropriate for healthy tooth surfaces, or surfaces with early forms of caries, to prevent or arrest the disease (**Fig. 9.5**). The control of plaque on approximal surfaces is, however, much more difficult

than on other tooth surfaces (see Chapter 10). The sealing and infiltration of caries are microinvasive measures that can be used to arrest the progression of noncavitated caries lesions. If an approximal lesion adjacent to a tooth is cavitated, restorative measures are indicated to enable the patient to clean the surface again. The poor accessibility frequently means that a large amount of enamel and dentin must be removed during the restoration to reach the diseased hard tissues.

NOTE

With occlusal and approximal lesions, cavitation in the surface is frequently an indication for restorative measures.

Therapeutic Options for Caries in Accessible Smooth Surfaces

Given the normally good accessibility of oral and buccal smooth surfaces, caries in these tooth surfaces is observed much less frequently today in populations with low caries prevalence than was the case in the pre-fluoridation era. Patients who have fixed orthodontic appliances and patients with poor oral hygiene may form an exception to this rule.

Lesions in accessible tooth surfaces are relatively easy to diagnose. In addition, easy accessibility renders noninvasive measures, such as plaque control or local fluoridation, very effective, and such lesions can frequently be stopped. The oral hygiene of patients who have fixed braces is often restricted due to the poor accessibility of the lesions, and

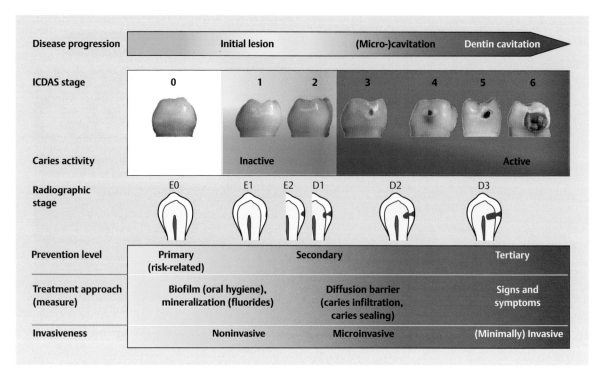

Disease progression	Initial lesion		(Micro-)cavitation	Dentin cavitation

Fig. 9.5   Therapeutic options for various stages in the caries process in approximal surfaces.

thus it is difficult to arrest the lesions using noninvasive measures. The esthetic appearance of the labial lesions is a special consideration. Whereas arresting the progression of noncavitated lesions in other tooth surfaces is considered a therapeutic success, for many patients, arresting lesions in this region is not enough due to their frequently unappealing appearance (brown or white spots).[32] Many patients therefore desire an esthetic rehabilitation, which is frequently associated with the loss of additional hard tooth substance.

NOTE

Even late-stage caries can be arrested by means of noninvasive measures in freely accessible smooth surfaces. For aesthetic reasons, however, microinvasive or minimally invasive procedures may be necessary.

Therapeutic Options for Root Caries

Today, root caries is found more frequently in older patients with a periodontal attachment loss and exposed cementum or dentin. The therapy for root caries primarily depends on the accessibility of the lesions. Easily accessible lesions, even in cavitated stages, can be arrested by appropriate noninvasive measures.[33] Here the regular removal of the biofilm is often successful. Since arrested root caries is frequently dark brown, esthetic considerations may also lead to additional restorative measures.

In contrast to freely accessible root caries lesions, those that are difficult to access (such as approximal or subgingival lesions, or lesions undermining the enamel) frequently cannot be successfully treated with noninvasive measures alone. Restorative measures are indicated in this case. Similar to approximal enamel caries, the restoration of approximal root caries is frequently associated with the loss of a large amount of healthy dentin and enamel due to the difficult access.

NOTE

Noninvasive measures are frequently successful when the root caries is freely accessible and the patient is compliant. In contrast, restorative measures are often required with root caries that is difficult to reach.

SUMMARY

The reduction of caries prevalence in many countries and improved knowledge of the etiology and pathogenesis of caries have caused the focus of dental treatment to shift over recent decades. Whereas dental treatment primarily used to consist of restoring caries lesions or replacing teeth destroyed by caries with prostheses, nowadays noninvasive and microinvasive therapeutic options that address etiological factors are gaining importance. The goal of these therapies is to heal or at least slow the progress of the disease. For this to occur, the disease must be diagnosed at an early stage. Today, in many countries, caries is generally diagnosed in screening or checkup visits. Beyond detecting caries in individual tooth surfaces, the clinical picture must be described with sufficient detail (assessment) to allow an appropriate intervention to be selected for the specific stage of caries. In addition to diagnosing caries lesions in individual teeth, individual risk factors need to be identified and weighted so that the causes of caries can be treated. This also provides an opportunity to address the patient's behavioral patterns that led to the disease.

REFERENCES

1. Baelum V. Caries management: technical solutions to biological problems or evidence-based care? J Oral Rehabil 2008;35(2):135–151
2. Pitts NB. Are we ready to move from operative to non-operative/preventive treatment of dental caries in clinical practice? Caries Res 2004;38(3):294–304
3. Merriam-Webster Online Dictionary. http//merriam-webster.com/dictionary/diagnosis (Accessed July 7, 2012)
4. Beck JD. Issues in assessment of diagnostic tests and risk for periodontal diseases. Periodontol 2000 1995;7:100–108
5. Bader JD, Shugars DA. Understanding dentists' restorative treatment decisions. J Public Health Dent 1992;52(2):102–110
6. Baelum V, Nyvad B, Gröndal HG, et al. The foundations of good diagnostic practice. In: Fejerskov O, Kidd EAM, eds. Dental Caries. The Disease and its Clinical Management. 2nd ed. Oxford: Blackwell Munksgaard; 2008:103–120
7. Brewer NT, Salz T, Lillie SE. Systematic review: the long-term effects of false-positive mammograms. Ann Intern Med 2007;146(7):502–510
8. Baelum V, Heidmann J, Nyvad B. Dental caries paradigms in diagnosis and diagnostic research. Eur J Oral Sci 2006;114(4):263–277
9. Ekstrand KR, Ricketts DN, Kidd EA. Occlusal caries: pathology, diagnosis and logical management. Dent Update 2001;28(8):380–387
10. Ekstrand KR, Zero DT, Martignon S, Pitts NB. Lesion activity assessment. Monogr Oral Sci 2009;21:63–90
11. Pitts NB. Modern concepts of caries measurement. J Dent Res 2004;83 (Spec C):C43–C47
12. Bader JD, Shugars DA. Variation in dentists' clinical decisions. J Public Health Dent 1995;55(3):181–188
13. Ismail AI, Hasson H, Sohn W. Dental caries in the second millennium. J Dent Educ 2001;65(10):953–959
14. Nyvad B. Diagnosis versus detection of caries. Caries Res 2004;38(3):192–198
15. Ekstrand KR, Ricketts DN, Kidd EA. Reproducibility and accuracy of three methods for assessment of demineralization depth of the occlusal surface: an in vitro examination. Caries Res 1997;31(3):224–231
16. Ismail AI. Visual and visuo-tactile detection of dental caries. J Dent Res 2004;83 (Spec C):C56–C66
17. Nyvad B, Machiulskiene V, Baelum V. Reliability of a new caries diagnostic system differentiating between active and inactive caries lesions. Caries Res 1999;33(4):252–260
18. Kidd EAM, van Amerongen JP. The role of operative treatment. In: Fejerskov O, Kidd EAM, eds. Dental Caries: The Disease and its Clinical Management. 2nd ed. Oxford: Blackwell Munksgaard; 2008:355–365
19. Hoffmann-La Roche AG. Roche Lexikon der Medizin. München: Urban und Fischer; 1999
20. Kidd EA, Fejerskov O. What constitutes dental caries? Histopathology of carious enamel and dentin related to the action of cariogenic biofilms. J Dent Res 2004;83 (Spec C):C35–C38
21. Kidd EAM. How 'clean' must a cavity be before restoration? Caries Res 2004;38(3):305–313
22. Zero DT, Moynihan P, Lingström P, et al. The role of dietary control. In: Fejerskov O, Kidd EAM, eds. Dental Caries. The Disease and its Clinical Management. 2nd ed. Oxford: Blackwell Munksgaard; 2008:329–349
23. Zero DT. Sugars – the arch criminal? Caries Res 2004;38(3):277–285
24. Mäkinen KK. Sugar alcohol sweeteners as alternatives to sugar with special consideration of xylitol. Med Princ Pract 2011;20(4):303–320
25. ten Cate JM, van Loveren C. Fluoride mechanisms. Dent Clin North Am 1999;43(4):713–742, vii
26. Bratthall D, Hänsel-Petersson G, Sundberg H. Reasons for the caries decline: what do the experts believe? Eur J Oral Sci 1996;104(4 (Pt 2)):416–422, discussion 423–425, 430–432
27. Stookey GK. The effect of saliva on dental caries. J Am Dent Assoc 2008;139(Suppl):11S–17S
28. Martignon S, Ekstrand KR, Ellwood R. Efficacy of sealing proximal early active lesions: an 18-month clinical study evaluated by conventional and subtraction radiography. Caries Res 2006;40(5):382–388
29. Splieth CH, Ekstrand KR, Alkilzy M, et al. Sealants in dentistry: outcomes of the ORCA Saturday Afternoon Symposium 2007. Caries Res 2010;44(1):3–13
30. Meyer-Lueckel H, Fejerskov O, Paris S. Novel treatment options for proximal caries [Article in German] Schweiz Monatsschr Zahnmed 2009;119(5):454–461
31. Paris S, Hopfenmuller W, Meyer-Lueckel H. Resin infiltration of caries lesions: an efficacy randomized trial. J Dent Res 2010;89(8):823–826
32. Mattousch TJ, van der Veen MH, Zentner A. Caries lesions after orthodontic treatment followed by quantitative light-induced fluorescence: a 2-year follow-up. Eur J Orthod 2007;29(3):294–298
33. Nyvad B, Fejerskov O. Active root surface caries converted into inactive caries as a response to oral hygiene. Scand J Dent Res 1986;94(3):281–284

Caries Management by Modifying the Biofilm

Sebastian Paris, Christof Doerfer, Hendrik Meyer-Lueckel

10

There's an old saying in dentistry that "a clean tooth never decays." Accordingly, the Keyes rings (**Fig. 2.1**, p. 22) illustrate plaque as an essential etiological factor of dental caries. If bacteria like *Streptococcus mutans* are one of the main causes of caries, it seems reasonable at first glance to eliminate as many of them as possible from the oral cavity by intense oral hygiene and chemical agents. However, this goal can neither be accomplished nor would it be helpful in maintaining oral health.

To understand better the role of oral hygiene in the etiology and treatment of caries, we should call to mind that bacteria have been with us since time immemorial. It is estimated that our body consists of ten times as many prokaryotic cells (bacteria) as eukaryotic (human) cells.[1] The physiological flora plays an important role in the physiology of the human body. It is involved in the digestion of nutrients and defense against potentially pathogenic microbes such as fungi. This also makes clear that a complete elimination of bacteria from the oral cavity is neither possible nor reasonable. Therefore, a control or beneficial modification rather than an elimination of bacteria/plaque seems to be the goal of our caries preventive strategies.

There are two classical ways of controlling plaque: first, by a **mechanical** disturbance of the biofilm; and second, by the **chemical** action of antimicrobial agents. Neither strategy is a human invention, since both have been established during our co-evolution with oral bacteria. The complex anatomy of the teeth and surrounding soft tissues allows a very efficient mechanical self-cleaning during mastication and movement of oral tissues. Moreover, the physiological exfoliation of oral epithelia limits the adhesion of bacteria. Besides these mechanical actions, the human body also provides a range of chemical agents with antimicrobial activity, including the innate and acquired immune system. In the past years a vast number of antimicrobial peptides has been identified,[2] and we are just beginning to understand what important roles these antimicrobial substances play in maintaining the ecological equilibrium between the host and the microorganisms.

Humans have always supported natural cleaning of the oral cavity by employing mechanical aids as well as chemical agents to keep their teeth healthy. The first known oral hygiene devices were tooth sticks (Miswak) that were already in use more than 5000 years ago (**Fig. 10.1**).[3] Antimicrobial substances derived from plants may have an even longer history in human culture.[4] In modern times, patients and dental professionals clean teeth with sophisticated mechanical techniques and use different antimicrobial agents to control growth and quality of dental plaque.

A third and more recent approach to control plaque arose from the idea that oral diseases such as caries and periodontitis are most probably caused by an ecological shift within the dental plaque (ecological plaque hypothesis). Consequently, **biological** approaches aim to alter the plaque composition by specific modification of the oral

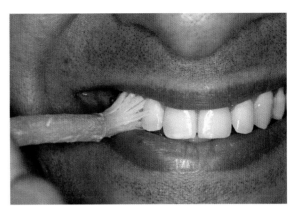

Fig. 10.1 Use of Miswak as a simple, natural toothbrush is still widespread in Africa and Arabic countries.

ecology, for example, by administration of harmless (probiotic) microorganisms that compete with pathogenic microbes.

This chapter aims to give the reader an insight into various strategies to prevent and treat caries by biofilm modification/control, and will cover:

- Dental plaque as a biofilm
- Methods to mechanically remove the oral biofilm
- Different chemical agents to control the oral biofilm
- Biological approaches for altering the biofilm composition

Dental Plaque as a Biofilm

The Dutch scientist Antonie van Leeuwenhoek first showed in 1683 that the sticky mass of dental plaque consists of tiny bacteria. He also showed that only the surface layers of bacteria were vulnerable, whereas the deeper layers resisted the vinegar he used to clean his teeth. Later, acid-producing bacteria in dental plaque like *S. mutans* were identified as being involved in caries initiation and consequently the reduction of dental plaque became one of the main strategies of caries prevention. In recent years new technologies have given scientists a deeper insight into the structure and microbiology of dental plaque, which has been shown to be much more complex than previously thought. In dental plaque, clusters of live and dead bacteria are embedded in an extracellular matrix of polymers, which are of host and bacterial origin.[5] The matrix gives mechanical stability and serves as an extracellular nutrition storage which helps bacteria to survive in times of starvation (see Chapter 11). Dental plaque shows a relatively open architecture with channels and voids that allow diffusion of liquids. A similar accretion of microorganisms can be found on many solid surfaces in nonsterile aqueous environments like rivers, aquaria, or the tubing systems of dental units. In biology these microbial aggregations are called "biofilms" and because many findings from biofilms in general can be transferred to dental plaque, today dental plaque is often referred to as an **oral biofilm**.

Bacteria associated in biofilms show different properties than planktonic (swimming, growing in liquid) bacteria with regard to their **gene expression profiles** and their **antimicrobial resistance**, which limits the informative value of studies on planktonic bacterial cultures vis-à-vis biofilms. Moreover, multispecies biofilms like dental plaque react differently compared to monospecies cultures which (for reasons of simplicity) are often used in laboratory experiments. The various microorganisms in dental biofilms show very complex interactions as they exchange signaling molecules and genetic information and thus can react better to environmental changes. Being protected in such biofilms, up to 300-fold concentrations of antibiotics are needed to kill those bacteria, exceeding by far in some cases the lethal dose for human beings.[6] Today, more than 700 different microbes and phylotypes have been identified in oral biofilms.[7] High throughput technologies showed more than 19000 different species in healthy mouths.[8] The composition of species varies between individuals and various tooth sites and even within different locations in the plaque. This complexity of oral biofilms should be considered whenever one thinks about approaches to eliminate dental plaque or to modify its composition and structure with the aim of caries prevention.

NOTE

Dental plaque is a complex oral biofilm. Bacteria associated in biofilms are highly resistant to antimicrobial substances, which limits the efficacy of chemotherapeutic approaches to control dental plaque.

Mechanical Biofilm Control

Correlation between Oral Hygiene and Caries

With regard to the etiology of caries one might assume a strong correlation exists between the oral hygiene of patients and the occurrence of dental caries. Indeed, it has been shown in several studies that children with good oral cleanliness tend to develop less caries than those with poor oral hygiene. However, interestingly, the differences were rather small.[9,10] This is not so surprising, if one takes into account the multifactorial nature of caries (see **Fig. 4.1**, page 67) in which oral hygiene is just one of the many factors. Significant differences in caries incidence between groups with good or bad oral hygiene were mainly observed for erupting teeth, free smooth surfaces, and front teeth, which are all relatively easy to clean,[11–15] whereas differences for approximal and occlusal surfaces

were rather small. It seems that good oral hygiene is efficacious at preventing caries only to a certain degree. Even if good oral hygiene is performed, the oral cavity is never free from microbial deposits and hence in many patients factors other than oral hygiene may play a dominant role, especially in tooth sites that are hard to clean, even by highly motivated individuals. This is important to consider, as oral hygiene education should be a major, but not the only, focus of caries prevention. Moreover, measures to improve oral hygiene should be focused on sites where the best preventive effect can be achieved.

In general, mechanical plaque control can be performed by the patient (**self-applied**) and by dental personnel (**professional** tooth cleaning).

NOTE

Oral hygiene is most effective in easily accessible sites such as buccal surfaces and front teeth. In tooth sites that are hard to reach (e.g., approximal surfaces) oral hygiene is less effective.

Self-Applied Mechanical Biofilm Control

Tooth Brushing

Tooth brushing with either manual or powered toothbrushes is the most common oral hygiene method in most countries. It is mostly performed using either manual or powered plastic brushes and in combination with a toothpaste.

It seems obvious that the quality of tooth brushing, that is, the efficacy of removing plaque, is important for its caries preventive effect. To evaluate whether the efficacy of tooth brushing can be improved, several studies investigated the effect of **supervision of tooth brushing** in children.[14,16,17] In these studies the overall effect on caries was modest and most apparent in front teeth and free smooth surfaces, since these were most easily reached by the brush[10] (**Fig. 10.2**). For scarcely accessible surfaces, however, only highly motivated individuals could maintain a high standard of plaque control by self-applied oral hygiene.[9]

Intensified oral hygiene has been shown to be efficacious in the occlusal surfaces of **erupting molars**.[18] During the eruption period the natural self-cleaning by occlusal mastication and anatomical shape, which keep most of the fissure and buccal surfaces free of plaque in fully erupted teeth, is often inefficient. Hence, during eruption particularly molars are susceptible to caries. Therefore, during this time special attention should be given to the cleaning. Brushing of erupting molars in a bucco-lingual direction (cross brushing) is often more efficacious than normal brushing techniques and should be advocated (**Fig. 10.3**).

Also during the **orthodontic treatment** with fixed appliances (self-) cleaning is often considerably impaired. To

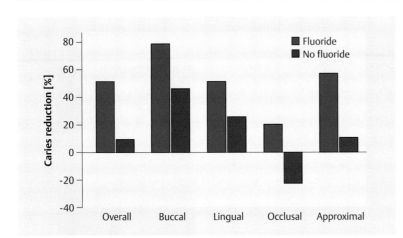

Fig. 10.2 Caries reduction by implementation of daily supervised tooth brushing in 9–11-year-olds over a 3-year period with and without the use of fluoridated toothpaste.[16] The caries preventive effect is more pronounced in easily accessible sites and in the group using fluoride toothpaste.

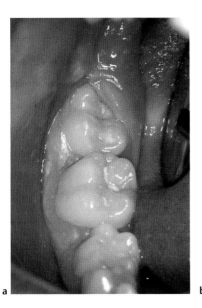
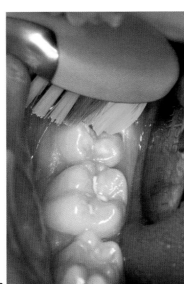

Fig. 10.3a, b Self-cleaning by mastication is impaired in erupting molars owing to the lack of occlusion (**a**). Moreover, manual brushing is often less efficacious because the brush does not reach the recessed occlusal surface during the normal brushing motion. Directed bucco-lingual "cross brushing" should be advised in these cases (**b**).

avoid an iatrogenic increase of caries risk it is necessary to compensate this impairment of self-cleaning with intensified oral hygiene during the treatment period. It has been shown that oral health education and promotion can improve oral hygiene in orthodontic patients at least in the short term.[19]

> **NOTE**
>
> Erupting molars and teeth under fixed orthodontic appliances are especially susceptible to caries, because (self-) cleaning is impaired. For these situations, special measures should be recommended.

Brushing Technique and Brush Used

The efficacy of plaque removal depends on the toothbrush and brushing technique used. In general today, a **multitufted brush** with a short head with end rounded plastic bristles is recommended. The use of natural brushes is discouraged because bristles tend to split, harbor many bacteria, and may even injure the gingiva.

In the past century, **several tooth brushing techniques** have been developed and advocated (summarized in **Table 10.1**). The plane bristle field of most manual brushes makes it difficult to reach the approximal areas. Therefore, most brushing techniques suggest holding the brush at about a 45° angle to better penetrate proximal areas (**Fig. 10.4**). Some advanced toothbrush models have cross-angulated bristles, which seems to slightly improve the approximal cleaning.[20] Although it has been shown that the employment of certain tooth brushing techniques results in better plaque removal compared with unstructured brushing,[21] such technical superiority with regard to caries prevention is yet to be demonstrated. Moreover, it should be kept in mind that most of the advocated techniques require a **high level of dexterity** and thus are not suitable for every patient.

For this reason **powered toothbrushes** have become more and more popular in recent years. Powered brushes

Table 10.1   Manual tooth brushing methods

Technique	Motion	
Modified Bass technique	• The filaments point toward roots of teeth at 45° angle • Short vibratory or circular movement while brushing forward and backward	
Modified Stillman technique	• The filaments point toward roots of teeth at 45° angle • Twisting of the brush (~45°) and proceeding to vibrate and roll against each tooth	
Charters technique	• The filaments point toward occlusal at 45° angle with half the bristles of the brush over the gingiva and half over the crown. • Vibratory movement along with a circular motion	
Fones technique	• The brush is placed perpendicular to teeth • Large circular motion of brush over occluded teeth to simultaneously cover both upper and lower teeth	

simulate parts of the brushing motion, thus reducing and simplifying the manual movements that are needed to clean the teeth. Early concerns that powered toothbrushes might injure the gingiva and lead to gingival recessions could be neither corroborated by clinical experience nor by scientific evidence. In addition, the efficacy of plaque removal could be significantly increased and different designs have been developed (**Fig. 10.5**).

Most powered toothbrushes seem to be at least as effective as manual brushing in reducing plaque and gingivitis, but fail to show superior results. Only powered brushes with a **rotating, oscillating/multidimensional motion** seem consistently to remove significantly more plaque than manual brushes.[22] However, keeping in mind the only modest association between oral cleanliness and the incidence of caries, it is still unclear whether the use of powered brushes also results in lower caries (and periodontitis) incidence compared with manual brushes. Moreover, it should be considered that most available studies investigated the tooth cleaning **efficacy** under the controlled conditions of clinical studies. The **effectiveness** (in real world conditions) of toothbrushes might differ from the efficacy, as patients' personal perceptions and preferences might also play an important role. For these reasons, no clear recommendations with respect to the superiority of either manual or powered toothbrushes can be made.[22] For the individual patient, personal preference should be considered as well as manual dexterity and adherence.

NOTE

Powered toothbrushes are more efficacious then manual brushes in removing dental plaque. However, it is unclear whether this results in lower incidence of caries and periodontitis.

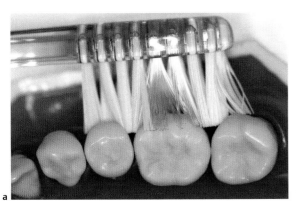
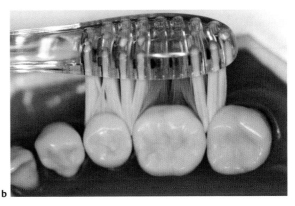

Fig. 10.4a, b Toothbrushes with a plane bristle field are ineffective at reaching the approximal surfaces when they are used perpendicularly to the teeth **(a)**. When the brush is inclined at about 45°, approximal areas are reached more easily **(b)**.

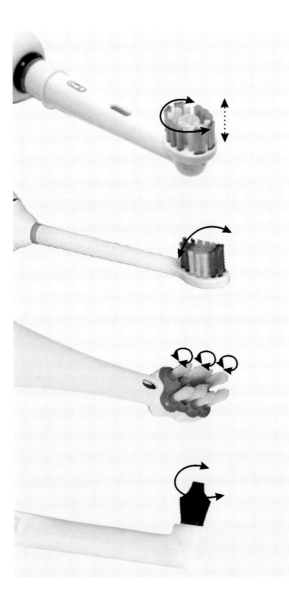

Fig. 10.5 Modes of action of various powered toothbrushes. The multidimensional motion is a further development of the rotating oscillating motion. Toothbrushes with multidimensional and (sonic) undirected motion are the most well known.
From top to bottom:
Rotating, oscillating/multidimensional motion (Professional Care 7000 [Braun Oral B]; Crest Spin Brush Pro [Procter & Gamble])
Undirected motion (Sonicare [Philips], Sonic Complete [Braun Oral B]
Counter oscillation (Interplak brush [Baush and Lomb Oral Care])
Circular motion (Rotadent [Professional Dental Technologies])

The Effect of Fluoride

In most countries tooth brushing is usually performed with fluoride toothpaste. Therefore, it is often not clear whether the caries preventive effect of tooth brushing is mainly due to the disturbance of plaque, or rather by the action of fluoride. In one study, which investigated the effect tooth brushing and fluoride separately, the caries increment of 9–11-year-old children was evaluated over a period of three years.[16] In one group, children brushed their teeth every school day under supervision using fluoride toothpaste. In a second group, children brushed their teeth with non-fluoride toothpaste also under supervision. In a control group, no intervention was performed and children carried on with their established oral hygiene (mainly non-fluoride toothpaste). To assess the effect of fluoride alone, in another control group, children only rinsed with 0.5% NaF solution fortnightly. In children brushing with non-fluoride toothpaste the relative reduction of caries incidence in the intervention compared with the control group was only modest (8%). When supervised brushing was performed with fluoride toothpaste, however, a significantly lower caries incidence (51% less compared with the nonsupervised control) was observed (**Fig. 10.6**). In conclusion, the **combination of tooth brushing with the local application of fluoride** (by using fluoride

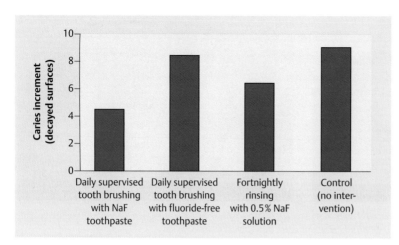

Fig. 10.6 Caries incidence (decayed surfaces) in 9–11-year-old children in a Swedish study over a 3-year period with different interventions.[16] The best caries preventive effect was achieved by the combination of supervised brushing and the use of fluoride toothpaste. Supervised brushing alone showed only very little preventive effect compared with the control. Also, regular rinsing with fluoride solution had a lower caries preventive effect than the combination of fluoride toothpaste and supervised brushing.

toothpaste) seems to be most effective in controlling caries.

NOTE

Tooth brushing is most effective in combination with fluoride toothpaste. Tooth brushing with fluoride-free toothpaste has only very limited caries preventive effect.

Tooth brushing: How Often, When, and How Long?

How often? It is widely recommended to brush the teeth at least twice daily. But what is the rationale behind it? Dental plaque grows quite slowly and the first subclinical tissue changes beneath plaque can be observed only after more than 24 hours of plaque accumulation.[23] As it seems unlikely that with an increase of brushing frequency the quality of brushing increases (see below), in consequence easily accessible sites are cleaned more often than necessary and plaque stagnation sites that are difficult to reach often remain untouched. As negative side effects of brushing, like wedge-shaped defects and erosion/abrasion (see below), may increase—for some highly motivated patients, too much oral hygiene is even detrimental. Besides cosmetic considerations, the recommendation to brush **twice daily** is mainly based on the fact that tooth brushing is the most efficient way to **apply fluorides** locally. It has been shown that patients brushing twice daily develop less caries compared with those brushing just once daily.[24,25]

When? It is often recommended to brush the teeth directly after meals[26] and especially before going to bed,[27] but there is no strong scientific evidence for this. On the one hand, brushing after meals might help to clear carbohydrates from the oral cavity but on the other hand removal of plaque before meals would leave no biofilm to ferment carbohydrates.[28] Brushing directly after acidic meals can trigger **erosion**, as the softened enamel is easily brushed away and has no time to remineralize.[28] With

regard to this, a safety period of more than one hour seems to be necessary before brushing after erosive meals.[29,30] However, there is little evidence behind these statements and it is currently doubted that such general advice is of any clinical relevance, as long as the teeth do not already show proven erosive damage. The rationale behind the recommendation to brush before going to bed is that salivary flow is decreased during sleep.[31] However, since at night usually no cariogenic food is consumed, it is questionable whether this has a clinical impact. As the main motivation of patients for tooth brushing is cosmetic, it makes sense to **support** this **intrinsic motivation** and to recommend that patients brush their teeth whenever they are most willing to in their daily routine. This might have a greater effect than theoretical considerations.

How long? Increasing the tooth brushing time more than one minute seems to have only limited effect on the quality of plaque removal, most probably because patients miss the same areas again.[32,33] However, when brushed professionally, manual brushing reaches its limit after six minutes, whereas brushing with oscillating–rotating brushes achieves this efficacy after **two minutes**. Longer brushing, however, also results in longer contact times with fluorides when fluoride toothpaste is used, which might be beneficial. Retention of fluoride in the mouth also depends on rinsing after brushing.[28] It has been shown that the caries preventive effect seems to be higher if less toothpaste is expectorated after brushing.[25,34] Thus, **mouth-rinsing** with water after brushing should be **reduced** to a minimum. The amount of toothpaste used, however, does not seem to have an important effect.[24]

NOTE

Most patients should brush their teeth twice daily with fluoride toothpaste. To enhance the fluoride effect the toothpaste slurry should not be rinsed with water. The individual's adherence should be considered when giving recommendations.

Interdental Hygiene

Flossing

Tooth brushing is usually not capable to remove interproximal plaque because the bristles may not penetrate the interdental areas.[9] Therefore, it is often recommended that patients should clean their interdental spaces regularly using dental floss. Interestingly, this recommendation is not supported by strong scientific evidence. There are only very few studies on the **efficacy of flossing**. In two studies in which the effect of supervised and unsupervised **self-performed flossing** was investigated in school children (10–13 years old), no preventive effect of flossing could be found.[35,36] For adults apparently no studies exist on the effectiveness of flossing, either alone or as an adjunct to fluorides.[37] This lack of evidence does not necessarily mean that flossing has no preventive effect. It could also be attributed to the small numbers of subjects as well as the design and quality of existing studies. However, it seems that the effect of self-applied flossing is not high enough to be easily detected in clinical trials. A caries preventive effect of flossing was only observed in a study where it was performed on a daily basis in schools by dental professionals in young children with poor tooth brushing habits and low fluoride exposure.[38,39] If professional flossing was performed only every third month, the preventive effect was lost.[36] This indicates that flossing per se may be efficacious (at least in high-risk groups) when it is performed meticulously and frequently enough. The use of fluoridated floss might also have some beneficial effect.[40] However, the difficulties in use and the high prevalence of local root concavities at approximal tooth surfaces, especially at the enamel–cementum interface, might easily overcome this effect.

Taking the limited evidence together it seems that efficacious flossing can only be performed by highly motivated patients or dental professionals and at convex approximal surfaces. The lack of evidence for the effectiveness of self-applied flossing calls the general recommendation to floss into question. Rather, before giving the instructions to floss regularly the dental professional should evaluate whether high-quality flossing is achievable in the individual patient. In addition, one should consider that the recommendation to floss may decrease the exposure time to caries preventive interventions that are supported by better evidence.[37]

> ### NOTE
>
> There is only limited evidence that flossing is efficacious and effective in reducing approximal caries incidence.

Interdental Brushes and Dental Sticks

As an alternative to flossing, the use of interdental brushes (**Fig. 10.7**) can be recommended, especially for patients with approximal restorations, periodontal attachment loss, and gingiva recessions. Interdental cleaning with

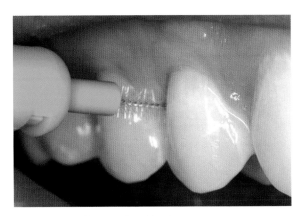

Fig. 10.7   Use of an interdental brush.

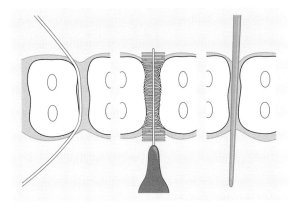

Fig. 10.8   Interdental brushes are more effective at cleaning anatomical grooves and concave surfaces compared with dental floss and dental sticks and therefore are more useful for patients with periodontal attachment loss.

floss is often ineffective because **anatomical recessions and grooves** at the tooth cervix and roots are not reachable by flossing (**Fig. 10.8**). Using interdental brushes, plaque removal is more efficacious than with tooth brushes alone,[41] and in patients with periodontitis it is more efficacious than dental floss.[42] Interdental brushes of very thin diameter are available, which may be used even in young patients with healthy periodontium. There are no studies on the long-term safety of interdental brushes, but there are concerns that frequent **injury of the col and dental papillae** might result in papilla recession. Therefore, it might be advisable to recommend the use of tiny interdental brushes only for patients with approximal lesions. In patients with periodontal attachment loss, where exposed cementum and dentin are especially susceptible to demineralization, interdental areas need special care not only to prevent further periodontal attachment loss, but also to prevent **root caries**. It has been shown that patients using interdental brushes exhibit less root caries than patients who do not perform interdental hygiene.[43] However, the size of the interdental brushes has to be adapted to the size of the interdental space to achieve optimal results.

Table 10.2 Effect of professional tooth cleaning trials

| Study | Age group (years) | Frequency of PTC | Intervention | | Length of time (years) | Caries increment | | Caries reduction |
			Test	Control		Test	Control	
Karlstad studies: Axelsson and Lindhe[49]	8–15	Fortnightly	PTC, OHI, 5% MFP	Monthly supervised brushing, 0.2% NaF	2	0.12	3.25	94%
Poulsen et al.[50]	7	Fortnightly	PTC, 0.2% NaF rinse	Fortnightly 0.2% NaF rinse	1	0.43	1.42	70%
Agerbaeck et al.[51]	8	Every 3rd week	PTC, 0.2% NaF rinse	Fortnightly 0.2% NaF rinse	1	1.40	2.09	33%
Hamp et al.[52]	7–16	Every 3rd week	PTC, 0.2% NaF rinse	Fortnightly 0.2% NaF rinse	3	2.10	4.17	51%
Karlstad studies: Axelsson and Lindhe[53]	35–50	Every 2nd/ 3rd month	PTC, OHI	–	3	0.00–0.03	0.13–1.53	98%–100%

PTC: Professional tooth cleaning; OHI: oral hygiene instructions; NaF: Sodium fluoride; MFP: Sodium monofluorophosphate. Source: Modified from ref. 10.

Dental sticks are popular in elderly patients, to clean interdental areas of food deposits after meals. Dental plaque, however, cannot be removed sufficiently with dental sticks and thus their effect is merely cosmetic or for convenience. Therefore, dental sticks should not be recommended as a substitute for dental floss or interdental brushes.

Professional Tooth Cleaning

The efficacy of professional tooth cleaning was extensively investigated for the first time in the so-called **Karlstad studies.** In this town in Sweden a group of schoolchildren received a preventive program which included fortnightly professional tooth cleaning with oral hygiene instructions, parent engagement, and diet counseling. In a control group children were examined just annually, and received oral hygiene and dietary education.[17,44] The program resulted in high levels of oral cleanliness in the children which recieved the preventive program and caries incidence fell to practically zero (**Table 10.2**). Later, when in the same group the originally fortnightly intervals were extended to monthly or two-monthly intervals, the effect did not diminish. However, when professional cleaning was substituted by supervised, self-performed oral hygiene, part of the caries preventive effect was lost.[45]

These results were confirmed in later studies, although caries reduction rates were not as high (**Table 10.2**). In schoolchildren, biannual professional cleaning did not

have an effect on oral hygiene, gingivitis, and caries.[46] The majority of these studies dealt with schoolchildren, but the effects on adolescents[47] and adults[48] were similar. In some of the trials fluoride was also professionally applied, so that the effect of professional tooth cleaning could be separated from the fluoride effect. In summary, professional tooth cleaning has a preventive effect and should be advocated, although its cost-effectiveness is a matter of debate.

NOTE

Regular, frequent professional tooth cleaning, especially in conjunction with oral hygiene instructions and fluoride application, is costly but highly efficacious in preventing caries.

Chemical Biofilm Control

Mechanical plaque removal requires manual dexterity and is time-consuming. Consequently, efforts have been made to use chemical agents in mouth rinses or dentifrices as adjuncts to mechanical tooth cleaning methods. There are many different chemotherapeutics used in oral hygiene products, which nearly all show rather unspecific antimicrobial effects and thus reduce both pathogenic and nonpathogenic bacteria.

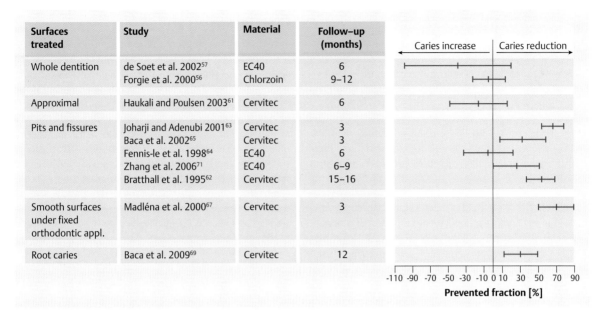

Fig. 10.9 Efficacy of chlorhexidine (CHX) varnish treatment at various tooth sites and after different periods. CHX varnishes show a caries preventive effect on pits and fissures, smooth surfaces under fixed orthodontic appliances, and root caries.

Chlorhexidine

The best studied and most effective antimicrobial agent used in dentistry is chlorhexidine (CHX),[54] which is a cationic bisbiguanide with hydrophilic and hydrophobic properties. Its mode of action is disruption of the microbial membrane by interaction with the hydrophobic part of the molecule. The positively charged molecule also binds on negatively charged groups in the oral mucosa, thus resulting in a **high substantivity** of the antimicrobial.[55]

While in periodontal therapy CHX is mainly used in the form of mouth rinses, in caries therapy professionally applied CHX varnishes are more common. Due to their local application, these varnishes do not show the common **side effects** of CHX mouth rinses, such as tooth discoloration, epithelial desquamation, and hairy tongue. The efficacy of CHX varnish application varies depending on the tooth site. When measuring the combined effect on all tooth surfaces, CHX varnish failed to show a beneficial effect.[56,57] Similarly, studies on the efficacy of CHX application on **approximal caries** showed no caries preventive effect.[58–61] In contrast, CHX varnishes seem to be efficacious to prevent fissure caries in **erupting molars**,[62–65] probably due to the high substantivity and slow release of the CHX from the retentive fissure system. Studies on the efficacy of CHX application on buccal caries lesions during orthodontic appliances showed conflicting results.[66,67] Studies on the effect of CHX application on reduction of **root caries** incidence found beneficial effects[68–70] (**Fig. 10.9**).

In summary, CHX varnishes seem to be efficacious in preventing caries at tooth sites at higher risk for caries, in particular when they are easy to apply. It seems rational that the effects of CHX varnish application depend on the frequency of application. In general, CHX seems to have a moderate caries-inhibiting effect when applied every three-to-four months and the protective effect seems to diminish after the last application.[71]

> **NOTE**
>
> Chlorhexidine varnish is efficacious in reducing caries incidence in high-risk patients. Preventive effects were found mainly for pits and fissures as well as for root caries lesions.

Xylitol

Xylitol is a noncariogenic sugar alcohol with antimicrobial properties. Its mode of action and its use will be extensively discussed in Chapter 11.

Triclosan/Copolymer

Triclosan is a nonionic bisphenol with hydrophilic and hydrophobic properties. In commercial products triclosan is solubilized in detergents such as sodium dodecyl sulfate (see below), which might also have an antimicrobial effect. The **substantivity** of triclosan is relatively poor and, therefore, either zinc chloride or a polyvinyl-methyl-ether maleic acid copolymer (PVM/MA) is added to commercial formulations to increase its efficacy.[55] When compared with a regular fluoride dentifrice, the use of triclosan/copolymer dentifrice improved the removal of plaque by 15%.[72] The anti-caries effect of triclosan, however, is not well documented. Since in laboratory experiments triclosan-resistant bacterial strains could be produced, concerns have been raised that the widespread use of triclosan might promote the development of **reduced susceptibility** to clinically important antimicrobials, due to either cross-resistance or co-resistance mechanisms.[73]

Essential Oil (Listerine)

Listerine is a hydro-alcohol solution of thymol, menthol, eucalyptol, and methyl silicate. It is one of the oldest mouth rinses and is highly popular, probably because of its "disinfectant" taste and its ability to dispel odors.[54] There are few disadvantages to Listerine. Patients seem to adapt to the unpleasant taste and smell. Moreover, only little staining and no enhancement of growth of pathogenetic microorganisms has been observed. Although plaque and gingivitis can be reduced by the regular use of Listerine,[74] there are no studies showing a caries preventive effect.

Sodium Lauryl Sulfate

Sodium lauryl sulfate (aka sodium dodecyl sulfate; SDS) is an anionic detergent with a hydrophobic organic part that has a high affinity for proteins. It seems to have a plaque inhibitory effect which is based on interaction of the SDS molecules with the microbial cell wall, which may lead to leakage of bacterial cell components. SDS also has strong protein-denaturing properties.[75,76] However, there is no study proving a cariostatic effect of SDS.[55] SDS is widely used as a detergent in mouth rinses and dentifrices. It inhibits the caries preventive effect of monofluorophosphate and also the antibacterial effect of CHX. Therefore, tooth brushing with SDS-containing dentifrice and rinsing with CHX solutions should be done at least 30 minutes apart.[54]

Metal Ions

Metal ions such as Cu^{2+}, Zn^{2+}, and Sn^{2+} show antimicrobial effects by interaction with anionic groups of bacterial enzymes and thus may inhibit bacterial metabolism. They may also alter the surface charge of microorganisms by replacement of Ca^{2+} and thus impair their adherence ability.[54,77] Similarly to CHX, metal ions bind to negatively charged groups of mucosa proteins and thus show a high substantivity. Zn^{2+} has furthermore the ability to react with odiferous sulfur containing compounds, which led to the widespread use of zinc salts in oral hygiene products.[55] Cu^{2+}, Zn^{2+}, and Sn^{2+} salts have been shown to reduce the acidogenicity of plaque.[78,79] The use of metallic ions is limited by their toxicity in higher concentrations as well as possible side effects such as metallic taste, feeling of dryness, and yellowish to brownish dental stain.[55] Moreover, evidence on the caries preventive effect of metals ions is scarce.

General Considerations

Except for xylitol, most of the aforementioned antimicrobial substances show **unspecific antimicrobial activity** and will therefore reduce both the pathogenic and the nonpathogenic (beneficial) microflora of the mouth. Moreover, any antimicrobial therapy will lead to an increased selection pressure within the biofilm. In patients with a cariogenic diet, the reduction of certain sensitive bacteria might even result to an overgrowth of aciduric species such as mutans streptococci and lactobacilli.[80] These considerations led to the general recommendation that any chemotherapeutic approach should be limited only to **patients with increased caries risk** and ongoing caries activity, and should always be accompanied by measures to **change the patient's diet**.[80–82]

CLINICAL PEARL

Any chemotherapeutic approach should be reserved for patients with increased caries risk and ongoing caries activity, restricted to a limited period, and always accompanied by measures to change the patient's diet.

Biological Biofilm Control

Most conventional dental therapies are primarily focused on the mechanical removal or chemical inhibition of plaque. However, since dental plaque consists of large amounts of commensal bacteria and only limited numbers of pathogens, this "remove-or-kill-all approach" may not be effective because it leaves exposed and noncompetitive surfaces that allow pathogens to repopulate the sites, if favoring factors such as a cariogenic diet remain.[83] Therefore, more recent approaches aim instead to **alter the ecology** of the plaque rather than to eliminate the bacteria.

In contrast, it has been shown that treatment with various biocides such as CHX, xylitol, iodine, antibiotics, and even simple mechanical tooth cleaning resulted in reduced *Streptococcus mutans* levels. This might be interpreted in the sense that persistence of *S. mutans* can easily be disturbed and 'specific reduction' of *S. mutans*, claimed for various agents, is more likely a result of a nonspecific response of *S. mutans* to an adverse environment from which other (noncariogenic) members of the oral flora can better recover, especially when other environmental factors are also changed. The flora might be beneficially modified by simply reducing the content of fermentable carbohydrate in the diet[84,85] (see Chapter 11). However, since a sustained change of dietary habits is strongly dependent on patient's adherence, and therefore is often hard to accomplish, there are also other approaches to modify the composition of the biofilm, such as vaccination and the use of probiotics.

Vaccination

In the past century great achievements have been made through vaccination against common (specific) infectious diseases like poliomyelitis and smallpox. This encouraged scientists to develop vaccines also against caries. If one considers caries as an infectious disease[86] associated with specific bacteria such as *S. mutans* (specific plaque hypothesis), it becomes almost "imperative" to develop a vaccine against these bacteria.[87]

There are two ways to achieve (enhanced) immune response against cariogenic bacteria: active and passive immunization. The administration of single or combined bacterial antigens aims to boost an **active immunization** against *S. mutans*. In animal studies this approach showed promising results.[87-89] In humans, however, so far only small-scale clinical trials with surrogate outcomes (not caries increment) have been performed,[90] and the caries preventive effect has not been corroborated so far. Moreover in humans, antibody production was only short-lived. **Passive immunization** aims to reduce bacteria levels by regular oral administration of antibodies against cariogenic bacteria such as *S. mutans*. While successfully tested in animal models, clinical trials with humans showed somewhat conflicting results.[91-94]

In general, the limited effects of vaccination thus far have had to be carefully balanced with safety and cost issues, especially because other safe and effective preventive options against caries (e.g., fluorides) do already exist. If caries is considered as a multifactorial rather than a classic infectious disease, the effectiveness of the vaccination approach is questionable—even more so, since other aciduric and acidogenic bacteria would most likely take over the role of *S. mutans*.

Probiotic Therapy

The ongoing paradigm shift toward an ecological plaque hypothesis supports new treatment strategies. The rationale of the probiotic approach is "to administer live microorganisms which confer a health benefit on the host."[95] The beneficial effects are thought to be caused by different modes of action ranging from direct inhibition of pathogenic microbes to improving the immune response of the host. Probiotics have been successfully used in the treatment of **gastrointestinal disorders** like Irritable Bowel Syndrome, virus induced diarrhea, and lactose intolerance, as well as allergies. More recently, the probiotic concepts have also been brought to bear on the oral cavity.

One probiotic approach is to regularly administer **non-pathogenic bacteria**, like *Lactobacillus rhamnosus*, which compete for their ecological niche with more pathogenic bacteria like *S. mutans*. It has been shown that long-term consumption of fluoridated milk containing probiotic *L.rhamnosus GG* strain reduced caries-associated factors (caries risk) and bacterially caused diseases like otitis media in children.[96] In other studies employing probiotic species like *L. reuteri* or *Bifidobacterium* strains the num-

bers of *S. mutans* could be reduced.[97-99] However, clinical studies showing a caries preventive effect are still lacking. Another probiotic approach is to administer genetically modified *S. mutans* strains which are only weakly acidogenic and compete with cariogenic wild-type strains. This concept has been proven in animal models,[100] but for safety reasons its efficacy in humans has not been shown yet.

Generally, there is still **little evidence** that probiotic therapy is efficacious in humans, and before the widespread use of probiotics some problems have to be solved. First, due to the complexity of live organisms, the safety of (eventually genetically modified) probiotic based commercial products is hard to evaluate. Second, live organisms usually have a short shelf-life and require complex storage conditions.[83] Thus, so far, no recommendation for the use of probiotics can be given to the dental practitioner.[101]

NOTE

Probiotic approaches aim to prevent caries by administration of noncariogenic microorganisms that have similar ecological niches to cariogenic microorganisms like *Streptococcus mutans*, thus promoting competition between the species and a reduction of pathogenic bacteria.

SUMMARY

Plaque is one essential causal factor for caries but the role of oral hygiene in caries etiology and prevention remains controversial. Dental caries can be prevented by highly efficient removal of plaque and the simplest way to achieve this is mechanical measures like brushing or flossing. Twice-daily brushing with fluoride toothpaste is probably the most effective caries preventive measure. However, in this regard the role of fluorides should not be underestimated. An oral hygiene level sufficient to prevent caries is difficult to maintain by self-performed oral hygiene, especially on scarcely accessible surfaces. Regular professionally applied oral hygiene seems to be very efficacious in preventing caries, but limited by the rather high costs. Chemotherapeutics are easy to apply but show only reduced efficacy on bacterial biofilms. The most efficient antimicrobial agent used in dentistry is chlorhexidine. For other plaque-regulating substances like triclosan or metal ions, the caries preventive effect is not very well documented. In general, the chemotherapeutic approach is always nonspecific and reduces both the pathogenic and the beneficial microflora, and therefore should be limited to patients in whom other measures are most likely ineffective. In recent years biological approaches like active or passive immunization or probiotic therapy have been discussed. But so far scientific data are too weak to support these approaches for the daily routine.

REFERENCES

1. Savage DC. Microbial ecology of the gastrointestinal tract. Annu Rev Microbiol 1977;31:107–133

2. Dale BA, Fredericks LP. Antimicrobial peptides in the oral environment: expression and function in health and disease. Curr Issues Mol Biol 2005;7(2):119–133

3. Hyson JM Jr. History of the toothbrush. J Hist Dent 2003;51(2):73–80

4. Cowan MM. Plant products as antimicrobial agents. Clin Microbiol Rev 1999;12(4):564–582

5. Marsh PD. Dental plaque as a microbial biofilm. Caries Res 2004;38(3):204–211

6. Larsen T. Susceptibility of Porphyromonas gingivalis in biofilms to amoxicillin, doxycycline and metronidazole. Oral Microbiol Immunol 2002;17(5):267–271

7. Zijnge V, van Leeuwen MB, Degener JE, et al. Oral biofilm architecture on natural teeth. PLoS ONE 2010;5(2):e9321

8. Keijser BJ, Zaura E, Huse SM, et al. Pyrosequencing analysis of the oral microflora of healthy adults. J Dent Res 2008;87(11):1016–1020

9. Andlaw RJ. Oral hygiene and dental caries—a review. Int Dent J 1978;28(1):1–6

10. Bellini HT, Arneberg P, von der Fehr FR. Oral hygiene and caries. A review. Acta Odontol Scand 1981;39(5):257–265

11. Marthaler TM. Reduction of caries, gingivitis and calculus after eight years of preventive measures—observations in seven communities. Helv Odontol Acta 1972;16(2):69–83

12. Sutcliffe P. A longitudinal clinical study of oral cleanliness and dental caries in school children. Arch Oral Biol 1973;18(7):765–770

13. Tucker GJ, Andlaw RJ, Burchell CK. The relationship between oral hygiene and dental caries incidence in 11-year-old children. A 3-year study. Br Dent J 1976;141(3):75–79

14. Vestergaard V, Moss A, Pedersen HO, Poulsen S. The effect of supervised tooth cleansing every second week on dental caries in Danish school children. Acta Odontol Scand 1978;36(4):249–252

15. Beal JF, James PM, Bradnock G, Anderson RJ. The relationship between dental cleanliness, dental caries incidence and gingival health. A longitudinal study. Br Dent J 1979;146(4):111–114

16. Koch G, Lindhe J. The state of the gingivae and the caries-increment in schoolchildren during and after withdrawal of various prophylactic measures. In: McHugh WD, ed. Dental Plaque. Edinburgh: Livingston; 1970:271–281

17. Lindhe J, Axelsson P. The effect of controlled oral hygiene and topical fluoride application on caries and gingivitis in Swedish schoolchildren. Community Dent Oral Epidemiol 1973;1(1):9–16

18. Carvalho JC, Thylstrup A, Ekstrand KR. Results after 3 years of non-operative occlusal caries treatment of erupting permanent first molars. Community Dent Oral Epidemiol 1992;20(4):187–192

19. Gray D, McIntyre G. Does oral health promotion influence the oral hygiene and gingival health of patients undergoing fixed appliance orthodontic treatment? A systematic literature review. J Orthod 2008;35(4):262–269

20. He T, Li S, Sun L. Clinical comparison of the plaque removal efficacy of a manual toothbrush with criss-cross bristle design. Am J Dent 2009;22(4):200–202

21. Poyato-Ferrera M, Segura-Egea JJ, Bullón-Fernández P. Comparison of modified Bass technique with normal toothbrushing practices for efficacy in supragingival plaque removal. Int J Dent Hyg 2003;1(2):110–114

22. Robinson PG, Deacon SA, Deery C, et al. Manual versus powered toothbrushing for oral health. Cochrane Database Syst Rev 2005;2(2):CD002281

23. Loe H, Theilade E, Jensen SB. Experimental Gingivitis in Man. J Periodontol 1965;36:177–187

24. Chesters RK, Huntington E, Burchell CK, Stephen KW. Effect of oral care habits on caries in adolescents. Caries Res 1992;26(4):299–304

25. Ashley PF, Attrill DC, Ellwood RP, Worthington HV, Davies RM. Toothbrushing habits and caries experience. Caries Res 1999;33(5):401–402

26. Fosdick LS. The reduction of the incidence of dental caries; immediate tooth-brushing with a neutral dentifrice. J Am Dent Assoc 1950;40(2):133–143

27. Sgan-Cohen HD. Oral hygiene: past history and future recommendations. Int J Dent Hyg 2005;3(2):54–58

28. Attin T, Hornecker E. Tooth brushing and oral health: how frequently and when should tooth brushing be performed? Oral Health Prev Dent 2005;3(3):135–140

29. Jaeggi T, Lussi A. Toothbrush abrasion of erosively altered enamel after intraoral exposure to saliva: an in situ study. Caries Res 1999;33(6):455–461

30. Attin T, Siegel S, Buchalla W, Lennon AM, Hannig C, Becker K. Brushing abrasion of softened and remineralised dentin: an in situ study. Caries Res 2004;38(1):62–66

31. Dawes C. Factors influencing salivary flow rate and composition. In: Edgar M, Dawes C, O'Mullane D, eds. Saliva and Oral Health. 3rd ed. London: British Dental Association; 2004:32–49

32. Huber B, Rüeger K, Hefti A. The effect of the duration of toothbrushing on plaque reduction. [Article in German] Schweiz Monatsschr Zahnmed 1985;95(10):985–992

33. Ashley P. Toothbrushing: why, when and how? Dent Update 2001;28(1):36–40

34. Sjögren K, Birkhed D. Factors related to fluoride retention after toothbrushing and possible connection to caries activity. Caries Res 1993;27(6):474–477

35. Granath LE, Martinsson T, Matsson L, Nilsson G, Schröder U, Söderholm B. Intraindividual effect of daily supervised flossing on caries in schoolchildren. Community Dent Oral Epidemiol 1979;7(3):147–150

36. Gisselsson H, Birkhed D, Björn AL. Effect of a 3-year professional flossing program with chlorhexidine gel on approximal caries and cost of treatment in preschool children. Caries Res 1994;28(5):394–399

37. Hujoel PP, Cunha-Cruz J, Banting DW, Loesche WJ. Dental flossing and interproximal caries: a systematic review. J Dent Res 2006;85(4):298–305

38. Wright GZ, Banting DW, Feasby WH. Effect of interdental flossing on the incidence of proximal caries in children. J Dent Res 1977;56(6):574–578

39. Wright GZ, Banting DW, Feasby WH. The Dorchester dental flossing study: final report. Clin Prev Dent 1979;1(3):23–26

40. Särner B, Birkhed D, Huysmans MC, Ruben JL, Fidler V, Lingström P. Effect of fluoridated toothpicks and dental flosses on enamel and dentine and on plaque composition in situ. Caries Res 2005;39(1):52–59

41. Slot DE, Dörfer CE, Van der Weijden GA. The efficacy of interdental brushes on plaque and parameters of periodontal inflammation: a systematic review. Int J Dent Hyg 2008;6(4):253–264

42. Christou V, Timmerman MF, Van der Velden U, Van der Weijden FA. Comparison of different approaches of interdental oral hygiene: interdental brushes versus dental floss. J Periodontol 1998;69(7):759–764

43. Takano N, Ando Y, Yoshihara A, Miyazaki H. Factors associated with root caries incidence in an elderly population. Community Dent Health 2003;20(4):217–222

44. Axelsson P, Lindhe J. The effect of a plaque control program on gingivitis and dental caries in schoolchildren. J Dent Res 1977;56(Spec No) C142–C148

45. Axelsson P, Lindhe J, Wäseby J. The effect of various plaque control measures on gingivitis and caries in schoolchildren. Community Dent Oral Epidemiol 1976;4(6):232–239

46. Ripa LW, Barenie JT, Leske GS. The effect on professionally administered bi-annual prophylaxes on the oral hygiene, gingival health, and caries scores of school children. Two year study. J Prev Dent 1976;3(1):22–26

47. Malmberg E. [The Tuve study. 3 years preventive treatment of 16 - 19 year olds]. Tandlakartidningen 1976;68(19):1087–1088

48. Axelsson P, Lindhe J, Nyström B. On the prevention of caries and periodontal disease. Results of a 15-year longitudinal study in adults. J Clin Periodontol 1991;18(3):182–189

49. Axelsson P, Lindhe J. The effect of a preventive programme on dental plaque, gingivitis and caries in schoolchildren. Results after one and two years. J Clin Periodontol 1974;1(2):126–138

50. Poulsen S, Agerbaek N, Melsen B, Korts DC, Glavind L, Rölla G. The effect of professional toothcleansing on gingivitis and dental caries in children after 1 year. Community Dent Oral Epidemiol 1976;4(5):195–199

51. Agerbaek N, Poulsen S, Melsen B, Glavind L. Effect of professional toothcleansing every third week on gingivitis and dental caries in children. Community Dent Oral Epidemiol 1978;6(1):40–41

52. Hamp SE, Lindhe J, Fornell J, Johansson LA, Karlsson R. Effect of a field program based on systematic plaque control on caries and gingivitis in schoolchildren after 3 years. Community Dent Oral Epidemiol 1978;6(1):17–23

53. Axelsson P, Lindhe J. Effect of controlled oral hygiene procedures on caries and periodontal disease in adults. J Clin Periodontol 1978;5(2):133–151

54. Adams D, Addy M. Mouthrinses. Adv Dent Res 1994;8(2):291–301

55. Scheie AA, Petersen FC. Antimicrobials in caries control. In: Kidd EAM, Fejerskov O, eds. Dental Caries. The Disease and its Clinical Management. 2nd ed. Oxford: Blackwell Munksgaard; 2008:265–277

56. Forgie AH, Paterson M, Pine CM, Pitts NB, Nugent ZJ. A randomised controlled trial of the caries-preventive efficacy of a chlorhexidine-containing varnish in high-caries-risk adolescents. Caries Res 2000;34(5):432–439

57. de Soet JJ, Gruythuysen RJ, Bosch JA, van Amerongen WE. The effect of 6-monthly application of 40% chlorhexidine varnish on the microflora and dental caries incidence in a population of children in Surinam. Caries Res 2002;36(6):449–455

58. Petersson LG, Magnusson K, Andersson H, Deierborg G, Twetman S. Effect of semi-annual applications of a chlorhexidine/fluoride varnish mixture on approximal caries incidence in schoolchildren. A three-year radiographic study. Eur J Oral Sci 1998;106(2 Pt 1):623–627

59. Twetman S, Petersson LG. Interdental caries incidence and progression in relation to mutans streptococci suppression after chlorhexidine-thymol varnish treatments in schoolchildren. Acta Odontol Scand 1999;57(3):144–148

60. Petersson LG, Magnusson K, Andersson H, Almquist B, Twetman S. Effect of quarterly treatments with a chlorhexidine and a fluoride varnish on approximal caries in caries-susceptible teenagers: a 3-year clinical study. Caries Res 2000;34(2):140–143

61. Haukali G, Poulsen S. Effect of a varnish containing chlorhexidine and thymol (Cervitec) on approximal caries in 13- to 16-year-old schoolchildren in a low caries area. Caries Res 2003;37(3):185–189

62. Bratthall D, Serinirach R, Rapisuwon S, et al. A study into the prevention of fissure caries using an antimicrobial varnish. Int Dent J 1995;45(4):245–254

63. Joharji RM, Adenubi JO. Prevention of pit and fissure caries using an antimicrobial varnish: 9 month clinical evaluation. J Dent 2001;29(4):247–254

64. Fennis-le YL, Verdonschot EH, Burgersdijk RC et al. Effect of a 6-monthly application of chlorhexidine varnish on incidence of occlusal caries in permanent molars: a 3-year study. J Dent 1998;26(3):233–238

65. Baca P, Muñoz MJ, Bravo M, Junco P, Baca AP. Effectiveness of chlorhexidine-thymol varnish for caries reduction in permanent first molars of 6-7-year-old children: 24-month clinical trial. Community Dent Oral Epidemiol 2002;30(5):363–368

66. Ogaard B, Larsson E, Glans R, Henriksson T, Birkhed D. Antimicrobial effect of a chlorhexidine-thymol varnish (Cervitec) in orthodontic patients. A prospective, randomized clinical trial. J Orofac Orthop 1997;58(4):206–213

67. Madléna M, Vitalyos G, Márton S, Nagy G. Effect of chlorhexidine varnish on bacterial levels in plaque and saliva during orthodontic treatment. J Clin Dent 2000;11(2):42–46

68. Brailsford SR, Fiske J, Gilbert S, Clark D, Beighton D. The effects of the combination of chlorhexidine/thymol- and fluoride-containing varnishes on the severity of root caries lesions in frail institutionalised elderly people. J Dent 2002;30(7-8):319–324

69. Baca P, Clavero J, Baca AP, González-Rodríguez MP, Bravo M, Valderrama MJ. Effect of chlorhexidine-thymol varnish on root caries in a geriatric population: a randomized double-blind clinical trial. J Dent 2009;37(9):679–685

70. Tan HP, Lo EC, Dyson JE, Luo Y, Corbet EF. A randomized trial on root caries prevention in elders. J Dent Res 2010;89(10):1086–1090

71. Zhang Q, van Palenstein Helderman WH, van't Hof MA, Truin GJ. Chlorhexidine varnish for preventing dental caries in children, adolescents and young adults: a systematic review. Eur J Oral Sci 2006;114(6):449–455

72. Davies RM, Ellwood RP, Davies GM. The effectiveness of a toothpaste containing triclosan and polyvinyl-methyl ether maleic acid copolymer in improving plaque control and gingival health: a systematic review. J Clin Periodontol 2004;31(12):1029–1033

73. Yazdankhah SP, Scheie AA, Høiby EA, et al. Triclosan and antimicrobial resistance in bacteria: an overview. Microb Drug Resist 2006;12(2):83–90

74. DePaola LG, Overholser CD, Meiller TF, Minah GE, Niehaus C. Chemotherapeutic inhibition of supragingival dental plaque and gingivitis development. J Clin Periodontol 1989;16(5):311–315

75. Jenkins S, Addy M, Newcombe R. Triclosan and sodium lauryl sulphate mouthwashes (I). Effects on salivary bacterial counts. J Clin Periodontol 1991;18(2):140–144

76. Jenkins S, Addy M, Newcombe R. Triclosan and sodium lauryl sulphate mouthrinses. (II). Effects of 4-day plaque regrowth. J Clin Periodontol 1991;18(2):145–148

77. Olsson J, Odham G. Effect of inorganic ions and surface active organic compounds on the adherence of oral streptococci. Scand J Dent Res 1978;86(2):108–117

78. Oppermann RV, Rölla G. Effect of some polyvalent cations on the acidogenicity of dental plaque in vivo. Caries Res 1980;14(6):422–427

79. Afseth J, Rølla G, Helgeland K, Oppermann RV. Aspects of Cu2 + and Zn2 + in mouth rinses with regards to dental health. Acta Pharmacol Toxicol (Copenh) 1986;59(Suppl 7):300–304

80. Twetman S. Antimicrobials in future caries control? A review with special reference to chlorhexidine treatment. Caries Res 2004;38(3):223–229

81. Kidd EA. Role of chlorhexidine in the management of dental caries. Int Dent J 1991;41(5):279–286

82. Rozier RG. Effectiveness of methods used by dental professionals for the primary prevention of dental caries. J Dent Educ 2001;65(10):1063–1072

83. He X, Lux R, Kuramitsu HK, Anderson MH, Shi W. Achieving probiotic effects via modulating oral microbial ecology. Adv Dent Res 2009;21(1):53–56

84. Wennerholm K, Birkhed D, Emilson CG. Effects of sugar restriction on Streptococcus mutans and Streptococcus sobrinus in saliva and dental plaque. Caries Res 1995;29(1):54–61

85. Beighton D. Can the ecology of the dental biofilm be beneficially altered? Adv Dent Res 2009;21(1):69–73

86. Shivakumar KM, Vidya SK, Chandu GN. Dental caries vaccine. Indian J Dent Res 2009;20(1):99–106

87. Taubman MA, Nash DA. The scientific and public-health imperative for a vaccine against dental caries. Nat Rev Immunol 2006;6(7):555–563

88. Xu QA, Yu F, Fan MW, et al. Protective efficacy of a targeted anti-caries DNA plasmid against cariogenic bacteria infections. Vaccine 2007;25(7):1191–1195

89. Li YH, Huang S, Du M, Bian Z, Chen Z, Fan MW. Immunogenic characterization and protection against Streptococcus mutans infection induced by intranasal DNA prime-protein boost immunization. Vaccine 2010;28(32):5370–5376

90. Childers NK, Tong G, Li F, Dasanayake AP, Kirk K, Michalek SM. Humans immunized with Streptococcus mutans antigens by mucosal routes. J Dent Res 2002;81(1):48–52

91. Hatta H, Tsuda K, Ozeki M, et al. Passive immunization against dental plaque formation in humans: effect of a mouth rinse containing egg yolk antibodies (IgY) specific to Streptococcus mutans. Caries Res 1997;31(4):268–274

92. Ma JK, Hikmat BY, Wycoff K, et al. Characterization of a recombinant plant monoclonal secretory antibody and preventive immunotherapy in humans. Nat Med 1998;4(5):601–606

93. Shimazaki Y, Mitoma M, Oho T, et al. Passive immunization with milk produced from an immunized cow prevents oral recolonization by Streptococcus mutans. Clin Diagn Lab Immunol 2001;8(6):1136–1139

94. Weintraub JA, Hilton JF, White JM, et al. Clinical trial of a plant-derived antibody on recolonization of mutans streptococci. Caries Res 2005;39(3):241–250

95. World Health Organization (WHO). Health and Nutritional Properties of Probiotics in Food including Powder Milk with Live Lactic Acid Bacteria. Report of a joint FAO/WHO Expert Consultation on Evaluation of Health and Nutritional Properties of Probiotics in Food including Powder Milk with Live Lactic Acid Bacteria. Cordoba: Food and Agriculture Organization of the United Nations, World Health Organization; 2001

96. Näse L, Hatakka K, Savilahti E, et al. Effect of long-term consumption of a probiotic bacterium, Lactobacillus rhamnosus GG, in milk on dental caries and caries risk in children. Caries Res 2001;35(6):412–420

97. Caglar E, Kavaloglu SC, Kuscu OO, Sandalli N, Holgerson PL, Twetman S. Effect of chewing gums containing xylitol or probiotic bacteria on salivary mutans streptococci and lactobacilli. Clin Oral Investig 2007;11(4):425–429

98. Caglar E, Kuscu OO, Selvi Kuvvetli S, Kavaloglu Cildir S, Sandalli N, Twetman S. Short-term effect of ice-cream containing Bifidobacterium lactis Bb-12 on the number of salivary mutans streptococci and lactobacilli. Acta Odontol Scand 2008;66(3):154–158

99. Cildir SK, Germec D, Sandalli N, et al. Reduction of salivary mutans streptococci in orthodontic patients during daily consumption of yoghurt containing probiotic bacteria. Eur J Orthod 2009;31(4):407–411

100. Hillman JD. Genetically modified Streptococcus mutans for the prevention of dental caries. Antonie van Leeuwenhoek 2002;82(1-4):361–366

101. Stamatova I, Meurman JH. Probiotics: health benefits in the mouth. Am J Dent 2009;22(6):329–338

Caries Management by Modifying Diet

Bennett T. Amaechi

11

As described in the previous chapters, caries occurs when the equilibrium between the teeth and the biofilm is in imbalance. Imbalance means that the pH in the biofilm frequently drops from neutral to below a critical range for dental hard tissues, resulting in net demineralization of the tooth's surface. The main factor that fosters this imbalance is the composition and mode of intake of the diet. In a consensus statement on diet, the FDI Second World Conference on Oral Health Promotion recognized food as being a complex mixture of macro- and micro- components. Following prolonged contact with the oral cavity, the diet can influence the oral microflora and can constitute a caries risk.[1] The major components of diet—carbohydrates, proteins, fats, fruits, vegetables, and various additives to foods—all modulate the caries process, playing either a promotional or inhibitory role. **Fermentable carbohydrates** play a promotional role in the development of dental caries. In particular, **sucrose** has been named as the "arch criminal" in the caries process.[2] Indeed, sucrose is the most cariogenic dietary carbohydrate, and diet with a high proportion of sucrose is known to increase the caries risk of an individual. Nonetheless, bacteria have the ability to ferment a wide variety of dietary carbohydrates to produce organic acids. Some proteins, fats, fruits, vegetables, and other food components may play a protective role in caries development. This chapter will describe the scientific basis of the influence of these food components on the caries process and caries risk of individuals. In particular this chapter will cover:

- The mechanisms of carbohydrate fermentation in the biofilm
- The role of sugar alcohols and intense sweeteners
- The mode of action of some protective food constituents
- Certain groups being at risk due to dietary patterns
- Guidelines for "tooth friendly" nutrition

Carbohydrates (Sugars) in the Caries Process

The evidence implicating carbohydrate as being essential in the etiology of dental caries is overwhelming. Several studies of adults between 30 and 50 years old, both longitudinal[3,4] and interventional,[5] showed a clear relationship between consumption of refined carbohydrate and the development of dental caries. The description of sugar (i.e., sucrose) as the "arch criminal" of dental caries[2] was based on these findings and also its unusual biochemical properties and the form in which it is consumed by humans. However, not all sugars are involved in the caries process. There are three types of sugars (**Table 11.1**): The **conventional sugars** consist of sucrose, lactose, glucose, fructose, and corn syrups, while the most widely used **sugar alcohols** (polyols) are xylitol, sorbitols, mannitol, lactitol, maltitol, and the products Lycasin and Palatinit. Among the **intense sweeteners** (synthetic or artificial sweeteners) are acesulfame-K, aspartame, neotame, saccharin, sucralose, and steviol glycosides. It is the conventional sugars and polyols, also referred to as nutritive sugars due to their calorific value, that play significant roles in the caries process, either promoting (conventional sugars) or inhibiting (sugar alcohols) the process.

Conventional Sugars

Monosaccharides (glucose and fructose) and **disaccharides** (sucrose, lactose, and maltose) constitute the readily fermentable carbohydrates, and are substantially more cariogenic than starch.[6,7] Starch is typically noncariogenic, because its molecules are too large to diffuse into the dental biofilm, but may be cariogenic in populations with high caries activity in that it can be hydrolyzed by salivary and plaque amylase into maltose, some glucose and dextrins. In rats a starch/sucrose mixture was shown to be more cariogenic than sucrose alone.[6] Although su-

Table 11.1 Types of sugars

Type of sugar	Class	Examples	Cal/g	Sweetness
Conventional sugars	Nutritive	Sucrose	4	1.0
		Lactose	4	0.2
		Glucose	4	0.7
		Corn syrups	3	0.9
		Fructose	4	1.7
Sugar alcohols (Polyols)		Sorbitols	2.6	0.6
		Mannitol	1.6	0.7
		Xylitol	2.4	1.0
		Maltitol	2.1	0.9
Intense (artificial) sweetners	Nonnutritive	Acesulfame-K	0	200
		Aspartame	4	200
		Neotame	0	8000
		Saccharin	0	300
		Sucralose	0	600
		Steviol glycosides	0	300

crose is regarded as the most cariogenic dietary carbohydrate,[8] probably because it is the most frequently ingested sugar, there is little difference in the cariogenicity of sucrose, glucose, and fructose.[9,10] Although cariogenic bacteria such as *Streptococcus mutans* can become established in the absence of sugar, the ingestion of sugar enhances the ability of these microorganisms to colonize tooth surfaces. Whereas in the absence of sucrose there is reversible adsorption of these bacteria to the tooth surface, in the presence of readily fermentable carbohydrate there is a stabilized attachment of the microorganisms to the tooth surface.[11]

NOTE

Although sucrose is regarded as the most cariogenic dietary carbohydrate, probably because it is the most frequently ingested sugar, there is little difference in the cariogenicity of sucrose, glucose, and fructose.

Sugar Metabolism and Acid Production by Cariogenic Microorganisms

A diet rich in readily fermentable carbohydrates promotes the development of dental caries due to the efficient metabolism of these sugars by cariogenic microorganisms, such as *S. mutans*. When a sucrose-rich diet is ingested, these bacteria do not only use the sugar as a primary energy source, but they also utilize it to initiate additional biochemical events which are responsible for the caries process. These biochemical activities occur through two major pathways: extracellular and intracellular (**Fig. 11.1**).[12] Because *S. mutans* is the best investigated cariogenic microorganism, sugar metabolism will be explained taking this bacterium as an example, although other caries-related microorganisms are thought to show similar metabolic patterns.

Intracellular Pathway

In the intracellular pathway, sucrose taken into the bacterial cell can be distributed within the cell in the following ways.

Direct phosphorylation. This proceeds via the glycolytic pathway into organic acid production (**Fig. 11.2**): Many oral microorganisms in plaque biofilm produce organic acids in the presence of sucrose.[13] All *S. mutans* strains are homolactic fermenters converting over 90% of hexose to lactic acid by the glycolytic pathway, since *S. mutans* does not possess the enzymes of the Krebs cycle or cytochromes. The ability of *S. mutans* to produce acid rapidly from sugar is the property most associated with the development of dental caries.[14,15] Each episode of fermentable sugar ingestion is followed by a rapid production of acid by microorganisms, which depresses the pH of the plaque, and values as low as 4 have been recorded.[16]

Glycogen production. Many cariogenic microorganisms have the capacity to produce and store intracellular polysaccharides (IPS) which are branched glycogens of the amylopectin type,[17] and are readily catabolized. A positive correlation has been reported between the numbers of IPS-containing microorganisms and the caries experience (DMFS).[18] Intracellular glycogen in the form of the extracellular polysaccharides (fructans and glucans, see below) serve as substrate reservoirs which the microorganisms may utilize for energy production as the exogenous supplies of readily metabolized carbohydrate are depleted. In this manner both types of polysaccharide may play a role in the survival of the microorganisms and in their poten-

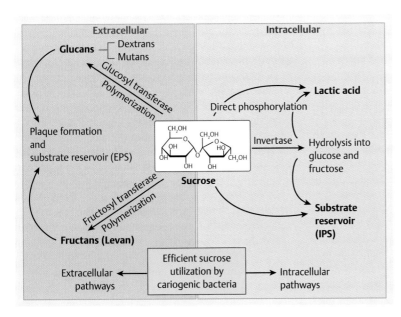

Fig. 11.1   Illustration of the efficient metabolism of sucrose by *Streptococcus mutans*. EPS: extracellular polysaccharides; IPS: intracellular polysaccharides.

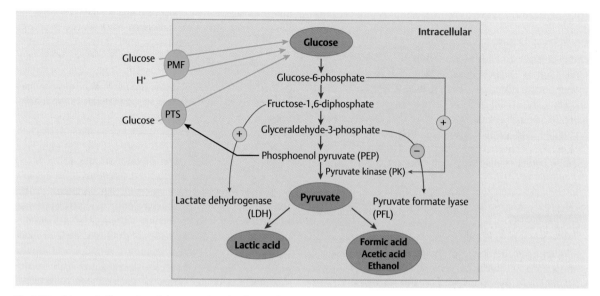

Fig. 11.2 Schematic Illustration of the anaerobic glycolytic pathway of bacterial metabolism. *Streptococcus mutans* can alter the acid profile in plaque according to the amount of sugar in the environment using a self-regulatory mechanism, which is facilitated by its dual metabolic systems, **proton motive force (PMF)** system, and **phosphotransferase (PTS)** system. The PMF is a low affinity sugar uptake system activated by a proton gradient, and operates at low pH. *Streptococcus mutans* uses this system to transport and metabolize sugars under high extracellular glucose concentrations such as during mealtimes. With excess intracellular glucose, the breakdown products of glucose in the glycolytic pathway—which include glucose-6-phosphate, fructose-1,6-diphosphate, glyceraldehyde-3-phosphate, and phosphoenol pyruvate (PEP)—will all be in excess. In the presence of excess glucose-6-phosphate, pyruvate kinase (which catalyses the conversion of PEP to pyruvate) is activated so that excess pyruvate is produced, limiting the amount of PEP available at any one time. In the presence of fructose-1,6-diphosphate, lactate dehydrogenase (LDH), which catalyses the conversion of pyruvate to lactate, is activated, so more lactate (lactic acid) is produced. At the same time, with excess glyceraldehyde-3-phosphate, pyruvate formate lyase (PFL) (which catalyses the conversion of pyruvate to formate, acetate, or ethanol) is inhibited, so little or none of these by-products is produced. The overall effect is that in the presence of high amounts of extracellular glucose, such as during and a few minutes after a meal of fermentable carbohydrates, more lactic acid is produced and less of other acids. The PTS, on the other hand, is a high affinity sugar uptake mechanism driven by PEP and operates at neutral pH. Under low extracellular sucrose concentrations such as between meals, *S. mutans* utilizes this system to transport the scarcely available sugar intracellularly. With limited sugar, the activating action of glucose-6-phosphate on pyruvate kinase will be withdrawn due to this metabolite's low concentration. This in effect will limit the conversion of PEP to pyruvate, resulting in accumulation of PEP. The increased PEP will trigger the PEP/PTS system to transport more glucose into the cell. At the same time, the inhibitory action of glyceraldehyde-3-phosphate on PFL will be withdrawn, favoring the production of formic acid, acetic acid, and ethanol. Thus the overall effect at low extracellular glucose concentration is production of formic acid, acetic acid, and ethanol within the plaque as a by-product of bacterial metabolism.

tial to prolong acid production via glycolysis well beyond meal time.

Invertase activity. Sucrose-adapted microorganisms possess significant levels of invertase, an enzyme which hydrolyzes sucrose intracellularly to free glucose and fructose. The glucose and fructose can either be directly phosphorylated to lactic acid or converted to intracellular polysaccharide (glycogen), as described above.

Extracellular Pathway

In the extracellular pathway, *S. mutans*, through its cell surface-associated enzymes, glucosyltransferases (Gtf) and fructosyltransferases (Ftf), polymerizes the glucose and the fructose moieties of sucrose to synthesize two types of extracellular polysaccharides (EPS): glucans and fructans, respectively.[19] These enzymes act by transferring glucosyl or fructosyl moieties from sucrose to primer molecules. No phosphorylated intermediates are involved, but the energy required for this activity is derived from the energy-rich disaccharide bond of sucrose, and this explains why this sugar is the essential substrate. The glucans provide binding sites for colonization by bacteria, promote the accumulation of microorganisms on the tooth surface (plaque formation), and contribute to the bulk and further development of the plaque biofilm.[20,21] The fructans synthesized by the *S. mutans* are also highly soluble and can be degraded by plaque bacteria, and therefore do not persist in plaque. The EPS serve as a reservoir of fermentable sugars for oral bacteria when extraneous sources are lacking (between meals),[22,23] with a consequent extended period of acid production and prolonged tooth tissue demineralization. EPS can also protect the microorganisms from the inimical influences of antimicrobials and other environmental assaults.[24,25]

A high sucrose diet places an individual at a high risk of developing dental caries. Through their fast and efficient metabolism of sucrose, cariogenic bacteria produce substantial amounts of organic acids. Moreover, they store extracellular and intracellular polysaccharides that serve as reservoirs of fermentable sugar for extended periods of acid production and prolonged tooth tissue demineralization.

Factors Modifying the Role of Sugars in Caries Development

As discussed above, each time cariogenic microorganisms come into contact with food or drink that contains readily fermentable sugars (monosaccharides or disaccharides) these are metabolized for energy and **organic acids** are produced as **metabolic by-products**. These acids are localized within the biofilm adjacent to the tooth tissue (enamel or dentin). The drop of pH leads to a demineralization of dental hard tissues (see Chapter 2) and demineralization proceeds as long as sufficient acid is available. In thick gel-plaque the pH drops within seconds of contact with dietary sugars, and it can stay low for up to 2 hours.

Frequency of Sugar Intake

The effect of frequency of sugar intake on the initiation and progression of caries can be better understood if we realize that caries does not develop by continuous cumulative loss of mineral, but its formation is a **highly dynamic process** characterized by alternating periods of demineralization and remineralization. Under neutral conditions, there is a well-balanced equilibrium between the two. However, this balance is lost when both dental plaque and sugar are frequently present in the oral cavity. As discussed above, ingestion of sugar in the oral cavity harboring cariogenic bacteria is followed by acid production and depression of plaque pH below the critical pH for tooth tissue dissolution. Time is needed for saliva to neutralize this acid through its buffering action to establish a neutral pH required for remineralization of the demineralized tissue. It is pertinent to mention that the time required to achieve this neutral environment varies from individual to individual, and can be as long as two hours in individuals with thick plaque due to poor oral hygiene. If sugar is ingested again before this required time lapse, the circle of acid production resumes again, thus the pH of the plaque remains below the neutral level, so preventing remineralization, or at worst, below the critical pH with continued demineralization. In this situation, demineralization will outweigh remineralization and caries begins and progresses. Caries therefore depends on the balance between demineralization and remineralization, that is, on the frequency of sugar intake. A frequent

and prolonged eating pattern therefore increases the caries risk of an individual. Studies have shown that both prevalence and incidence of dental caries are related to the frequency of ingestion of readily fermentable sugars.[26-29] The result of a Swedish study showed that a group of subjects who consumed only 85 kg of sugar per year, 15 kg of which were ingested **between meals**, developed substantially more caries than their counterparts who consumed 94 kg with meals.[5] Similarly, infants who suck for prolonged periods on **bottles filled with syrup** or other sugary solutions develop rampant caries.[30-32] It has also been demonstrated that the frequency of consumption of a carbohydrate solution needed to exceed seven times a day before significant demineralization was observed in situ in volunteers using fluoride toothpaste.[33]

A frequent and prolonged eating pattern increases the caries risk of an individual. In a frequent-eating condition, such as snacking with sugary food between meals, the pH is seldom allowed to return to neutrality. So demineralization continues and remineralization cannot keep pace with mineral loss, which leads to induction and progression of dental caries.

Consistency of the Sugary Food

The physical nature of the sugary food determines the rate of its clearance from the oral cavity, and influences its cariogenicity.[34] Sugar clearance, determined by the consistency of the food as well as salivary flow rate, may be important in determining cariogenicity of foodstuffs and the caries risk of individuals. The level of dental caries is directly related to the **duration** for which sugar is present in the mouth.[5] Sugar solutions are significantly less cariogenic than sugar ingested in solid form.[35] The influence of the consistency of the sugary food in the caries process is similar to the effect of the frequency of sugar intake. It was easily understandable when subjects who chewed **sticky** toffees developed more caries than those who ingested a comparable amount of sugar in a nonsticky form (**Fig. 11.3**).[5] The toffee sticks on and between the teeth for a long time, leading to a steady supply of fermentable sugar to the microorganisms, with consequent continued acid production similar to frequent sugar consumption. Thus, it is not necessarily the frequency of ingestion of sugars per se that is related to development of caries, but the duration that sugars are available to microorganisms in the mouth, and in particular those in the plaque.[36]

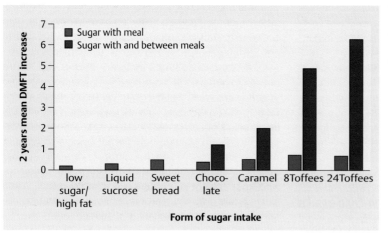

Fig. 11.3 Results of the Vipeholm-Study. Caries increased significantly when sucrose-containing foods were ingested between meals. Sticky or adhesive forms of sucrose-containing foods, which can maintain high sugar levels in the mouth, were more cariogenic than those forms that were rapidly cleared (the Vipeholm study[5]).

> **NOTE**
>
> The intake of a sticky, sugary food is much like frequent eating. The food sticks on and between the teeth for a long time, leading to a steady supply of fermentable sugar to the microorganisms, with consequent continued acid production over a prolonged period.

Amount of Sugar Intake

The relative importance of the amount as opposed to the frequency of consumption of carbohydrates for the development of dental caries remains controversial within the scientific community. Examination of published data and systematic reviews has also failed to convincingly show a positive correlation between the total amount of consumption and caries incidence.[37,38] Weak correlation was observed between the amount of sugar consumed and caries occurrence.[37] In a further analysis of data from the National Diet and Nutrition Survey of Children aged 1.5–4.5 years in the UK,[39] the association between the amount of sugar consumed and caries was only evident in children whose teeth were brushed less than twice a day, so it was suggested that tooth brushing frequency has a stronger impact on dental caries development than the amount of sugar intake.

Investigation of cariogenic potential of foods by measurement of plaque pH has shown that a relationship exists between acidogenic/cariogenic potential of food and the presence of sugars, but much less their amount or concentration.[30,32,33,40] Logically, the **amount of carbohydrate may not have a significant effect** in caries development provided adequate time is given for saliva to neutralize the acid produced in one episode of sugar ingestion before the next one. Consumption of sugar even at high levels was not importantly positively with caries increment when the sugar was taken up to four times a day with meals.[5] The burden of cariogenic food depends more on frequency of intake than on total amount, although both may be directly related.[41]

> **NOTE**
>
> The frequency of sugar consumption is more important than the amount of sugar, since the frequency of intake determines the duration that sugars are available to microorganisms in the mouth, and hence the duration of acid production and the consequent demineralization.

Thickness and Age of the Plaque

The ingestion of fermentable sugar enhances the proliferation of cariogenic microorganisms, such as *S. mutans*, and the development of dental plaque through the **bacterial synthesis of EPS**. Elevated amounts of EPS increase the stability, thickness, and the chemical nature of the plaque's matrix from a liquid to a sticky, gel-like matrix. Thick gel-plaque allows the development of an acid environment against the tooth surface, while limiting the movement of charged ions needed for acid buffering, remineralization, and antimicrobial effects from saliva and other exogenous agents.[42] Thus a thick and older plaque predisposes the teeth to longer periods of demineralization (and hence more demineralization) by prolonging the time it takes the saliva to penetrate the entire depth of the plaque to neutralize the acid produced by the large number of bacteria enmeshed within the thick plaque. Poor oral hygiene, therefore, predisposes an individual to the risk of dental caries, as a small quantity of sugar intake will tend to produce significant demineralization. Similarly, an oral cavity with thick plaque harbors a higher proportion of bacteria capable of synthesizing and storing EPS and IPS, which as stated previously serve as carbohydrate storage compounds for extended periods of acid production and demineralization, even when the ingestion of carbohydrate has stopped. It is also known that these bacteria utilize more environmental substrate (carbohydrates) and produce acid at higher rates than mutants defective in IPS synthesis. Thick plaque harbors a higher proportion of S. mutans in persons with poor oral hygiene.

NOTE

Thick gel-plaque allows the development of an acid environment against the tooth surface, while limiting movement of charged ions needed for acid buffering, remineralization, and antimicrobial effects from saliva and other exogenous agents. Thus poor oral hygiene predisposes an individual to the risk of dental caries, as a small quantity of sugar intake can result in a significant demineralization.

Sugar Alcohols

The sugar alcohols (polyols) that are most frequently used as substitutes for sucrose are xylitol, sorbitol, and maltitol.

Xylitol

The most studied of the polyols is xylitol, which occurs naturally in many fruits, berries, and vegetables,[43] and has been used as a sugar substitute for many years in confectionery.[44] Xylitol has long been known to be **noncariogenic** in humans and animals,[45] as demonstrated in clinical studies by its use in chewing gum,[46–49] oral syrup,[50] and in candies such as gummy bears.[51] The noncariogenicity of xylitol is based on the inability of the oral microorganisms to metabolize this sucrose substitute. The reduction of the prevalence and incidence of dental caries by xylitol is believed to be due its ability to decrease the number of mutans streptococci in saliva and inhibit formation of dental plaque.[52,53] Reductions in S. mutans and S. sobrinus levels were observed after 6 weeks of gummy bear snack consumption containing xylitol at 11.7 or 15.6 g/day divided among three exposures.[51] This effect of xylitol is strongly dependent on daily dose and frequency of consumption. Xylitol **inhibits the growth and acid production** of S. mutans in the presence of glucose by the mechanisms depicted in **Fig. 11.4**.[54–57]

The habitual consumption of xylitol by mothers can prevent dental caries in their children propably by suppression of mother–child transmission of S. mutans.[58,59] This may be associated with the report that habitual consumption of xylitol can initiate an ecological shift in the plaque in favor of xylitol-resistant strains of S. mutans with impaired adhesion properties, that is, they shed easily into the saliva from plaque.[60,61] Frequent use of xylitol by mothers, caregivers, and potential playmates of an unborn infant may endow this group of people

with mutans streptococci that are incapable of adhering to the tooth surface, so when transmitted into the oral cavity of the infant following birth, the flora can hardly establish itself.

Xylitol has been reported by some scientists to facilitate remineralization of early caries,[47,62–64] and to arrest the progress of caries.[64,65] These two functions were attributed to two factors: a) **salivation stimulation**[66] causing increased salivary flow with consequent acid neutralization providing a suitable environment and providing the necessary ions for remineralization; b) xylitol, in high concentration, has been shown to possess the ability to **form complexes with calcium and phosphate ions**,[67] and to penetrate into demineralized enamel, where it can interfere with the transport of dissolved ions from the lesions to the demineralizing solution. Based on this fact, it is speculated that xylitol could participate in caries prevention by acting as calcium ion carrier and an agent that can concentrate calcium, but still there is no clinical evidence for this.

Two main reasons limit the use of xylitol as a substitute for simple sugars. First, xylitol is relatively expensive as a bulk sweetener. Second, it is poorly hydrolyzed in and/or absorbed from the small intestine and thus may cause osmotic diarrhea and flatulence when consumed in high amounts.[68,69]

NOTE

The noncariogenicity of xylitol is based on the inability of cariogenic bacteria to metabolize this sugar substitute. Xylitol in gums and candies has been shown to have a caries-preventive effect which is probably based on stimulation of salivary flow, although an antimicrobial effect cannot be excluded. Its use, however, is limited due to adverse events such as diarrhea and its relatively high costs.

Sorbitol

Sorbitol is only slowly metabolized by S. mutans,[70] with formic acid and ethanol as the end product of this metabolic process,[71,72] and hence the noncariogenicity of this sugar.[73,74] There is evidence of slight increases of sorbitol-fermenting organisms in the mouths of frequent sorbitol consumers,[75] thus raising the suggestion that its consumption is associated with the hazard of enriching the plaque with S. mutans.[75,76] However, humans consuming large amounts of sorbitol show no evidence of an increase in caries.[75,77]

Although the results of several clinical trials, that either tested chewing gums sweetened with xylitol or with sorbitol suggested a somewhat higher caries reduction with xylitol, this superiority was not confirmed in three out of five trials that directly compared the caries preventive effect of gums containing either sweetener.[78,79]

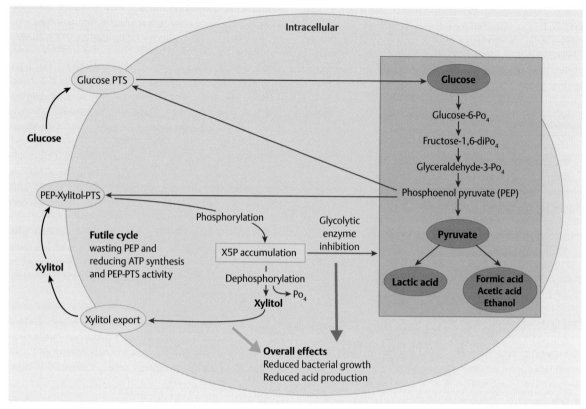

Fig. 11.4 Schematic illustration of the effect of xylitol on bacteria growth and acid production. Xylitol is transported and phosphorylated as xylitol-5-phosphate (X5P) by a phosphoenolpyruvate–xylitol phosphotransferase system (PEP–xylitol PTS) into *Streptococus mutans* cells in the presence of glucose. The PEP–xylitol PTS functions ultimately at the expense of the primary energy reserve of the cell. The accumulated X5P is dephosphorylated to xylitol by an intracellular phosphorylase and then xylitol is expelled from the cell. This rapid expulsion of xylitol also requires a source of energy. The ability of the bacteria cells to (i) import xylitol via a specific PTS, (ii) dephosphorylate the transport product to xylitol, and (iii) expel free

xylitol provides these organisms with all of the components necessary to drive a cycle mechanism that pumps xylitol into and out of the bacteria cells. This phosphorylation–dephosphorylation cycle of xylitol has been termed a "futile cycle," where PEP is wasted.[57] Since PEP is a phosphoryl donor for ATP synthesis and an energy source for PEP–sugar PTS, the existence of the futile cycle effectively depletes intracellular energy stores, and decreases bacterial growth and acid production. Also the intracellular accumulation of X5P poisons the glycolysis of fermentable carbohydrates by inhibiting the activity of bacterial glycolytic enzymes, resulting in reduction of acid production and inhibition of the growth of *S. mutans*.[53,55–57]

Maltitol

This sugar is included in a fairly wide range of food products. Maltitol is especially used in the **production of sweets**, including sugarless hard candies, chewing gum, chocolates, baked goods, and ice cream. Consumption of gummy bear snacks containing maltitol sugar three times daily for 6 weeks at a total daily dose of 45 g was effective in reducing *S. mutans and S. sobrinus* levels.[51] There is also some previous evidence of its relatively minimal cariogenicity and poor fermentability.[80] However, due to its slow absorption, excessive consumption can have a laxative effect and produce intestinal gas, bloating, and diarrhea.

Intense Sweeteners

These are non-natural (artificial, synthetic) or natural sugar substitutes commonly used in flavored beverages and foods due to their low or noncaloric characteristics. They are compounds with **sweetness** that is **many times that of sucrose**, but with negligible to zero energy contribution. Although it is generally believed that these compounds play no part in the caries process as they are neither fermented by nor have any deleterious effect on the microflora of the dental plaque,[81] logically the simple substitution of conventional sugars by intense sweeteners may translate to lower intake of cariogenic diet and thus less caries. Most widespread are aspartame, cyclamate, saccharin, sucralose, neotame, and acesulfame-K (**Table 11.1**).

Based on early findings in animal experiments, concerns about **potential carcinogenicity** of some sugar substitutes arose, leading to the ban on saccharin and cyclamate in some countries like the United States. However, recent reviews concluded that safety concerns about saccharin and cyclamate lack evidence.[82] More recently, several sugar substitutes derived from extracts of the natural plant *Stevia rebaudiana* (steviol glycosides) have been patented and promoted as natural intense sweeteners.[83] Trademarks are Rebiana, Truvia, and PureVia. Also due to safety concerns. Stevia products are still banned in some countries.

Other Food Components

Proteins

The physiological strategies for oral biofilm control include reduction of the frequency of low pH in plaque by: i) promoting alkali generation from arginine or urea supplements; and ii) replacing cariogenic with noncariogenic dietary components. Proteins in the diet provide the urea in saliva, which is hydrolyzed by the enzyme urease to produce **ammonia**[84]. Ammonia is highly alkaline and causes a rise in pH within the plaque environment. Deamination of certain amino acids in foods and saliva such as the arginine-rich peptides and pyridoxine (vitamin B_6) also results to ammonia production.[85] Similarly, decarboxylation of amino acids in foods and saliva leads to production of amines with the loss of CO_2 leading to a rise in pH.[86] Arguably, increasing the amount of protein and reducing the percentage of fermentable carbohydrates in diet may reduce caries in an individual through reduction in the amount of cariogenic dietary components and promotion of neutralization of plaque acid.

Milk and milk products contain a variety of agents, such as protein buffers, calcium and phosphate ions, and non-phosphorylated proteins (whey proteins) which can suppress caries progression, and phosphopeptides derived from casein which can exert caries preventive effects.[87] Lactose, which is the major monosaccharide in human breast milk (7.2%), bovine (cow) milk (4.5%) and infant formula (7.0%), is poorly cariogenic,[88,89] except when supplemented with sucrose[90] or consumed very frequently as in breast-feeding at will.[91] A large body of evidence has shown that phosphoproteins from both saliva and diet can influence the mineralization of hydroxyapatite.[92] **Casein phosphopeptides (CPP)** have been shown to reduce the rate of hydroxyapatite dissolution through protein binding to the surface of hydroxyapatite.[93] Complexes of CPP and amorphous calcium phosphate (CPP-ACP) have been shown to exert anti-cariogenic effects in human in-situ caries models.[93] The proposed mechanism of anticariogenicity is that these complexes localize ACP in dental plaque and substantially increase the level of calcium phosphate, which in turn serves as a reservoir for free calcium and phosphate ions. The net effect is that the plaque fluid (and saliva) is maintained in a state of supersaturation with respect to tooth enamel for both calcium and phosphate ions, which suppresses demineralization and enhances remineralization. The protective effect of milk and milk products demonstrated in several studies reflects the impact of CPP. Casein phosphopeptides are known to become incorporated into pellicle and to suppress the adhesion of mutans streptococci.[94] These effects of CPP have been exploited commercially by adding CPP-ACP complexes into acidic or cariogenic foodstuff as well as products targeted to suppress demineralization and promote remineralization.

Cheeses have been shown in several studies to have anticariogenic and antiacidogenic effects,[95–98] and this is believed to be due to various components in the cheese. Calcium lactate, a known component of cheese, has been shown to have a caries-protective effect.[99] Fatty acids in cheese may play all the roles discussed below for inhibition of demineralization. Micelles in cheese may retain calcium and phosphates that may serve as a slow-release reservoir for these minerals to promote remineralization and protect the tooth surface against demineralization. Obviously, the salivation-stimulating effect of the texture and flavor of cheeses, like in other foods and drinks, cannot be underestimated. When milk or cheese products are consumed at the end of a meal, the proteins they contain can buffer pH changes induced by acidogenic foodstuffs, and can also exert a topical effect through CPP.

Fats

Fat may decrease both caries activity and incidence by formation of fatty films that act as a physical barrier on the tooth surface, and thus preventing demineralization. Fat may also reduce sugar solubilization. Certain fatty acids in the diet are known to have antimicrobial action.[100,101] Contact between fermentable carbohydrates and bacteria may be reduced in the presence of fat. Fats, if they replace carbohydrates in the diet, may have indirect benefit derived from reduced consumption of carbohydrates. It was reported that a low carbohydrate, high fat diet depressed caries activity to practically nil.[5] However, the suggestion is to choose fats in diet wisely to reduce the risk of chronic disease and still benefit from fat adherence to the tooth surface to prevent demineralization.

Food Preservatives

Some food preservatives such as benzoates and sorbates have been shown to inhibit the growth and metabolism of cariogenic microflora.[102,103] Research data suggest that these preservatives have an effect on cytoplasmic acidification, just like fluoride and several weak acids.[104] Cytoplasmic acidification leads to inhibition of enolase and other enzymes in the glycolytic pathway of carbohydrate metabolism.[105,106] The dose of sodium benzoate required to achieve this effect (662 mg) can be obtained from 660 mL (2 cans) of **carbonated beverages**, the reported average quantity consumed daily by an individual.[107] Benzoate occurs naturally in **cranberries**, prunes, cinnamon, and ripe olives,[108] and cranberry has been shown to have multiple inhibitory effects on the development of *S. mutans* biofilm, especially the glucan-mediated processes.[109] It was suggested that the increased usage of preservatives and their availability in foods could be contributing to the decline in prevalence of dental caries,[110] but this is yet to be proven clinically.

Fresh Fruits, Vegetables, and Other Dietary Components

Cranberries are rich sources of **phenolics**, and have anti-microbial and antioxidant actions. For example cranberry polyphenols show inhibitory effects on formation and acidogenicity of *S. mutans* biofilms.[109,111] Fresh fruits and vegetables increase salivary flow rate as well as provide a source of antioxidants. A perception nurtured for a long time was that raisins promote caries; however, oleanolic acid, oleanolic aldehyde, and 5-(hydroxymethyl)-2-furfural in raisins was found to inhibit the growth of *S. mutans* at concentrations ranging from ca. 200 to 1000 μg/mL. At a concentration of 31 μg/mL, oleanolic acid also blocked *S. mutans* adherence to tooth surfaces.[112]

Fluoride tends to accumulate in **leaves of the tea plant** and concentrations are higher in tea bags than tea leaves, and in black more than green tea.[113,114] A few studies have investigated tea's therapeutic potential in oral health, and reported preventive effect against dental caries based on its antimicrobial properties and as a source of fluoride.[115–117] Tannin in tea has been shown to inhibit hydrolysis of starch by amylase,[118] thereby reducing the cariogenic effect of starches retained in the oral cavity that act as slow-release substrate reservoirs for plaque bacteria.

Influence of Nutritional Deficiencies in the Caries Process

Caries of the primary dentition has been associated with early childhood malnutrition, and this has been attributed to enamel hypoplasia, salivary glandular hypofunction, and saliva compositional changes.[119] Hypocalcemia associated with vitamin D deficiency has been associated with enamel hypoplasia, a condition predisposing the affected teeth to dental caries.[120] There is evidence that severe nutritional deficiencies in experimental animals are known to affect the development of teeth and salivary glands and increase their susceptibility to dental caries.[121]

Population Groups with Raised Caries Risk Due to Dietary Pattern

Generally all individuals with frequent sugar consumption are susceptible to caries. But there are two special groups of individuals that mostly suffer the direct effect of dietary

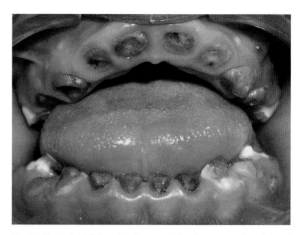

Fig. 11.5 Early childhood caries caused by frequent and prolonged exposure of plaque-coated teeth to fermentable sugar.

influence on caries, namely **children and the elderly**. These two groups of people share a common characteristic of depending on others to care for them, dictating their diet, food choice, and oral care provision, and hence may fall victim to the ignorance and poor practice of others.

Children

A typical problem in children caused by dietary pattern is **early childhood caries** (nursing caries, baby's bottle tooth decay, or rampant caries), a form of severe dental decay that affects the primary teeth of infants and toddlers (**Fig. 11.5**). The primary cause of early childhood caries is frequent and prolonged exposure of teeth to sugar.[89] This exposure is often the result of a child going to bed with a bottle or drinking at will from a bottle during the day. While improper nursing bottle feeding habits are the most frequently cited cause of this condition, it may also occur in children who are breast-fed at will, and in those who are given sweetened pacifiers, sweetened medications, or sweetened fruit drinks. Particularly harmful is putting a child to bed with a sugar-sweetened bottle at night, when the child is likely to fall asleep while nursing, and when reparative salivary flow is diminished. Depending on the frequency of use, rampant caries may also occur in children using inhalers for **asthma** treatment due to the lactose content of the spray. Steroid inhalers are more acidogenic than the others, especially the dry powder varieties.[122,123]

Although the lactose component of bovine milk and human breast milk is poorly cariogenic,[88,89] addition of sucrose[90] and high frequency of ingestion[89] can lead to aggressive caries. Soy-protein formula is free of lactose but, depending on the brand, may contain equivalent concentrations of fermentable carbohydrates, usually sucrose. Natural fruit juices and soft drinks contain significant concentrations of sugar, and their improper use in infant feeders also may cause dental decay. Many studies have shown that children with nursing caries have been given bottles of liquids to which sugar or other cariogenic sweetening agents have been added. In general, at any age, sugary foods are appealing to children, and they reach for them at the slightest opportunity.

Attitudes Predisposing Children to Early Childhood Caries

Early childhood caries is caused by frequent and prolonged exposure of teeth to fermentable sugar amid poor oral hygiene. The following practice of the caregiver can predispose the child to early childhood caries.
• Going to bed with a bottle filled with cariogenic drink
• Drinking at will from a bottle filled with cariogenic drink
• Prolonged breast-feeding at will
• Giving sucrose-sweetened pacifiers
• Using inhalers for asthma treatment
• Giving sucrose-sweetened medications
• Developmental defects (hypoplasia)

The Elderly

The level of dependence of an elderly individual can also be a factor that influences dietary habits, oral care, and hence the caries risk.[124] Two groups of elderly people are most at risk. The first group is the sick elderly who are **dependent on carers**. It has been shown that knowledge of oral care among carers for elderly people in residential and nursing homes can be poor.[125] Evidence from the United Kingdom National Diet and Nutritional Survey showed that residents of long-term care institutions are subjected to nearly eight sugar intakes per day, often in the form of sweetened beverages,[126] and this obviously increases their caries risk (**Fig. 11.6**). The second group is elderly people who are partially dependent, requiring little support and/or living on low income, but mainly choosing their own diet and oral care habit. **Poverty and lack of support** for shopping may influence this group to buy cheaper and light-to-carry foods, which are often cariogenic, whereas less cariogenic foods such as fruits and fresh vegetables are heavier to carry.[127] Their food choice may also be influenced by the ease of preparation as well as the ease of mastication, especially if the elderly person has poor dentition or poorly fitting dentures. The overall consequence of these problems is exposure to high caries risk, and in the elderly the commonest manifestation is root surface caries (**Fig. 11.6**), which may be complicated by **xerostomia** caused by the multiple medications being taken by most of these senior citizens. Root caries is caused by exposure of exposed root surfaces to cariogenic diet amid inadequate oral hygiene due to lack of manual dexterity and loss of muscle tone around oral musculature required for adequate tooth brushing. Their poorly-designed or ill-fitting removable partial dentures[128] may also encourage plaque accumulation.

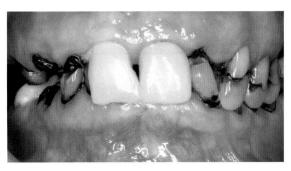

Fig. 11.6   Root and coronal caries in an elderly person.

Behavioral Factors Influencing the Cariogenicity of Diet

In order of importance:
• Frequency of intake of simple sugars
• Form of simple sugars (liquid or retentive)
• Time of ingestion of simple sugars
• Total intake of simple sugars
• Starch-rich foods are retained for a prolonged period
• Combining cariogenic foods with noncariogenic foods

Dietary Guidance for Prevention of Dental Caries

While dietary advice should be offered to those who need it, it is important to acknowledge the difficulty in changing the long-term dietary habits of individuals owing to their social or cultural backgrounds.

APPLICATION

The following basic dietary principles may help to reduce the risk for dental caries:
• Eat a diet that is low in retentive carbohydrates.
• Reduce the frequency of eating or drinking fermentable carbohydrates: cooked and processed forms should be combined with natural foods.
• Do not eat cariogenic snacks.
• When eating, combine acidogenic foods with basic foods to maintain all nutrients in the diet.
• Include foods of firm or hard texture.
• Choose fats in the diet wisely to reduce risk of chronic disease yet still benefit from fat adherence to the tooth surface.
• Chew sugarless gum after eating for 15–20 minutes to increase salivary benefits.
• Combine and sequence foods to encourage chewing and saliva production.
• Only eat candies with noncariogenic sweeteners.

Table 11.2 Basic advice on snacking between meals

Avoid	Snack on:
Sugar	Fresh fruits and vegetables
Honey	Breads or crackers with margarine or peanut butter
Corn syrup	Low fat (or filled milk) cheese
Candies	Lean meats
Jellies	Skimmed milk
Jam	
Sugared breakfast cereals	
Cakes	
Sugared chewing gum	
Sucrose sweetened drinks	
Sweetened fruit juice	
Fruit-flavored drinks	

Snacking Habit

Although considerable evidence exists that between-meal snacks favor development of dental caries,[129] it is often not possible to gain the compliance of people when asking them to avoid snacking. Alternatively, patients can be advised to snack smartly by choosing nonsugary, low-fat snack foods such as raw vegetables, fresh fruits, or wholegrain crackers, or bread with margarine or peanut butter, low fat (or filled milk) cheese, lean meats, or skimmed milk (**Table 11.2**).

Diet and Erosion

Frequent and prolonged ingestion of acidic dietary products has been reported as causing dental erosion.[130,131] Such products as acidic fruit-flavored candies, citrus and other acidic fruit juices, citrus fruits, and other acidic fruits, acidic carbonated beverages, acidic sports drinks, wines, cider, salad dressing, and some herbal teas. Erosion may manifest through such dietary attitude as habitual intake of these products, dieting with citrus fruits and fruit juices, drinking during strenuous sporting activities, bed-time use in reservoir feeder, or continuous use in baby bottle feeding as a comforter. Erosion is not only caused by acidic dissolution of tooth minerals, but also by calcium-chelation. The chelating properties of citric

acid of citrus fruits/juices (for example) can enhance the erosive process in vivo by interacting with saliva as well as directly softening and dissolving tooth mineral. The properties of food and beverages that influence their erosive potential include pH, titratable acidity, type of acid (pK_a), calcium chelating properties, concentration of inorganic element (calcium, phosphate, and fluoride), physical and chemical properties affecting adherence to the enamel surface and stimulation of salivary flow.[131] Steps such as the **addition of calcium and phosphate** salts or reduction of carbonation have been taken to modify the composition of dietary products with the aim of reducing their erosive potential.[132] Some of these steps have been found to affect the flavor as well as pH of drinks, depending on the type of salt used and its concentration.[133]

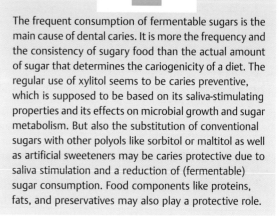

SUMMARY

The frequent consumption of fermentable sugars is the main cause of dental caries. It is more the frequency and the consistency of sugary food than the actual amount of sugar that determines the cariogenicity of a diet. The regular use of xylitol seems to be caries preventive, which is supposed to be based on its saliva-stimulating properties and its effects on microbial growth and sugar metabolism. But also the substitution of conventional sugars with other polyols like sorbitol or maltitol as well as artificial sweeteners may be caries protective due to saliva stimulation and a reduction of (fermentable) sugar consumption. Food components like proteins, fats, and preservatives may also play a protective role.

REFERENCES

1. König KG. Diet and oral health. Int Dent J 2000;50(3):162–174
2. Newbrun E. Sucrose, the arch criminal of dental caries. ASDC J Dent Child 1969;36(4):239–248
3. Toverud G. Decrease in caries frequency in Norwegian children during World War II. J Am Dent Assoc 1949;39(2):128–136
4. Fisher FJ. A field survey of dental caries, periodontal disease and enamel defects in Tristan da Cunha. Br Dent J 1968;125(10): 447–453
5. Gustafsson BE, Quensel CE, Lanke LS, et al. The Vipeholm dental caries study; the effect of different levels of carbohydrate intake on caries activity in 436 individuals observed for five years. Acta Odontol Scand 1954;11(3-4):232–264
6. Green RM, Hartles RL. The effect of uncooked and roll-dried wheat starch, alone and mixed in equal quantity with sucrose, on dental caries in the albino rat. Br J Nutr 1967;21(4):921–924
7. Shaw JH, Krumins I, Gibbons RJ. Comparison of sucrose, lactose, maltose and glucose in the causation of experimental oral diseases. Arch Oral Biol 1967;12(6):755–768
8. Brown AT. The role of dietary carbohydrates in plaque formation and oral disease. Nutr Rev 1975;33(12):353–361
9. Guggenheim B, König KG, Herzog E, Mühlemann HR. The cariogenicity of different dietary carbohydrates tested on rats in relative gnotobiosis with a Streptococcus producing extracellular polysaccharide. Helv Odontol Acta 1966;10(2):101–113

10. Colman G, Bowen WH, Cole MF. The effects of sucrose, fructose, and a mixture of glucose and fructose on the incidence of dental caries in monkeys (M. fascicularis). Br Dent J 1977;142(7):217–221

11. Krasse B. Human streptococci and experimental caries in hamsters. Arch Oral Biol 1966;11(4):429–436

12. Loesche WJ. Role of Streptococcus mutans in human dental decay. Microbiol Rev 1986;50(4):353–380

13. Beighton D. The complex oral microflora of high-risk individuals and groups and its role in the caries process. Community Dent Oral Epidemiol 2005;33(4):248–255

14. Stephan RM. pH and dental caries. J Dent Res 1947;26(4):340

15. Kleinberg I. Regulation of the acid-base metabolism of the dento-gingival plaque and its relation to dental caries and periodontal disease. Int Dent J 1970;20(3):451–471

16. Graf H. The glycolytic activity of plaque and its relation to hard tissues pathology—recent findings from intraoral pH telemetry research. Int Dent J 1970;20(3):426–435

17. van Houte J, Winkler KC, Jansen HM. Iodophilic polysaccharide synthesis, acid production and growth in oral streptococci. Arch Oral Biol 1969;14(1):45–61

18. Loesche WJ, Henry CA. Intracellular microbial polysaccharide production and dental caries in a Guatemalan Indian Village. Arch Oral Biol 1967;12(2):189–194

19. Wood JM, Critchley P. The extracellular polysaccharide produced from sucrose by a cariogenic streptococcus. Arch Oral Biol 1966;11(10):1039–1042

20. Schilling KM, Bowen WH. Glucans synthesized in situ in experimental salivary pellicle function as specific binding sites for Streptococcus mutans. Infect Immun 1992;60(1):284–295

21. Rozen R, Steinberg D, Bachrach G. Streptococcus mutans fructosyltransferase interactions with glucans. FEMS Microbiol Lett 2004;232(1):39–43

22. van Houte J, Jansen HM. Levan degradation by streptococci isolated from human dental plaque. Arch Oral Biol 1968;13(7):827–830

23. Wood JM. The state of hexose sugar in human dental plaque and its metabolism by the plaque bacteria. Arch Oral Biol 1969;14(2):161–168

24. Rolla G, Mathiesen P. The adsorption of salivary proteins and dextrans to hydroxyapatite. In: McHugh WD, ed. Dental Plaque. Edinburgh: Livingston;1970:129–155

25. Bowen WH. Dental caries. N Y State J Med 1978;78(14):2278–2279

26. Read T, Knowles EA. Study of the diets and habits of school children in relation to freedom from or susceptibility to dental caries. Br Dent J 1938;64:185–191

27. Green RM, Hartles RL. The effect of diets containing different mono- and disaccharides on the incidence of dental caries in the albino rat. Arch Oral Biol 1969;14(3):235–241

28. König KG, Larson RH, Guggenheim B. A strain-specific eating pattern as a factor limiting the transmissibility of caries activity in rats. Arch Oral Biol 1969;14(1):91–103

29. Frostell G, Baer PN. Effects of sucrose, starch and a hydrogenated starch derivative on dental caries in the rat. Acta Odontol Scand 1971;29(3):253–259

30. Syrrist A, Selander P. Some aspects on comforters and dental caries. Odontol Tidskr 1953;61(4):237–251

31. Winter GB, Hamilton MC, James PM. Role of the comforter as an aetiological factor in rampant caries of the deciduous dentition. Arch Dis Child 1966;41(216):207–212

32. Goose DH. Infant feeding and caries of the incisors: an epidemiological approach. Caries Res 1967;1(2):166–173

33. Duggal MS, Toumba KJ, Amaechi BT, Kowash MB, Higham SM. Enamel demineralization in situ with various frequencies of carbohydrate consumption with and without fluoride toothpaste. J Dent Res 2001;80(8):1721–1724

34. Caldwell RC. Physical properties of foods and their caries-producing potential. J Dent Res 1970;49(6):1293–1298

35. Sognnaes RF. Experimental rat caries; production of rat caries in the presence of all known nutritional essentials and in the absence of coarse food particles and the impact of mastication. J Nutr 1948;36(1):1–13

36. Bowen WH, Amsbaugh SM, Monell-Torrens S, Brunelle J. Effects of varying intervals between meals on dental caries in rats. Caries Res 1983;17(5):466–471

37. Woodward M, Walker AR. Sugar consumption and dental caries: evidence from 90 countries. Br Dent J 1994;176(8):297–302

38. Burt BA, Pai S. Sugar consumption and caries risk: a systematic review. J Dent Educ 2001;65(10):1017–1023

39. Gibson S, Williams S. Dental caries in pre-school children: associations with social class, tooth brushing habit and consumption of sugars and sugar-containing foods. Further analysis of data from the National Diet and Nutrition Survey of children aged 1.5-4.5 years. Caries Res 1999;33(2):101–113

40. Nikiforuk G. Posteruptive effects of nutrition on teeth. J Dent Res 1970;49(6):1252–1262

41. Burt BA, Eklund SA, Morgan KJ, et al. The effects of sugars intake and frequency of ingestion on dental caries increment in a three-year longitudinal study. J Dent Res 1988;67(11):1422–1429

42. Rorem ES. Uptake of rubidium and phosphate ions by polysaccharide-producing bacteria. J Bacteriol 1955;70(6):691–701

43. Aminoff C, Vanninen E, Doty T. Xylitol—occurrence, manufacture and properties. Oral Health 1978;68(4):28–29

44. Voirol F. [Alternatives to sugar. Sweet substances and sweetening agents]. Schweiz Rundsch Med Prax 1982;71(51):1977–1984

45. Larmas M, Mäkinen KK, Scheinin A. Turku sugar studies. III. An intermediate report on the effect of sucrose, fructose and xylitol diets on the numbers of salivary lactobacilli, candida and streptococci. Acta Odontol Scand 1974;32(6):423–433

46. Makinen KK. Latest dental studies on xylitol and mechanism of action of xylitol in caries limitation. In: Grenby TH, ed. Progress in Sweeteners. London: Elsevier; 1989:331–362

47. Tanzer JM. Xylitol chewing gum and dental caries. Int Dent J 1995;blank;45(1, Suppl 1):65–76

48. Ly KA, Milgrom P, Roberts MC, Yamaguchi DK, Rothen M, Mueller G. Linear response of mutans streptococci to increasing frequency of xylitol chewing gum use: a randomized controlled trial [ISRCTN43479664]. BMC Oral Health 2006;6:6

49. Milgrom P, Ly KA, Roberts MC, Rothen M, Mueller G, Yamaguchi DK. Mutans streptococci dose response to xylitol chewing gum. J Dent Res 2006;85(2):177–181

50. Milgrom P, Ly KA, Tut OK, et al. Xylitol pediatric topical oral syrup to prevent dental caries: a double-blind randomized clinical trial of efficacy. Arch Pediatr Adolesc Med 2009;163(7):601–607

51. Ly KA, Riedy CA, Milgrom P, Rothen M, Roberts MC, Zhou L. Xylitol gummy bear snacks: a school-based randomized clinical trial. BMC Oral Health 2008;8:20

52. Trahan L. Xylitol: a review of its action on mutans streptococci and dental plaque—its clinical significance. Int Dent J 1995;45(1, Suppl 1):77–92

53. Ly KA, Milgrom P, Rothen M. Xylitol, sweeteners, and dental caries. Pediatr Dent 2006;28(2):154–163; discussion 192–198

54. Assev S, Vegarud G, Rölla G. Growth inhibition of Streptococcus mutans strain OMZ 176 by xylitol. Acta Pathol Microbiol Scand [B] 1980;88(1):61–63

55. Hausman SZ, Thompson J, London J. Futile xylitol cycle in Lactobacillus casei. J Bacteriol 1984;160(1):211–215

56. Trahan L, Néron S, Bareil M. Intracellular xylitol-phosphate hydrolysis and efflux of xylitol in Streptococcus sobrinus. Oral Microbiol Immunol 1991;6(1):41–50

57. Kakuta H, Iwami Y, Mayanagi H, Takahashi N. Xylitol inhibition of acid production and growth of mutans Streptococci in the presence of various dietary sugars under strictly anaerobic conditions. Caries Res 2003;37(6):404–409

58. Söderling E, Isokangas P, Pienihäkkinen K, Tenovuo J. Influence of maternal xylitol consumption on acquisition of mutans streptococci by infants. J Dent Res 2000;79(3):882–887

59. Thorild I, Lindau B, Twetman S. Effect of maternal use of chewing gums containing xylitol, chlorhexidine or fluoride on mutans streptococci colonization in the mothers' infant children. Oral Health Prev Dent 2003;1(1):53–57

60. Söderling EM, Hietala-Lenkkeri AM. Xylitol and erythritol decrease adherence of polysaccharide-producing oral streptococci. Curr Microbiol 2010;60(1):25–29

61. Trahan L, Söderling E, Dréan MF, Chevrier MC, Isokangas P. Effect of xylitol consumption on the plaque-saliva distribution of mutans streptococci and the occurrence and long-term survival of xylitol-resistant strains. J Dent Res 1992;71(11):1785–1791

62. Vissink A, Gravenmade EJ, Gelhard TB, Panders AK, Franken MH. Rehardening properties of mucin- or CMC-containing saliva substitutes on softened human enamel. Effects of sorbitol, xylitol and increasing viscosity. Caries Res 1985;19(3):212–218

63. Smits MT, Arends J. Influence of extraoral xylitol and sucrose dippings on enamel demineralization in vivo. Caries Res 1988; 22(3):160–165

64. Amaechi BT, Higham SM, Edgar WM. Caries inhibiting and remineralizing effect of xylitol in vitro. J Oral Sci 1999;41(2):71–76

65. Mäkinen KK, Mäkinen PL, Pape HR Jr, et al. Stabilisation of rampant caries: polyol gums and arrest of dentine caries in two long-term cohort studies in young subjects. Int Dent J 1995;45(1, Suppl 1):93–107

66. Aguirre-Zero O, Zero DT, Proskin HM. Effect of chewing xylitol chewing gum on salivary flow rate and the acidogenic potential of dental plaque. Caries Res 1993;27(1):55–59

67. Mäkinen KK, Söderling E. Solubility of calcium salts, enamel, and hydroxyapatite in aqueous solutions of simple carbohydrates. Calcif Tissue Int 1984;36(1):64–71

68. Ziesenilz SC, Siebert G. The metabolism and utilization of polyols and other bulk sweeteners compared with sugar. In: Grenby TH, ed. Developments in Sweeteners. London: Elsevier; 1987: 109–149

69. Manning RH, Edgar WM, Agalamanyi EA. Effects of chewing gums sweetened with sorbitol or a sorbitol/xylitol mixture on the remineralisation of human enamel lesions in situ. Caries Res 1992;26(2):104–109

70. Guggenheim B. Streptococci of dental plaques. Caries Res 1968;2(2):147–163

71. Dallmeier E, Bestmann HJ, Kröncke A. [The degradation of glucose and sorbit by plaque streptococci]. Dtsch Zahnarztl Z 1970; 25(9):887–898

72. Brown AT, Patterson CE. Ethanol production and alcohol dehydrogenase activity in Streptococcus mutans. Arch Oral Biol 1973; 18(1):127–131

73. Clark R, Hay DI, Schram CJ, et al. Removal of carbohydrate debris from the teeth by salivary stimulation. Br Dent J 1961;111: 244–248

74. Cornick DE, Bowen WH. The effect of sorbitol on the microbiology of the dental plaque in monkeys (Macaca irus). Arch Oral Biol 1972;17(12):1637–1648

75. Birkhed D, Svensäter G, Kalfas S, Edwardsson S. The risk of adaptation of the oral microflora to Sorbitol. Dtsch Zahnarztl Z 1987;42(10, Suppl 1): S141–S144

76. Loesche WJ. The effect of sugar alcohols on plaque and saliva level of Streptococcus mutans. Swed Dent J 1984;8(3):125–135

77. Glass RL. A two-year clinical trial of sorbitol chewing gum. Caries Res 1983;17(4):365–368

78. Van Loveren C. Sugar alcohols: what is the evidence for caries-preventive and caries-therapeutic effects? Caries Res 2004; 38(3):286–293

79. Splieth CH, Alkilzy M, Schmitt J, Berndt C, Welk A. Effect of xylitol and sorbitol on plaque acidogenesis. Quintessence Int 2009; 40(4):279–285

80. Imfeld TN. Identification of low caries risk dietary components. Monogr Oral Sci 1983;11:1–198

81. US Food and Drug Administration (FDA). Artificial sweeteners: no calories … sweet! FDA Consum. 2006;40(4):27–28

82. Weihrauch MR, Diehl V. Artificial sweeteners—do they bear a carcinogenic risk? Ann Oncol 2004;15(10):1460–1465

83. Carakostas MC, Curry LL, Boileau AC, Brusick DJ. Overview: the history, technical function and safety of rebaudioside A, a naturally occurring steviol glycoside, for use in food and beverages. Food Chem Toxicol 2008;46(Suppl 7):S 1–S 10

84. Burton SA, Prosser JI. Autotrophic ammonia oxidation at low pH through urea hydrolysis. Appl Environ Microbiol 2001;67(7): 2952–2957

85. van Hall G, van der Vusse GJ, Söderlund K, Wagenmakers AJ. Deamination of amino acids as a source for ammonia production in human skeletal muscle during prolonged exercise. J Physiol 1995;489(Pt 1):251–261

86. Chappelle EW, Luck JM. The decarboxylation of amino acids, proteins, and peptides by N-bromosuccinimide. J Biol Chem 1957;229(1):171–179

87. Walsh LJ. Anti-cariogenic actions of milk and cheese produces, and their clinical application. ADA News Bulletin 2000;278: 17–20

88. Jenkins GN, Ferguson DB. Milk and dental caries. Br Dent J 1966; 120(10):472–477

89. Pearce EI, Sissons CH. On the cariogenicity of lactose. N Z Dent J 1987;83(372):32–36

90. Erickson PR, Mazhari E. Investigation of the role of human breast milk in caries development. Pediatr Dent 1999;21(2):86–90

91. Iida H, Auinger P, Billings RJ, Weitzman M. Association between infant breastfeeding and early childhood caries in the United States. Pediatrics 2007;120(4):e944–e952

92. Reynolds EC. Anticariogenic complexes of amorphous calcium phosphate stabilized by casein phosphopeptides: a review. Spec Care Dentist 1998;18(1):8–16

93. Reynolds EC, del Rio A. Effect of casein and whey-protein solutions on caries experience and feeding patterns of the rat. Arch Oral Biol 1984;29(11):927–933

94. Schüpbach P, Neeser JR, Golliard M, Rouvet M, Guggenheim B. Incorporation of caseinoglycomacropeptide and caseinophosphopeptide into the salivary pellicle inhibits adherence of mutans streptococci. J Dent Res 1996;75(10):1779–1788

95. Harper DS, Osborn JC, Hefferren JJ, Clayton R. Cariostatic evaluation of cheeses with diverse physical and compositional characteristics. Caries Res 1986;20(2):123–130

96. Silva MF, Jenkins GN, Burgess RC, Sandham HJ. Effects of cheese on experimental caries in human subjects. Caries Res 1986; 20(3):263–269

97. Jenkins GN, Hargreaves JA. Effect of eating cheese on Ca and P concentrations of whole mouth saliva and plaque. Caries Res 1989;23(3):159–164

98. Jensen ME, Wefel JS. Effects of processed cheese on human plaque pH and demineralization and remineralization. Am J Dent 1990;3(5):217–223

99. Kashket S, Yaskell T. Effectiveness of calcium lactate added to food in reducing intraoral demineralization of enamel. Caries Res 1997;31(6):429–433

100. Kabara JJ, Vrable R. Antimicrobial lipids: natural and synthetic fatty acids and monoglycerides. Lipids 1977;12(9):753–759

101. Williams KA, Schemehorn BR, McDonald JL Jr, Stookey GK, Katz S. Influence of selected fatty acids upon plaque formation and caries in the rat. Arch Oral Biol 1982;27(12):1027–1031

102. Leikanger S, Bjertness E, Scheie AA. Effects of food preservatives on growth and metabolism of plaque bacteria in vitro and in vivo. Scand J Dent Res 1992;100(6):371–376

103. Amaechi BT, Saldana VM. Inhibitory effect of sodium benzoate on the growth of cariogenic microorganisms. J Dent Res 2003;82 Spec Iss A: Abstract 671

104. Belli WA, Buckley DH, Marquis RE. Weak acid effects and fluoride inhibition of glycolysis by Streptococcus mutans GS-5. Can J Microbiol 1995;41(9):785–791

105. Eklund T. Inhibition of growth and uptake processes in bacteria by some chemical food preservatives. J Appl Bacteriol 1980;48(3):423–432

106. Marquis RE. Diminished acid tolerance of plaque bacteria caused by fluoride. J Dent Res 1990;69(Spec No):672–675, discussion 682–683

107. Standard and Poor's Food and Non-Alcoholic Beverages Handbook. New York: Standard and Poor's Corporation; 1998

108. Chichester D, Tanner FW. Antimicrobial food additives. In: Furia TE, ed. CRC Handbook of Food Additives. Cleveland: Chemical Rubber Co; 1968:142–157

109. Koo H, Nino de Guzman P, Schobel BD, Vacca Smith AV, Bowen WH. Influence of cranberry juice on glucan-mediated processes involved in Streptococcus mutans biofilm development. Caries Res 2006;40(1):20–27

110. Davis BA, Raubertas RF, Pearson SK, Bowen WH. The effects of benzoate and fluoride on dental caries in intact and desalivated rats. Caries Res 2001;35(5):331–337

111. Duarte S, Gregoire S, Singh AP, et al. Inhibitory effects of cranberry polyphenols on formation and acidogenicity of Streptococcus mutans biofilms. FEMS Microbiol Lett 2006;257(1):50–56

112. Rivero-Cruz JF, Zhu M, Kinghorn AD, et al. Antimicrobial constituents of Thompson seedless raisins (Vitis vinifera) against selected oral pathogens. Phytochem Lett 2008;1:151–154

113. Cabrera C, Artacho R, Giménez R. Beneficial effects of green tea—a review. J Am Coll Nutr 2006;25(2):79–99

114. Cao J, Zhao Y, Li Y, Deng HJ, Yi J, Liu JW. Fluoride levels in various black tea commodities: measurement and safety evaluation. Food Chem Toxicol 2006;44(7):1131–1137

115. Kavanagh D, Renehan J. Fluoride in tea—its dental significance: a review. J Ir Dent Assoc 1998;44(4):100–105

116. Hamilton-Miller JM. Anti-cariogenic properties of tea (Camellia sinensis). J Med Microbiol 2001;50(4):299–302

117. Gardner EJ, Ruxton CH, Leeds AR. Black tea—helpful or harmful? A review of the evidence. Eur J Clin Nutr 2007;61(1):3–18

118. Zhang J, Kashket S. Inhibition of salivary amylase by black and green teas and their effects on the intraoral hydrolysis of starch. Caries Res 1998;32(3):233–238

119. Psoter WJ, Reid BC, Katz RV. Malnutrition and dental caries: a review of the literature. Caries Res 2005;39(6):441–447

120. Fraser D, Nikiforuk G. The etiology of enamel hypoplasia in children—a unifying concept. J Int Assoc Dent Child 1982;13(1):1–11

121. Navia JM. Nutrition in dental development and disease. In: Winick M, ed. Human Nutrition: A Comprehensive Treatise. New York: Plenum Publishing; 1979:333–340

122. Milano M. Increased risk for dental caries in asthmatic children. Tex Dent J 1999;116(9):35–42

123. Amaechi BT, Jan J, Lozano-Pineda J. Association of asthma medications and caries among children in South Texas. Caries Res 2008;42:185–238

124. Warren JJ, Cowen HJ, Watkins CM, Hand JS. Dental caries prevalence and dental care utilization among the very old. J Am Dent Assoc 2000;131(11):1571–1579

125. Preston AJ, Kearns A, Barber MW, Gosney MA. The knowledge of healthcare professionals regarding elderly persons' oral care. Br Dent J 2006;201(5):293–295, discussion 289, quiz 304

126. Steele JG, Sheiham A, Marcenes W, et al. National Diet and Nutrition Survey: People aged 65 and over. Vol 2: Report of the Oral Health Survey. London: HMSO; 1998

127. Hawkins RJ. Functional status and untreated dental caries among nursing home residents aged 65 and over. Spec Care Dentist 1999;19(4):158–163

128. Shay K. Dental management considerations for institutionalized geriatric patients. J Prosthet Dent 1994;72(5):510–516

129. Weiss RL, Trithart AH. Between-meal eating habits and dental caries experience in preschool children. Am J Public Health Nations Health 1960;50:1097–1104

130. Amaechi BT, Higham SM, Edgar WM. Factors influencing the development of dental erosion in vitro: enamel type, temperature and exposure time. J Oral Rehabil 1999;26(8):624–630

131. Lussi A, Jaeggi T, Zero D. The role of diet in the aetiology of dental erosion. Caries Res 2004;38(Suppl 1):34–44

132. Hughes JA, West NX, Parker DM, Newcombe RG, Addy M. Development and evaluation of a low erosive blackcurrant juice drink. 3. Final drink and concentrate, formulae comparisons in situ and overview of the concept. J Dent 1999;27(5):345–350

133. Grenby TH. Lessening dental erosive potential by product modification. Eur J Oral Sci 1996;104(2 (Pt 2)):221–228

Caries Management by Influencing Mineralization

Svante Twetman, Kim R Ekstrand

12

Fluoride has been proven to play a significant role in preventing and controlling the caries disease.[1] Therefore, this chapter gives a thorough description of fluoride, how it works, its dangers, and side effects. The clinical use and caries-preventive effectiveness of fluoride are reviewed. A novel remineralization technology (CPP-ACP) is also described.

In detail this chapter will cover:
- nature and occurrence of fluoride;
- absorption and distribution of fluoride in humans;
- safety aspects of fluoride at various ages;
- mechanisms of fluoride action in the plaque–enamel interface;
- population-based fluoride strategies;
- fluoride in patient-based caries management; and
- alternative methods for lesion repair.

What is Fluorine/Fluoride?

Fluorine is one of 118 chemical atomic elements in the periodic system. In its pure form, it is a poisonous pale yellowish brown gas. Fluorine is placed as number 9 in the periodic table, as it has 2 electrons in the inner shell and 7 electrons in the outer shell. Fluorine belongs to the group of chemical elements called halogens, which refers to their ability to form salts in union with a metal. Halogens, and in particular fluorine, are highly reactive being one electron short of a full outer shell. This electron can be gained by reacting with, for example, calcium, forming calcium fluoride (CaF_2). Thus, fluoride is the term used when fluorine is combined with a positively charged counterpart. The complexes often consist of crystalline ionic salts such as fluorapatite ($Ca_{10}[PO_4]_6F_2$).

NOTE

Fluorine is an atom with 7 electrons in the outer shell, thus it is very reactive to other atoms such as calcium and sodium.

Units of Measure

Fluoride content is commonly expressed in **parts per million (ppm)** (**Table 12.1**), which is equivalent to 1 mg fluoride per kilogram or liter of water. Thus, 1 ppm fluoride in the water supply corresponds to 1 mg fluoride per liter of water. Similarly, 1450 ppm fluoride toothpaste corresponds to 1450 mg fluoride per kg toothpaste. We use about 1 g toothpaste for normal tooth brushing, which contains around 1.45 mg fluoride.[2]

When fluoride is combined with sodium, for example, in a 2% NaF solution, we have to include the molecular weight (mol wt) of Na^+ and F^- to calculate the final concentration of fluoride in the solution. The mol wt of Na is about 23 g

and for F it is 19 g; together, 42 g per mole. Thus, 2% NaF contains $19/42 \times 2\%$ $F^- = 0.9047\%$ $F^- = 9047$ ppm F^-.

The concentration of fluoride in human enamel is also often expressed as ppm. However, a more relevant measure is how much of the hydroxyapatite (HAP) is replaced by fluorapatite (FAP) or fluorhydroxyapatite (FHAP) (see Chapter 2) when the enamel contains, for example, 2500 ppm F^-. This requires that we know the mol wt for HAP which is 500. The following formula can be used:

$$2500 \text{ ppm } F^- \times 500/19 \times 10^6 = 0.0657$$

which corresponds to 6.57% of the enamel containing FAP/FHAP while 93.43% is HAP.

Fluoride in Our Surroundings

Fluoride occurs in nature as a constituent of natural minerals in the soil and more than 150 fluoride-containing minerals have been described.[3] For example, cryolite contains aluminum fluoride and fluorspar contains calcium fluoride. As many of the minerals in the soil are soluble in water, fluoride is found in varying concentrations in the groundwater. Data from Denmark show that the concentration of **fluoride in piped drinking water** varies across the country between 1.4 ppm to 0.01 ppm with a mean value of 0.3 ppm.[4] Values higher than 1.4 ppm are noted in local wells. Similar variations in fluoride concentration exist in many other countries around the world. The recommended upper limit of the World Health Organization (WHO) for fluoride in drinking water is 1.5 mg/L (1.5 ppm F) and a high probability of excessive concentrations is found in the mountainous regions of South America, the Middle East, and Central Asia. In Kenya and South Africa, the levels can exceed 25 ppm, and in India, concentrations up to 38.5 ppm have been reported. The concentration of fluoride in food varies (**Table 12.2**) and is dependent on the water content of fluoride and the places where the dietary sources have originated.

NOTE

- Fluoride is a natural mineral in soil and water.
- The fluoride concentration is commonly expressed as parts per million (ppm).

Fluoride in Humans

Acute Toxicity

The normal daily intake of fluoride is rather low and estimated to be 1–3 mg per day in adults.[5] The intake in newborns is much less at about 0.32 mg F per day, but increases rapidly to 1.23 mg at the age of 4–6 months.[5] Intake of high amounts of fluoride can be toxic, however,

Table 12.1 Fluoride products for oral use

Product	F content (ppm)	Comments
Toothpaste < 0.05% F⁻	< 500	Self-administered daily procedure
Toothpaste 0.1% F⁻	1100	Self-administered daily procedure
Toothpaste 0.15% F⁻	1500	Self-administered daily procedure
Toothpaste 2.8 mg F⁻/g	2800	High-risk patients
Toothpaste 5.0 mg F⁻/g	5000	High-risk patients
0.05% NaF solution*	~250	Home-based, daily rinsing
0.2% NaF solution*	~1000	Home-based, weekly rinsing
0.1% Fluor Protector	1000	For professional application
2% NaF solution*	9047	For professional application
5% Duraphat-varnish (NaF, 2.26% F⁻)	22600	For professional application
6% Bifluoride-varnish (NaF/CaF₂, ~2.8% F⁻)	28000	For professional application
Chewing gum 0.1–0.25 mg F⁻/unit	100–250	High-risk patients
Gels for trays 0.2%–1% F⁻	2000–10000	High-risk patients
Tablets 0.25, 0.50 and 0.75 mg F⁻ pr. Tablet	0.25–0.75	For children at risk
Salt (table salt, 90–250 mg F⁻/kg)	90–250	Population approach
Drinking water: 0–1.4 mg F⁻/L	From 0 to 1.4	Population approach

* Sometimes F⁻ is present with Na, sometimes alone. If present with Na halve the concentration because the mol weight of fluoride and Na is nearly the same

Table 12.2 Fluoride content in different food products

Dietary source	F⁻ content (ppm)
Human milk	0.01–0.02
Cow's milk	0.02
Rice	1.0
Potatoes	0.5
Fish and shellfish	1.5–50
Beef	0.4
Chicken	0.6
Tea	0.8–3.4

although very rarely lethal. The **probably toxic dose** (PTD) sufficient to produce severe poisoning (including death, in some individuals) in humans is estimated to be around 5 mg F⁻/kg body weight. Thus, for a 1-year-old child with a weight of 8 kg, eating 8 g of 5000 ppm F⁻ toothpaste (~ 1/6 of the content of the tube containing 51 ml) on an empty stomach could be critical. The symptoms of **acute toxicity** occur rapidly, with diffuse abdominal pain, diarrhea, vomiting, excess saliva, and thirst. The **immediate treatment** when a toxic dose is suspected is to induce vomiting. Second, milk should be swallowed to reduce fluoride absorption. Then, without delay the person should be referred to medical/toxicological attendance. Chronic toxicity due to high intakes of fluoride over an extended period of time will be covered later in this chapter.

Fluoride Absorption and Distribution

The major route of fluoride absorption in the human body is via the gastrointestinal tract. The compound's physical and chemical properties will influence the amount that eventually enters the systemic circulation. The level of **fluoride in the blood plasma** averages between 0.01 and 0.05 ppm, but the concentration increases considerably after an intake of compounds with high fluoride content. Let us use ingested fluoride-containing toothpaste as an example. The degree of absorption of fluoride from toothpaste is almost 100% for sodium fluoride (NaF)-containing dentifrices and somewhat less for monofluorophosphate (MFP) toothpaste when ingested on the fasting stomach,[6]

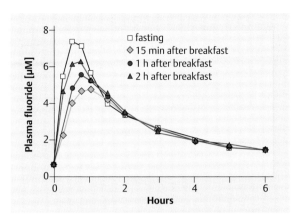

Fig. 12.1 Mean plasma fluoride concentration after swallowing 3 mg of MFP-toothpaste on the fasting stomach and 15 minutes after breakfast (modified after Ekstrand and Ehrnebo[6]).

where the peak concentration is reached within 30 minutes (**Fig. 12.1**). When fluoride is ingested after a meal this peak is reduced, delayed, and extended (**Fig. 12.1**). This knowledge is important in particular for young children who swallow a great proportion of the toothpaste used because they are unable to spit. Therefore, in young children a limited amount of toothpaste should be used (pea size) and tooth brushing should be performed after a meal to reduce the chance of developing dental fluorosis (see below).

When the fluoride has reached the blood plasma it is circulated around in the body and distributed to the various organs before it is eliminated (about 50% is eliminated) from the body. The major route for the removal of fluoride is via the kidneys. The distribution of fluoride that is not eliminated within the different organs is related to the blood supply of the individual organs. Organs with high blood flow accumulate more fluoride than organs with low blood flow. However, 99% of the fluoride in the body is eventually accumulated in the **bones**. This is related to the fact that mineralized tissues consist of hydroxyapatite (HAP) and fluoride has, due to its size and negative charge, a high affinity to replace the hydroxyl ion and to form fluorhydroxyapatite (FHAP) (see Chapter 2). It is important to understand that fluoride is not irreversibly bound to the bone. If the plasma concentration drops over a long time, for example, when a person moves from a place with high concentration of fluoride in the water supply to a place with no or low concentration of fluoride in the water, fluoride will leave the bone.

> **NOTE**
> - Fluoride is absorbed via the gastrointestinal tract and accumulated in the bones.
> - The probable toxic dose in humans is about 5 mg/kg body weight.
> - Acute overdose symptoms are abdominal pain, diarrhea, vomiting, and thirst.

Fluoride in Teeth

In the dental hard tissues, fluoride is distributed in a very characteristic way. In **surface enamel**, the concentration of fluoride is quite high, about 2500 ppm, and as mentioned earlier, about 7% of the surface enamel consists of FAP/FHAP. This is in sharp contrast to the **subsurface enamel** which contains only around 50–100 ppm. In the dentin, especially in the pulpal part, the fluoride levels are higher than in the enamel. The highest concentration is seen in the cementum. The explanation is that dentin and cementum form during one's entire lifetime in contrast to enamel (see Chapter 1). The elevated levels of fluoride in the surface enamel are related to the following facts:

- Access to fluoride (in plasma) is greater at the surface of the enamel compared with the deeper layers during the entire mineralization process (pre-eruptive period).
- Fluoride can further accumulate in the surface enamel during and after eruption due to maturation and in particular remineralization (post-eruptive period).

Fluoride in Saliva and in Plaque

The fluoride concentration in resting whole saliva is low, ranging between 0.005 and 0.05 ppm. The fluoride concentration in the secreted saliva is, however, influenced by the amount of fluoride in the environment. One important factor is the systemic ingestion of fluoride. A study from Sweden[7] showed that people living in an area with 1.2 ppm **fluoride in the drinking supply** had a three-times-higher concentration of fluoride (mean 0.02 ppm F⁻) in their saliva during the whole day compared with those living in areas with low fluoride levels in the water. In plaque, the fluoride concentration is much higher than in saliva (5–10 ppm), but the major part is bound in complexes, for example as CaF_2.[8]

Fluoride concentrations in whole saliva and in plaque are significantly elevated after, for example, tooth brushing with **fluoride toothpaste** or after topical applications of fluoride.[9,10] Concerning toothpaste, the peak concentration and the clearance time are related to the amount of fluoride in the formula. For example, during tooth brushing with 1500 ppm toothpaste, a peak concentration of 150 ppm can be seen that rapidly drops to 0.2 ppm after 20–40 minutes. If 500 ppm toothpaste is used, the peak concentration is limited to 60 ppm.

> **NOTE**
> Regular use of fluoride toothpaste or other vehicles for fluoride provides elevated fluoride concentrations in saliva as well as in plaque, with a clear dose–response relationship.

From Mottled Enamel (Colorado Stained Teeth) to Dental Fluorosis

The dentist F. S. McKay from Colorado discovered in 1901 that many of his patients had permanent stains on their teeth (**Fig. 12.2**). He termed it **"Colorado stain"** or "stain mottled enamel." The visual appearance varied between "minute white flecks, yellow or brown spots or areas, scattered irregularly over the surface of a tooth, or it may be a condition where the entire tooth surface is of a dead paper-white, like the color of a china dish." G. W. Black (the "father of dentistry") examined the teeth histologically and stated that there was an "endemic imperfection of the enamel (hypocalcification) of the teeth heretofore unknown in the literature of dentistry".[11] Some of the conclusions concerning mottled enamel were:

- Not related to class of people
- Also seen in parts of the world other than Colorado
- Restricted to localized areas
- Only natives from the area had mottle enamel
- Newcomers older than 10 years did not have it
- Families, whether rich or poor, were affected

F. S. McKay in 1916[12] stated "that mottled conditions, in itself, does not seem to increase the susceptibility of teeth to caries, which is perhaps contrary to what might be expected, because the enamel surface is much more corrugated and rougher than normal enamel."

During the 1920s, analyses of the water in some areas where mottled enamel was prevalent showed very high levels of fluorine, between 2.0 and 13.7 ppm.[13] Through findings from histological studies on rats and humans[14] it was finally possible in the beginning of the 1930s to establish that fluoride was the reason for mottled enamel and the term **"dental fluorosis"** was introduced.

H. T. Dean developed a six-step clinical classification system for dental fluorosis in the beginning of the 1940s: no fluorosis, questionable, very mild, mild, moderate, and severe fluorisis.[15] Later, in 1978, Thylstrup and Fejerskov[16] suggested a new classification based on histological examinations and operated with 10 classifications (the TF-index, **Fig. 12.2**). This refined system contributed strongly to the understanding of the pathogenesis of dental fluorosis. The tooth surface index of fluorosis is yet another index,[17] focusing more on the esthetic aspects of tooth surfaces. In one study from Brazil,[18] data indicated that the three **fluorosis indices** mentioned above found similar prevalences when the same measuring methods for clinical examination were used. For further reading on this subject we refer to the review by Rozier.[19]

Numerous investigations have tried to explore and establish a **threshold level for the development of dental fluorosis** in humans,[20,21] but without conclusive results. In fact, any level over zero milligrams of fluoride per kilogram body weight per day can induce dental fluorosis, but an intake exceeding 0.04 mg/kg per day increases the risk for the mild forms of fluorosis significantly (TF-index 1–2). An intake above 0.1 mg/kg per day would almost certainly result in more severe (TF-index ≥ 3) and esthetically compromising forms of the condition.[2] The risk for developing dental fluorosis that is visible on the permanent incisors is greatest during the first three years of life.

NOTE

- Dental fluorosis can affect both dentitions.
- There is a linear dose–response relationship between fluoride ingestion and dental fluorosis.
- There is only a risk of developing dental fluorosis when the dentitions are developing.
- Dental fluorosis is an impairment of mineral acquisition into the enamel during the long-lasting and complex process of maturation. This results in increasing enamel porosity along the striae of Retzius and along the entire tooth surface.[22]

Prevalence of Dental Fluorosis

Numerous epidemiological studies have been performed around the world over the years to investigate the prevalence and severity of dental fluorosis and its relation to the use of fluoride in any form. The prevalence of dental fluorosis (TF-index ≥ 1) among 8-year-olds from 7 different European study sites was found to be between 51% and 89%.[23] However, fewer than 5% had stages of dental fluorosis where professionals regarded it as a **cosmetic problem** (TF-index ≥ 3). The prevalence of fluorosis has increased in some countries during the later years of the last century. In the United States, for example, an increase in prevalence of definite stages of dental fluorosis (corresponding to TF-index ≥ 3) in children from **North America** from 1% in 1938–44 to 5% for 1982–88 was reported.[24] In **Germany** an increase in prevalence of dental fluorosis in 12-year-old children from 7% in 1993 to 15% in 1997 was reported; however, the majority of cases were of very mild degree (TF-index 1 and 2).[25] In some parts of **Australia** the prevalence of dental fluorosis has dropped during recent years from about 35% (TF-index ≥ 1) of children born in 1989/90 to 22% of children born in 1993/94.[26] This reduction was, according to the authors, a result of implementing a new policy in South Australia in 1992/93 which focused on a reduction in exposure to fluoride, particularly from fluoride toothpaste.

Figure 12.3 shows data from **Denmark** on the prevalence of dental fluorosis in 12-year-olds related to areas with different fluoride concentration in the water supply. It appears that hardly anyone had dental fluorosis of TF-index ≥ 3. Furthermore, around 80% had no dental fluorosis, or fluorosis which required air drying (TF-index 1) in order to be diagnosed. The **fluoride politics** in Denmark has been to maximize the benefit of fluoride on caries and to minimize the risk of getting dental fluorosis. As the

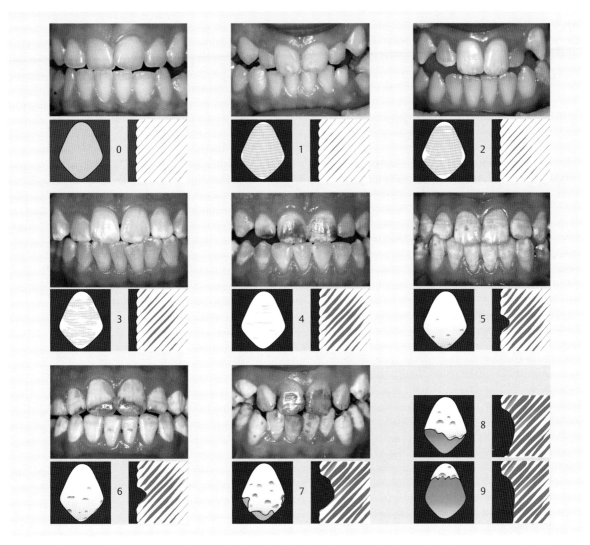

Fig. 12.2 Illustration of the associations between the clinical and histological stages of the first eight of the 10 stages in the Thylstrup–Fejerskov index.[16]

natural level of fluoride in the water supply is low in Denmark (average 0.3 ppm[3]) and no other systemic fluoride supplements are offered, the focus of attention has been on fluoride toothpaste: 1050–1100 ppm is recommended from the time when the first tooth erupts (~8 months, see Chapters 1 and 21). With increasing age (> 3 years) the parents are recommended to use 1450–1500 ppm fluoride toothpaste for their children. The amount of toothpaste used for young children should correspond to the size of the fingernail of the child. If tooth brushing is performed twice a day the amount of toothpaste should correspond to one-half of the child's fingernail. In contrast, local application of fluoride has been undertaken by professionals when they found indications for doing so (active caries or risk of active caries).[27]

The effect of fluoride on teeth is cumulative, meaning that the longer the teeth undergo mineralization, the more likely that severe dental fluorosis will appear fol-

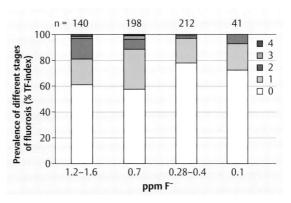

Fig. 12.3 Prevalence and severity of dental fluorosis in 12-year-old Danes in 2006 in relation to fluoride concentration in the water supply. The colors indicate the stages of TF-index.

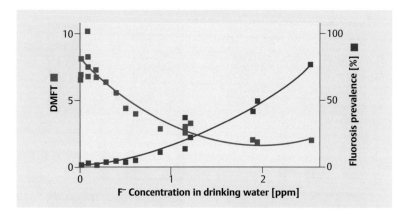

Fig. 12.4 The relation between DMFT, fluoride concentration in the water supply, and severity of dental fluorosis (very mild to severe).[29]

lowing a constant dose of fluoride.[28] Posterior teeth are therefore more severely attacked by dental fluorosis than anterior teeth.[16]

NOTE

- Dental fluorosis is impaired mineral acquisition that occurs during tooth development.
- There is a linear dose–response relationship between fluoride ingestion and fluorosis but there is no safe threshold level.
- The mild forms of fluorosis display increasing prevalence in many countries, albeit cosmetic problems are rare.

Effects of Water Fluoridation on Caries and Dental Fluorosis: Pre- or Posteruption?

In the beginning of the 1940s H.T. Dean and his co-workers [15,29,30] mapped the caries data of various communities ($n = 21$) with regard to their respective concentration of fluoride in the water supply as well as with prevalence of dental fluorosis (**Fig. 12.4**). Under conditions at that time, when no fluoride toothpaste or fluoridated tablets, etc. were available, it was concluded that an optimal caries reduction would be seen at around 1 ppm fluoride, a level at which the harmful effects (dental fluorosis) were still considered to be acceptable.

The original data were collected from cross-sectional study designs for which cause–effect relationships cannot be established. During the 1940s, several prospective intervention studies were performed to investigate the influence of **water fluoride** on the prevalence of dental caries. In general, it was established that fluoride in the water supply at a level of 1 ppm versus no fluoride reduced the number of decayed, missing, and filled teeth by 50%.[31,32] These studies resulted in some communities ar-

tificially adding fluoride to their water supply. WHO has several times stated that "fluoridation of communal water supplies, where feasible, should be the cornerstone of any national programme of dental caries prevention."[33]

From the early water fluoridation studies done in the 1940s, it was assumed, notably by McKay in 1952, that the preventive effect of fluoride on caries was related to a **pre-eruptive** action.[34,35] The theory was that incorporation of fluoride into the enamel during enamel formation increased the size of the apatite crystals and made them more well-formed, which was supposed to decrease their solubility.[36] The concept of pre-eruptive effect of fluoride led to the development of fluoride tablets and fluoride drops intended for infant use. Histological examinations, however, revealed a very small difference (1%) in the fluoride content of surface enamel from persons raised in areas with high fluoride content in the water (1 ppm) compared with persons that had grown up in low-fluoride areas (0.2 ppm).[37] Furthermore, clinical observations showed that children who were raised in a low-fluoride area and moved to areas with higher fluoride content experienced a significant reduction in dental caries prevalence.[38] This was confirmed by findings that children exposed to naturally fluoridated water since birth had significantly less caries than children from areas with no fluoridated water (control group), also as adolescents.[39] Moreover it was found that children of the same age who only had consumed fluoridated water for the last two years had less DMFS (decayed, missing, fillings in the tooth surfaces; see also Chapter 8) than the control group (**Fig. 12.5**). Today, it is generally accepted that the pre-eruptive effect of fluoride is of little importance compared with the more significant **post-eruptive effect**.[40–43]

NOTE

The main beneficial effect of fluorides on caries is post-eruptive.

How Fluoride Interacts with the Caries Process

An often cited expression concerning the caries-preventive action of fluoride is that "fluoride affects the caries process by diminishing demineralization and enhancing remineralization." This section will elaborate on this statement.

Chapters 1 and 2 have dealt with the dissolution, precipitation, and remineralization of relevant ions on the crystal surfaces of the dental hard tissues during a drop and subsequent rise of pH in the plaque/saliva interface. This section will combine the knowledge gleaned from those chapters with current understanding of the role of fluoride in the caries process.[8,42,44]

The pre-eruptive incorporation of fluoride into the crystals occurs both at the surface and in the core of the crystals. The concentration is dependent upon the fluoride intake during enamel development. Studies have shown that fluoride incorporation into the crystals does not significantly affect their dissolution rate.[42] In contrast, the presence of fluoride in the fluid surrounding the crystals **decreases the solubility** of the crystals in response to acids, and this is what happens locally (Chapter 2).

We will initially describe the de- and remineralization process as it occurs in the absence of fluoride, which is far from the in-vivo conditions, but it is hoped that this will facilitate the understanding. At pH 7, saliva is supersaturated with respect to HAP. Indeed this should result in precipitation of the ions according to the law of Le Chatelier. However, the saliva/plaque fluid contains some **calcium-binding proteins** (e.g., statherin) that inhibit such a spontaneous precipitation with respect to calcium phosphate salts. When the pH drops as a result of metabolic activity in the plaque, the buffers in the saliva will initially neutralize the acid (H$^+$). The **buffers** are effective in the range of pH 7.0–5.5. If the pH drops below that, phosphate ions and the hydroxyl ions will be undersaturated in the saliva/plaque fluid. Under such circumstances, HAP will become soluble and investigations have shown that a pH-value around 5.5 is the **critical point** for dissolution of the enamel.[45] When the pH drops below 5.5 the mineral is lost from the surface and subsurface of the enamel. However, when pH increases again to above 5.5, **precipitation of HAP** can take place, primarily at the surface.[44] Precipitation is possible because the protein inhibitors (e.g., statherin) are inactivated by the acids produced in the cariogenic plaque and are totally or partially dysfunctional.

Even with low concentrations of fluoride (< 0.1 ppm), plaque is a supersaturated solution with respect to fluorhydroxyapatite (FHAP) at slightly acidic pH, down to 4.0. Thus, when the pH drops below 5.5 (the critical point) and HAP is dissolved, FHAP is precipitated at the surface of the crystals and this continues when the pH rises again. Put differently, small amounts of fluoride, as low as 0.01–0.1 ppm,[42] in the plaque/saliva interface reduce min-

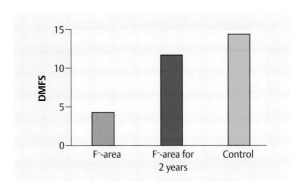

Fig. 12.5 Mean DMFS data on children (12.5–16 years old) from three different areas: Fluoride (F$^-$)-area from birth, F$^-$-area in the past 2 years, and control (no F$^-$ in the water supply). (Data from Hellwig and Klimek.[39])

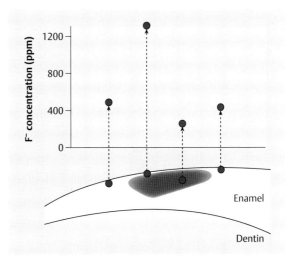

Fig. 12.6 Principle illustration of the early caries lesion in enamel and the content of fluoride in the lesion and in the surrounding sound enamel. The fluoride content in carious enamel, in particular at the surface lesion, is much higher than content in the sound enamel (data based on Weatherell et al.[46]).

eral loss, as FHAP is formed at the same time as HAP is dissolved, but also at the same time as HAP is precipitated (when the pH rises again). This precipitation or re-mineralization (repair) of both HAP and FHAP results in the outer part of the lesion being more mineralized than immediately below the surface. The evidence for this process is seen when the fluoride concentration in carious enamel is investigated and compared with sound enamel; the concentration of FAP/FHAP is significantly higher in carious enamel than in sound enamel[46] (**Fig. 12.6**).

Formation of Calcium Fluoride

As mentioned at the beginning of this chapter, fluoride is very reactive: when it comes into contact with the dental hard tissue or the plaque/saliva fluid, fluoride will combine with calcium. The amount of calcium fluoride (CaF$_2$)

formed is proportional to the concentration of fluoride.[8] Consequently, the amount of calcium fluoride is larger after local application of 2% sodium fluoride than after application of 1% sodium fluoride. The calcium fluoride acts as a local depot or reservoir of fluoride that dissolves when the pH drops. The subsequently released fluoride can result in the formation of FHAP as explained above.

NOTE

- Small amounts of fluoride present in the plaque/enamel interface reduce mineral loss and facilitate remineralization.
- Topical application of fluoride results in local calcium fluoride reservoirs.

Influence of Fluoride on Microbial Metabolism

Yet another possibility on how fluoride may interfere with the caries process has been considered, namely the influence on the colonization and metabolism of several microorganisms. Fluoride can interfere with **enolase**, an enzyme which is used by bacteria in the fermentation of carbohydrates. Studies, however, indicate that it requires quite a high concentration of fluoride (> 20 ppm) which is not very often achieved in dental plaque.[44] Thus, fluoride may have an influence on the metabolic activity of plaque bacteria, but the clinical effect is not likely to be significant.

Discussion of Classical Data

We conclude this part of the chapter by presenting and discussing very important and classical data, because they provide further evidence as to how fluoride interferes with the caries process and why fluoride needs to be combined with other caries preventive/controlling methods.

Table 12.3 shows data from the famous study conducted by Baker Dirks and his colleagues in Holland from the

1950s onward.[32,47] Two towns were included: in Tiel, the water supply was artificially fluoridated to 1.1 ppm and in Culemborg, the water naturally contained 0.1 ppm. The caries reduction obtained was different on different tooth surfaces. The lowest caries reduction, expressed as a percentage, was seen on surfaces with pits and fissures (36%) and the highest was found on gingivally located (86%) and approximal (75%) lesions. Thus, in terms of percentage reduction, it seemed that some teeth or sites received better protection due to fluoride than others. However, the results are actually logical when seen in the light of how fluoride influences caries. It is important to remember that fluoride **does not totally inhibit** mineral dissolution; it merely slows down the rate at any sites where it is available. Therefore, if no preventive interventions other than fluoridated water are initiated, tooth surfaces with fast caries progression (pits and fissures) will be cavitated earlier or faster than surfaces with slow caries progression rate (smooth surfaces).

Figure 12.7 shows longitudinal data in subjects from 7 years of age in the Tiel/Culemborg study. In **Fig. 12.7a** the traditional way of expressing caries experience at the cavity level discloses a >50% caries reduction both at approximal surfaces and at pits and fissures of inhabitants in Tiel (water fluoridated) compared with those in Culemborg (water not fluoridated). The corresponding data in **Fig. 12.7b** take into account all lesions, noncavitated as well as cavitated. Apparently, at this level of caries recording, there are no major differences in the prevalence of caries between the two towns. Again, as fluoride slows down the caries progression rate, the cavity development is obviously delayed or even avoided (**Fig. 12.7a**). Noncavitated lesions still develop in areas with fluoridated water, but significantly later than in fluoride-deficient areas (**Fig. 12.7b**). Thus, the following statements about fluoride can be made:
- Fluoride can prevent caries from becoming clinically detectable, if the progression rate is slow.
- Fluoride reduces caries progression (from early stages to more mature stages), irrespective of whether the progression rate is slow, moderate, or fast. Decades ago, the average time for a lesion to progress through

Table 12.3 Fluoride and caries data (at the age of 15 years) from the Culemborg/Tiel study in Holland (adopted from refs. 32, 47)

	Culemborg	Tiel	Differences	Reduction (%)
ppm F⁻ in water	0.1	1.0		
DMFT	13.9	6.8	7.1	51
DMFS occlusal	12.9	8.2	4.7	36
DMFS approximal	10.1	2.5	7.6	75
DMFS cervical	3.6	0.5	3.1	86
DMFS total	26.6	11.2	15.4	58

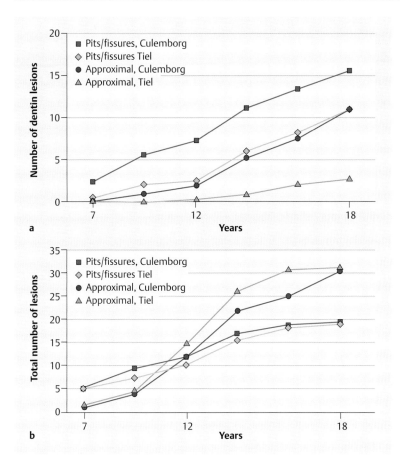

Fig. 12.7 a, b
a Number of **dentinal lesions** only in pits and fissures and on approximal surfaces of inhabitants in a fluoridated (Tiel) and a nonfluoridated (Culemborg) area in Holland (from Groeneveld et al.[47]). Note the ~35% difference in number of pits and fissure lesions and the ~75% difference in number of approximal lesions between the two areas
b Number of **enamel and dentinal lesions** in pits and fissures and on approximal surfaces of inhabitants in a fluoridated (Tiel) and nonfluoridated (Culemborg) area in Holland. When both enamel and dentinal lesions are combined there are no significant differences in number of lesions between the two areas (from Groeneveld et al.[47]).

enamel was about 3 years. Today, with multiple sources of fluoride, cavity formation can be delayed further.

This is a very important principle because, **strictly speaking**, fluoride cannot completely prevent caries, but it can effectively delay its progression, and even keep lesions at an inactivated or a subclinical level. An immediate consequence is that preventive programs should not solely rely on fluoride. The use of fluoride should ideally be combined with other preventive initiatives which deal with the etiology of caries according to the common risk factor approach (see Chapters 4, 7, 13, and 21).

Clinical Effectiveness of Fluoride

The effectiveness of measures to prevent or control caries must be evaluated in prospective intervention studies with at least two parallel groups (one "treatment" and one "control") and the most reliable estimations come from **randomized placebo-controlled trials (RCTs)**. A common way to express the outcome of clinical trials is the **prevented fraction** (PF) which is the difference in mean caries increment between the treatment and control groups, expressed as the percentage of the mean caries

in the control group. Unfortunately, this system reflects only the number of new lesions adequately, and it is not optimal for measuring the progression (or regression) of existing lesions over time.

Systematic reviews are compilations of several quality-assessed RCTs that are selected on the basis of defined criteria and constitute the top of the hierarchy of evidence. From such systematic reviews, it is obvious that the majority of the clinical trials with fluoride have been performed with the goal of preventing caries, while few have been designed to evaluate the effect of fluoride on caries control. The main reasons are probably problems in quantifying early caries lesions, and the fact that reliable methods to select patients with active caries are lacking. Consequently, there is a strong body of evidence supporting the caries-preventive effectiveness of fluoride, especially during childhood, while the evidence for caries control is limited or even insufficient. This intriguing fact is quite likely to contribute to the preservation of conservative restorative thinking, and holds back the nonoperative management of caries. However, bearing the fluoride mechanism of action in mind, a cautious extrapolation of the findings from caries prevention to caries control may be justified.

Table 12.4 Options to apply fluorides either on a community or individualized level

Mode of application	Community-based	Individually applied	
		Professionally applied	Self-applied
Fluoride sources	• Water • Salt • Milk	• Varnishes • Solutions • Gels	• Toothpaste • Tablets • Mouth rinses • Gels

Systemic and Topical Fluorides

There is a global consensus that regular use of fluoride constitutes a cornerstone in preventive dentistry. By tradition, fluoride administration has been divided into I) **systemic measures** such as fluoridated water, milk or salt, and II) **topical measures**. However, with the current understanding that the primary effect of fluoride is posteruptive, it is important to stress that systemic and topical fluoride act essentially by the same mechanism, viz. locally at the plaque–enamel interface. Due to this discrepancy another classification has been proposed (**Table 12.4**). The strength of the **community-based methods** is that they have a broad reach in the population, are less expensive than most of the individually applied methods, and that they rely less on active compliance.

Community-Based Fluoride Application

Water Fluoridation (After Introduction of Fluoride Toothpaste)

Water is an efficient vehicle for delivering a low concentration of fluoride to saliva and plaque at high frequency.[48] A systematic review of 77 trials has concluded that fluoridation of drinking water remains the most effective and socially equitable means of achieving community-wide exposure to the caries preventive effects of fluoride.[49] The median prevented fraction in communities before and after water fluoridation was 15% (ranging from 64% reduction to a 5% increase in dmft/DMFT [see Chapter 8]). A concentration in the range of **0.6–1.1 ppm F⁻**, depending on the climate, was considered as optimal to balance reduction of dental caries and occurrence of dental fluorosis.[50] However, the conclusions were mainly based on older observational studies and, as such, were deemed to be lower in quality from an evidence point of view. It should also be emphasized that artificial fluoridation of water is an ethical and political issue today and the legal framework does not allow water fluoridation in many European countries.

Fluoridated Milk and Salt

With regard to the frequently raised safety concerns (see below), the advantage of milk or salt fluoridation is that individuals may choose to use it or not, which is not possible with water fluoridation. According to the WHO, fluoridated milk and fluoridated salt may be considered as cost-effective alternatives to water fluoridation in communities or countries in which other preventive measures are not feasible.[51] However a systematic review has concluded that there are insufficient studies of good quality examining the effects of fluoridated milk in preventing dental caries.[52] The investigations that finally were included in the review suggested, however, that programs serving fluoridated milk in schools were beneficial to children, especially to their permanent dentition.

The use of table salt supplemented with about 250 ppm fluoride is another way to achieve an "automatic" increase in the amount of fluoride in the oral environment, especially for adolescents and adults. Fluoridated salt is available for consumers in several European countries and has an increasing share of the salt market. In Germany, for example, over 60% of the table salt is fortified with 250 ppm fluoride. Although significant caries reductions have been demonstrated in cohorts and case-control studies from areas with and without domestic fluoride salt, no firm conclusions can be drawn due to possible bias and confounding factors.[53] Therefore, further research concerning the caries-preventive effectiveness of fluoridated milk and salt is urgently needed.

Individual Fluoride Application: Professionally Applied Fluorides

Fluoride Varnishes

Fluoride varnishes have since the 1970s had a strong tradition in Europe as a professional caries-preventive measure for children and adolescents. The concept is that a high content of fluoride (0.1%–6%) is incorporated into a resin-based solution that sets hard after application onto dried teeth (**Fig. 12.8**). The main advantage of fluoride varnishes has been ascribed to the prolonged slow-release feature, but also the easy application technique and relative independence of patient compliance are enhancing factors. Systematic reviews have unveiled mod-

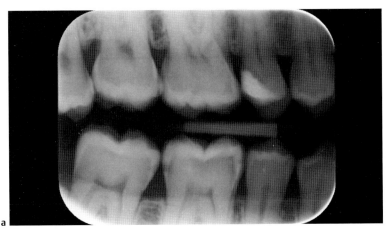

a

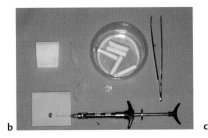

b

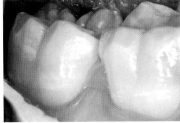

c

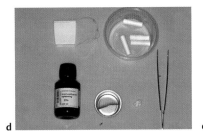

d

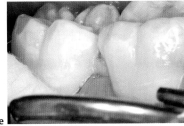

e

Fig. 12.8a–e Local fluoridation using fluoride varnish and 2% sodum fluoride solution.

a The bitewing radiograph shows proximal lesions mesial 47 and distal 46. Clinically, no cavitation could be detected, but the adjacent papilla showed bleeding after gentle probing. Diagnosis: *Caries progressiva superficialis*. The decision whether the quite deep lesion 46 distal should be treated restoratively was made later during excavation of occlusal caries. At this appointment both lesions were fluoridated.

b Equipment used for local application of Duraphat (~22 600 ppm fluoride)

c Duraphat treatment. After cleaning (floss) and drying (compressed air, cotton rolls) a small amount of the varnish is placed locally. The patient is asked not to rinse, drink or eat for a couple of hours to allow the release of fluoride and formation of calcium fluoride.

d Equipment used for local application of 2% sodium fluoride (~10 000 ppm fluoride)

e Two-percent sodium fluoride treatment: After cleaning (floss) and drying (compressed air, cotton rolls), a small cotton pellet is placed proximally and soaked with the solution for 45 secs, removing the pellet after a further 15 secs. No restrictions are given to the patient in terms of eating and drinking as the formation of calcium fluoride is an immediate reaction.

erate to strong evidence of effectiveness from studies conducted in pre-school children, schoolchildren, and adolescents provided that the varnish is applied at least twice a year.[54] The prevented fraction was estimated at 40% in a Cochrane review (**Table 12.5**) but few studies were included. A later systematic review based on 24 trials suggested a 30% reduction in caries increment when compared with placebo varnish treatments.[54]

The superior action in caries-prone surfaces such as occlusal and approximal sites is often used as an argument for professional fluoride varnish applications. There are no head-to-head comparisons between the different fluoride varnish brands. From a health-economics standpoint, caries prevention by fluoride varnish is more costly than self-applied methods, since the method is time-consuming and requires follow-up recalls. Recent studies indicate that a fluoride varnish program can be cost-effective,[55] especially when undertaken by auxiliaries. Therefore, focusing on high caries-risk patients after risk assessment, and school-based applications in deprived areas, are strategies being implemented economically.

Table 12.5 Cochrane reviews[53] on the caries preventive effectiveness of topical fluorides versus placebo expressed as prevented fraction (PF, %) and confidence interval

Topical fluoride	Number of trials	PF (95% CI)
Fluoride toothpaste	70	24 (21–28)
Fluoride varnish	3	40 (9–72)
Fluoride gel	13	21 (14–28)
Fluoride rinse	30	26 (22–29)

Fluoride Solutions

Professional applications of fluoride solutions, such as 2% NaF and 1.23% acidulated phosphate–fluoride (APF) solution, to teeth with caries or teeth at risk have been a commonly used strategy in some countries in Europe and in the United States. The solutions are less expensive alternatives to fluoride varnishes. According to a systematic review, this treatment has been evaluated in seven clinical trials in schoolchildren and adolescents.[1] The level of evidence was rated as limited, but the prevented fraction was estimated at 30% when the treatment was performed twice per year.

Fluoride Gels

Fluoride gels have been the method of choice in many countries outside Europe. The method involves the use of a flavored gel with around 1% NaF, which is applied into a standard or custom-made tray and covers the tooth surfaces for 4 minutes. The professional gels are either neutral or acidulated (APF-gels) to enhance fluoride uptake but there are also low-fluoride gels available for home use based on amino-fluoride (AmF). There is a body of evidence from controlled trials of a significant caries-preventive effect (preventive fraction, 28%) in the young permanent dentition when compared with placebo.[56] However, the American Dental Association has recently compared the clinical use of fluoride gel and fluoride varnish.[57] Their guidelines favor the fluoride varnish due to the decreased risk of swallowing and for its superior outcome in the primary dentition. It was concluded that fluoride varnish takes less time, creates less patient discomfort, and achieves greater patient acceptability, especially in preschool children. Furthermore, there is a lack of clinical studies on fluoride gel for high-risk patients.

Individual Fluoride Application: Self-Applied Fluorides

Fluoride Toothpaste

There are different fluoride formulations available in toothpaste, the most common being sodium fluoride (NaF), sodium monofluorophosphate (Na_2PO_3F; MFP) and amine fluoride (AmF). Although several clinical trials have suggested a somewhat greater anti-caries effectiveness in caries-prone children with a sodium fluoride dentifrice, there is no definite scientific proof of the superiority of one fluoride compound over another. It should therefore be stressed that all fluoride compounds contrib-

ute to the maintenance of dental health and the possible differences from a clinical point of view are not to be considered as meaningful.

Toothpaste is probably the **most readily available form of fluoride**, and tooth brushing is a convenient and accepted habit in most cultures. In fact, a global survey revealed that experts addressed fluoride toothpaste as the main reason for the dramatic decline in caries during the last decades of the 20th century.[58] More than a half a century of research suggests that regular use of fluoride toothpaste is associated with a clear reduction in caries increment.

The prevented fraction was 24%–25% (**Table 12.5**) in the two most comprehensive systematic reviews to date.[59,60] The outcome varied with the level of disease in the population and was most favorable in communities with a high level of the disease.[59] The number needed to treat (NNT) was 1.6, which means that almost two individuals have to use fluoride toothpaste to avoid one lesion. The absolute caries reduction was 0.6 surfaces per year in a population with an average caries increment of around 2.5 decayed, missing and filled surfaces (DMFS) per year. In populations with a lower caries increment, the NNT increased to 3.7 and the annual saving decreased to 0.3 DMFS in the permanent dentition. Thus, the tooth brushing is more cost-effective in high-caries areas. It is also important to stress that the use of fluoride toothpaste reduces caries regardless of water fluoridation and other sources of fluoride exposure. The systematic reviews have also concluded that the caries-preventive effect of fluoride toothpaste increases when the use is supervised by an adult and by moving from brushing once a day to twice a day (**Table 12.6**).

The effect is also boosted by a higher concentration of fluoride in the toothpaste with good evidence up to around 2500 ppm.[61] On the other hand, it is also clear that the caries preventive effect of low-fluoride toothpastes intended for children (< 1000 ppm) is inferior compared with the adult products.[60,61] Consequently, the benefits of caries prevention must be balanced with the risk of fluorosis for children under 6 years old. High-fluoride toothpastes with 2500–5000 ppm fluoride are available upon prescription in some countries and intended for caries-active individuals over 16 years of age and for patients with special needs. There is emerging evidence

Table 12.6 Factors influencing the caries-preventive effect of fluoride toothpaste as displayed in systematic reviews. Caries reduction is expressed as prevented fraction (PF, %) with confidence interval (CI).[56]

Intervention	Control	Number of trials	PF (95% CI)
Supervised brushing	Nonsupervised brushing	70	11 (4–18)%
Brushing twice per day	Once per day	70	14 (6–22)%
1450–1500 ppm F⁻	1000–1100 ppm F⁻	69	8 (1–16)%
F⁻-toothpaste + additional topical F⁻*	F⁻-toothpaste	9	10 (2–17)%

* Fluoride varnish, fluoride gel, or fluoride rinsing.

that high-fluoride toothpaste may promote root caries arrest in frail elderly people and reduce progression of approximal caries in caries-active adolescents.[62,63]

Fluoride Mouth Rinses

Fluoride mouth rinses were one of the first public caries-preventive measures introduced for schoolchildren in classroom settings back in the 1960s. However, with decreasing caries prevalence, their use as a population-based strategy came into question and the method is less commonly utilized today. About 10 mL of sodium fluoride solution (0.05%–0.2%, 230–900 ppm F, see **Table 12.1**) is used for thorough rinsing during 1–2 minutes before it is spat out. The frequency varies from once daily to once weekly but there is no evidence to recommend one frequency over the other. Due to the risk of swallowing, fluoride rinsing is not advocated to children below 6 years of age. The prevented fraction has been calculated at 26% when compared with placebo rinses.[59] Notably, however, inconclusive evidence was found regarding the effect of fluoride mouth rinses in schoolchildren and adolescents exposed to additional fluoride sources such as daily use of fluoride toothpaste.[64] Consequently, the current primary indication for fluoride rinses is likely to be vulnerable citizens in low-socioeconomic areas or districts where tooth brushing is not a commonly accepted habit. For older adults, as well as frail elderly people, there was limited evidence to suggest a caries-preventive effect of fluoride rinses on root caries development.

Fluoride Tablets and Chewing Gums

Before the era of modern fluoride toothpastes, fluoride tablets were the main exposure to fluoride in fluoride-deficient areas and were widely prescribed to infants from the age of 6 months. A pre-eruptive effect was anticipated through an increased incorporation of fluoride during the mineralization of the permanent teeth. The pioneering clinical trials were, however, performed in cohorts with or without control groups during the 1970s, which limits any generalization applicable to the present caries situation. In fact, due to the methodological shortcomings, a systematic review has concluded that the body of evidence for a caries preventive effect of fluoride tablets was poor.[1] One problem with the method was the generally low compliance and the families that complied best were those with the least need. Nevertheless, fluoride lozenges with 0.5 mg F may still be an alternative for caries-active adolescents or adults as a part of a comprehensive preventive program.[65] Fluoride-containing chewing gums have the benefit of stimulating saliva (see Chapter 1) and, at best, enhance compliance, but clinical trials addressing the sole effect of fluoride chewing gums are as yet not available.

Other Fluoride-Containing Products and Devices

Fluoride has been incorporated in several dental products and devices with the aim of increasing the amount of fluoride in the biofilm environment close to the enamel. Examples are wooden toothpicks, dental floss, and adhesives. Studies have also shown that attachment of slow-releasing fluoride devices on the buccal surfaces of molar teeth may have a cariostatic effect.[66] It is important to bear in mind that distribution of fluoride from the approximal use of toothpicks and sustained-release devices is very local and a generally beneficial effect cannot be anticipated. Moreover, the level of evidence for clinical efficacy still is incomplete but the slow-release concept must be regarded as promising.

> **NOTE**
>
> - The clinical effectiveness of fluoride is expressed as a prevented fraction.
> - Water, salt, and milk are examples of systemic vehicles for community-based fluoride administration.
> - Toothpaste is the most readily available form of self-applied fluoride.
> - Strong scientific evidence suggests that topical fluorides can prevent, control, and reduce progression of crown and root caries at all ages.
> - Daily use of fluoride toothpaste is the most cost-effective way to prevent cavities.
> - Fluoride varnish, gel, and mouth rinses are effective adjuncts for groups and individuals with increased caries risk.

Safety of Fluorides

It is well known that the use of fluoride in very young children is a potential risk factor for **dental fluorosis** (see above). The first 3 years of life seem to be most critical and the risk of fluorosis is related to the dose ingested, which is a function of both the amount of systemic or topical fluoride ingested and its fluoride concentration. Most data on the prevalence of fluorosis on the upper incisors emanates from systemic fluorides and, unfortunately, more limited data on the possible harm of topical fluorides can be found in the literature. It seems clear nevertheless that the prevalence of the very mild forms of dental fluorosis has increased along with the increased use of topical fluorides over the last decades. A meta-analysis has found a consistent and strong association between the use of fluoride supplements and the risk for developing dental fluorosis.[67] Experiences from Australia have shown that introduction of low-fluoride toothpaste (400–550 ppm F) and use of smaller amounts of toothpaste restricted the risk of fluorosis associated with early tooth-

Table 12.7 Clinical guidelines for use of topical fluorides

- Basic fluoridation (self-applied, for all individuals)
  - Pre-school children have to be assisted with tooth brushing by an adult twice a day. The amount of fluoride toothpaste ($\leq$1100ppm F^- at least to age 3 years) should be very limited corresponding to a pea or less per day. If there is no or only limited systematic use of fluoride then 1450–1500 ppm F^- toothpaste can be recommended from the age of 3½ years. Again the amount of toothpaste used per tooth brushing should be limited.
  - Children age 6 years and over are advised to brush their teeth with toothpaste containing 1450–1500 ppm F^- for 2 min, and twice a day (before or after breakfast and before bedtime). A small amount of water to remove the waste toothpaste slurry is recommended

- Intense fluoridation (professionally applied, for high-risk caries patients)
  - Fluoride varnish or a fluoride solution should be applied to the dentition at least twice yearly in caries-active patients and in patients assessed as being at risk of future caries, regardless of age
  - Other topical fluorides should only be prescribed or recommended by dental practitioners on an individual basis after comprehensive risk assessment

paste use.[26] Yet it has to stressed that the prevalence of "merging and irregular cloudy areas of opacity" (TF-index 3) on the upper front teeth does not exceed 2% in the population. Thus, evaluation of the risk–benefit balance is a true pivotal point in the formulation of appropriate guidelines concerning fluoride toothpaste use in infants and toddlers.

Guidelines

Evidence-based guidelines or clinical recommendations should assist the clinician in decision-making—to do the right thing in the right way. In fact, the **"best available evidence"** must be balanced with the practitioner's expertise and skills as well as the individual patient's preferences and willingness to pay. The clinical decision is also influenced by factors such as the background fluoride exposure, socioeconomic level of the community, and the patient's caries risk. One must also remember that lack of evidence is not necessarily the same as lack of effect. Thus, the **fluoride guidelines** presented in **Table 12.7** should be looked upon as suggestive and not directive. As mentioned above, further research is needed, especially concerning the effectiveness of fluoride to slow down caries progression in caries-active patients and in more mature age groups.

Other Remineralization Agents

Remineralization is the natural repair of early caries lesions and occurs when calcium and phosphate re-crystallize on the surfaces of existing crystal remnants. These minerals come primarily from saliva but may be insufficient in highly caries-active individuals and in persons with reduced salivary function. Therefore, enhanced calcium and phosphate delivery is an alternative avenue to improve hard tissue repair and several technologies including **nanotechnology** have been suggested, solely or as an adjunct to fluoride treatment.[68] For example, there are today toothpastes and mouth-rinsing solutions on the market which contain carbonate hydroxylapatite nanoparticles which, according to the companies, should be able to fill up microdefects developed due to caries or erosions. However, documentation of clinically relevant effects for these products is still lacking.[69] Up till now the most data available are for the **casein phosphopeptide – amorphous calcium phosphate (CPP-ACP)** system which will be described below.

CPP-ACP

The compound **casein phosphopeptide** is a milk derivative that has the ability to stabilize and preserve high concentrations of calcium and phosphate ions to form amorphous or soluble nanocomplexes (1.5 nm radius) at the tooth surfaces by binding to pellicle and plaque.[70] These ions are freely **bioavailable** to diffuse down concentration gradients into enamel subsurface lesions, thereby promoting remineralization. It is also claimed that the CPP-ACP technology may enhance the buffering capacity of saliva.

CPP-ACP can be added to sugar-free chewing gums, lozenges, mouth rinses, and filling materials but is most readily available as a topical self-applied paste. Since an additive and enhancing interaction with fluoride is suggested, several products offer a combination of the CPP-ACP nanocomplexes and fluoride.[71] Elevated levels of calcium and phosphate have been shown in both dental plaque and saliva after topical applications. Several in-vitro and in-situ studies have demonstrated that CPP-ACP can inhibit enamel and dentin demineralization and promote remineralization.[70] Furthermore, an ability to slow down approximal caries progression[72] and reverse white spot lesions after orthodontic treatment has been demonstrated in randomized clinical trials.[73,74] It should be noted, however, that conflicting results are also available, suggesting that CPP-ACP has no additive beneficial effect compared with fluoride alone.[75,76] Therefore, the evidence is currently not strong enough for clinical guidelines and further studies are needed to establish the clinical efficacy. Nevertheless, CPP-ACP may be regarded as an adjunct to fluoride in the noninvasive management of early caries lesions.

SUMMARY

One way to look at the caries disease is that demineralization of the dental hard tissues due to bacterial acidic waste products outweighs the remineralization potential of the plaque/saliva (see Chapter 2). Calcium, phosphate, and in particular fluoride affect the caries process by diminishing demineralization and enhancing remineralization. The positive effect of calcium, phosphate, and fluoride requires that these ions be present in the plaque/saliva environment during periods of pH drops and recoveries. Increasing levels of calcium, phosphate, and fluoride in the plaque saliva environment can be achieved by means of systemic or topical approaches. Examples of the former are adding fluoride to the drinking water, salt, and milk; and of the latter are adding fluoride, calcium, and phosphate to rinsing solutions and toothpaste. Numerous studies show that the caries preventive effect of fluoride is clinically significant; so far the effect of calcium and phosphate is more theoretical, but all three ions together seem to boost the caries preventive effect. The side effect of too much fluoride is dental fluorosis. The whole idea behind fluoride treatment is to maximize its effect toward caries and to minimize its side effects, mainly in the form of dental fluorosis. It is important to understand that fluoride cannot completely prevent caries, but it can effectively delay its progression and even keep lesions on a subclinical level. Consequently, if we want to control caries disease fluoride should ideally be combined with other noninvasive measures which address etiological factors of caries.

REFERENCES

1. The Swedish Council on Technology Assessment in Health Care. [Att förebygga karies]. http://www.sbu.se. Accessed January 31, 2011
2. Ellwood R, Fejerskov O. Clinical use of fluoride. In: Fejerskov O, Kidds E, eds. Dental caries: The disease and its clinical management. Copenhagen: Blackwell/Munksgaard; 2003:189–219
3. Smith FA, Ekstrand J. The occurrence and the chemistry of fluoride: In: Fejerskov O, Ekstrand J, Burt BA, eds. Fluoride in dentistry. Copenhagen: Munksgaard; 1996:17–26
4. Ekstrand KR, Christiansen MEC, Qvist V. Influence of different variables on the inter-municipality variation in caries experience in Danish adolescents. Caries Res 2003;37(2):130–141
5. Mellberg JR, Ripa LW. Fluoride metabolism. In: Mellberg JR, Ripa LW, eds. Fluoride in preventive dentistry. Chicago: Quintessence; 1983, 81–95
6. Ekstrand J, Ehrnebo M. Absorption of fluoride from fluoride dentifrices. Caries Res 1980;14(2):96–102
7. Oliveby A, Twetman S, Ekstrand J. Diurnal fluoride concentration in whole saliva in children living in a high- and a low-fluoride area. Caries Res 1990;24(1):44–47
8. Larsen MJ, Bruun C. Enamel/saliva – inorganic chemical reactions. In: Thylstrup A, Fejerskov O,eds. Textbook of Cariology. Copenhagen: Munksgaard; 1986:181–202
9. Bruun C, Lambrou D, Larsen MJ, Fejerskov O, Thylstrup A. Fluoride in mixed human saliva after different topical fluoride treatments and possible relation to caries inhibition. Community Dent Oral Epidemiol 1982;10(3):124–129
10. Bruun C, Givskov H, Thylstrup A. Whole saliva fluoride after tooth brushing with NaF and MFP dentifrices with different F concentrations. Caries Res 1984;18(3):282–288
11. Black GW, McKay FS. Mottled enamel. An endemic developmental imperfection of the teeth, heretofore unknown in the literature of dentistry. Dent Cos 1916;58:129–156
12. McKay FS, Black GW. An investigation of mottled teeth (I). Dent Cos 1916; 58:477–484
13. Churchill HV. Occurrence of fluorides in some waters of the United States. Ind Eng Chem 1931;23:996–998
14. Smith MC, Lantz EM, Smith HV. The cause of mottled enamel, a defect of human teeth. Agricultural Experimental Station University of Arizona. Techn Bull 1931;32:253–282
15. Dean HT, Arnold FA, Elvove E. Domestic water and dental caries V. Additional studies of the relation of fluoride domestic waters to dental caries experience in 4,425 white children age 12–14 years of 13 cities in 4 states. Public Health Rep 1942;57(32):1155–1179
16. Thylstrup A, Fejerskov O. Clinical appearance of dental fluorosis in permanent teeth in relation to histologic changes. Community Dent Oral Epidemiol 1978;6(6):315–328
17. Horowitz HS, Driscoll WS, Meyers RJ, Heifetz SB, Kingman A. A new method for assessing the prevalence of dental fluorosis—the Tooth Surface Index of Fluorosis. J Am Dent Assoc 1984;109(1):37–41
18. Pereira AC, Moreira BH. Analysis of three dental fluorosis indexes used in epidemiologic trials. Braz Dent J 1999;10(1):29–37
19. Rozier RG. Epidemiologic indices for measuring the clinical manifestations of dental fluorosis: overview and critique. Adv Dent Res 1994;8(1):39–55
20. Fejerskov O, Manji F, Baelum V. The nature and mechanisms of dental fluorosis in man. J Dent Res 1990;69(Spec No):692–700, discussion 721
21. Fejerskov O, Larsen MJ, Richards A, Baelum V. Dental tissue effects of fluoride. Adv Dent Res 1994;8(1):15–31
22. Aoba T, Fejerskov O. Dental fluorosis: chemistry and biology. Crit Rev Oral Biol Med 2002;13(2):155–170
23. Cochran JA, Ketley CE, Arnadóttir IB, et al. A comparison of the prevalence of fluorosis in 8-year-old children from seven European study sites using a standardized methodology. Community Dent Oral Epidemiol 2004;32(Suppl 1):28–33
24. Rozier RG. The prevalence and severity of enamel fluorosis in North American children. J Public Health Dent 1999;59(4):239–246
25. Momeni A, Neuhäuser A, Renner N, et al. Prevalence of dental fluorosis in German schoolchildren in areas with different preventive programmes. Caries Res 2007;41(6):437–444
26. Do LG, Spencer AJ. Risk-benefit balance in the use of fluoride among young children. J Dent Res 2007;86(8):723–728
27. www. nexodent.com (accessed 21st June 2011)
28. Larsen MJ, Kirkegård E, Fejerskov O, Poulsen S. Prevalence of dental fluorosis after fluoridegel treatment in a low-fluoride area. J Dent Res 1985;64(8):1076–1079
29. Dean HT, Arnold FA, Elove, E. Domestic water and dental caries V. Additional studies of the relation of fluoride domestic waters to dental caries experience in 4,425 white children aged 12–14 years of 13 cities in 4 states. Public Health Rep 1942;57:1155–79
30. Hodge HC. The concentration of fluorides in the drinking water to give the point of minimum caries with maximum safety. J Am Dent Assoc 1950;40:436–439

31. Arnold FA, Dean HT, Knutson JW. Effect of fluoridated public water supplies on dental caries prevalence. Public Health Rep 1953;68(2):141–148

32. Dirks OB. The benefits of water fluoridation. Caries Res 1974; 8(0, Suppl 1)2–15

33. Murray JJ, Rugg-Gunn AJ, Jenkins GN. Fluorides in caries prevention. 3rd ed. Oxford: Butterworth-Heinemann, 1991

34. Arnold FA. A discussion of the possibility of reducing dental caries by increasing fluoride ingestion. J Am Coll Dent 1945;12:61–62

35. McKay FS. The study of mottled enamel (dental fluorosis). J Am Dent Assoc 1952;44(2):133–137

36. Gron P, Spinelli M, Trautz O, Brudevold F. The effect of carbonate on the solubility of hydroxylapatite. Arch Oral Biol 1963;8:251–263

37. Kidd EAM, Thylstrup A, Fejerskov O, Bruun C. Influence of fluoride in surface enamel and degree of dental fluorosis on caries development in vitro. Caries Res 1980;14(4):196–202

38. Arnold FA Jr. The use of fluoride compounds for the prevention of dental caries. Int Dent J 1957;7:54–72

39. Hellwig E, Klimek J. Caries prevalence and dental fluorosis in German children in areas with different concentrations of fluoride in drinking water supplies. Caries Res 1985;19(3):278–283

40. Fejerskov O, Thylstrup A, Larsen MJ. Rational use of fluorides in caries prevention. A concept based on possible cariostatic mechanisms. Acta Odontol Scand 1981;39(4):241–249

41. Thylstrup A. Clinical evidence of the role of pre-eruptive fluoride in caries prevention. J Dent Res 1990; 69 (Spec Iss)742–750, discussion 820–823

42. ten Cate JM, Featherstone JDB. Physicochemical aspects of fluoride-enamel interactions. In: Fejerskov O, Ekstrand J, Burt BA, eds. Fluoride in dentistry. Copenhagen: Munksgaard; 1996:252–272

43. Fejerskov O. Changing paradigms in concepts on dental caries: consequences for oral health care. Caries Res 2004;38(3):182–191

44. Larsen MJ, Bruun C. Caries chemistry and fluoride – mechanisms of action. In: Thylstrup A, Fejerskov O, eds. Textbook of clinical cariology. Copenhagen: Munksgaard; 1994:231–252

45. Larsen MJ. Dissolution of enamel. Scand J Dent Res 1973; 81(7):518–522

46. Weatherell JA, Deutsch D, Robinson C, Hallsworth AS. Assimilation of fluoride by enamel throughout the life of the tooth. Caries Res 1977;11(Suppl 1):85–115

47. Groeneveld A, Backer Dirks O. Fluoridation of drinking water, past, present and future. In: Ekstrand J, Fejerskov O, Silverstone LM, eds. Fluoride in dentistry. Copenhagen: Munksgaard; 1988:229–251

48. Kumar JV. Is water fluoridation still necessary? Adv Dent Res 2008;20(1):8–12

49. Yeung CA. A systematic review of the efficacy and safety of fluoridation. Evid Based Dent 2008;9(2):39–43

50. McDonagh MS, Whiting PF, Wilson PM, et al. Systematic review of water fluoridation. BMJ 2000;321(7265):855–859

51. Petersen PE, Lennon MA. Effective use of fluorides for the prevention of dental caries in the 21st century: the WHO approach. Community Dent Oral Epidemiol 2004;32(5):319–321

52. Yeung CA, Hitchings JL, Macfarlane TV, Threlfall AG, Tickle M, Glenny AM. Fluoridated milk for preventing dental caries. Cochrane Database Syst Rev 2005;20(3):CD003876

53. Meyer-Lueckel H, Satzinger T, Kielbassa AM. Caries prevalence among 6- to 16-year-old students in Jamaica 12 years after the Introduction of salt fluoridation. Caries Res 2002;36(3):170–173

54. Petersson LG, Twetman S, Dahlgren H, et al. Professional fluoride varnish treatment for caries control: a systematic review of clinical trials. Acta Odontol Scand 2004;62(3):170–176

55. Sköld UM, Petersson LG, Birkhed D, Norlund A. Cost-analysis of school-based fluoride varnish and fluoride rinsing programs. Acta Odontol Scand 2008;66(5):286–292

56. Marinho VC. Evidence-based effectiveness of topical fluorides. Adv Dent Res 2008;20(1):3–7

57. American Dental Association Council on Scientific Affairs. Professionally applied topical fluoride: evidence-based clinical recommendations. J Dent Educ 2007;71(3):393–402

58. Bratthall D, Hänsel-Petersson G, Sundberg H. Reasons for the caries decline: what do the experts believe? Eur J Oral Sci 1996;104(4 (Pt 2)):416–422, discussion 423–425, 430–432

59. Marinho VC, Higgins JP, Logan S, Sheiham A. Topical fluoride(-toothpastes, mouthrinses, gels or varnishes) for preventing dental caries in children and adolescents. Cochrane Database Syst Rev 2003;(4):CD002782

60. Twetman S, Axelsson S, Dahlgren H, et al. Caries-preventive effect of fluoride toothpaste: a systematic review. Acta Odontol Scand 2003;61(6):347–355

61. Walsh T, Worthington HV, Glenny AM, Appelbe P, Marinho VC, Shi X. Fluoride toothpastes of different concentrations for preventing dental caries in children and adolescents. Cochrane Database Syst Rev 2010;(1):CD007868

62. Ekstrand K, Martignon S, Holm-Pedersen P. Development and evaluation of two root caries controlling programmes for home-based frail people older than 75 years. Gerodontology 2008;25(2):67–75

63. Nordström A, Birkhed D. Preventive effect of high-fluoride dentifrice (5,000 ppm) in caries-active adolescents: a 2-year clinical trial. Caries Res 2010;44(3):323–331

64. Twetman S, Petersson L, Axelsson S, et al. Caries-preventive effect of sodium fluoride mouthrinses: a systematic review of controlled clinical trials. Acta Odontol Scand 2004;62(4): 223–230

65. Hausen H, Seppä L, Poutanen R, et al. Noninvasive control of dental caries in children with active initial lesions. A randomized clinical trial. Caries Res 2007;41(5):384–391

66. Toumba KJ. Slow-release devices for fluoride delivery to high-risk individuals. Caries Res 2001;35(Suppl 1):10–13

67. Ismail AI, Bandekar RR. Fluoride supplements and fluorosis: a meta-analysis. Community Dent Oral Epidemiol 1999;27(1): 48–56

68. Cochrane NJ, Cai F, Huq NL, Burrow MF, Reynolds EC. New approaches to enhanced remineralization of tooth enamel. J Dent Res 2010;89(11):1187–1197

69. Hanning M, Hanning C. Nanomaterials in preventive dentistry. Nat Nanotechnol 2010;83:1–5

70. Reynolds EC. Casein phosphopeptide-amorphous calcium phosphate: the scientific evidence. Adv Dent Res 2009;21(1):25–29

71. Reynolds EC, Cai F, Cochrane NJ, et al. Fluoride and casein phosphopeptide-amorphous calcium phosphate. J Dent Res 2008; 87(4):344–348

72. Morgan MV, Adams GG, Bailey DL, Tsao CE, Fischman SL, Reynolds EC. The anticariogenic effect of sugar-free gum containing CPP-ACP nanocomplexes on approximal caries determined using digital bitewing radiography. Caries Res 2008;42(3):171–184

73. Andersson A, Sköld-Larsson K, Hallgren A, Petersson LG, Twetman S. Effect of a dental cream containing amorphous cream phosphate complexes on white spot lesion regression assessed by laser fluorescence. Oral Health Prev Dent 2007;5(3):229–233

74. Bailey DL, Adams GG, Tsao CE, et al. Regression of post-orthodontic lesions by a remineralizing cream. J Dent Res 2009;88(12): 1148–1153

75. Azarpazhooh A, Limeback H. Clinical efficacy of casein derivatives: a systematic review of the literature. J Am Dent Assoc 2008;139(7):915–924, quiz 994–995

76. Yengopal V, Mickenautsch S. Caries preventive effect of casein phosphopeptide-amorphous calcium phosphate (CPP-ACP): a meta-analysis. Acta Odontol Scand 2009;67:321–332

Oral Health Promotion: Implementation of Noninvasive Interventions and Health-Related Behaviors to Control the Caries Process

Hendrik Meyer-Lueckel, Sebastian Paris

13

So far in this book the pathogenesis of caries, its diagnosis, epidemiology, and possible noninvasive interventions to prevent either disease occurrence (primary preventive level) or disease progression (secondary preventive level) have been presented. Moreover, we have proposed a feasible way for professionals in daily clinical practice to document the findings detected and assessed during the diagnostic process (Chapters 9 and 24). The goal of this procedure is to provide dentists with the most useful information to enable informed decision-making (Chapter 20) with respect to non-, micro-, or minimally invasive interventions, taking into account the patient's wishes, needs, and also economic circumstances.

Whereas micro- and minimally invasive interventions are solely performed by dental professionals, noninvasive ones can be adopted either by professionals or by the patients themselves. **Professional noninvasive interventions** backed by acceptable levels of clinical evidence include fluoride (Chapter 12) or chlorhexidine varnish application (Chapter 10) as well as special brushing techniques for single erupting teeth (Chapter 10, 21), whereas many other interventions / health-related behaviors that modify the biofilm, nutrition, or the mineralization process can only be successful if patients adhere to the proposed regimens as advocated by dental professionals (**Fig. 13.1**). Although professional interventions seem to be efficacious in certain groups and for certain tooth surfaces, **self-applied noninvasive interventions** are the cornerstone of patient-centered caries management.

NOTE

The noninvasive interventions to prevent occurence and progression of severe carious decay include the classical triad.
Modification of:
- Biofilm
- Diet
- Mineralization

Microinvasive interventions comprise sealing of mainly occlusal pits and fissures as well as approximal sealing or caries infiltration.

On the one hand, given boundless fiscal or private resources, one might conceive that all caries can be prevented from progressing to a stage where drilling and filling are necessary to save the tooth. Nonetheless, even under such circumstances this presumption is utopian, since it does not take into account people's behaviors and attitudes as well as socioeconomic and cultural backgrounds. This means that not all people are "ready" to adhere to proposed noninvasive measures wholeheartedly. Moreover, their efforts are somehow counteracted by "false attitudes" with respect to sugar consumption in their social surroundings. On the other hand, for some people **basic noninvasive measures**—that is, tooth brushing with fluoride toothpaste plus use of either fluoridated salt or water as well as a balanced diet (**Fig. 13.1**), as established in many countries—are sufficient to protect the teeth from severe decay, at least in those of a younger age. Nonetheless, most people need to adopt some additional behaviors

"Patient level"

	Modification:	Biofilm	Diet	Mineralization	Diffusion	
Basic		Tooth brushing	Avoidance of sugar	Salt or water fluoridation		Self-applied
Basic			Sugar substitution	Fluoride toothpaste		Self-applied
Basic				Chewing gum (saliva stimulation)		Self-applied
Risk-related		Special brushing techniques and tools		Fluoride gel/rinse		Self-applied
Risk-related		(Probiotics)		(Remineralization pastes)		Self-applied
	"Tooth level"					
Risk-related		Professional cleaning		Fluoride varnish, gel, solution	Sealing	Prof.
Risk-related		Chlorhexidine varnish			Infiltration	Prof.

Fig. 13.1 Noninvasive interventions (modification of biofilm, diet, or mineralization) can be applied either by professionals or by patients themselves ("self-management"). The self-applied interventions can be subdivided into basic and additional (risk-related) measures. These interventions should be advocated and performed in relation to a certain caries-risk on either particular (e.g., lateral brushing of erupting permanent molars) or numerous (e.g., general tooth cleaning) tooth sites. Efficacy of those interventions in parentheses still needs further elaboration. Microinvasive interventions in order to establish a diffusion barrier, such as sealing of occlusal surfaces and infiltration of approximal surfaces, can only be performed by dental professionals (Prof.).

or **see the dental professional** to have additional interventions done to control tooth decay. All these efforts should be related to the local and general caries risk (**risk-related noninvasive interventions**).

Another aspect in this field of **cariology / public dental health** is the implementation of primary/secondary preventive strategies, that is, the way that information and techniques are made available to the people: the major ones are **population-, community- and practice-based strategies.**

In detail, this chapter will cover:

- Strategies of how noninvasive and microinvasive interventions can be implemented
- Theories to explain adoption of health-related behavior
- Evidence for the effectiveness of oral health education and noninvasive interventions with respect to caries prevention

Implementing Strategies of Prevention

Prevention—What Does This Mean?

The synonyms "prevention" and "prophylaxis" are used by many dental professionals to describe any measure that is not linked to „drilling and filling." Thus, rather differing interventions which either alter the tooth surface macroscopically (sealing) or microscopically (e.g., fluoride application), as well as efforts to change oral health-related behaviors, are brought together under the heading "prevention." Literally, preventing illness means that some stage of disease occurrence in the future is anticipated and measures (including therapeutic ones) are applied to avoid this stage (Chapter 9). Therefore, it is not surprising that the original publication in the 1960s introducing three **levels of prevention** presented a broad range of disease conditions that can be approached "preventively."[1] A fourth level, which actually comes first with respect to disease occurrence, is called primordial prevention. This level aims to change underlying risk factors leading to the cause of a disease.

NOTE

Levels of Prevention
- **Primordial level:** The aim is to avoid conditions that might trigger causative factors for a disease.
- **Primary level:** The aim is to prevent a disease occurring by keeping conditions at a prepathologic state.
- **Secondary level:** The aim is to identify disease or specific conditions at an early stage and to apply prompt intervention to prevent advanced stages.
- **Tertiary level:** The aim is to stop the disease process of advanced stages.

Source: Modified from ref. 1

For cariology this means that avoiding transfection of cariogenic bacteria, if possible, would be prevention on the **primordial level**. Noninvasive interventions such as oral hygiene education or regular low-concentration fluoride applications are efficacious preventions on the **primary level**, but also on the **secondary level**. Microinvasive interventions such as caries infiltration or fissure-sealing fulfill the criteria of a measure that is **secondary level**. Inserting a restoration into a decayed tooth can be seen as **tertiary level** prevention.[2] Even replacing fillings or larger restorations can still be seen in the sense of this tertiary level, before prosthetic measures, such as replacement of teeth come into play. From this wider perspective on prevention it becomes clear that noninvasive interventions and dental health education are important parts of **prevention**, but not the only ones.

Why Do People Get Sick?

Before an answer can be given to the question of how to implement preventive interventions some theoretical thoughts on how a chronic disease, such as caries, is determined need to be discussed.

A dental professional having a preventive attitude, after working for several years might wonder why his or her efforts to maintain teeth as sound as possible are not successful every time in a single person and/or in certain subgroups of patients. When looking at the caries models (Chapters 4 and 21) it becomes clear that caries is influenced by direct and more distant determinants. The latter cannot be easily changed by an individual, but have also to be seen in the social context.

An example. If a child is born into a family that is living on social benefits, it might not be the family's first concern to buy toothpaste and toothbrushes on a regular basis. Moreover, their social surroundings might not be supportive to "make the healthy choice" with respect to food, meaning that a cariogenic nutrition would be favored. This would not be a good choice with respect to weight control, either. Thus, the child will be at a higher risk of obesity and in consequence for cardiovascular disease and diabetes. In addition, due to many other more severe problems in life, the importance of oral hygiene might only be considered subordinate to other things that are better supported in the setting the child is living in. All in all, this unfavorable social context might trigger a high prevalence of caries. This means caries cannot only be seen as a personal problem, but also it is a result of structural and contextual influences.[4]

The thinking that the dental professional is repairing the sequels of unfavorable social contexts has been allegorized by an **upstream–downstream model** (**Fig. 13.2**), which was first proposed for cardiovascular patients.[5] For caries, people are either pushed *upstream* into the "caries river" by the confectionery industry that sells sugar-containing foods, or fall into it if they are "blind" with respect to oral health-related behavior. People are

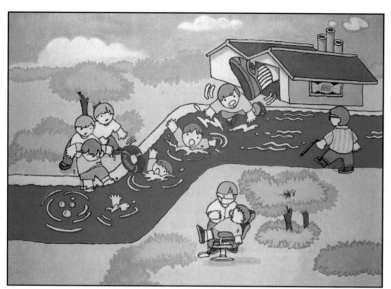

Fig. 13.2 The upstream–downstream model gives an idea of how unfavorable contexts may support occurrence of a diseaselike caries (for explanation see text). (Adapted with permission from Baelum V, Sheiham A, Burt BA. Caries control for populations. In: Fejerskov O, Kidd EAM, eds. Dental Caries: The Disease and its Clinical Management. 2nd ed. Oxford: Blackwell Wiley; 2008: p. 509.)

only able to "swim" for a while, meaning that adopted oral hygiene behavior is not sufficient to prevent development of cavitated caries lesions, although fluorides ("lifebelts") are offered on their way *downstream*, to "rescue the victims." Thus, most people need to be saved further *downstream* from drowning in the "caries river" by dental professionals who refer the "victim" to rehabilitation by a dentist.[6] This allegory gives the idea that if "unhealthy choices would be made more difficult (and healthy choices easier),"[6] for example, by governmental regulation, caries prevalence at the dentinal level would decrease. Nonetheless, it should be kept in mind that necessary changes in the society as a whole only occur slowly.

A Little More Upstream: Setting-Approaches

A realistic way to implement health promotion further **upstream** is to choose approaches that take into account the **setting** of an individual. The roots of this approach can be traced back to the first International Conference on Health Promotion in 1986. Its publication is known as the **Ottawa-Charter**.[7] It was said:

"Health promotion is the process of enabling people to increase control over, and to improve, their health. To reach a state of complete physical, mental and social well-being, an individual or group must be able to identify and to realize aspirations, to satisfy needs, and to change or cope with the environment. Health is, therefore, seen as a resource for everyday life, not the objective of living. Health is a positive concept emphasizing social and health personal resources, as well as physical capacities. Therefore, health promotion is not just the responsibility of the health sector, but goes beyond healthy life-styles to well-being."

Besides others, two key **health promotion action means** were defined:
- Creation of health supporting environments
- Development of personal skills

Both these key action means are covered by **setting-approaches**. Here, low-threshold, systematic interventions in real living conditions (school, neighborhood, etc.) are implemented by involving all stakeholders. The focused group should be empowered to actively assume responsibility for health-related issues. This approach is somehow in contrast to the situation where the individual or a group is just the recipient of offers and messages being supportive for one's health. Setting-approaches are considered as being appropriate to diminish restricted health chances due to social inequities.[8]

An example. A young mother from a low socioeconomic background shows some of the unfavorable behaviors (see previous example) that set the child at a higher risk to develop severe tooth decay. Her surroundings do not reflect her attitudes and behaviors as being "false"; the common offers by dental professionals are either ignored or the mother cannot adopt suggestions to improve her and/or the child's oral health. In this case a more educated member belonging to the *setting* the young mother lives in might be the only person to get the message across, since the young mother will identify herself with this person to a greater extent than with a dental professional coming from a high socioeconomic stratum or different cultural background.

> **NOTE**
>
> The **setting-approach** seems to fulfill the call for a paradigm shift in oral health promotion "away from the biomedical and behavioral approach to one which addresses the underlying social determinants of oral health through a combination of complementary public health strategies".[9]

Most Upstream: the Population-Based Common Risk Factor Approach

As will be outlined a little later, current efforts in dental health promotion mainly focus on the prevention of either one of the two most prevalent diseases in the oral cavity, namely caries and periodontitis. This is quite a narrow approach to maintaining health, since many risk factors are related to several diseases and vice versa—some diseases have similar risk factors in common. If oral health programs are implemented in isolation from other general or specific health programs, this bears the risk of conflicting messages that might overburden the public. Therefore, a **common risk factor** implemented through a comprehensive health promotion strategy has been proposed.[10] Examples are considerable changes in **Food Policy** and the **Health Promoting School Initiative**. The latter was originally linked to preventing injuries,[10] but can be easily extended to obesity, caries, or cancer prevention.[11] All these efforts on changing policy in surroundings or even countries depend on collaborative working among several stakeholders. For the **Health Promoting School Initiatives** this means that staff, students, parents, education authorities, local government, and health professionals coming from various backgrounds have to agree and work together.[10]

With respect to the implementation of upstream approaches a lot can be learned from the field of tobacco control, "where in many parts of the westernized world significant success has been achieved".[9] Smoking has been known as a strong risk factor for many diseases for many decades. To change smoking habits, as a first step, awareness of smoking being the cause of many health problems had to be conveyed to policy makers. A pre-requisite for this was high-quality epidemiological studies. Then, policies (e.g., taxation, labeling packages with health warnings) and environmental measures (e.g., smoking restrictions in various places) were introduced. As a result, the "manufacturers of illness,"[9] the tobacco industries, were regulated. This seemed to have more impact on smoking habits than more downstream options such as health campaigns or individualized preventive measures (i.e., behavior change under the unfavorable contexts) to control diseases related to smoking.[9] Nonetheless, with respect to caries prevention, changing food policy seems to be rather difficult as shown in an analysis on "reported commitments and practice of 25 of the world's largest food companies" in response to recommendations on nutrition.[12]

Despite of all these *New Public Health* approaches, it should be kept in mind that not everybody will be willing and able to refrain from falling into the "caries river," even under more desirable social circumstances. In addition, those who have already fallen into the river, can no longer be rescued in the sense of a restitutio ad integrum. These patients will still need individualized (re-)dentistry, at least in the next decades.

> **NOTE**
>
> A **common risk factor** approach aims at changing things mostly upstream to prevent people from contracting more than one disease. Examples in cariology are considerable changes in **Food Policy** and the **Health Promoting School Initiative**.

Contemporary Strategies to Improve Oral Health

High-Risk versus Population-Based

As presented thoroughly in Chapter 8, caries experience is very unequally distributed throughout the population. It is skewed in particular for children, meaning that the majority do not have any or only low numbers of affected teeth and that a minority shows most of the affected teeth. In a graphic showing cumulative percentages of children in relation to DMFT, the typical picture of a "mountain" on the left and a "tail" on the right is depicted (**Fig. 13.3**). Large variations with respect to the extent of this **caries polarization** exist between countries and also within countries such as Denmark, for example. In 1999, the lowest and highest DMFS scores for the 15-year-olds were 0.88 and 8.73, respectively, with a national mean of 3.52. The proportion of individuals with no cavitated caries (D3-level plus filled and extracted teeth due to caries) ranged from 10% to 71%.[13]

This distribution with relatively low numbers of children having several affected tooth surfaces calls for the so-called **high-risk strategies** that concentrate on those presumably being at a high risk for further caries development. This strategy comprises the need to identify those who are at a high risk, which is sometimes not so easy (Chapter 7) at affordable cost without making an unreasonable number of errors as is the case with any screening procedure that relies on the rules of testing statistics. Depending on the validity of the screening procedure, there will inevitably be false positives (wrongly allocated to the high-risk group) and false negatives (wrongly missed out of the high-risk group). In addition, the individual protection for the high-risk patients must be efficient enough to justify the effort of screening.[14]

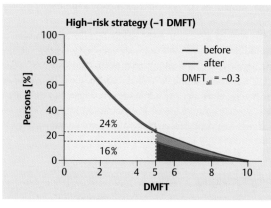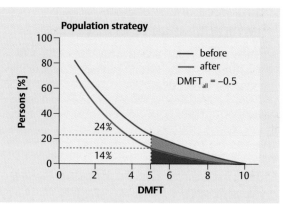

Fig. 13.3   Shift in the distribution of DMFT by either a hypothetical population-based intervention (right) that drops the DMFT from 3.2 to 2.7 or a by hypothetical high-risk intervention (left) that is capable of dropping down the DMFT by 1 for only those 24% who are considered to be at higher risk for caries (those having DMFT ≥ 5) (Modified according to Baelum et al.[4]) With the assumption that everyone at high-risk will be identified correctly during screening and referred thereafter to interventional treatment, the mean reduction for the whole population would only be 0.3 DMFT. The high-risk approach "pushes" only 8% of all people into the low risk group compared to 10% with the population strategy.

Table 13.1   Caries experiences of the two hypothetical scenarios of preventive interventions described in **Fig. 13.3** ("high risk −1 DMFT" and "population-based") as well as more favorable scenario for the high-risk group (DMFT −2) are given

Strategy	DMFT all	DMFT HR prev.	DMFT HR new	% reached
Population	−0.5	−1.3 (24%)	−0.5 (14%)	81%
HR (−1 DMFT)	−0.3	−1.0 (24%)	−0.2 (16%)	24%
HR (−2 DMFT)	−0.6	−2.0 (24%)	−0.5 (9%)	24%

On the contrary, **population-based strategies** aim "to shift the risk distribution of the entire population to a more favorable level. If such efforts are successful, the average risk of the population decreases and the frequency distribution of disease and risk is pushed to the left. Even a smallish decrease in the average level of a risk factor may result in a considerable reduction in the incidence of a health problem".[14] Thus, the main difference is that the population approach steps in more "upstream," whereas high-risk approaches are trying to protect diseased individuals from developing more disease further "downstream," by changing their risk factors.[15] Several other advantages and disadvantages can be defined for both strategies within the field of caries prevention,[4] according to the basic publication on preventive medicine of Rose.[16] In general, the efficacy, effectiveness, and efficiency of the high-risk strategy has been be challenged (**Table 13.1** and **Fig. 13.3**).

The **directed population strategy** tries to combine the elements of the high-risk and population strategies. This strategy seeks "sick communities" or well-definable groups according to underlying determinants of oral health, such as lower socioeconomic status. For example, in Germany students that attend a secondary school orientated to the world of work, which is compulsory for all pupils (Hauptschule), can be defined as a group with lower socioeconomic status and referred to particular preventive measures as a whole, with no previous screening. Thus, for those being defined as "high-risk" by their social determinants, the principles of the whole population strategy can be applied.[14]

Current strategies being implemented differ from country to country and even within countries, mainly due to high-quality scientific evidence at a higher level being missing with respect to the effectiveness of the several interventions or their combinations, as well as due to varying political and historical backgrounds. In this clinical textbook we will focus in due course on the existing evidence from epidemiological studies with respect to caries prevention. Later on, an individualized population strategy for children will be introduced separately (Chapter 21).

NOTE

Primary and secondary preventive measures can be implemented according to various strategies:
- High-risk
- Population-based
- Directed population-based
- Individualized population-based

Noninvasive Interventions versus Behavioral Change in Caries Prevention

As outlined so far the effectiveness of an oral health-related program seems to rely to some extent on the strategy employed. Within the chosen strategy various options can be adopted for differing recipients: as whole populations, as certain communities or groups in a specific setting, as well as in a one-to-one situation. For prevention of caries, the various applicable options can be divided into **noninvasive (medical) interventions** and **educational** ones. **Medical** means that the intervention mainly focuses on mineralization or biofilm modification on a tooth surface level. **Educational** options subsume *oral health education*, as teaching oral hygiene techniques and giving recommendations for use of self-applied fluorides, but also *mass campaigns* to change the diet of individuals as well as (teacher) *supervised tooth brushing* (**Table 13.2**). At least supervised tooth brushing and oral health education focus on the prevention of gingivitis, as well. Most of the time, oral (dental) health-related programs rely on various options.

Is it Possible to Change Oral Health-Related Behaviors?

This subchapter will briefly give some information on the underlying psychological issues that come into play when a dental professional tries to change oral health–related behaviors. In contrast, to the professional application of "medical" methods (e.g., fluoride varnish or sealants) it is more difficult to achieve sustainable effects in oral-health related behaviors by the means of one-to-one advice, oral health education, or empowerment.

Definition

Health-related behaviors are influenced by both internal and external factors and are conceptualized apart from risky behaviors. They may be defined thus: "Any activity undertaken by an individual regardless of actual or perceived health status, for the purpose of promoting, protecting or maintaining health, whether or not such behavior is objectively toward the end."[17]

Models

Proposed models to explain change of (oral-)health-related behaviors seem to be rather complex and are somehow impracticable to use for the dental professional in daily practice. Nonetheless, models might give an idea about the complexity and trigger interest in this topic.

The so called **KAB-model** relies on the assumption that **K**nowledge should be adopted to change the **A**ttitude and in consequence the **B**ehavior. This rather static model does not take into account that people (patients) do not all have the same level of education, and that their levels may change in time. Even if the dental professional considers differences between individuals, behavioral change by only providing knowledge is rather ineffective, although necessary in the first place. Although the patients feel some cognitive dissonance they keep on with their unfavorable behaviors or seem to ignore good advice given by dental professionals.

There are several more complex behavioral models available:
- Health belief model
- Theory of action planned behavior
- Theory of self-determination
- Theory of self-efficacy
- Transtheoretical model

Table 13.2 Educational (red) and medical (black) noninvasive options of oral health programs

Recipient	Population only	Community/setting	One-to-one
Strategy	• Population/directed population	• High-risk • Directed population	• High-risk
	Mass campaigns (e.g., diet regulations)	Oral health education (hygiene techniques, self-applied fluorides, diet)	
	Fluoridated water	Supervised tooth brushing	Professional cleaning
	Fluoridated salt	Professionally applied fluorides (gel/varnish) or CHX	
		Fluoride rinse program	
		Fluoridated school milk	
	Free fluoride toothpaste		
	Fluoride tablets		

For more detailed information we refer to other textbooks on cariology[18,19] or the original literature. As an example, the patient-centered transtheoretical model[20] is presented here. According to this theory, individuals can be sorted to five stages.

- **Precontemplation:** Patient is not aware that a certain behavior leads to a disease.
- **Contemplation:** The patient is aware and weighs the pros and cons of a behavioral change to change susceptibility or symptoms of a disease.
- **Preparation:** Small changes are made, but patients are prone to relapse, which should be recorded by the counselor.
- **Action:** Most ambivalence with the behavioral change is resolved and the behavioral is consistently adopted.
- **Maintenance:** The "new" behavior is no longer new, but part of everyday lifestyle.

At any time the individual might relapse to a previous stage or completely. The dental professional should be aware and consider this theory in their efforts to advocate oral health related behaviors.

Effectiveness of Contemporary Programs for Caries Prevention

Before an assortment of oral health programs are presented as examples with respect to their effectiveness, the role of regular dental checkups on a community basis (screenings) to avoid caries progression will be discussed. For both, oral health programs as well as screenings, measurement of efficacy is much more difficult compared with the setting of a randomized clinical trial studying a new fluoride product to reduce caries. Thus, good quality data on the efficacy of oral health programs, and in particular on those with educational aspects, are scarce. Moreover, as explained later in this book (Chapter 20), effectiveness and efficacy are not the same. This is in particular true for the medical approaches that might "work" in a randomized clinical trial, but not when applied under real-life conditions, as in a high-risk group.

Role of Routine Serial Examinations in Communities

In many countries, for caries as well as other oral diseases, routine serial examinations are undertaken for surveillance and generation of cross-sectional data. Moreover, regular dental check-ups also play a considerable (financial) role in oral health programs and their effectiveness needs to be considered with respect to seeking out a dentist not only when active caries lesions are detected but also in the broader aspect to reduce caries prevalence.

The available evidence is, however, restricted to investigations of elementary school children in England over a period of 2–4 months after completion of a mass screen-

ing. One investigation concerned the frequency of dental appointments after a mass screening, and one was a study of the incidence of caries. On the one hand, a positive effect of the mass screening on the frequency of dental appointments was demonstrated (test: 46%, control: 28%) in children with caries from all social strata. Since the frequency of visits to the dentist depends in particular on the previous appointment frequency of both children and their parents, it was recommended above all to include children in mass screenings who have a corresponding predisposition (the parents do not go to the dentist).[21] On the other hand, the effect of screenings on the prevalence of caries and frequency of subsequent dental visits was relatively small in a significant number of children.[22] This was particularly true for children from the lower social stratum.[23] In considering all the children from the corresponding groups, no positive effect from the screening was identified in comparison to a control group in regard to the subsequent frequency of dental appointments and caries incidence. The authors concluded that the conventional screening practice in England must be reassessed, especially since only one-half of the investigated children who were recommended to undergo treatment actually underwent full treatment.[22] Nevertheless, mass screenings are important for the surveillance of the oral health of the population.

Population-Based Approaches

Mass Campaigns to Change Behavior

As pointed out with respect to the common risk factor approach earlier in this chapter, *upstream strategies* seem to be effective in reducing prevalence of risk factors or even disease. To support necessary policies and environmental measures, mass campaigns might be supportive, at least to inform the population. With respect to the effects of mass media on promoting knowledge or behavior change, no specific conclusion could be drawn.[24]

Fluoridated Water

Fluoridation of water is an effective and efficient method for reducing the incidence of caries (for details, see Chapter 12). However, the effects are doubtless not as striking today as before the introduction of fluoride toothpaste. Nevertheless, in many countries there exists a broad consensus that the population should be offered one of the two population-based fluoridation methods, that is, drinking water or salt.

Fluoridated Salt

In addition to fluoride toothpaste, the use of fluoridated salt for seasoning food is one alternative to the fluoridation of water. Fluoridated seasoning salt can be obtained in many countries (e.g., Switzerland, France, Germany, and a few Latin American countries). Since, nonfluoridated salt is also available, as is the case in Germany, fluoridated salt does not reach the entire population. Prospective cohort studies on the reduction of the incidence of caries by using fluoridated table salt have been performed on Hungarian[25] and Colombian[26] populations (children and adolescents). These populations had a higher prevalence of caries than present-day adolescents, and they did not use other fluoridated products such as toothpaste or mouth washes. In addition, no group prophylactic programs were introduced in kindergarten and elementary schools parallel to the introduction of salt fluoridation. According to these older studies, the isolated caries-reducing effect of salt fluoridation is estimated to be 50%. Similar to the fluoridation of water, the costs are very low (less than one cent/year/person) so that this type of fluoridation is considered to be very efficient.[27]

Approaches for Communities: Medical Options

Fluoride Tablets

Given the awareness that children from regions with a low level of fluoride in drinking water have a comparatively high prevalence and incidence of caries, the "missing fluoride" was supplemented with fluoridated tablets to be swallowed, lozenges, and drops.[28] These recommendations are based on the paradigm that optimal fluoridation should be performed, and that caries can in a sense be considered a manifestation of fluoride deficiency.[29] In the early 1980s, randomized prospective studies of young children,[30–32] schoolchildren,[33,34] and seniors were performed to determine the efficacy of fluoridation through supplements (especially tablets).[35] Some of these studies had a high dropout rate,[30,33] and they also revealed a low incidence of caries in the examined population.[32] In general, a reduction in the incidence of caries was noted after fluoride supplementation. Only one-half of the cited studies investigated the prevalence of caries and fluorosis at the same time.[32,33,36,37] However, most of these studies were performed more than 20 years ago when there was significantly higher incidence of caries than today. One current, retrospective cohort study was able to demonstrate a reduction in the caries incidence accompanied by an increase in fluorosis resulting from supplementation. This was particularly the case in children who also consumed fluoridated table salt.[38] Even though tablet fluoridation is effective, there are a few disadvantages in comparison to early training in tooth brushing and the use of fluoride toothpaste:

- Tooth brushing with fluoride toothpaste is not only effective against caries, as are fluoride supplements, but it also counteracts gingivitis.
- Older children, adolescents, and adults only manifest a limited degree of compliance when instructed to take fluoride tablets; tooth brushing in contrast is an established practice in all age classes.

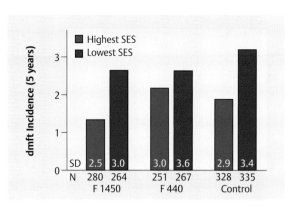

Fig. 13.4   The free provision of fluoridated toothpaste to children starting at 1 year of age reduces the incidence of caries over the next four years. Children from the lowest social stratum (SES) profit from using toothpaste containing both low and high levels of fluoride (F), whereas children in the highest social stratum only benefit from toothpaste with high fluoride content.[39]
SD = standard deviation, N = number

- Taking tablets in childhood conveys the idea of favoring a medical approach to preventing disease in general, resulting in pedagogic options becoming of secondary psychological importance.

Providing Free Fluoride Toothpaste

The provision of free toothpaste was the subject of a series of studies carried out in England with the aim of illustrating the effectiveness of this approach. Free toothpaste was offered over a period of 4–5 years starting at the age of 1 year. A reduction of caries by about 15% in comparison to control children was observed[39] when toothpaste containing 1450 ppm F[−] or 440 ppm F[−] was offered, without a significant increase in the prevalence of fluorosis.[40] This only occurred in children from a high socioeconomic stratum when the toothpaste contained 1450 ppm F[−][41] (**Fig. 13.4**); a significantly higher prevalence of fluorosis was also noted in these children[42] (**Fig. 13.5**). According to these studies an expenditure of £80 over 4 years would be required to prevent carious teeth, whereas £425 would be needed for a child to remain caries-free.[40] However, there was no significant decrease in the incidence of caries for all children in the community.[43,44]

> **NOTE**
>
> Providing free, highly fluoridated toothpaste (1450 ppm) is an effective means of reducing the incidence of caries. However, the costs of doing so are relatively high.

Other Methods of Fluoride Application

The effectiveness of various medical approaches (use of fluoride varnish, gel, mouthwash, and chlorhexidine varnish) have been systematically investigated numerous

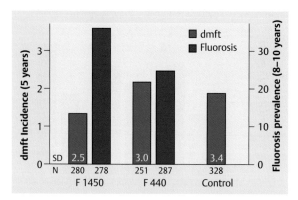

Fig. 13.5 Providing free toothpaste with a high level of fluoride to young children (1- to 5-year-olds) in the highest socioeconomic stratum reduces the incidence of caries but also elevates the prevalence of fluorosis.[41] SD = standard deviation, N = number

times.[45–55] In particular, the efficacy of fluoride varnishes has been demonstrated in several survey articles and meta-analyses.[45,56–58] The compiled results of the Cochrane Reviews are presented here in brief:

- Using **toothpaste** by itself is just as effective as using only fluoridated mouthwash or fluoride varnish applications.[52]
- The use of **toothpaste** together with fluoridated **mouthwashes** or **fluoride varnish** is only moderately more effective than using toothpaste by itself.[51]
- The use of **fluoride gels** reduces caries by 21%; this means that given an annual caries incidence of 0.2 DMFS, 24 children must use fluoride gel to prevent one DMFS unit in one child.[46]
- Given an annual caries incidence of 0.25 DMFS, one DMFS unit would be prevented if 16 children were to use a **fluoridated mouthwash** twice a day.[48]
- The use of **fluoride varnish** reduces caries by 33%.[45]
- Due to the anticipated poorer efficacy when the risk of caries is low, **fluoride varnish should be applied** when the incidence of caries is > 2 DMFS.[59]

These meta-analyses frequently make reference to randomized clinical trials that allow the efficacy on the study participants to be analyzed, but only permit limited conclusions about the effectiveness of a measure within a population. It is therefore quite possible that fluoride varnish applications from twice a year to quarterly (and also other in frequently applied fluorides) are only slightly effective in reducing the caries incidence, especially within populations of a low socioeconomic stratum,[60] since a sufficient degree of involvement is not always manifested by every child, and not every child participates in the follow-up examinations. The same observation holds true when these measures are complemented.

Another reason why this measure is modestly effective is the lack of compliance in showing up for appointments at the dentist or health care center for the professional **fluoride applications.** Nonetheless, even if compliance is poor, a certain reduction in the incidence of caries can be achieved by the biannual application of fluoride varnishes.[61,62] However, the cost-effectiveness of applying fluoride-containing gels or varnishes has been called into question, at least for populations with a low risk of caries,[63] although this issue has not yet been conclusively resolved.[64]

Chlorhexidine varnish (Chapter 11) can also be effectively employed to reduce the incidence of caries.[65] However, the efficacy under everyday conditions (effectiveness) in a larger cohort has not been confirmed, and the efficiency is highly questionable.

Approaches for Communities: Oral Health Education

Oral health education is offered on an individual basis in dental offices, and it is also presented in oral health programs for groups. The difficulty of lasting change has already been noted in the discussion of the aforementioned behavioral modification models. This section presents examples of **oral health education with behavioral modification** that are offered for groups. However, only a limited amount of high-level evidence exists on this topic (see Chapter 20).[24,66–69]

Supervised Tooth Brushing

The incidence of caries in first molars could be significantly reduced by supervised brushing twice daily over 2.5 years.[70] In particular, the frequency of brushing appeared to be the primary reason for the effectiveness of the approach in this Scottish health program. Convincing parents of the necessity for adequate oral hygiene was a key factor in reducing the caries incidence.[71] Interestingly, a significant reduction in the caries incidence of first molars was noted in comparison to the control even 4.5 years after the program had concluded.[72] A comparable reduction of caries did not appear to be achievable in older children; however, the prevalence of gingivitis was significantly reduced over four years by supervised twice-a-day brushing.[73]

> **NOTE**
>
> Brushing twice a day under the supervision of a teacher, especially with the cooperation of parents, appears to be an effective and lasting[72] method for reducing the incidence of caries.[70,71,74]

Programs Relying on Oral Health Education

It is difficult to provide a summary of studies that evaluate **purely educational approaches**, since the different methods that were pursued vary significantly. Consequently, two programs will be discussed below that exemplify the general possibilities and were sufficiently researched.

A **motivational program** that included both the teachers and parents of 13-year-old schoolchildren (3.5 hours contact time) appeared to be significantly more effective than traditional oral hygiene training programs (1.5 hours of contact time) in reducing the amount of plaque and gingival bleeding.[75] After being informed about the etiology and prevention of tooth diseases, the parents of the children involved in the intensive program were asked to actively support the oral hygiene of their children at home. The children were also taught in small groups and trained how to self-diagnose gingivitis, plaque, and initial caries. In addition, the children performed active oral hygiene exercises (brushing, flossing) and were asked to include these practices in their daily routine ("linking method"). These measures were repeated after two days and then monthly (months 1–4) and quarterly (months 5–12). The group with the motivational program manifested a significantly lower incidence of caries in comparison to the control group.[76] The children's dental knowledge and behavior had improved[77] after 3 years of the study; after 5 years, only their knowledge had improved.[78]

In a British program, the mothers of 1-year-old children from a **lower socioeconomic stratum** were educated during home visits regarding adequate nutrition and oral hygiene. After three years of the study, 33% of children of an uninstructed control group had caries lesions and 16% had gingivitis, whereas there was almost no incidence of caries or gingivitis in the intervention groups. Increasing the frequency of instruction (once a year or quarterly) did not have any apparent influence.[79]

NOTE

In general, it can be concluded that short-term improvements in knowledge and behavioral changes can influence the plaque level through group education in oral hygiene as well as individual instruction which is frequently offered chairside in the dental office. A lasting change in the approach to oral health by this methodology is considered critical.

Setting-Approaches

In **setting-approaches**, low-threshold, systematic interventions in real living conditions (school, neighborhood, etc.) are implemented by involving all stakeholders. The focused group is empowered to actively assume responsibility for health-related issues. The individual or the group is not just the recipient of offers and messages being supportive for one's health.[8]

A health-promoting environment is established in emulation of **WHO health promoting schools.** With the participation of teachers, students are informed monthly about the anatomy of the oral cavity, various oral hygiene measures, and the etiopathogenesis of caries and gingivitis.[80] The mothers are motivated to supervise tooth brushing. A study on the efficacy of these measures over a 2.5-year period revealed in particular an improvement in behavior affecting oral hygiene and a reduction in gingival bleeding in comparison to the control. The mothers and teachers also profited from the program in regard to their knowledge and attitude toward oral hygiene.

In a study of another health program for generating independent initiative (**motivational interviewing approach**), the caries incidence in children as young as 1 year was significantly reduced after one[81] and two years[82,83] in comparison to a program that only offered explanations of oral hygiene in a brochure and video. The extensive program consisted of a 45-minute informational session for the parents that was held by women with a comparable immigrant background. Direct confrontation outlining potentially harmful behavior was avoided, and an attempt was made to create an open atmosphere supportive of self-reflection. Differences between the desired goal (child with healthy dentition) and conventional behavior were illustrated in a manner based on mutuality. Over the following months, attempts were made to further enhance the parents' oral health skills in several telephone calls and mailings.

The positive results of setting approaches may also be explained by the creation of stable, positive beliefs regarding oral hygiene behavior that can reduce the plaque level and tooth loss over the long term.[84]

NOTE

The oral health of children from the lower socioeconomic stratum can apparently be promoted using the setting-approach, which avoids triggering defense mechanisms by not stigmatizing both parents and children as victims of society and refraining from accusations of poor behavior.

Approaches for Communities: Combining Medical Options and Oral Health Education

Behavior-shaping (pedagogical) elements are frequently combined with "medical" measures (noninvasive interventions). The cited combinations mean that instruction about oral health behavior and nutrition is offered besides "medical" interventions as examinations and, for example, fluoridation measures. Generally, these complex interventions target high-risk groups since the greatest reduction of the individual incidence of caries can be anticipated through these measures. As outlined above, **high-risk strategies** concentrate on those presumably being at a higher risk for further caries development. This implies that those are reliably identified at affordable costs.[85] In addition, the individual protection for the high-risk patients must be efficient enough to justify the effort.[14] Some examples are given to show that high-risk ap-

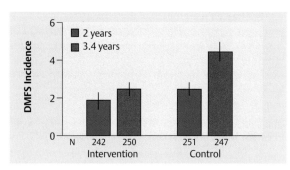

Fig. 13.6 A program for high-risk children including multiple measures reduced the caries increment considerably within 3.4 years in caries-active individuals (Hausen et al. [89]). Error bars (|) represent 95% confidence intervals.

proaches are challenging and somehow questionable with respect to effectiveness and efficiency

Several **Finnish** randomized controlled trials have studied the efficacy of **high-risk approaches**. Unfortunately, no significant improvement of caries increment in high-risk children could be observed in earlier studies.[86,87] For children at high risk, the intensified prevention program monitored by dental authorities was no more successful than prevention planned by individual dentists.[86] Another even more intensive program (counseling, F-varnish applications, F-lozenges, sealants, chlorhexidine) also failed to show more beneficial effects compared with counseling plus one F-varnish application per year.[88]

> **NOTE**
>
> The described **high-risk approaches** might not have been successful in preventing caries, due the missing mutual understanding between dental personnel and patients.

Therefore, in a subsequent program focusing on 11- to 12-year-olds, sessions were performed by experts trained in patient- and empowerment-centered counseling with emphasis on enhancing use of the children's own resources in everyday life. Toothbrushes, fluoride toothpaste, fluoride, and xylitol lozenges were distributed to the children, and fluoride/chlorhexidine varnish was applied. These multiple measures reduced the caries increment considerably within 3.4 years in caries-prone children living in an area where the overall level of caries experience was low[89] (**Fig. 13.6**). Cost-effectiveness increased with longer duration of the program; it would have been even better if dental nurses had conducted the preventive procedures.[90]

Other programs reveal contradictory results regarding the efficacy of **high-risk approaches**. Traditional oral hygiene education apparently does not reduce the incidence of caries in comparison to a control group without instruction. Additional professional tooth cleaning and chlo-

rhexidine mouthwashes were also not much more effective.[91] Following an observation period of 2.5 years, a significant reduction in the caries incidence of 3-year-old Russian kindergarten children was observed in comparison to the control group where only the parents were offered instruction. More intensive measures such as professional tooth cleaning, the use of fluoride varnish and risk-oriented fissure sealing in 6-year-olds and 11-year-olds led to a strong reduction in the incidence of caries in comparison to control groups without instruction.[92] Other programs which included risk-oriented fissure sealing also revealed a marked reduction in caries incidence[93,94] (see also Chapters 15 and 20).

In a Swedish study of the general population and children with a high risk of caries which exclusively offered instruction in proper tooth brushing, the application of fluoride varnish or the taking of fluoride tablets did not strongly reduce the incidence of caries, even after observation periods extending up to 5 years.[61,62] A relatively comprehensive program in Scottish communities with a low socioeconomic status that was based on the **principles of the Ottawa Charter** (see above) had a positive influence on the caries incidence of 3–5-year-olds. Changes in nutrition and tooth brushing habits were established in kindergarten and elementary schools. Fluoride toothpaste and toothbrushes were provided free of charge, and oral health education was offered in a broad local effort in the community.[95,96] Another concept (individualized population-based approach) of reducing caries incidence, also in high-risk children, will be presented later in this book (Chapter 21).

> **NOTE**
>
> Providing free, highly fluoridated toothpaste is an effective means for reducing the incidence of caries. However, the costs of doing so are relatively high.

There is little available scientific evidence from clinical studies on the reduction of the incidence of caries in **age groups above 18 years.** Biannual oral health programs by themselves appear to be inferior to the additional use of other strategies (combination of fluoride and chlorhexidine varnish and the smoothing of root surfaces).[97] In this study, senior adults over 60 years old from the lower socioeconomic stratum were investigated for three years with regard to the incidence of extractions, fillings, and caries.

One-to-One Situation in Dental Practice

The concerns with regard to the effectiveness of the high-risk approaches in communities hold true for the one-to-one situation in dental practice as well. Nonetheless, high-quality studies still need to be undertaken to elucidate the efficacy of oral health counseling for individuals. Fluoride/chlorhexidine varnish application is considered as being efficacious, although their efficiency can be questioned. Professional tooth cleaning seems to be efficacious (Chapter 10), although only on a regular basis taking into account psychological issues as outlined above. Some more practical aspects will be given in the second part of this book (Chapters 25 and 26).

SUMMARY

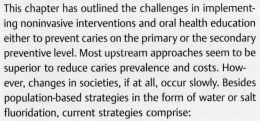

This chapter has outlined the challenges in implementing noninvasive interventions and oral health education either to prevent caries on the primary or the secondary preventive level. Most upstream approaches seem to be superior to reduce caries prevalence and costs. However, changes in societies, if at all, occur slowly. Besides population-based strategies in the form of water or salt fluoridation, current strategies comprise:

- Routine serial examinations
- Prescription of fluoride tablets/lozenges
- Application of fluorides (varnish, gel) or chlorhexidine
- Providing free-fluoride toothpaste
- School programs including fluoride milk or mouth rinse
- Teacher-supervised tooth brushing
- Oral health counseling in communities, settings, or for the individual in dental practice

Many medical options as fluoride applications either for populations (water/salt), self-administered (toothpaste/rinse), or professionally applied (varnish/gel) seem to be efficacious. Nonetheless, the effectiveness and efficiency of professionally applied fluorides has been challenged. For oral health counseling, scientific evidence still needs to be improved, which is true in particular for oral health promotion in certain settings.

In addition, the following suggestions can be made with respect to oral health promotion to reduce caries incidence:

- Teacher-supervised tooth brushing including the parents is efficacious.
- Providing free fluoride toothpaste is efficacious, but costly.
- It is possible to change knowledge and attitudes concerning oral health in the short term, but in the long run it is hard to change unfavorable behaviors.
- High-risk approaches where oral health counseling by empowerment is combined with risk-related fluoride and/or sealant applications seem to be most beneficial.
- A directed population approach will result in greater caries reductions compared with a high-risk approach.
- For certain communities with low socioeconomical background, provision of oral health counseling by a person who is accepted by people of the respective setting seems to be successful.

REFERENCES

1. Leavell HR, Clark EG. Preventive Medicine for the Doctor in his Community: An Epidemiological Approach. New York: McGraw-Hill; 1965

2. Fejerskov O, Nyvad B. Is dental caries an infectious disease? Diagnostic and treatment consequences for the practitioner. In: Schou L, ed. Nordic Dentistry 2003 Yearbook. Copenhagen: Quintessence Publishing; 2003:141–151

3. Fejerskov O, Manji F. Risk assessment in dental caries. In: Bader J, ed. Risk Assessment in Dentistry. Chapel Hill: University of North Carolina; 1990:215–217

4. Baelum V, Sheiham A, Burt BA. Caries control for populations. In: Fejerskov O, Kidd EAM, eds. Dental Caries: The Disease and its Clinical Management. 2nd ed. Oxford: Blackwell Wiley; 2008: 505–526

5. McKinlay JB. A case for refocusing upstream: the political economy of illness. In: Enelow A, Henderson J, eds. Applying Behavioural Science to Cardiovascular Disease. Washington DC: American Heart Association; 1975:7–17

6. Baelum V, Nyvad B, Grondahl HG, et al. The underpinnings of good diagnostic practice. In: Fejerskov O, Kidd EAM, eds. Dental Caries: The Disease and its Clinical Management. 2nd ed. Oxford: Wiley Blackwell; 2008:103–118

7. World Health Organization (WHO). The Ottawa Charter for Health Promotion. Geneva: World Health Organization; 1986

8. Siebert D, Hartmann T. Arbeitskreis Gesundheitsfördernde Hochschulen. Basiswissen Gesundheitsförderung – Historische Entwicklung und gesetzliche Grundlagen. http://www.gesundheitsfoerdernde-hochschulen.de/HTML/B_Basiswissen_GF/B1_-Historische_Entwicklung_und_gesetzliche_Grundlagen. Published June 21, 2010. Accessed July 28, 2011

9. Watt RG. From victim blaming to upstream action: tackling the social determinants of oral health inequalities. Community Dent Oral Epidemiol 2007;35(1):1–11

10. Sheiham A, Watt RG. The common risk factor approach: a rational basis for promoting oral health. Community Dent Oral Epidemiol 2000;28(6):399–406

11. Kwan SY, Petersen PE, Pine CM, Borutta A. Health-promoting schools: an opportunity for oral health promotion. Bull World Health Organ 2005;83(9):677–685

12. Lang T, Rayner G, Kaelin E. The Food Industry, Diet, Physical Activity and Health: A Review of Reported Commitments and Practice of 25 of the World's Largest Food Companies. London: City University Centre for Food Policy; 2006

13. Ekstrand KR, Christiansen ME, Qvist V. Influence of different variables on the inter-municipality variation in caries experience in Danish adolescents. Caries Res 2003;37(2):130–141

14. Sheiham A. Public health approaches to promoting dental health. Z Gesundheitswiss 2001;9:100–112

15. Sheiham A, Foffe M. Public dental health strategies for identifying and controlling dental caries in high and low risk populations. In: Johnson NW, ed. Risk Markers for Oral Diseases. Vol l. Dental Caries: Markers of High and Low Risk Groups and Individuals. Cambridge: Cambridge University Press; 1991:445–481

16. Rose G. Strategy of Preventive Medicine. Oxford: Oxford University Press; 1992

17. Nutbeam D. Health promotion glossary. Health Promot 1986; 1(1):113–127

18. Kay EJ, Craven R. Promoting oral health in populations. In: Fejerskov O, Kidd EAM, eds. Dental Caries: The Disease and its Clinical Management. 2nd ed. Oxford: Wiley Blackwell; 2008:475–486

19. Freeman R, Ismail A. Assessing patients' health behaviours. In: Pitts NB, ed. Detection, Assessment, Diagnosis and Monitoring of Caries. Basel: Karger; 2009:113–127

20. Prochaska JO, di Clemente CC. Transtheoretical therapy: towards a more integrative model of change. Psychoth Theory Res Pract 1982;19:276–288

21. Donaldson M, Kinirons M. Effectiveness of the school dental screening programme in stimulating dental attendance for children in need of treatment in Northern Ireland. Community Dent Oral Epidemiol 2001;29(2):143–149

22. Milsom K, Blinkhorn A, Worthington H, et al. The effectiveness of school dental screening: a cluster-randomized control trial. J Dent Res 2006;85(10):924–928

23. Milsom KM, Threlfall AG, Blinkhorn AS, Kearney-Mitchell PI, Buchanan KM, Tickle M. The effectiveness of school dental screening: dental attendance and treatment of those screened positive. Br Dent J 2006;200(12):687–690, discussion 673

24. Kay EJ, Locker D. A systematic review of the effectiveness of health promotion aimed at improving oral health. Community Dent Health 1998;15(3):132–144

25. Toth K. Caries Prevention by Domestic Salt Fluoridation. Budapest: Akadémiai Kiadó; 1984

26. Marthaler TM, Mejía R, Tóth K, Viñes JJ. Caries-preventive salt fluoridation. Caries Res 1978;12(Suppl 1):15–21

27. Gillespie GM, Marthaler TM. Cost aspects of salt fluoridation. Schweiz Monatsschr Zahnmed 2005;115(9):778–784

28. Dean HT, Arnold FA, Elove E. Domestic water and dental caries. V. Additional studies of the relation if fluoride domestic waters to dental caries experience in 4425 white children aged 12–13 years of 13 cities in 4 states. Public Health Rep 1942;57:1155–1179

29. Ellwood R, Fejerskov O, Cury JA, et al. Fluorides in caries control. In: Fejerskov O, Kidd EAM, eds. Dental Caries: The Disease and its Clinical Management. 2nd ed. Oxford: Blackwell Munksgaard; 2008:287–327

30. Driscoll WS, Heifetz SB, Brunelle JA. Caries-preventive effects of fluoride tablets in schoolchildren four years after discontinuation of treatments. J Am Dent Assoc 1981;103(6):878–881

31. Reich E, Schmalz G, Bergmann RL, et al. Kariesbefall von Kindern nach unterschiedlich langer Applikation von Fluoridtabletten. Dtsch Zahnarztl Z 1992;47:232–234

32. Leverett DH, Adair SM, Vaughan BW, Proskin HM, Moss ME. Randomized clinical trial of the effect of prenatal fluoride supplements in preventing dental caries. Caries Res 1997;31(3):174–179

33. Allmark C, Green HP, Linney AD, Wills DJ, Picton DC. A community study of fluoride tablets for school children in Portsmouth. results after six years. Br Dent J 1982;153(12):426–430

34. Gülzow HJ, Strübig W. Need for the continuous ingestion of fluoride tablets. [Article in German] Dtsch Zahnarztl Z 1984;39(7):512–514

35. Fure S, Gahnberg L, Birkhed D. A comparison of four home-care fluoride programs on the caries incidence in the elderly. Gerodontol 1998;15(2):51–60

36. de Liefde B, Herbison GP. Prevalence of developmental defects of enamel and dental caries in New Zealand children receiving differing fluoride supplementation. Community Dent Oral Epidemiol 1985;13(3):164–167

37. Wang NJ, Riordan PJ. Fluoride supplements and caries in a non-fluoridated child population. Community Dent Oral Epidemiol 1999;27(2):117–123

38. Meyer-Lueckel H, Grundmann E, Stang A. Effects of fluoride tablets on caries and fluorosis occurrence among 6- to 9-year olds using fluoridated salt. Community Dent Oral Epidemiol 2010;38(4):315–323

39. Davies GM, Worthington HV, Ellwood RP, et al. A randomised controlled trial of the effectiveness of providing free fluoride toothpaste from the age of 12 months on reducing caries in 5-6 year old children. Community Dent Health 2002;19(3):131–136

40. Davies GM, Worthington HV, Ellwood RP, et al. An assessment of the cost effectiveness of a postal toothpaste programme to prevent caries among five-year-old children in the North West of England. Community Dent Health 2003;20(4):207–210

41. Ellwood RP, Davies GM, Worthington HV, Blinkhorn AS, Taylor GO, Davies RM. Relationship between area deprivation and the anticaries benefit of an oral health programme providing free fluoride toothpaste to young children. Community Dent Oral Epidemiol 2004;32(3):159–165

42. Tavener JA, Davies GM, Davies RM, Ellwood RP. The prevalence and severity of fluorosis in children who received toothpaste containing either 440 or 1,450 ppm F from the age of 12 months in deprived and less deprived communities. Caries Res 2006;40(1):66–72

43. Davies GM, Duxbury JT, Boothman NJ, Davies RM, Blinkhorn AS. A staged intervention dental health promotion programme to reduce early childhood caries. Community Dent Health 2005;22(2):118–122

44. Davies GM, Duxbury JT, Boothman NJ, Davies RM. Challenges associated with the evaluation of a dental health promotion programme in a deprived urban area. Community Dent Health 2007;24(2):117–121

45. Marinho VC, Higgins JP, Logan S, Sheiham A. Fluoride varnishes for preventing dental caries in children and adolescents. Cochrane Database Syst Rev 2002;3(3):CD002279

46. Marinho VC, Higgins JP, Logan S, Sheiham A. Fluoride gels for preventing dental caries in children and adolescents. Cochrane Database Syst Rev 2002;2(2):CD002280

47. Marinho VC, Higgins JP, Logan S, Sheiham A. Topical fluoride (toothpastes, mouthrinses, gels or varnishes) for preventing dental caries in children and adolescents. Cochrane Database Syst Rev 2003;4(4):CD002782

48. Marinho VC, Higgins JP, Logan S, Sheiham A. Fluoride mouthrinses for preventing dental caries in children and adolescents. Cochrane Database Syst Rev 2003;3(3):CD002284

49. Marinho VC, Higgins JP, Sheiham A, Logan S. Fluoride toothpastes for preventing dental caries in children and adolescents. Cochrane Database Syst Rev 2003;1(1):CD002278

50. Twetman S, Axelsson S, Dahlgren H, et al. Caries-preventive effect of fluoride toothpaste: a systematic review. Acta Odontol Scand 2003;61(6):347–355

51. Marinho VC, Higgins JP, Sheiham A, Logan S. Combinations of topical fluoride (toothpastes, mouthrinses, gels, varnishes) versus single topical fluoride for preventing dental caries in children and adolescents. Cochrane Database Syst Rev 2004;1(1):CD002781

52. Marinho VC, Higgins JP, Sheiham A, Logan S. One topical fluoride (toothpastes, or mouthrinses, or gels, or varnishes) versus another for preventing dental caries in children and adolescents. Cochrane Database Syst Rev 2004;1(1):CD002780

53. Twetman S, Petersson L, Axelsson S, et al. Caries-preventive effect of sodium fluoride mouthrinses: a systematic review of controlled clinical trials. Acta Odontol Scand 2004;62(4):223–230

54. van Rijkom HM, Truin GJ, van't Hof MA. Caries-inhibiting effect of professional fluoride gel application in low-caries children initially aged 4.5-6.5 years. Caries Res 2004;38(2):115–123

55. Hiiri A, Ahovuo-Saloranta A, Nordblad A, Mäkelä M. Pit and fissure sealants versus fluoride varnishes for preventing dental decay in children and adolescents. Cochrane Database Syst Rev 2006;4(4):CD003067

56. Helfenstein U, Steiner M. Fluoride varnishes (Duraphat): a meta-analysis. Community Dent Oral Epidemiol 1994;22(1):1–5

57. Bader JD, Shugars DA, Bonito AJ. A systematic review of selected caries prevention and management methods. Community Dent Oral Epidemiol 2001;29(6):399–411

58. Strohmenger L, Brambilla E. The use of fluoride varnishes in the prevention of dental caries: a short review. Oral Dis 2001;7(2):71–80

59. Marinho VC. Evidence-based effectiveness of topical fluorides. Adv Dent Res 2008;20(1):3–7

60. Hardman MC, Davies GM, Duxbury JT, Davies RM. A cluster randomised controlled trial to evaluate the effectiveness of fluoride varnish as a public health measure to reduce caries in children. Caries Res 2007;41(5):371–376

61. Källestål C. The effect of five years' implementation of caries-preventive methods in Swedish high-risk adolescents. Caries Res 2005;39(1):20–26

62. Källestål C, Fjelddahl A. A four-year cohort study of caries and its risk factors in adolescents with high and low risk at baseline. Swed Dent J 2007;31(1):11–25

63. Seppä L. The future of preventive programs in countries with different systems for dental care. Caries Res 2001;35(Suppl 1):26–29

64. Källestål C, Norlund A, Söder B, et al. Economic evaluation of dental caries prevention: a systematic review. Acta Odontol Scand 2003;61(6):341–346

65. Zhang Q, van Palenstein Helderman WH, van't Hof MA, Truin GJ. Chlorhexidine varnish for preventing dental caries in children, adolescents and young adults: a systematic review. Eur J Oral Sci 2006;114(6):449–455

66. Kay EJ, Locker D. Is dental health education effective? A systematic review of current evidence. Community Dent Oral Epidemiol 1996;24(4):231–235

67. Petersen PE, Kwan S. Evaluation of community-based oral health promotion and oral disease prevention—WHO recommendations for improved evidence in public health practice. Community Dent Health 2004; 21(4, Suppl):319–329

68. Watt RG. Strategies and approaches in oral disease prevention and health promotion. Bull World Health Organ 2005;83(9):711–718

69. Meyer-Lückel H, Schiffner U. Effektivität und Effizienz verhaltensmodifizierender gruppenprophylaktischer Maßnahmen bei Kindern. Dtsch Zahnarztl Z 2009;64:152–167

70. Curnow MM, Pine CM, Burnside G, Nicholson JA, Chesters RK, Huntington E. A randomised controlled trial of the efficacy of supervised tooth brushing in high-caries-risk children. Caries Res 2002;36(4):294–300

71. Pine CM, McGoldrick PM, Burnside G, et al. An intervention programme to establish regular tooth brushing: understanding parents' beliefs and motivating children. Int Dent J 2000;Suppl Creating A Successful (Suppl.):312–323

72. Pine CM, Curnow MM, Burnside G, Nicholson JA, Roberts AJ. Caries prevalence four years after the end of a randomised controlled trial. Caries Res 2007;41(6):431–436

73. Suomi JD, Peterson JK, Matthews BL, Voglesong RH, Lyman BA. Effects of supervised daily dental plaque removal by children after 3 years. Community Dent Oral Epidemiol 1980;8(4):171–176

74. You BJ, Jian WW, Sheng RW, et al. Caries prevention in Chinese children with sodium fluoride dentifrice delivered through a kindergarten-based oral health program in China. J Clin Dent 2002;13(4):179–184

75. Albandar JM, Buischi YA, Mayer MP, Axelsson P. Long-term effect of two preventive programs on the incidence of plaque and gingivitis in adolescents. J Periodontol 1994;65(6):605–610

76. Axelsson P, Buischi YA, Barbosa MF, Karlsson R, Prado MC. The effect of a new oral hygiene training program on approximal caries in 12-15-year-old Brazilian children: results after three years. Adv Dent Res 1994;8(2):278–284

77. Buischi YA, Axelsson P, Oliveira LB, Mayer MP, Gjermo P. Effect of two preventive programs on oral health knowledge and habits among Brazilian schoolchildren. Community Dent Oral Epidemiol 1994;22(1):41–46

78. Mayer MP, de Paiva Buischi Y, de Oliveira LB, Gjermo O. Long-term effect of an oral hygiene training program on knowledge and reported behavior. Oral Health Prev Dent 2003;1(1):37–43

79. Kowash MB, Pinfield A, Smith J, Curzon ME. Effectiveness on oral health of a long-term health education programme for mothers with young children. Br Dent J 2000;188(4):201–205

80. Petersen PE, Peng B, Tai B, Bian Z, Fan M. Effect of a school-based oral health education programme in Wuhan City, Peoples Republic of China. Int Dent J 2004;54(1):33–41

81. Weinstein P, Harrison R, Benton T. Motivating parents to prevent caries in their young children: one-year findings. J Am Dent Assoc 2004;135(6):731–738

82. Weinstein P, Harrison R, Benton T. Motivating mothers to prevent caries: confirming the beneficial effect of counseling. J Am Dent Assoc 2006;137(6):789–793

83. Harrison R, Benton T, Everson-Stewart S, Weinstein P. Effect of motivational interviewing on rates of early childhood caries: a randomized trial. Pediatr Dent 2007;29(1):16–22

84. Broadbent JM, Thomson WM, Poulton R. Oral health beliefs in adolescence and oral health in young adulthood. J Dent Res 2006;85(4):339–343

85. Burt BA. Concepts of risk in dental public health. Community Dent Oral Epidemiol 2005;33(4):240–247

86. Seppä L, Hausen H, Pöllänen L, Kärkkäinen S, Helasharju K. Effect of intensified caries prevention on approximal caries in adolescents with high caries risk. Caries Res 1991;25(5):392–395

87. Hawkins RJ, Zanetti DL, Main PA, et al. Oral hygiene knowledge of high-risk Grade One children: an evaluation of two methods of dental health education. Community Dent Oral Epidemiol 2000;28(5):336–343

88. Hausen H, Kärkkäinen S, Seppä L. Application of the high-risk strategy to control dental caries. Community Dent Oral Epidemiol 2000;28(1):26–34

89. Hausen H, Seppa L, Poutanen R, et al. Noninvasive control of dental caries in children with active initial lesions. A randomized clinical trial. Caries Res 2007;41(5):384–391

90. Hietasalo P, Seppä L, Lahti S, et al. Cost-effectiveness of an experimental caries-control regimen in a 3.4-yr randomized clinical trial among 11-12-yr-old Finnish schoolchildren. Eur J Oral Sci 2009;117(6):728–733

91. Axelsson P, Kristoffersson K, Karlsson R, Bratthall D. A 30-month longitudinal study of the effects of some oral hygiene measures on Streptococcus mutans and approximal dental caries. J Dent Res 1987;66(3):761–765

92. Ekstrand KR, Kuzmina IN, Kuzmina E, Christiansen ME. Two and a half-year outcome of caries-preventive programs offered to groups of children in the Solntsevsky district of Moscow. Caries Res 2000;34(1):8–19

93. Bagramian RA, Graves RC, Srivastava S. A combined approach to preventing dental caries in schoolchildren : caries reductions after 3 years. Community Dent Oral Epidemiol 1978;6(4):166–171

94. Lalloo R, Solanki GS. An evaluation of a school-based comprehensive public oral health care programme. Community Dent Health 1994;11(3):152–155

95. Blair Y, Macpherson LM, McCall DR, McMahon AD, Stephen KW. Glasgow nursery-based caries experience, before and after a community development-based oral health programme's implementation. Community Dent Health 2004;21(4):291–298

96. Blair Y, Macpherson LM, McCall DR, McMahon A. Dental health of 5-year-olds following community-based oral health promotion in Glasgow, UK. Int J Paediatr Dent 2006;16(6):388–398

97. Powell LV, Persson RE, Kiyak HA, Hujoel PP. Caries prevention in a community-dwelling older population. Caries Res 1999;33(5):333–339

Basics in Adhesion Technology

Bart Van Meerbeek, Yasuhiro Yoshida

14

Although noninvasive interventions might be successful in inhibiting the development or further progression of a caries lesion, their success is dependent on the adherence of the patient (Chapter 13). Thus, self-management of the caries disease is of limited sustainability, which is reflected by the number of dentinal caries lesions that can still be observed worldwide (Chapter 8). In former days, amalgam and, if affordable for the patient, gold cast restorations were placed in the teeth mainly for the purpose of providing the patient with a functioning dentition. In recent years, more esthetic solutions have been demanded, which has been accompanied by a discussion on the biocompatibility of restorative materials, with the consequence that amalgams, at least, have lost some of their status in modern dentistry. **Tooth-colored filling materials** can be mainly divided into cements (glass-ionomers) and resin-based materials (composites) (Chapter 19), the latter being in need of a pretreatment procedure before they can be applied. This procedure comprises the use of several chemical agents to allow for a durable interface between tooth hard substances and the resin-based material. This intriguing step in invasive dentistry has been referred to as **adhesion technology**.

Adhesive technology has evolved rapidly since it was introduced nearly 60 years ago. The main challenge for dental adhesives is to provide an equally effective bond to two substrates of different nature. Bonding to enamel has proven to be durable. Reliable bonding to dentin is more intricate and can apparently only be achieved when rather complicated and time-consuming application procedures are followed. Consequently, today's adhesives are often regarded as technique-sensitive with the smallest error in the clinical application procedure being penalized, either by rapid de-bonding or by early marginal degradation. As a consequence, the demand for simpler, more user-friendly and less technique-sensitive adhesives has been high, urging manufacturers to develop new adhesives at a rapid pace.

In detail, this chapter will cover:
- A critical review on the laboratory and clinical performance of dental adhesive technology that dentists can use today in their practice
- The basic mechanisms of bonding to enamel and dentin
- The strengths and weaknesses of the two major bonding approaches, being the **etch-and-rinse** and the **self-etch** (or **etch-and-dry**) bonding strategies
- The more challenging bonding to caries-affected dentin
- Clear guidelines for predictable, reliable, and durable bonding to enamel and dentin, both separately and jointly

Evolution of Adhesive Technology in Generations

Early Days

After observing the industrial use of phosphoric acid to improve adhesion of paints and resin coatings to metal surfaces, Buonocore, in 1955,[1] applied acid to teeth to "render the tooth surface more receptive to adhesion". Imitating his **enamel acid-etch technique**, Brudevold et al. reported in 1956[2] that glycerophosphoric acid dimethacrylate (GPDM) could bond to hydrochloric acid-etched dentinal surfaces. The bond strength attained with this primitive adhesive technique was only 2–3 MPa, in contrast to the common 15–20 MPa bond strength obtained to acid-etched enamel. Predating the experiments of Buonocore, other investigators used the same monomer, GPDM, in the early 1950s with the introduction of Sevriton Cavity Seal (Amalgamated Dental Company).[3]

After the failures of this early **dentin acid-etch technique**, numerous dentin adhesives with complex chemical formulas were designed and developed with the objective of promoting chemical adhesion. So-called **dentin bonding agents** were no longer unfilled resins intended purely to better wet the dentinal surface prior to the application of a stiff resin composite. They became bifunctional monomers with specific reactive groups that were claimed to react chemically with the inorganic calcium-hydroxyapatite and/or organic collagen component of dentin.[4] The development of N-phenylglycine glycidyl methacrylate (NPG-GMA) was the basis of the first commercially available dentin bonding agent, Cervident (SS White).[5] This **first generation** dentin bonding agent theoretically bonded to enamel and dentin through chelation with calcium. Clearfil Bond System F (Kuraray), introduced in 1978, was the first product of a large **second generation** of dentin adhesives, such as Bondlite (Kerr/Sybron), J&J VLC Dentin Bonding Agent (Johnson & Johnson Dental), Dentin Adhesit (Vivadent), and Scotchbond (3 M), among others. These products were based on phosphorous esters of methacrylate derivatives for enhanced surface wetting as well as ionic interaction with calcium.[6] Clinically, they failed rather early, as these adhesives primarily bonded to the weak smear layer. The basis for the **third generation** of dentin adhesives was laid when the Japanese philosophy of etching dentin to remove the smear layer gained acceptance.[7] This had earlier been discouraged in America and Europe until the end of the 1980s because of pulpal inflammation concerns.[8] Based on this **total-etch concept**, Clearfil New Bond (Kuraray) was introduced in 1984, which contained 2-hydroxyethyl methacrylate (HEMA) and 10-methacryloyloxy decyl dihydrogenphosphate (10-MDP). Another approach, at that time unique, to deal with the cavity smear layer was the use of Scotchprep (3 M), which was an aqueous HEMA solution containing also maleic acid at low concentration; it was followed by the application of an unfilled adhesive resin, Scotchbond 2 (3 M), which contained bisphenol A diglycidyl dimethacrylate (Bis-GMA) and HEMA. In this way, this acidic primer simultaneously etched and impregnated the dentinal surface and was in fact the precursor of the current **self-etch adhesives**. At that time, Scotchprep (3 M) was, however, advocated to be used solely on dentin. Other systems, such as Superlux Universalbond 2 (DMG), and Syntac (Ivoclar-Vivadent), followed this smear layer-dissolving approach.

Breakthrough in Adhesion Technology

Significant advances in adhesive dentistry were made with the development of the multistep **fourth generation** adhesives in the early-to-mid 1990s. They are today referred to as **three-step etch-and-rinse adhesives**, and are considered as the "gold standard" and consequently still widely used. Essential is the pretreatment of dentin with **conditioners** and **primers** that make the heterogeneous and hydrophilic dentin substrate more receptive to bonding. Although etchants formerly contained **phosphoric acid** at a concentration well below 30%, or contained alternative milder acids (such as maleic, nitric or oxalic acid), today the fourth generation adhesives generally come with 30%–40% phosphoric-acid gels. An important final step in this multistep approach, regarding interface sealing and thus bond stability, involves the separate application and light curing of a hydrophobic adhesive resin. Representative adhesives in this group are All-Bond 3 (Bisco), OptiBond Fl (Kerr), Permaquik (Ultradent) and Scotchbond Multi-Purpose (3 M).

Because of the alleged complexity of the fourth generation systems, the **fifth generation** adhesives involve a separate etch-and-rinse phase followed by a combined application of a primer-adhesive resin or so-called **one-bottle**. Although most of these **two-step etch-and-rinse** adhesives have somewhat fallen short of achieving at least similar or even improved bonding with fewer bottles, this generation has been adopted very well in routine clinical practice. Representative commercial products of this generation are Excite (Ivoclar-Vivadent), iBond Total Etch (Hereaus-Kulzer), One-step (diverse versions, Bisco), OptiBond Solo (diverse versions, Kerr), Prime&Bond (diverse versions, Dentsply), Scotchbond 1 (diverse versions, 3 M ESPE), and TECO (DMG).

No Separate Etching?

The **sixth generation** is one of **self-etch adhesives** that can be further subdivided into **two-step self-etch** and **one-step, two-component self-etch** adhesives, depending respectively on whether a separate self-etching primer is provided or not. To ensure etching, the presence of water as an ionizing medium is necessary. The bonding performance attained by the sixth generation adhesives varies a great deal, depending on the actual composition and more specifically on the actual functional monomer included in

the adhesive formulation. Representative of the two-step self-etch adhesives are AdheSE (Ivoclar-Vivadent), Clearfil SE Bond and Protect Bond (Kuraray), Contax (DMG), and OptiBond Solo Plus Self-Etch (Kerr). Representative of the one-step, two-component self-etch adhesives are Adper Prompt L-Pop (3 M ESPE), One-up Bond F (Tokuyama), and Xeno III (Dentsply).

The latest and **seventh generation** comprises **single-component, one-step self-etch** adhesives, or the only true one-bottle or all-in-one adhesives; they combine conditioning, priming, and application of adhesive resin, but do not require mixing. These most simple-to-use adhesives are intricate mixes of hydrophilic and hydrophobic components, and have been abundantly documented as having several shortcomings (see box). Representative (single-component) one-step self-etch adhesives are Adper Easy Bond and Scotchbond Universal (3 M ESPE), Bond Force (Tokuyama), Clearfil S 3 Bond Plus (Kuraray), G-Bond and G-aenial Bond (GC), iBond Self Etch (Hereaus-Kulzer), and Xeno V (Dentsply).

> **NOTE**
>
> Shortcomings of simple-to-use adhesives (all-in-one)[9–13]:
> - Reduced immediate and long-term bonding effectiveness
> - Increased interfacial nanoleakage
> - Enhanced water sorption for adhesives that are rich in HEMA
> - Phase-separation for HEMA-free/poor adhesives
> - Reduced shelf-life
> - Especially, less favorable clinical performance

Modern Classification of Adhesives

Classifying dental adhesives into different categories is not straightforward, because of the great supply and vast turnover of manufactured adhesives. Although the classification in **generations** was referred to above, this chronological classification is not logical, lacks scientific background with regard to the bonding strategy followed, is often commercially misused, and most importantly does not provide any clear information to practitioners with regard to their correct use.[14] Classifying adhesives into **etch-and-rinse adhesives, self-etch adhesives,** and **glass-ionomers** is simple, reliable and consistent, because of which this classification has been internationally accepted (**Fig. 14.1**). **Further subdivisions** are/can be made based on the number of application steps, the number of components (that need to be mixed), and especially with regard to the self-etch systems on the basis of their **interaction intensity** as self-etch adhesives (**Fig. 14.2**).[15]

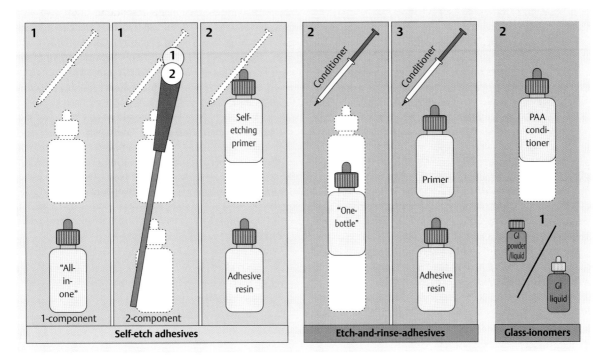

Fig. 14.1 Classification of adhesives and number of application steps for each method.

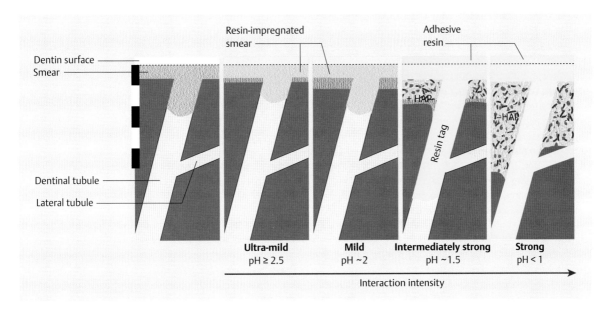

Fig. 14.2 Schematic illustration of the differential interaction of self-etch adhesives with dentin depending on the pH of the self-etching solution.[15] HAP: hydroxyapatite.

- *strong* (pH < 1)
- *intermediately strong* (pH ~1.5)
- *mild* (pH ~2)
- *ultra-mild* (pH ≥ 2.5)

NOTE

Internationally accepted classification of adhesives:
- Etch-and-rinse
- Self-etch
- Glass-ionomers

Interaction with Hydroxy-apatite-Based Tissues

The fundamental mechanism of bonding to enamel and dentin is essentially based on an exchange process, in which minerals removed from the dental hard tissues are replaced by resin monomers that upon polymerization become micromechanically interlocked in the created porosities.[4,14] This so-called **hybridization** is thus a process primarily based upon diffusion. While the resultant micromechanical interlocking is needed to achieve good bonding in clinical circumstances, the potential benefit of additional chemical interaction between functional monomers and tooth substrate components is thought to particularly improve bond durability.[14,16,17]

The way molecules interact with hydroxyapatite-based tissues has been described in the so-called **AD-concept** or **Adhesion–Decalcification concept** (**Fig. 14.3**).[18] This model dictates that initially all acids bond chemically (ionically) to the calcium of hydroxyapatite (Phase I). Whether the molecule will remain bonded (Phase II, Option 1), or will de-bond (Phase II, Option 2), depends on the stability of the formed bond, or in other words on the stability of the respectively formed calcium salt.

More specifically, molecules like 10-MDP (as functional monomer in a mild self-etch adhesive), but also polyalkenoic acids (as functional polymers in conventional and resin-modified glass-ionomers), will readily bond chemically to the calcium of hydroxyapatite (Phase II, Option 1). They form stable calcium-phosphate and calcium-carboxylate salts, respectively, along with only a limited surface decalcification effect. Mild self-etch adhesives and glass-ionomers only superficially interact with enamel and dentin, and hardly dissolve hydroxyapatite crystals, but rather keep them in place (within a thin, submicron hybrid layer; see below). In this way, the hydroxyapatite remains to protect the more vulnerable collagen fibrils.

On the contrary, molecules like phosphoric and maleic acid, but also strongly etching monomers like HEMA-phosphate (as in specific strong self-etch adhesives), will initially bond to calcium of hydroxyapatite (Phase I), but will readily de-bond (Phase II, Option 2) with the negatively loaded phosphate or carboxylate ions, taking the positively loaded calcium ions with them. This results in a severe decalcification or etching effect, as is best known for phosphoric acid which is used as the etchant as part of the etch-and-rinse approach (see below). Because the calcium phosphate/carboxylate bond originally formed (Phase I) at the enamel/dentin surface is not stable, the bond will dissociate, leading to a typical etch pattern at the enamel and a relatively deep (thick) hybrid layer at the dentin that no longer contains any hydroxyapatite crystals.

> **NOTE**
>
> The AD-concept or Adhesion–Decalcification concept describes the way molecules interact with hydroxyapatite-based tissues.

Current Strategies for Bonding to Enamel

On enamel, phosphoric-acid etching selectively dissolves the enamel rods, thereby providing micro-etch pits that increase the surface energy so much that an ordinary hydrophobic bonding agent is readily sucked in by capillary attraction (**Fig. 14.4**).[19] Without doubt, this micromechanical interlocking of multiple, tiny resin tags within the acid-etched enamel surface is still today the best achievable bond to enamel (**Figs. 14.5, 14.6**).[14] It not only effectively seals the restoration margins in the long term, but also protects the more vulnerable bond to dentin against degradation.[20]

> **NOTE**
>
> The micromechanical interlocking of multiple, tiny resin tags within the acid-etched enamel surface is still today the best achievable bond to enamel.

While **strong self-etch adhesives** generally perform not that unfavorably at enamel, bonding of **mild self-etch adhesives** to enamel (and certainly to aprismatic enamel) remains so far unsatisfactory (**Fig. 14.6**).[21] Clinical research has clearly revealed that restoration defects develop rather quickly at the enamel margins, whereas the dentin margins appear to maintain their marginal integrity for much longer (**Fig. 14.7**).[22,23] This is somewhat odd, since one might expect that the chemical bonding potential to hydroxyapatite (that can be achieved with specific mild self-etch adhesives that contain functional monomers like 10-MDP) should also show its benefit at the

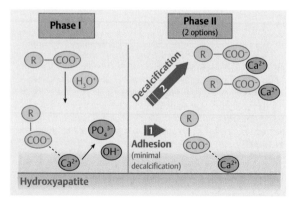

Fig. 14.3 Schematic illustration of the AD-concept, dictating whether molecules after initial attachment (Phase I) either remain bonded (Phase II, Option 1) or decalcify hydroxyapatite-based hard tissues (Phase II, Option 2).[17,18]

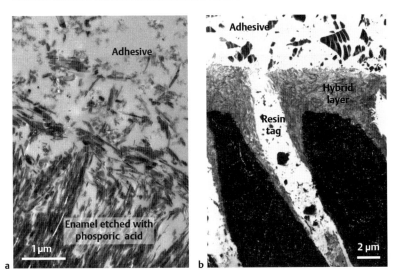

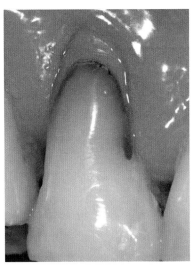

Fig. 14.4a, b Collage of TEM photomicrographs illustrating the interfacial ultrastructure of an etch-and-rinse adhesive at enamel (**a**) and dentin (**b**).

Fig. 14.5 Typical 5-year-old Class-V restoration illustrating a well-maintained marginal integrity at enamel versus severe marginal discoloration at the dentin.

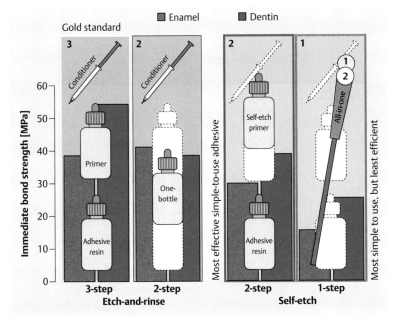

Fig. 14.6 General trends in micro-tensile bond strength of the different classes of adhesives to enamel and dentin (taken from pooled data for different adhesives per class, as tested at KU Leuven following a standard protocol). Note that the higher bond strength to dentin than to enamel should not be literally interpreted as "higher," but rather should be ascribed to the brittleness of enamel, which leads to the measurement of lower values in micro-tensile bond-strength experiments.

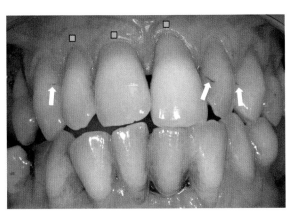

Fig. 14.7 Clinical examples of Class-V composite restorations (3-year-old) either bonded with an etch-and-rinse (green boxes, cervical) or a self-etch adhesive (white arrows). While a smooth enamel margin was obtained with the etch-and-rinse adhesive, a less optimal marginal adaptation with slight discoloration can be observed at the enamel margin when a mild self-etch adhesive was employed.

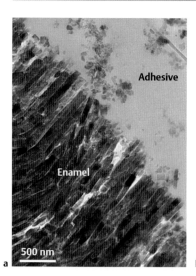 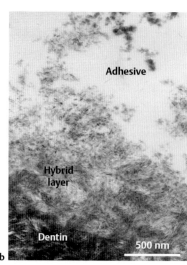

Fig. 14.8a, b   Collage of TEM photomicrographs illustrating the interfacial ultrastructure of a mild self-etch adhesive at enamel (**a**) and dentin (**b**).

enamel, which even contains much more hydroxyapatite than dentin does. Hence, the specific enamel hydroxyapatite crystal must be less receptive to primary chemical interaction than the dentin hydroxyapatite crystal. This enigma quite obviously demands further in-depth investigation.

Obstacles in Bonding to Dentin

The more reliable that adhesion to enamel is, the less predictable and durable the bonding to dentin is—still today! The main hindrance is due to **the mixed inorganic/organic nature** of dentin, with dentinal hydroxyapatite deposited on a mesh of collagen.[4] In addition, dentin is intimately connected with pulpal tissue by means of numerous fluid-filled tubules, which i.e. transverse through dentin from the enamel–dentin junction to the pulp. This constant outward fluid flow renders the exposed dentin surface naturally moist and thus intrinsically hydrophilic. This hydrophilic character definitely represents one of the major challenges for modern adhesives to durably interact with dentin, and has in essence led to the different bond strategies today available.

The presence of cutting debris on instrumented dental surfaces in the form of a smear layer and smear plugs that obstruct the dentin tubules is another clinical factor that may seriously interfere with bonding.[24,25] As regards the evolution in adhesive technology, surface smear formation precluded the intimate interaction of early **dentin bonding agents** with the underlying tooth tissue, which led to the low bond strengths and totally unsatisfactory clinical performances in the 1980s.[4] The first bonding protocol that revealed a clinically acceptable outcome involved complete removal of the smear layer by the **etch-and-rinse** approach (**Fig. 14.4b**).[14] The **self-etch** (or **etch-and-dry**) approach only dissolves the smear layer (but does not remove it, as there is no rinse phase) and

embeds the dissolved calcium phosphates within the interfacial transition zone (**Fig. 14.8b**).[4] Especially for the relatively high-pH self-etch adhesives, rather thick and compact smear layers may negatively influence their bonding effectiveness.[25,26]

> **NOTE**
>
> Two main factors are responsible for lower durability of dentin bonding compared with enamel bonding:
> * Mixed inorganic/organic nature of dentin
> * Presence of cutting debris on instrumented dental surfaces in the form of a smear layer and smear plugs that obstruct the dentin tubules

Bonding to Dentin through the Etch-and-Rinse Approach

Following an etch-and-rinse approach, acid etching demineralizes dentin over a depth of 3–5 µm, thereby exposing a scaffold of collagen fibrils that is almost totally depleted of hydroxyapatite (**Fig. 14.4b**).[4] According to the three-step procedure, the subsequently applied primer contains specific **monomers with hydrophilic properties**, such as HEMA, that with the help of organic solvents (acetone, ethanol, and/or water) can diffuse rapidly into the microporous collagen network to individually envelop collagen fibrils with resin. The functional monomers within etch-and-rinse primers basically need good diffusion (and no chemical bonding) potential. The primer solvent functions to carry the monomers deeply into the collagen network, but needs to be evaporated thoroughly afterward. In this way, the primer prepares the acid-etched dentin for the final infiltration of the solvent-free adhesive resin in the third and last application step. Micro-mechanical interlocking is then achieved through thick hybrid-layer formation in combination with resin tags that seal the opened dentin tubules (**Fig. 14.4b**). Interestingly, neither the thickness of the hybrid layer, nor the length of the resin tags is a principal factor determining bonding effectiveness.[27]

Simplified **two-step etch-and-rinse** adhesives, though being slightly more user-friendly, tend to perform inferiorly when compared to their three-step "gold-standard" counterparts.[28,29] Besides suboptimal hybridization due to blending primer and bonding components into a single solution,[14] the solvent-rich and hydrophilic nature of these adhesives render them more susceptible to water sorption and consequently to hydrolytic bond-degradation processes.[30,31] The solvent provided to the interface with these **one-bottle adhesives** can also be more difficult to evaporate, and therefore more of it easily remains entrapped within the hybrid and adhesive layer upon polymerization.[28]

NOTE

The etch-and-rinse approach at the dentin comprises three steps:
1. Acid etching demineralizes dentin, exposing a scaffold of collagen fibrils.
2. Monomers with hydrophilic properties diffuse rapidly into the micro-porous collagen network, with the help of organic solvents (acetone, ethanol and/or water).
3. Infiltration of the solvent-free adhesive resin.

Shortcomings of Etch-and-Rinse Technology and Potential Solutions

The major weakness of the etch-and-rinse approach is that dentinal collagen is almost completely depleted from hydroxyapatite (**Fig. 14.9**). Collagen molecules keep extracellular fluid bonded, whereby acid-etched dentin gets its highly hydrophilic state. Therefore, although primary chemical bonding is the most stable form of intermolecular interaction and is thus highly desirable, an intrinsically hydrophobic medium like the methacrylate-based dental adhesive can hardly link chemically to this hydrophilic dentinal surface. Some chemical interaction of monomers with dentinal collagen has been demonstrated,[32,33] but mainly involves hydrogen bonding and possibly van der Waals forces that are expected to be too weak to contribute much to bond durability. To achieve long-term bond durability, the exposed collagen fibril network should therefore be filled with resin as completely as possible.

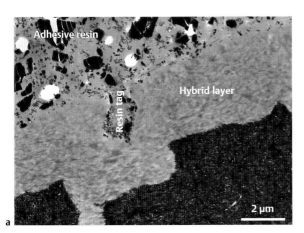

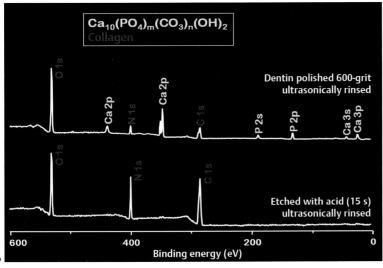

Fig. 14.9a, b TEM photomicrograph and XPS surface analysis of dentin etched with either phosphoric or maleic acid, demonstrating ultra-morphologically and chemically that an etch-and-rinse approach completely removes hydroxyapatite from dentin up to a depth of 3–5 µm.

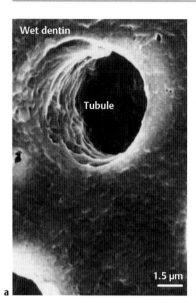

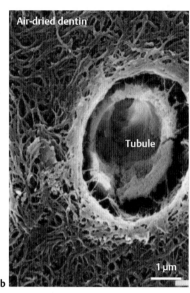

Fig. 14.10a, b Scanning electron microscopic photomicrographs illustrating the effect of a water wet-bonding technique (**a**) versus a gentle air-drying technique (**b**). While water wet-bonding is mandatory for an acetone-based etch-and-rinse adhesive, a water/ethanol-based etch-and-rinse adhesive is less technique-sensitive and can be applied using a gently air-drying technique (involving automatic re-wetting).

Wet Bonding—How Moist is Wet?

It has been well documented that especially the post-etching handling of surface water is crucial for the success of the etch-and-rinse protocol. Ideally, the etched collagen network must be kept loosely arranged during adhesive procedures to allow proper resin–monomer infiltration (**Fig. 14.10**).[34] A certain amount of surface water is needed to prevent the collagen network from collapsing, a methodology commonly referred to as (water) **wet bonding**.[35,36] This wet-bonding application procedure definitely makes the etch-and-rinse approach rather technique-sensitive and exacting in clinical use.

Adhesives containing hydrophilic monomers dissolved in acetone were found to produce a higher bond strength when acid-conditioned dentin was left visibly moist (**Fig. 14.10**).[37] Owing to their relatively high volatility, solvents such as acetone and to a lesser degree ethanol displace the surface water that has been left after etching, allowing the primer monomers to effectively fill the 20–30 nm interfibrillar spaces within the exposed collagen network.[34] Although sufficient surface moisture clinically manifests as a uniformly shiny dentin surface, the **window of opportunity** between over-dry and over-wet conditions is narrow; therefore in clinical circumstances, especially in complex cavity configurations, pooling of water might be difficult to avoid.[37] In the latter over-wet condition, the residual water will cause phase separation between hydrophobic and hydrophilic components of the adhesive, resulting in the formation of water-filled blisters at the adhesive–dentin interface, which definitely will weaken the interfacial strength.[38] Furthermore, excess moisture decreases resin polymerization, and thereby reduces the mechanical properties of the adhesive layer.[39]

CLINICAL PEARL

Clinically, a wet surface can best be achieved by removing excess water with a short air blast or, even better, using a dry cotton pellet so that the surface looks still rather glossy, but visibly without a clear film of water being present.

Rewetting

Interestingly, water-based primers have shown a potential self-rewetting effect on gently air-dried dentin (**Fig. 14.10**).[34] Their water content re-hydrates the air-dried and thus collapsed collagen network, transforming it into a loosely arranged structure that allows the hydrophilic primer monomers to infiltrate. Over-drying—meaning that the acid-etched dentin surface gets severely dehydrated—should of course be avoided at any time during the clinical application procedure. Therefore, the surface should be gently dried until the etched enamel presents its white-frosted appearance and dentin loses its shine and turns dull. The major drawback of this (gentle) **dry-bonding technique** is that additional water is delivered to the interface by the water-based primers. Self-evidently, it should be removed as much as possible during the 15-second priming time, that is, once its job as re-wetting agent and monomer carrier is completed. To facilitate solvent-evaporation in water-based adhesives, ethanol and acetone can be used in conjunction with water as co-solvents.[40,41] This implies the formation of hydrogen bonds between water and ethanol/acetone molecules, resulting in a solvent that is more easily evaporated. In this way, multistep etch-and-rinse adhesives that provide water-based primers are less technique-sensitive to variations in the bonding protocol as far as the wetness of the acid-etched dentinal surface is concerned.[34,37] Applied

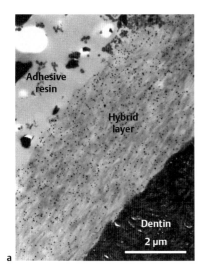
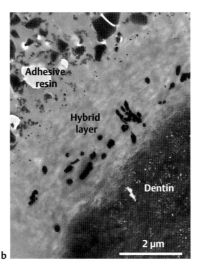

Fig. 14.11a, b Transmission electronic photomicrographs illustrating that nanoleakage (upon application of ammonium silver nitrate in the pulp chamber [**a**], or complete immersion of the tooth in ammonium silver nitrate [**b**]) is also detected at the interface of dentin with a gold-standard, three-step etch-and-rinse adhesive.

following the classic **three-step etchant-primer-bonding procedure,** adhesives like OptiBond FL (Kerr) and Syntac Classic (Ivoclar-Vivadent) have been granted the **gold-standard label** by virtue of their repeatedly documented superior performance.[14,42] This status has been vindicated through many laboratory studies as well as clinical trials conducted at independent research institutes worldwide.

> **NOTE**
>
> Multi-step etch-and-rinse adhesives that provide water-based primers are less technique-sensitive to variations in the bonding protocol. This seems to be the main reason for their repeatedly documented superior performance both in the laboratory and in clinical use.

Nanoleakage

Unfortunately, complete hybridization of the exposed collagen network seems to be practically unattainable, even with these three-step etch-and-rinse adhesives. Numerous papers have described nanoleakage, i.e., the presence of nanometer-sized voids within and/or beneath the hybrid layer (**Fig. 14.11**).[43] They originate from spaces around collagen fibrils that were not completely enveloped by resin, and/or from discrepancies between the etching and subsequent resin-infiltration depth. The clinical impact of these findings is not clear, however.

Recent Developments

More recent attempts to improve infiltration efficiency have involved the use of a new solvent known as **tert-butanol**, resulting in an innovative two-step etch-and-rinse adhesive, commercialized by Dentsply as XP-Bond. This adhesive is much less technique-sensitive with regard to maintaining the appropriate surface wetness after etching, as compared with its acetone-based precursors.[44]

It is clear that the current etch-and-rinse bonding protocol requires adhesives that are hydrophilic enough to interact with the intrinsically moist acid-etched dentin. This prerequisite is somewhat contradictory given the need for more hydrophobic adhesives to extend bond longevity. Nevertheless, less water will then be absorbed from both the host dentin and the oral environment, and render the interface more resistant to water-degradation effects.[30,31] One interesting attempt to optimize infiltration of more hydrophobic resins into acid-etched dentin has more recently been introduced as an **ethanol wet-bonding** technique.[45] It basically involves the intermediate application of a highly concentrated ethanol solution (duration at least 1 minute) to replace most water within the exposed collagen fibril network, thereby dehydrating the acid-etched dentin as well as transforming it into a more hydrophobic state. In this way, the acid-etched dentinal substrate is better prepared to receive more hydrophobic and thus less water-absorbing resin monomers. Hence, a more hydrophobic resin–dentin interface is formed that is expected to absorb less water over time and offer better resistance against degradation. This unfortunately laborious and therefore perhaps clinically less practical technique originated in the laboratory-processing of samples for electron microscopy. In particular for transmission electron microscopy (TEM), specimens typically undergo a gradual and thus slow dehydration process using increasing concentrations of ethanol prior to embedding procedures with highly hydrophobic epoxy resins. As mentioned by the proponents of this technique, "the bonding of BisGMA to acid-etched dentin should be viewed as a proof of concept for hydrophobic dentin-bonding, rather than as the development of a clinically applicable bonding technique."[45] There is a striking similarity in performance of this experimental ethanol wet-bonding technique with that of the above-mentioned "gold-standard" three-step etch-and-rinse adhesive, OptiBond FL (Kerr), which also provides an ethanol/water-based primer. This research has therefore definitely established that ethanol is the better solvent within an etch-and-rinse primer. It may be confirming the overall superior effectiveness of the above-mentioned gold-standard adhesive.

Another elegant approach to potentially *repair* etch-and-rinse hybrid layers that are incompletely resin-infiltrated has been proposed through the so-called *guided-tissue remineralization*. This technology involves a relatively long exposure of the adhesive interface to a highly concentrated calcium-phosphate remineralization medium.[46] Within 2–4 months, areas within the hybrid layers that were initially poorly infiltrated by adhesive resins appeared to have remineralized to a certain extent. Now that the working principle of this guided-tissue remineralization has been proven,[46] research effort is being spent toward development of methodologies that are clinically applicable. Although for instance such a remineralization liner could be effective to heal caries tissue that was intentionally left at the cavity bottom (thereby minimizing cavity preparation and potentially avoiding pulp exposure), combining bonding procedures with liners (to repair deficient hybrid layers) appears perhaps clinically less feasible.

Bonding to Dentin through the Self-Etch Approach

In contrast to etch-and-rinse adhesives, self-etch adhesives do not require a separate etching step, as they contain acidic monomers that simultaneously condition and prime the dental substrate.[4] Consequently, this approach has been claimed to be more user-friendly and less technique-sensitive, thereby resulting, though very product dependent, in a clinically reliable performance.[22,47] Some self-etch adhesives have indeed been proven to perform quite satisfactorily, both in vitro and in vivo, leading to a growing popularity of self-etch adhesives in modern dental practices.

> **NOTE**
>
> *Self-etch* adhesives contain acidic monomers that simultaneously condition and prime the dental substrate.[4] Consequently, this approach has been claimed to be more user-friendly and less technique-sensitive, but not all *self-etch* adhesives have in practice performed satisfactorily.

Nomenclature

As mentioned before, the morphological features of the adhesive–dentin interface produced by self-etch adhesives depend to a great extent on the manner in which their functional monomers interact with the dental substrate. In part depending on the pH of the self-etch solutions, the actual interaction depth of self-etch adhesives in dentin differs from) a few hundred nanometers following **an ultra-mild self-etch approach** (pH > 2.5), often being referred to as nanointeraction,[48] like AdheSE One (Ivo-

clar-Vivadent), Clearfil S³ Bond Plus (Kuraray), G-genial (GC), and Bond Force (Tokuyama), b) an interaction depth of around 1 μm for a **mild self-etch approach** (pH ≈2) like Clearfil SE (Kuraray) (see **Fig. 14.8**) and Contax (DMG), c) an interaction depth between 1 and 2 μm for an **intermediately strong self-etch approach** (pH 1–2) like AdheSE (Ivoclar-Vivadent) and OptiBond Solo Self-etch (Kerr), and d) to an interaction of several micrometers deep for a strong self-etch approach (pH ≤ 1) like Adper Prompt L-Pop (3 M ESPE).

Strong self-etch adhesives such as Adper Prompt L-pop (3 M ESPE) or Non-rinse Conditioner (Dentsply) in combination with Prime&Bond NT (Dentsply) demineralize dentin rather deeply. The interfacial ultrastructure produced by these adhesives resembles that of the etch-and-rinse systems (deep, 2–3 μm hybrid layer), the difference being that the dissolved calcium phosphates are not rinsed away, but embedded within the hybrid layer. These strong self-etch adhesives follow Option 2 of Phase II in the AD-model (see above), namely massive decalcification of dentin, since their bond to hydroxyapatite during Phase I in the AD-model is not stable. The calcium phosphates produced are not very hydrolytically stable, explaining their weak bonding effectiveness to dentin (despite the fact that they bond reasonably well to enamel). This was confirmed clinically, when both above-mentioned strong self-etch adhesives presented relatively high loss rates over the short term for Class-V composite restorations.[47]

Mild Self-Etch Adhesives

The future lies mostly in the further development of mild self-etch adhesives that demineralize dentin only partially (see **Fig. 14.8**). Following the AD-concept, stable chemical bonding of the functional monomer to hydroxyapatite goes together with only a limited decalcification effect (Phase II, Option 1). This keeps the vulnerable collagen protected with hydroxyapatite, to which the functional monomer can bond ionically.[17]

At the dentin, the resultant interfacial ultrastructure is similar for both mild self-etch adhesives and glass-ionomers.[4,14] A thin, submicron hybrid layer is formed that still contains abundant hydroxyapatite (see **Figs. 14.2** and **14.8**). According to the AD-concept (see **Fig. 14.3**), polyalkenoic acid is a polymer with a multitude of carboxyl functional groups that act as "chemical hands," as it were, and grab individual calcium ions along the mineral substrate. This chemical bonding along with micro-mechanical interlocking through shallow hybridization explains the successful self-adhesiveness of glass-ionomers (even without any form of initial pretreatment). Glass-ionomers do have the lowest annual failure rate with regard to Class-V composite restorations.[47] Likewise, as part of a self-etch adhesive, the functional monomer 10-MDP bonds through its phosphate groups to hydroxyapatite and has been demonstrated to even form a self-assembled layered structure at the hydroxyapatite surface, being referred to as **nano-layering** (see **Fig. 14.3**).[49] This additional chemical bonding of mild self-etch adhesives is believed to be especially advantageous in terms of bond durability.[50]

In addition, mild and ultramild self-etch adhesives hardly form resin tags at all, or at maximum slightly demineralize and subsequently infiltrate the tubule smear plugs with resin. This effect is believed to contribute greatly to the significantly lower risk of postoperative sensitivity of patients' teeth, typically recorded for mild self-etch adhesives, and in contrast to the more frequent postoperative sensitivity reported by clinicians for etch-and-rinse adhesives.

Further progress in adhesive technology should therefore be expected from synthesizing functional monomers that are not only capable of chemically and durably bonding to dentin, but also to enamel.[51] Enamel bonding is the major weak point of mild self-etch adhesives. As mentioned before, today's adhesives still require a certain minimal degree of micro-mechanical interlocking at enamel through some kind of etching process (which current mild self-etch adhesives may not provide enough of) (**Figs. 14.7** and **14.8a**). A combined enamel etch-and-rinse and enamel/dentin self-etch approach seems to be the best alternative and has already frequently been applied in routine practice.[22]

CLINICAL PEARL

Selective etching of enamel margins with phosphoric acid followed by a mild self-etch treatment of both enamel and dentin should today be regarded as the most successful adhesive approach.[51] It basically turns a two-step into a three-step adhesive.

Mechanisms of Bond Degradation

Several currently available dental adhesives have been shown to bond reliably over the short term, but not always long term.[30,31] Current literature has proved that immediate bond-strength values do not always correlate with **long-term bond stability**.[42] The longevity of bonded restorations is to a large extent related to the resistance of the adhesive interface against degradation. This may occur in a relatively short term, depending on the way the adhesive has been manipulated, the actual adhesive approach, and the adhesive composition. In fact, none of the current adhesives or techniques is able to produce an interface that is absolutely resistant to degradation. Therefore, many research efforts are currently devoted to improving bond durability. The hybrid layer seems to be the most susceptible part of the composite restoration as far as degradation is concerned. Two degradation patterns can be observed within the hybrid layer: loss of resin from interfibrillar spaces, and disorganization of unpro-

tected collagen fibrils.[30,31] Such degradation may result from the hydrolysis of resin and/or collagen, thereby weakening the physical properties of the resin–dentin interface.

NOTE

The current challenge in adhesive dentistry is to create a more stable bonding interface that is less prone to degradation, thereby rendering restorative treatment more predictable in terms of clinical performance in the long term.

Degradation of collagen within the hybrid layer does not occur only due to activity of collagenases produced in vivo by bacteria, but also due to host-derived enzymes that are released and iatrogenically activated by specific adhesive procedures.[52] Such collagenolytic and gelatinolytic activities are triggered by endogenous enzymes, which are naturally present in the mineralized dentin matrix and known as **matrix metalloproteinases** (MMPs). During bonding procedures, acid etching of dentin has been shown to release and activate such MMPs,[53,54] which may in part digest nonresin-enveloped collagen within the hybrid layer. Phosphoric acid probably denatures the MMP activity rapidly as it becomes exposed, so that the resultant gelatinolytic activity is very low. pH values near to zero seem to destroy whatever gelatinolytic activity is exposed by acid etching.[53] On the other hand, mild self-etch adhesives (pH ≥ 2) may activate MMPs far above the nonactivity level, but may not be acidic enough to denature MMPs.[55] A simple method to protect the interface against such enzymatic degradation is the use of MMP inhibitors, of which chlorhexidine is already commonly used in dentistry and seems effective in vitro as well as in vivo.[56,57] However, how long this inhibition would be effective remains to be determined. However, the actual relevance of this enzymatic breakdown of the hybrid layer may be less important clinically than has been suggested in some papers. The levels of such endogenous enzymes gradually decrease with age, commonly disappearing before one reaches the age of 40 years.[58]

NOTE

Strategies to render the adhesive interface more resistant against degradation:
- Intensify the chemical monomer–tooth component interaction
- Improve resin impregnation into demineralized dentin
- Decrease the permeability of the bonding interface
- Optimize the degree of resin polymerization
- Avoid the occurrence of phase separation
- Inhibit the activation of endogenous collagenolytic enzymes

Bonding to Carious Dentin

Except for traumatic injuries where teeth need to be restored or corrected esthetically, adhesive tooth restoration mostly involves bonding to caries-affected dentin. As mentioned above, today's adhesives bond effectively to sound dentin through hybridization, but this bonding mechanism remains vulnerable in the long term. Bonding to caries-affected dentin is even less predictable and durable. In general, the presence of carious dentin results in a lower bond strength.[59] This is related to the alterations that occur in this substrate as a consequence of caries progression. Reduction in mineral content and loss of crystallinity of the remaining mineral phase, coupled to the changes in the secondary structure of collagen, result in a dentin substrate with a lower hardness and modulus of elasticity (than those of sound dentin), by which it consequently performs more poorly in mechanical tests. Moreover, the deposition of mineral casts, namely of β-tricalcium phosphates (so called whitlockites) in the dentin tubules during caries progression, also alters the etch pattern and thus the penetration capacity of resin monomers into the tubules. In fact, the bond strength of adhesives to carious dentin has been reported to be inversely proportional to the degree of caries progression, with **infected dentin** presenting the lowest bond strength. The latter should obviously be related to its extremely low cohesive strength, due both to its low degree of mineralization and to its collagen-matrix disorganization. Bonding to severely caries-infected and soft dentin is clinically seldom indicated, except when the aim is to prevent further caries progression in an uncooperative patient. However, the effect of bonding to partially removed carious dentin on the durability of the bond or the restoration in teeth is not clear. Therefore, step-wise excavation using cements seems to be the better choice compared with sealing of the soft dentin in deep carious lesions, as long as clinical evidence is missing (Chapter 18).

> **NOTE**
>
> Reasons for lower bond strengths in carious compared to bound dentin:
> - Lower hardness and modulus of elasticity leading to poorer performance in mechanical testing
> - Deposition of mineral casts in the dentin tubules alters the etching pattern

Altogether, irrespective of the caries-excavation method chosen, it remains clinically recommended to finish the cavity margins in clean/sound tooth tissue to achieve the best performance of adhesives, while at the same time being minimally invasive with regard to caries excavation and most conservative with regard to sound-tissue preservation.

Clinical Performance

Despite the importance of laboratory studies attempting to predict clinical performance of biomaterials, clinical trials remain the ultimate way to collect scientific evidence on the clinical afficacy and effectiveness of a restorative treatment.[47] The **popularity of in-vitro studies** in the field of adhesive dentistry may in part be ascribed to the rapid evolution of dental adhesive technology and the resultant high commercial turnover of adhesives. This often tempts manufacturers to release a successor product on the market even before its precursor has been clinically evaluated, at least in the long term. By carrying out in-vivo studies, all possible aging factors come into play at the same time, thereby disclosing whether an adhesive is truly reliable for routine clinical practice. Retention, marginal integrity, and clinical micro-leakage are usually the key parameters recorded to judge the clinical effectiveness of adhesives.

> **NOTE**
>
> Clinical trials remain the ultimate way to collect scientific evidence on the efficacy of a restorative treatment. However, recently quite reasonable correlation between aged bond-strength data and 5-year Class-V retention rates have been revealed in two meta-analyses.[42]

As mentioned before, the best clinical performance with regard to retention (the most objective criterion to judge upon clinical efficacy) has so far been achieved by **glass-ionomers** (**Fig. 14.12**).[47] Despite their excellent clinical performance in terms of retention in class V cavities, glass-ionomers commonly present with lower esthetic features and poorer physico-mechanical properties that may clinically require them to be replaced more rapidly than resin-based restorative materials as is the case for Class I and II restorations.

Besides glass-ionomers, **three-step etch-and-rinse adhesives** have exhibited good clinical efficacy (**Fig. 14.12**).[47] The clinical durability of three-step etch-and-rinse adhesives confirms their generally superior laboratory results, in which they are considered as the gold-standard and employed as the benchmark against which to compare the performance of new-generation adhesives.

According to the same standard, **mild two-step self-etch adhesives** tend to approach three-step etch-and-rinse adhesives in terms of low annual failure rates (**Fig. 14.12**).[47] Their ability to provide a shallow but uniform hybrid layer, along with their capability to bond chemically to the dentin substrate seems to play an important role in resisting long-term hydrolytic degradation. Commonly, the clinical performance of such self-etch adhesives does not vary substantially from one study to another, which is indicative of their rather low technique sensitivity. Considering

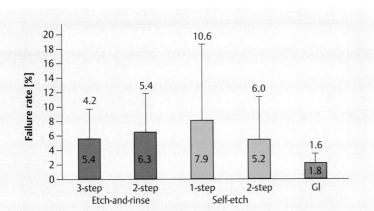

Fig. 14.12 Mean annual failure rates (restoration losses) of the different adhesive approaches when applied in Class-V composite restorations.[47]

solely mild self-etch adhesives, their annual failure rate is as low as that of glass-ionomers.[42]

In general, two-step etch-and-rinse adhesives have performed less favorably than the conventional three-step version.[47] Laboratory studies have corroborated these results, ascribing their poorer performance to their higher hydrophilicity and reduced hybridization potential. So far, rather inefficient clinical performance has been noted for the newest generation of one-step adhesives. Widely varying retention scores have been recorded, indicating their high technique sensitivity despite their favorable user-friendliness (**Fig. 14.12**). Such lower bonding performance must be ascribed to the many concerns advanced earlier.

NOTE

It is noteworthy that irrespective of the number of application steps, acetone-based etch-and-rinse adhesives have performed less satisfactorily than their water/ethanol-based alternatives. The above-mentioned high technique sensitivity of acetone-based adhesives must be the reason for their compromised long-term clinical data.

Epilogue

The design and synthesis of functional monomers is definitely a worthwhile pathway toward new and improved adhesive technology. Many studies on dental adhesive technology are nowadays empirical, basically testing the bond strength of different cocktails of adhesive solutions to enamel and dentin in the laboratory. The adhesive formulation that scores best commonly makes it rapidly to the market, after which the superior laboratory performance of the product is hopefully confirmed in independent randomized controlled clinical trials. Much knowledge on the underlying mechanisms of adhesion to enamel and dentin has been provided by numerous studies that imaged adhesive–tooth interfaces with all

sorts of microscopes. On the other hand, the actual molecular interactions at the interface have hardly been explored. Many basic questions still remain unanswered, like for instance why certain functional monomers have better bonding potential than others, and why mild self-etch adhesives with additional chemical bonding do not perform better with enamel. Thus, fundamental for future design and development of dental adhesives is the further unraveling of the **molecular interfacial interactions**.

SUMMARY

Adhesive technology has undergone great progress in the last decade. In the light of the major drawbacks attributed to all-in-one self-etch adhesives, **conventional three-step etch-and-rinse adhesives** and **two-step self-etch adhesives** are still the benchmark for dental adhesion in routine clinical use. When bonding to enamel, an etch-and-rinse approach is definitely preferred, indicating that simple micro-mechanical interaction appears sufficient to achieve a durable bond to enamel. When bonding to dentin, a mild self-etch approach is superior, as it keeps hydroxyapatite around the collagen and additionally chemically interacts. Such intimate chemical intermolecular interaction should definitely contribute most to bond durability.

Along with the fast evolution of multistep adhesives toward one-step adhesives, delete composites to adhesively lute indirect ceramic restorations underwent a similar evolution toward simple-to-use and less technique-sensitive one-step luting agents. Hence, these self-adhesive delete composites do not need any kind of pretreatment of the tooth substrate, thereby bringing the development of self-adhesive composites closer to reality.

When bonding to both enamel and dentin, a three-step approach is advocated:
1. Selective etching of enamel.
2. Application of a two-step self-etch adhesive, including a self-etching primer with chemical bonding potential.

3. Separate solvent-free bond agent as final sealer to both the pre-etched enamel and unetched dentin. This approach currently appears to be the best choice to effectively and durably bond adhesives to tooth tissue.

REFERENCES

1. Buonocore MG. A simple method of increasing the adhesion of acrylic filling materials to enamel surfaces. J Dent Res 1955; 34(6):849–853

2. Brudevold F, Buonocore M, Wileman W. A report on a resin composition capable of bonding to human dentin surfaces. J Dent Res 1956;35(6):846–851

3. McLean JW, Kramer IRH. A clinical and pathological evaluation of a sulphinic acid activated resin for use in restorative dentistry. Br Dent J 1952;18(93):255–269

4. Van Meerbeek B, Van Landuyt K, De Munck J, et al. Adhesion to enamel and dentin. In: Summit J, Robbins J, Hilton T, Schwartz R, eds. Fundamentals of Operative Dentistry. 3rd ed. Chicago: Quintessence Publishing; 2006:183–260

5. Bowen RL. Adhesive bonding of various materials to hard tooth tissues. II. Bonding to dentin promoted by a surface-active co-monomer. J Dent Res 1965;44(5):895–902

6. Eliades GC, Caputo AA, Vougiouklakis GJ. Composition, wetting properties and bond strength with dentin of 6 new dentin adhesives. Dent Mater 1985;1(5):170–176

7. Fusayama T, Nakamura M, Kurosaki N, Iwaku M. Non-pressure adhesion of a new adhesive restorative resin. J Dent Res 1979; 58(4):1364–1370

8. Stanley HR, Going RE, Chauncey HH. Human pulp response to acid pretreatment of dentin and to composite restoration. J Am Dent Assoc 1975;91(4):817–825

9. Van Landuyt KL. Optimization of the Chemical Composition of Dental Adhesives. Towards a Simplified and Durable, Universal Enamel/Dentin Adhesive [PhD thesis]. Leuven: Katholieke Universiteit Leuven; 2008

10. Van Landuyt KL, De Munck J, Snauwaert J, et al. Monomer-solvent phase separation in one-step self-etch adhesives. J Dent Res 2005;84(2):183–188

11. Van Landuyt KL, Snauwaert J, De Munck J, et al. Origin of interfacial droplets with one-step adhesives. J Dent Res 2007;86(8): 739–744

12. Tay FR, Pashley DH, Suh BI, Carvalho RM, Itthagarun A. Single-step adhesives are permeable membranes. J Dent 2002;30(7-8): 371–382

13. Nishiyama N, Tay FR, Fujita K, et al. Hydrolysis of functional monomers in a single-bottle self-etching primer—correlation of 13C NMR and TEM findings. J Dent Res 2006;85(5):422–426

14. Van Meerbeek B, De Munck J, Yoshida Y, et al. Buonocore memorial lecture. Adhesion to enamel and dentin: current status and future challenges. Oper Dent 2003;28(3):215–235

15. De Munck J. An in Vitro and in Vivo Study on the Durability of Biomaterial-Tooth Bonds [PhD thesis]. Leuven: Katholieke Universiteit Leuven; 2004

16. Yoshida Y, Van Meerbeek B, Nakayama Y, et al. Evidence of chemical bonding at biomaterial-hard tissue interfaces. J Dent Res 2000;79(2):709–714

17. Yoshida Y, Nagakane K, Fukuda R, et al. Comparative study on adhesive performance of functional monomers. J Dent Res 2004; 83(6):454–458

18. Yoshida Y, Van Meerbeek B, Nakayama Y, et al. Adhesion to and decalcification of hydroxyapatite by carboxylic acids. J Dent Res 2001;80(6):1565–1569

19. Gwinnett AJ, Matsui A. A study of enamel adhesives. The physical relationship between enamel and adhesive. Arch Oral Biol 1967;12(12):1615–1620

20. De Munck J, Van Meerbeek B, Yoshida Y, et al. Four-year water degradation of total-etch adhesives bonded to dentin. J Dent Res 2003;82(2):136–140

21. Perdigão J, Geraldeli S. Bonding characteristics of self-etching adhesives to intact versus prepared enamel. J Esthet Restor Dent 2003;15(1):32–41, discussion 42

22. Peumans M, De Munck J, Van Landuyt KL, Poitevin A, Lambrechts P, Van Meerbeek B. Eight-year clinical evaluation of a 2-step self-etch adhesive with and without selective enamel etching. Dent Mater 2010;26(12):1176–1184

23. Van Landuyt KL, Kanumilli P, De Munck J, Peumans M, Lambrechts P, Van Meerbeek B. Bond strength of a mild self-etch adhesive with and without prior acid-etching. J Dent 2006;34(1): 77–85

24. Pashley DH, Tao L, Boyd L, King GE, Horner JA. Scanning electron microscopy of the substructure of smear layers in human dentine. Arch Oral Biol 1988;33(4):265–270

25. Ermis RB, De Munck J, Cardoso MV, et al. Bond strength of self-etch adhesives to dentin prepared with three different diamond burs. Dent Mater 2008;24(7):978–985

26. Cardoso MV, Coutinho E, Ermis RB, et al. Influence of dentin cavity surface finishing on micro-tensile bond strength of adhesives. Dent Mater 2008;24(4):492–501

27. Yoshiyama M, Carvalho R, Sano H, Horner J, Brewer PD, Pashley DH. Interfacial morphology and strength of bonds made to superficial versus deep dentin. Am J Dent 1995;8(6):297–302

28. Van Meerbeek B, Van Landuyt K, De Munck J, et al. Technique-sensitivity of contemporary adhesives. Dent Mater J 2005;24(1): 1–13

29. Finger WJ, Balkenhol M. Practitioner variability effects on dentin bonding with an acetone-based one-bottle adhesive. J Adhes Dent 1999;1(4):311–314

30. De Munck J, Van Landuyt K, Peumans M, et al. A critical review of the durability of adhesion to tooth tissue: methods and results. J Dent Res 2005;84(2):118–132

31. Breschi L, Mazzoni A, Ruggeri A, Cadenaro M, Di Lenarda R, De Stefano Dorigo E. Dental adhesion review: aging and stability of the bonded interface. Dent Mater 2008;24(1):90–101

32. Nishiyama N, Suzuki K, Komatsu K, Yasuda S, Nemoto K. A 13C NMR study on the adsorption characteristics of HEMA to dentinal collagen. J Dent Res 2002;81(7):469–471

33. Xu J, Stangel I, Butler IS, Gilson DF. An FT-Raman spectroscopic investigation of dentin and collagen surfaces modified by 2-hydroxyethylmethacrylate. J Dent Res 1997;76(1):596–601

34. Van Meerbeek B, Yoshida Y, Lambrechts P, et al. A TEM study of two water-based adhesive systems bonded to dry and wet dentin. J Dent Res 1998;77(1):50–59

35. Kanca J III. Improving bond strength through acid etching of dentin and bonding to wet dentin surfaces. J Am Dent Assoc 1992;123(9):35–43

36. Tay FR, Gwinnett AJ, Pang KM, Wei SH. Resin permeation into acid-conditioned, moist, and dry dentin: a paradigm using water-free adhesive primers. J Dent Res 1996;75(4):1034–1044

37. Tay FR, Gwinnett JA, Wei SH. Micromorphological spectrum from overdrying to overwetting acid-conditioned dentin in water-free acetone-based, single-bottle primer/adhesives. Dent Mater 1996; 12(4):236–244

38. Ikeda T, De Munck J, Shirai K, et al. Effect of evaporation of primer components on ultimate tensile strengths of primer-adhesive mixture. Dent Mater 2005;21(11):1051–1058

39. Wang Y, Spencer P. Hybridization efficiency of the adhesive/dentin interface with wet bonding. J Dent Res 2003;82(2):141–145

40. Moszner N, Salz U, Zimmermann J. Chemical aspects of self-etching enamel-dentin adhesives: a systematic review. Dent Mater 2005;21(10):895–910

41. Van Landuyt KL, Snauwaert J, De Munck J, et al. Systematic review of the chemical composition of contemporary dental adhesives. Biomaterials 2007;28(26):3757–3785

42. Van Meerbeek B, Peumans M, Poitevin A, et al. Relationship between bond-strength tests and clinical outcomes. Dent Mater 2010;26(2):e100–e121

43. Tay FR, Pashley DH. Water treeing—a potential mechanism for degradation of dentin adhesives. Am J Dent 2003;16(1):6–12

44. Van Meerbeek B, De Munck J, Van Landuyt KL, et al. Dental adhesives and dental performances. In: Curtis RV, Watson TF, eds. Dental Biomaterials. Imaging, Testing and Modelling. Cambridge: Woodhead Publishing; 2008:81–111

45. Tay FR, Pashley DH, Kapur RR, et al. Bonding BisGMA to dentin—a proof of concept for hydrophobic dentin bonding. J Dent Res 2007;86(11):1034–1039

46. Tay FR, Pashley DH. Guided tissue remineralisation of partially demineralised human dentine. Biomaterials 2008;29(8):1127–1137

47. Peumans M, Kanumilli P, De Munck J, Van Landuyt K, Lambrechts P, Van Meerbeek B. Clinical effectiveness of contemporary adhesives: a systematic review of current clinical trials. Dent Mater 2005;21(9):864–881

48. Koshiro K, Sidhu SK, Inoue S, Ikeda T, Sano H. New concept of resin-dentin interfacial adhesion: the nanointeraction zone. J Biomed Mater Res B Appl Biomater 2006;77(2):401–408

49. Yoshihara K, Yoshida Y, Nagaoka N, et al. Nano-controlled molecular interaction at adhesive interfaces for hard tissue reconstruction. Acta Biomater 2010;6(9):3573–3582

50. Van Meerbeek B, Yoshihara K, Yoshida Y, Mine A, De Munck J, Van Landuyt KL. State of the art of self-etch adhesives. Dent Mater 2011;27(1):17–28

51. Inoue S, Koshiro K, Yoshida Y, et al. Hydrolytic stability of self-etch adhesives bonded to dentin. J Dent Res 2005;84(12):1160–1164

52. Pashley DH, Tay FR, Yiu C, et al. Collagen degradation by host-derived enzymes during aging. J Dent Res 2004;83(3):216–221

53. Nishitani Y, Yoshiyama M, Wadgaonkar B, et al. Activation of gelatinolytic/collagenolytic activity in dentin by self-etching adhesives. Eur J Oral Sci 2006;114(2):160–166

54. De Munck J, Van den Steen PE, Mine A, et al. Inhibition of enzymatic degradation of adhesive-dentin interfaces. J Dent Res 2009;88(12):1101–1106

55. De Munck J, Mine A, Van den Steen PE, et al. Enzymatic degradation of adhesive-dentin interfaces produced by mild self-etch adhesives. Eur J Oral Sci 2010;118(5):494–501

56. Gendron R, Grenier D, Sorsa T, Mayrand D. Inhibition of the activities of matrix metalloproteinases 2, 8, and 9 by chlorhexidine. Clin Diagn Lab Immunol 1999;6(3):437–439

57. Carrilho MR, Geraldeli S, Tay F, et al. In vivo preservation of the hybrid layer by chlorhexidine. J Dent Res 2007;86(6):529–533

58. Martin-De Las Heras S, Valenzuela A, Overall CM. The matrix metalloproteinase gelatinase A in human dentine. Arch Oral Biol 2000;45(9):757–765

59. de Almeida Neves A, Coutinho E, Cardoso MV, Lambrechts P, Van Meerbeek B. Current concepts and techniques for caries excavation and adhesion to residual dentin. J Adhes Dent 2011;13(1):7–22 10.3290/j.jad.a18443

Fissure Sealing

Hafsteinn Eggertsson

15

It is over four decades since the introduction of sealants into dentistry in the form of research that also ushered in adhesive dentistry.[1] Because of its impact on restorative and preventive dentistry, adhesive dentistry must be ranked among the major breakthroughs in the dental profession (Chapter 14 and 19), similar to the advent of radiographs or high-speed handpieces. Moreover, concepts have changed regarding how we view disease management, how we treat our patients, and how dental services are provided at population level.

The **pits and fissures** are vulnerable sites on the teeth for formation of caries lesions. They can be difficult to keep clean, which easily leads to **plaque stagnation**. The concept of halting or preventing caries from forming at these sites was addressed in various ways in the late 19th and early 20th century.[2] Ideas were proposed such as eradicating the fissures (a procedure termed "prophylactic odontotomy"), by removing enough of the tooth structure so that plaque would not collect in them,[3] or by placing "small fillings in the grooves of those teeth, irrespective of whether they were carious or noncarious, as soon as practicable after eruption."[4] **Figure 15.1** shows such **amalgam "sealants"** which are more than half a century old, and fulfill all requirements we can ask of sealants as a means of preventing potential damage of the teeth due to caries. The fact that these procedures were adopted as routine practice in clinics around the world, based on the unscientific assumption that 98% of these grooves eventually become carious, has been criticized.[5]

In this atmosphere Buonocore started his pursuit of finding ways to make a material that would adhere directly to the occlusal enamel (see Chapters 14 and 19). In his own words: "With such a material, there would be no need for retention and resistance form in cavity preparation, and effective sealing of pits, fissures, and superficial caries lesions could be realized."[6] Silicate cement and copper cement were among materials that had been tried, along with several other means of blocking the fissures. Buonocore's innovation was of preparing the enamel surface with a weak acid, and then to penetrate it with a thin organic plastic sealant that was then polymerized. The first sealants introduced in 1967 used cyanoacrylate.[7] The material did not adhere well and deteriorated under the hydrated conditions in the mouth. Those were replaced with Bis-GMA resins,[8] with the first generation of sealants being cured by ultraviolet light, and a second generation using chemically cured resin material. Subsequent generations have used **light activated sealants**, which are the sealants most commonly used today. Other materials have also been used, mainly based on glassionomer, either by themselves or combined with resin.

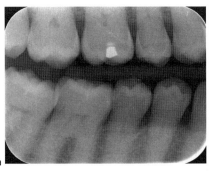
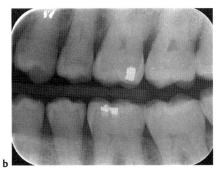
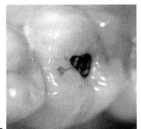
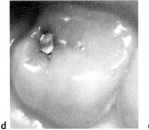
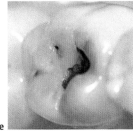

Fig. 15.1 a–e These small amalgam fillings, or amalgam "sealants," were placed as a preventive measure due to perceived risk of caries, and have lasted for more than 60 years. (Courtesy of Dr. S. Fischman.)
The bitewing radiographs reveal the slight extension of the amalgam into dentin. Although margins seem not to be „perfect" (c–e), no radiolucencies in dentin can be observed on the x-rays (a + b).
a Bitewing right side.
b Bitewing left side.
c Tooth 16.
d Tooth 26.
e Tooth 36.

NOTE

Many materials were tried as sealants, including silicate cement, copper cement, and cyanoacrylate (super glue). The first successful material was Bis-GMA resin.

This chapter will cover in detail:

- Similarities and differences between sealing and restorative procedures
- The anatomy of the pit and fissure system, either carious or not, as a substrate for resin bonding
- The pros and cons of therapeutic use of sealants for patients with high caries risk
- The effectiveness of sealants
- The arguments as to whether sealants are a cost-effective preventive option at either individual or population level

Caries Prevalence on Occlusal Surfaces

The occlusal surfaces constitute only around 12% of all the surfaces in the mouth, and yet they often account for 80%–90% of all the decay in younger populations.[9,10] Although a net reduction of occlusal caries has occurred over the last decades, the proportion of occlusal decay has increased, mainly due to increased use of fluoride (Chapter 12). The pit and fissure system has been proportionally less affected by the caries preventive effect of fluoride than approximal or smooth surfaces. **Figure 15.2** shows the considerable variation in shape found in the fissures. The pit and fissure system is usually the first site on the **erupting tooth** to be subject to caries, often because of lack of hygiene during the eruption period.[11] Although the caries status of the erupting teeth can be affected, it takes a vigorous program of hygiene instruction, coupled with application of fluorides, to keep those teeth free of decay. Initial active lesions detected during the eruption period often revert to a status of inactivity once the teeth have reached full occlusion.[12]

NOTE

The eruption period is a particularly susceptible time for caries in the life of a tooth.

While the occlusal surfaces are usually the first sites to show signs of caries, this may give the impression that 90% of caries could be successfully treated by sealant placement. This would be an overly optimistic assumption. The prevalence numbers are based on studies that use the methodology of visual examination, usually performed without prior cleaning of the teeth, and on a population

of 12–15-year-old children. The occlusal lesions usually progress rapidly, and they lend themselves easily to direct visual examination, while progress of approximal lesions, for example, is more gradual, and their early development necessitates radiographic examination to be detected. The risk of caries formation is a stepwise process, whereby the sites of a group within the dentition with similar resistance for caries get affected as the patient's individual defenses against the caries process become overwhelmed.[13] Placing of sealants only assists with the risk of the pit and fissure system, and continued care is needed to protect other areas and sites of the dentition. There is no evidence so far of sealants reducing the risk of other surfaces, although hypotheses have been formed related to reduction in retention sites for oral bacteria. Even so, it is clear that sealants are an indispensable part of caries preventive strategies in clinical practice and in community programs.

NOTE

The proportion of caries on occlusal surfaces in relation to the whole caries burden is high in children and adolescents.

The Sealant–Restoration Spectrum

There is a long tradition among dental professionals to view sealants as separate entities from fillings. The distinction was made on the basis of materials and procedures, since almost no tooth substance would be removed for the placement of a sealant. However, progress in materials and concepts of treatment has blurred this distinction. Really, it is best to regard sealants as almost **noninvasive (microinvasive) therapy**, as they are placed with no or very little mechanical modification of the surface. Nonetheless, the procedures and materials are similar to those used when a restoration is placed. Therefore, sealants require the same care and attention to detail as do fillings. Just as mishandling of filling procedures can compromise the adaptation and longevity of a restoration, the same applies to sealant placement: it is important to respect the advantages and limitations of the procedures and the materials that go toward making sealing into a successful caries-preventing procedure.

Historically, the reason for this separation is easy to understand. By the time sealants became available for use on occlusal surfaces of posterior teeth, the only other option was to place a **class I amalgam** restoration. The amalgam required technical skills, mechanical preparation with rotary instruments, understanding of engineering principles, good understanding of materials science, and an artistic touch in adapting and carving the material into a functional filling. The **sealants**, however, seemed

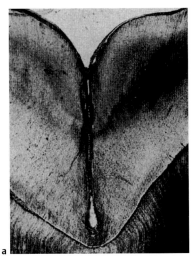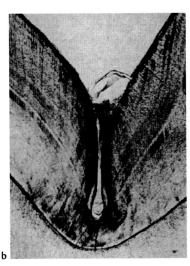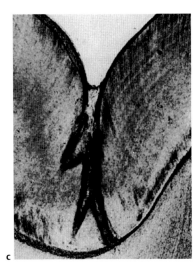

a b c

Fig. 15.2 a–c Variations in the shape of fissures. These cross-sectional images show well the great diversity that can be found in the forms and shapes that the fissures can take. (With permission from Sage Publications. From Gillings B, Buonocore M. Thickness of enamel at the base of pits and fissures in human molars and bicuspids. J Dent Res 1961;40:119–133)

simple and required little else but cleaning of the tooth surface, a little etching, and then the sealing material would flow into place. Indeed the procedure seemed so simple that the task could be referred to auxiliary members of the dental team. Dental hygienists and assistants could even offer sealants in school-based programs without the direct oversight of a dentist. Excellent staff and good training have proved the last statement to be true, but it is also recognized that the procedure requires attention to detail and adherence to certain principles to be successful.

Today the picture is a little more complicated. A myriad of materials has been marketed for use as sealants. The different types of material make up an entire spectrum, from being **unfilled resin materials**, to resins with varying degrees of filler content, through various stages of **compomers, resin-modified glass-ionomers**, and **glass-ionomers** (see Chapters 14, 19). Fluoride is sometimes incorporated into some of these materials, and bonding agents may also be used. Even **flowable composites** are used by some dentists as sealant material. The procedure itself offers many options for how to place sealants, how to clean the surface, how to prepare the surface, and various other factors, as discussed below. The only clear procedural difference between placement of sealants and fillings lies in the preparation of the dental hard tissues.

NOTE

Clinical procedures for sealing are similar to those used when placing adhesive restorations. A major difference refers to the mechanical preparation of the tooth surface: sealing requires only etching.

A hybrid technique, so-called **preventive resin restoration,** was already advocated in the 1970s.[14] Whether used in conjunction with amalgam or resin, this calls for removal of the caries-affected part of the lesion only and sealing of the rest of the fissure system, the sealing treatment becoming the predominant part of the operation. Sealants applied with amalgam fillings have also been shown to add to the longevity of the fillings.[15] This sealant–restoration spectrum gives us many options to apply the correct treatment in various situations (Chapter 20).

NOTE

Classical sealing nomenclature:
- *Preventive sealing*: Sealing sound fissures
- *Therapeutic sealing*: Sealing fissures with initial caries lesions
- *Preventive resin restoration*: Local invasive treatment + sealing of neighboring, nonprepared fissures (either sound or decayed)

Epidemiological considerations

A consequence of this blurred interface between sealants and fillings is how they are scored in clinical studies. In **epidemiological studies** there is now a problem in distinguishing sealants from small restorations underneath part of the sealant. The distinction is important in reporting of data, for example, national data measured with the **DMFT index**, as the sealed teeth would be regarded as sound, but filled teeth would contribute to the perceived disease burden of the participants (see Chapter 8). A few years ago, the sealants would have been either clear or white, but with the use of tooth-colored materials for the routine sealing, even that distinction has become blurred. More

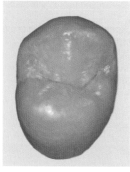 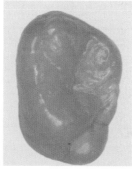

a   b

Fig. 15.3 a, b Premolars do not show so many fissures as molars, although in premolars these might be rather deep. Not all molars have deep fissures, which makes it more easy for biofilm control by tooth brushing.

viscous materials do not flow as well into the fissures, and the proportion of overfilled fissures seems high.

The same problem is faced in clinical trials and other longitudinal studies. A surface with an overfilled tooth-colored sealant may resemble a filling at baseline, but with wear of the overfilled portion it may become clear that it was placed as a sealant. This would be counted as a reversal in the data set, and potentially obscure the effect of the treatment being tested.

Fissure Morphology

The fissures are **developmental grooves**, mainly in the occlusal surfaces of the teeth. They are considered to be faults which arose during development of the cuspal enamel, caused by the failure of the enamel lobes to coalesce perfectly during the formative stages, with their location based on the developmental lobes of the tooth formation (**Fig. 15.2**). Although most common in molar teeth, the premolars have such grooves too (**Fig. 15.3**). Also for palatal surfaces of upper anterior teeth, pits and fissures might be found. Since many of those pits and fissures become very narrow, they easily lead to **plaque stagnation**, which can then lead to lesion formation.

As part of risk assessment used to justify sealant placement, the phenomenon of "deep" fissures is commonly mentioned. In the North Carolina risk assessment study,

one of the three risk predictors found to significantly correlate with subsequent caries formation was fissure morphology (deep fissures – high caries risk).[16] Other studies have also linked deep fissures with prevalence of caries[17–19] and dentists' perception of the caries risk of deep fissures.[20]

> **NOTE**
>
> - The fissures are faults that arise during the development of the tooth morphology.
> - Having deep fissures is cited as one of the main risk factors for the development of caries.

Several methods have been used to examine fissure morphology. Serial sectioning,[19,21,22] fissure splitting,[23] resin replicas infused under vacuum[24,25] and 3-D computer reconstruction of resin impregnated sections following dye infusion.[26] Although there have been attempts to classify the different morphological types of fissure—into V-shaped, U-shaped, I-shaped, or combinations of these[18,26]—there are great variations in the shape, size, and width of fissures.[21,22,27]

The fissure system may not be an open canyon through the center of the teeth, but rather resembles a series of pits separated by cols that may change continuously as one travels along the system. It becomes obvious that those systems are vulnerable to plaque accumulation and caries formation (**Figs. 15.4** and **15.5**).

The thickness of the enamel at the bottom of the fissures in the upper premolars is estimated to be around 0.2–0.35 mm.[24] This varies to the extent that in rare cases some fissures can be found as having a very thin enamel covering at the bottom. The following dimensions on maxillary first premolars have been reported:[27]

- Fissure depth: 120–1050 µm
- Width in the middle part of the fissure: 40–156 µm
- Thickness of the enamel at the bottom of the fissure: 270–1000 µm

Thus, it can be stated that there is great variation in the shape and depth of the fissure system from one part to the next within the same surface, and it is likely that only some parts will need to be covered by sealants to reduce the caries risk.

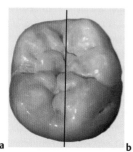 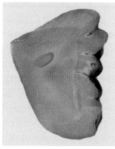 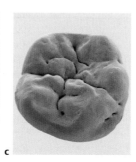

a   b   c

Fig. 15.4a–c The shape of the fissure system may resemble a series of pits separated by cols (**a**, **c**). These narrow grooves may be affected by caries (**b**), if a cariogenic biofilm is frequently established.
a Molar where cut is indicated.
b Cut surface.
c Scanning electron microscopic image.

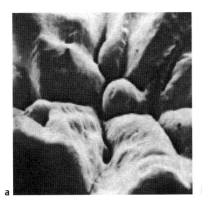
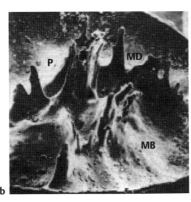

a

b

Fig. 15.5 a, b The shape of the fissure system, shown here as a resin replica of the fissure system. Scanning electron micrograph (SEM) of an intact occlusal surface (a). SEM of a vinyl replica showing the details of an upper molar (b). (Reproduced with permission from Elsevier Ltd., from Galil and Gwinnett.[24])

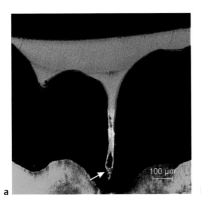
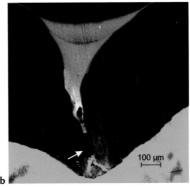

a

b

Fig. 15.6 a Confocal microscopic images of sealed fissures. Organic and anorganic substances collect in deep fissures, and removing them with a toothbrush is difficult (arrow). As a result the sealing material (red) cannot penetrate completely into the fissure (red). In deep fissures the enamel is often only a few μm thick.

Fig. 15.6 b The goal is to make sealant penetration into the fissures as complete as possible; nonetheless, with these materials no penetration into the lesion body can be expected.

NOTE

- The fissure system is a series of pits, separated by cols.
- Thickness of enamel at the bottom of the pits is below 0.5 mm, whereas the thickness of occlusal enamel is otherwise more than 1 mm.

A **limitation of scientific studies** concerning morphology of fissures is that they mostly refer to either third molars, which are known for their rich variation in anatomy and structure, or premolars extracted for orthodontic reasons. Extrapolating those results to the teeth most commonly recommended for sealing—that is, the first and second molars—needs to recognize this limitation, although the challenge is obvious: to be able to clean those narrow spaces, dry them, and get the sealant material to penetrate as far as possible downward into the fissure space. However, caries formation takes place at the upper part of the fissures, so penetration to the full depth of the fissure may not be needed.

The Fissure as Substrate for Resin Bonding

A fundamental question in planning placement of a sealant is to consider what the sealant is binding to. In this regard we must consider both the **microscopic composition** of the enamel, the **morphological formation** of the fissures, and the **organic material** found occupying the fissure space. At the time of eruption the fissures are filled with remnants of enamel protein, protein from tissue and blood fluids, and cellular remnants, forming a loose organic mesh inside the fissure (**Fig. 15.6**).[22] As soon as the tooth penetrates the mucosal lining, salivary proteins are added to the mix, forming acquired pellicle along with organic and inorganic ions from the saliva. At that time there is also an influx of bacteria, laying the foundation of the dental biofilm.[19] Food debris gets compacted into the fissures, and calcifications can be seen within the fissures. After several weeks the **biofilm** has taken on a more distinct structure with successive layers of microorganisms and extracellular material.

In most cases sealants are placed on the teeth within a few months to a few years after their eruption. During this time there are changes taking place in the inorganic content of the enamel, and in the organic material that attaches to the enamel. When the enamel is formed it is immature, not all spaces are occupied by ions, there are intercrystalline spaces, remnants of enamel forming protein, and impurities. Also, a hypomineralized area has been described descending from the bottom of the fissure although its role in caries formation is not regarded as crucial.[28] The enamel in the fissure does not all possess the regular keyhole structure found on smooth surfaces, but often a thin amorphous layer lines the fissure enamel that is different from the regular crystalline enamel rods.[29] The importance of this must be understood in the context of using **acid etching** to create microscopic tags in the enamel for **micromechanical retention** of the sealant material.

With the fissure enamel constantly covered by biofilm and bathed in saliva, the enamel slowly transforms during the **maturation phase**, for up to two years, increasing the content of fluoride and the hardness of the enamel. The importance of the biofilm to sealant placement is that the phosphoric acid has poor capabilities for removing the biofilm, and therefore etching the enamel when it is covered by the biofilm may turn out to be incomplete. Studies also show that the organic content of the fissure is very hard to clean out,[23] and that the methods of cleaning, mainly with pumice or prophylactic paste, can leave some of the cleaning agent in the fissure.[29] Moreover, the fissures might be lined with remnant aprismatic enamel.[30] In the last-cited study no full penetration of resins into the bottom of the fissures or gap-free interfaces could be observed in any of the specimens. Phosphoric acid did not penetrate well into the fissures and although hybridization of the etched **aprismatic enamel** was observed, etching was inconsistent and gaps were frequently observed. Entrapment of bacteria within the fissure walls was frequently seen.[30]

The goal is to make sealant penetration as complete as possible. The combination of three factors results in possible interference not only with enamel etching, but also with sealant penetration and therefore the proportion of the fissure that is filled with the sealant material:

- The microscopic structure of enamel
- The macroscopic fissure configuration
- The constant presence of a biofilm

Drying will be incomplete, and due to incompatibility of resin materials with hydrated environment, sealant penetration is suspect. This will result in fissures being at best partially filled,[29] and in some cases with only limited retention available at the opening of the fissure.

NOTE

- For sealant placement it is important to keep in mind that the etching has to deal with some amorphous and aprismatic enamel.
- The etchant does not dissolve the biofilm or organic contents of the fissure.

Cleaning of Fissures Prior to Sealant Placement

Several methods have been recommended over the years. Initially, using a rotary instrument such as a rubber cup or a rotating brush was considered necessary, often with the aid of pumice or prophylactic paste. This can actually load the pumice or the paste into the fissures and reduce retention. Hydrogen peroxide has also been suggested, but carries the risk of bubble formation underneath the sealants. Vigorous cleaning with air-water spray, and running the explorer gently along the fissure prior to acid etching has shown just as good retention as the mechanical removal. Similarly with **simple brushing** of the teeth with a toothbrush, either dry or with toothpaste, and either supervised or done by the operator. The simple recommendation to use only toothbrush cleaning before sealant placement is therefore all that seems to be needed.[31]

CLINICAL PEARL

The simple method of cleaning teeth with a toothbrush, or by running an explorer along the length of the fissures, along with vigorous rinsing with an air-water spray, seems to be enough to clean the surface before sealant placement.

Should Mechanical Preparation Be Routine?

No current guidelines recommend the use of mechanical removal of fissure enamel, either by bur or air-abrasion. Although briefly described here, the empirical evidence is that no routine opening of the fissures is needed in order for sealing to be successful. Sealant retention is not improved, and the limited number of existing studies gives conflicting results.

If the clinician decides that removal of fissure enamel is needed, this essentially changes the procedure to an **invasive treatment**, which is sometimes called "preventive resin restoration." Fissure preparation should then be done with very fine burs, where the shape of the bur and its use result in minimal removal of tooth structure.[32] Fissure preparation may assist in two ways. First, by providing a more predictable surface for bonding of sealant material by removing unsupported carious enamel, the amorphous enamel layer, and some of the organic material in the fissure.[33] Second, due to the widening of the fissure space, the sealant will penetrate more easily and deeper than in an unprepared fissure.[34] On the other hand, if fissure preparation is performed, the dentist might consider using a filled resin such as a flowable resin for replacement of the lost structure, since unfilled resin is not likely to show good wear characteristics in the widened fissure. This means that a restoration, though being rather small, is placed and not only sealing of the surface performed (Chapter 19).

The selection of procedures and materials often draws a fine line between definitions of a filling and a sealant. The American Dental Association (ADA) definition for this threshold is that the procedure becomes a filling when a bur preparation extends into the **dentin**. This threshold is well selected to prevent simple **enameloplasty** being regarded as the same level in patient treatment as excavation of dentinal caries. However, due to the anatomy of the fissure system, where only a few hundred micrometers of enamel may be situated at the bottom of the fissure, invasive intervention will very likely end up in the dentin. Therefore, these kinds of invasive treatments should be preferably called a *restoration* and clearly be distinguished from *sealing*. The hybrid is the so called *preventive resin restoration* which means that neighboring nondrilled fissures are sealed, whereas the small cavity is filled.

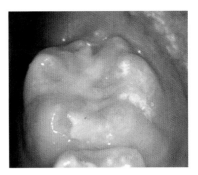

Fig. 15.7 Glass-ionomer cements may be used for fissure sealing. Nonetheless, these show inferior adhesion to enamel, which may result in partial loss and subsequent development of a caries lesion at the margin (with courtesy of U. Schiffner).

NOTE

- The removal of enamel as a routine before sealant placement is not supported by the limited number of studies available.
- It may appear that removing enamel should remove aprismatic enamel, remove organic content from fissure walls, remove possible decay, improve binding, improve penetration of sealant, and allow for better drying, but studies show that it is not necessary for successful prevention of caries.

NOTE

- Glass-ionomer sealants have low retention rates. They are recommended in areas where moisture control is suspect, such as newly erupted teeth that are partially covered by the oral mucosa. Here, in most cases it is more advisable to wait some months and to use a resin-based sealant.

Glass-Ionomer Sealants

The retention rate of glass-ionomer sealants is consistently found to be low. The caries preventive effect is often found to be equivalent to resin-based sealants.[35],[36] This is most probably attributed to remnants of the glass-ionomer being found deep within the fissure, although no visible remnant is found on the surface.[37] However, they are recommended only in situations where conventional resin sealants cannot be successfully used, such as erupting teeth, where complete moisture control may not be achieved, or where only part of the surface has erupted but is considered to need the protection of a sealant, and then as an interim measure[38] (**Fig. 15.7**).

Preventive versus Therapeutic Sealants

Sealants can be placed on the posterior teeth shortly after eruption, on occlusal surfaces of the molars, with the intention of preventing development of caries lesions. These are called **preventive sealants**. In other cases lesion formation may already have started, or the dentist may suspect that lesions may be present. In those cases sealants may still be appropriate and effective treatments, but in those situations they are properly termed **therapeutic sealants**. However, it may be hard to distinguish clearly between sound and initially decayed fissures (**Fig. 15.8**) (see Chapter 5).

When should preventive sealants be placed? The answer is based on the potential risk of an individual surface. Sealants may be most beneficial shortly after eruption of the teeth, and the time frame is often mentioned as 2–4 years after eruption. However, studies on college students and army recruits showed that those groups are still forming primary caries lesions on occlusal surfaces[40] (**Fig. 15.9**). This emphasizes that though majority of pit and fissure caries occurs within the first few years after eruption,[41] the development of decay may continue through adolescence and well into young adulthood.

Recent recommendations leave the decision of placing a sealant to the clinical judgment of the dentist.[38] Therefore, sealants can be prescribed for adults and for primary teeth, when the dentist judges that there is **sufficient risk of caries development** or progression in that partic-

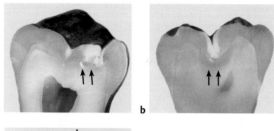

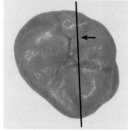

Fig. 15.8a–c In the cross-sections (**a**, **c**) caries lesions extending (histologically) into dentin are visible, although the signs of the caries process seen from the occlusal aspect were very little (**b**).

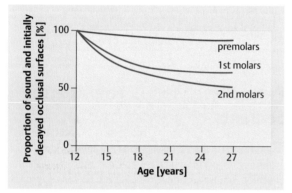

Fig. 15.9 Proportion of occlusal surfaces on different tooth types to develop caries lesions: 1st and 2nd molars, and premolars. There is less risk for premolars to form cavitated lesions (ICDAS 5+6) than for molars.[39]

ular tooth. This has extended the use of sealants; however, most sealants are placed within the first few years after eruption.

> **NOTE**
>
> - Sealants should be placed in all teeth that are at potential risk of developing caries.
> - This is usually within 2–4 years after eruption of the teeth.
> - Based on risk, primary teeth should be considered for sealant placement, and so should young adults, or any other group which is experiencing an increased risk.

Application of preventive sealants should only be performed when the dentist has a reasonable suspicion that a caries lesion may form in a given fissure system, and must be based on a detailed assessment of the risk for the patient (Chapters 7 and 24), following the gathering of information along with careful observation of the condition and morphology of the tooth under consideration. Therapeutic use of sealants has been practiced consciously in many cases, and probably inadvertently in many more cases. Treatment is always based on **four levels of assessment**: first, processing the information of the individual tooth surface, then examining the rest of the dentition, followed by estimation of the patients' risk factors, and finally estimation of the population factors. The summation of the professional evaluation on all these factors by the dentist leads to a decision on how to treat—in other words, information from the data gathering has to be filtered through the brain of the dentist before being applied to the treatment (Chapter 9). Accurate detection of the caries status of the surface is important, as can be achieved using the ICDAS criteria. Additional methods can be used, but care must be taken that a greater amount of information is also likely to result in overestimation of the caries.[42]

> **NOTE**
>
> Sealants could, and also should, be placed on active noncavitated lesions as a therapeutic measure. Those who say they would never seal-in caries have probably inadvertently done so many times.

Sealing over Caries?

A crucial question for a profession that bases its livelihood on removing demineralized tooth structure is whether a sealant can be placed over existing lesions. The predominant notion is that this has probably often happened, owing to imprecision in the diagnostic procedures. According to two recent statement papers, sealants are effective in reducing progression of noncavitated lesions.[43,44] Crucial to such therapeutic use of sealants is to assess the activity level of the lesion. If a noncavitated lesion is not active there is probably no need for any further treatment. For an **active lesion** (Caries progressiva superficialis) placement of a sealant may provide an excellent treatment for the patient. The things that matter here are the extent of the lesion, the level of porosity within the lesion, and the strength of the remaining tooth structure.

The sealant has to do exactly what the name implies, that is, to seal off the lesion and prevent influx of nutrients to bacteria in the fissure, or diffusion of acids into the existing lesion. If cut off from the oral environment, such lesions will not progress.[15] For lesions of grade ICDAS 1 (see Chapter 5), sealants would easily accomplish such a goal. For many grade ICDAS 2 lesions, this goal may also be reached, and even for lesions of grades ICDAS 3 and -4, sealants may still be a good alternative to invasive treatment, if there is only a minimal break in the surface, small enough for the sealant to cover (**Fig. 15.10**). Potential problems may arise if the lesion extends so far up along the cuspal inclines that a safely sealed margin cannot be assured. Also, if the progression of the lesion has severely weakened the remaining enamel which is needed to provide bonding of the resin to the tooth. Such a **weakened structure** may not be able to withstand the forces of occlusal contact or the contraction during polymerization.

However, many sealants never penetrate far enough into the fissures, so only about half of the fissure space can reasonably be expected to be filled with resin material.[29] **Penetration** may be enhanced by using bonding agents, due to its hydrophilic properties, although bond strength is not enhanced unless it is used on surfaces which are subject to moisture contamination.[45–47]

Overall, the risk of sealing over caries is minimal, and even if the sealant fails by losing its retention, the tooth is at no greater risk than before.[48]

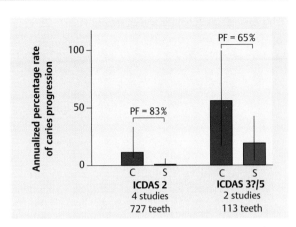

Fig. 15.10 Sealing over caries. The prevented fraction (PF) for sealed ICDAS 2 lesions was determined at 83%. This means that after 1 year, caries progression in 5 out of 6 teeth will have been stopped by sealants compared with non-sealing. For cavitated caries, lesion sealing still works, but here a composite restoration seems to be the better choice.[43] S = sealed; C = control

> **NOTE**
>
> - Sealants are effective in halting progression of existing carious lesions.
> - As long as the sealant effectively seals off the lesion, there is no reason to suspect any lesion progression.
> - If a sealant placed on top of lesions fails, the tooth is at no greater risk than if it had never been sealed.

> **NOTE**
>
> - Although rubber dam isolation gives the best means for moisture control, routine use of rubber dam has not been recommended.

Factors influencing decision for or against fissure sealing are summarized in **Table 5.1**.

Moisture Control

Good moisture isolation is a "must" for placing a sealant successfully. Sealants placed while using a **rubber dam** tend to show slightly better retention than those without. However, placing a rubber dam is not always necessary or feasible, and even if the dam can be placed, the procedure frequently requires administration of a local anesthetic to prevent discomfort of the clasp. If other more invasive procedures are planned in the same area, sealing of indicated teeth can be done under excellent conditions while the rubber dam is in place. This is particularly true for partially erupted teeth, where there is still operculum covering part of the occlusal surface. In those cases the clasp and the rubber dam may actually assist in keeping the soft tissue out of the way while the sealant is being placed. This would require the patient to be anesthetized, and doing so for only the purpose of sealing a newly erupted molar is not indicated. Another alternative would be the use of a glass-ionomer sealant as a temporary measure. To ensure good moisture control, four-handed delivery (two operators) is recommended over two-handed delivery (one person), as it has shown a superior retention rate of 9%.[49]

Are Sealants Working Clinically?

The success of sealant treatment has been measured mainly as the **retention rate** of sealants. Retention after 1 year is usually greater than 90%, and then gradually tapers off, to around 80% after 3–5 years. Simonsen[50] reported retention rates of surfaces after 15 years to be 28% complete retention, and 35% partially retained. Other long-term clinical observations have reported similar results: 22% complete and 35% partial retention, respectively, also 15 years after placement.[51] In a group of 148 patients followed up on average for 11.6 years, 41% sealants were fully retained, but 11% had been replaced by a restoration.[52] The long-term performance of sealants depended on the restoration profile of the patient, with higher failure rates in high restoration-profile patients. It is expected that 5%–10% of sealants lose retention per year. It is therefore recommended to monitor them and **replace** lost sealant. Retention of sealants is used as a surrogate for effectiveness, since it is ethically nowadays not possible to compare the success of sealants in caries reduction in one group of patients or teeth to a group that does not receive the benefits of sealant treatment.

The key question regarding sealants is whether they actually **reduce development of caries lesions**. This ques-

Table 15.1 Pros and cons for sealant placement

Pros
- Deep, retentive pits and fissures
- Stained pits and fissures with appearance of demineralization (ICDAS 1 and 2)
- Caries or restorations in other primary or permanent teeth
- No evidence of dentinal approximal caries on teeth to be sealed
- Non-invasive treatment applied to inhibit approximal caries
- Adequate moisture control possible
- Less than 4 years from tooth eruption, unless clinical judgment indicates risk of caries development

Cons
- Well-coalesced, self-cleaning pits and fissures
- Approximal caries in the tooth that needs a restoration
- Approximal caries in other teeth and no compliance by the patient to adapt non invasive self-applied interventions on a regular basis
- Partially erupted teeth, or moisture control not possible
- Teeth showing no signs of caries after 4 years in the oral cavity, and patient is at low risk for caries

tion has been answered recently in several excellent systematic reviews.[36,43,53,54] The unanimous conclusion is that sealants are effective in reducing caries. A Cochrane review found the **effectiveness** to be 87% at 1 year, and 60% at 4.0–4.5 years for preventive sealants.[36] (**Table 15.1**) Another review found the reduction to be slightly lower with an average effect of 33%.[54]

The prevented fraction in four randomized clinical trials was 71% at 5 years after placement for sealants over noncavitated caries lesions[43] (**Fig. 15.11**). The outcome is unequivocally that sealants can reduce caries progression. Furthermore, the sealing of noncavitated caries in permanent teeth was found to be effective in reducing caries progression.

NOTE

- Sealant retention rates are usually over 90% after 1 year, and greater than 80% after 3 years.
- The efficacy in reducing caries on occlusal surfaces is 87% at 1 year and 60% after 4 years.

Sealant Failures and Maintenance

Retention rates of sealants are usually above 90% after 1 year, and above 80% after 3–5 years. But why and how do sealants fail? And what are the consequences of such failures? There can be many reasons for failure of sealants. **Moisture control** is of great importance and lack thereof will have a detrimental effect on the sealant success rate.

Occlusal forces constitute one of the biggest challenges to sealants. Overfilled fissures expose the unfilled resin material to high occlusal forces that may help to dislodge the sealant. The low retention rate of sealants on buccal pits and lingual grooves is probably due to high shearing forces in those locations. It is important to apply just enough sealant to fill the fissures, and not to extend the material far up on the lateral aspects of the cusps.

When sealants are either partially or totally lost, it is important to maintain the tooth surface by **re-applying the sealant**. Risk assessment of the surface should be done, and if there is still need for protection against caries, a sealant can be placed on the location where it was lost. Therefore it is good practice to monitor sealed teeth on a yearly basis. In the case where monitoring is not practicable, such as in community programs, the lack of monitoring should not prevent children from benefitting from the caries-reducing effect of sealants, since teeth with lost sealants are not at increased risk compared with teeth that never received the treatment.[48,55]

NOTE

- Sealant failures are mostly attributed to lack of moisture control, to occlusion forces on the sealant, or to case selection (high caries risk).
- Re-application of lost sealants should be based on risk assessment, as would be done for any sealant placement.

Cost-Effectiveness of Sealants

Although the efficacy and effectiveness of sealants are well established in the scientific literature, there has long been a need for well-designed and well-conducted cost–benefit and cost–utility analyses. The earlier studies did not consider the advantages of a sound tooth in the calculation of a budget.[56] Comparisons revolve around how much the application of sealants costs, and how many of those sealed teeth are actually saved from developing caries lesions. In a simple form the **cost of a sealant** ($45) can be compared with the lifecycle of a molar tooth over a long period; through increasingly bigger restorations, adding a root canal treatment, crown, and finally an extraction, for the total cost of $2346. That is to assume that all teeth will go down that road. The longer the time span, the more cost-effective it is for the individual to have the first filling delayed for as long as possible. In the short term the comparison will be with number of lesions and restorations within the early years of the life of an individual.

Several studies have looked into this topic. Comparisons have included strategies of **not sealing**, versus strategies of **sealing all teeth** or applying a **risk-based sealant strategy**. Risk-based strategies (see also Chapter 13) usually after the least cost while still reducing caries, but as the caries risk of the population increases, a **seal-all strategy** becomes more cost-effective.[57] Similarly, another study found that a risk-based seal-all strategy improved outcome over not sealing, and that the strategy further improved the outcome of reducing caries, but at an increased cost.[58] In a low-risk population it is not surprising that risk-based strategies are found to be more cost-effective.[59] Under such conditions indiscriminate application of sealants to all patients is both unnecessary and expensive. More recently it could be shown that a publicly funded program in the public sector was more cost-effective than a universal publicly funded private practice.[60] However, it was also found that the cost of such arrangements varied with the incidence of decay and proportion of high-risk children. Thus, in all instances the option of sealing was more cost-effective than the option of not sealing, even in a low-risk population.

NOTE

- The cost of sealing is far less than the costs of a typical lifetime treatment for a tooth, through repeated fillings, crowns, root canals, and extractions.
- Sealants are more cost effective in higher risk populations.
- Risk-based strategies are recommended in low and medium risk populations.
- When appropriately executed, the option of sealing is more cost-effective than not sealing, even in low risk populations.

Widespread Use of Sealants

Although supportive scientific evidence for the health benefits associated with sealants has been published for a long time, their adoption has been slow. In the **United States** in 1990, just under 20% of young people aged 5–17 years had at least one sealant,[61] although that percentage 10 years later was over 30%.[62] Many reasons may lie behind this slow adoption, but some relate it to lack of **reimbursement by a third party payer**. Obstacles for implementation may lie in the reimbursement or funding arrangements. In the United States these have now been overcome, as most insurance and public health programs provide fees for sealant placement, which has proved to be a powerful incentive.[63] According to the Centers for Disease Control and Prevention (CDC) National Oral Health Surveillance System, the percentage of 3rd grade students with dental sealants on at least one permanent molar varied among states from 20% to 66%; however, some states did not report their sealant usage.[64] In most states this falls short of the goal of 50% set by the US Department of Health and Human Services for Healthy People 2010. Sealant usage also shows significant ethnic and income disparities.[10] An increase in using sealants as an inexpensive and easy way to improve health and relief

Table 15.2 Relative risks of developing a caries lesion of an occlusal surface (i. e., molars) that has not been sealed compared with a sealed one

Time (years)	No. of studies	Risk ratio (95% CI)
1	3	7.7 (5–11)
2	3	4.5 (2.9–6.7)
3	3	3.3 (2.5–4.5)
4.5	3	2.5 (2–3.2)
9	1	2.9 (1.8–4.5)

CI = confidence interval.
Source: ref. [36].

disparities is being advocated through federal and state agencies, as well as in school-based programs.[55]

The use of sealants in other countries is both widespread and long-standing. Recent reports indicated that in **Denmark**, two-thirds of 15-year-olds have at least one molar sealed, although sealant use varied by municipality,[65] while **Iceland** reported 88% of the same age group having at least one sealed surface.[66] Indeed, half of all molar occlusal surfaces in 12- and 15-year-old children were scored as having a sealant (H. Eggertsson, unpublished data). In **Finland**, sealants have been widely used since 1970, and their use continues to be high.[67] Comparison between population samples in **Sweden** and Finland showed that 80%–90% of molars in Finnish adolescents were sealed, while a risk-based strategy used in Sweden reported 30% sealed.[68] In **Germany**, prevalence of at least one fissure sealing in 12-year-olds has increased from 50% in 1997 to 70% in 2005.[69] In a recent survey of dental schools in 13 countries in **Europe**, indications on when to use sealants varied considerably among pediatric departments. Only 6% of universities applied sealants routinely, while most used risk-based strategies. And most were hesitant to apply sealants to noncavitated dentinal lesions.[70] Thus the use of sealants can depend on availability of service, risk-based need, population strategies, and re-imbursement policies.

NOTE

- Use of sealants has been widely accepted in some countries for a long time, while their adaption has been more gradual in other countries.
- Usage is highest in countries with national health policies advocating their use through public health programs.
- Risk-based strategy is most commonly advocated.
- Their usage also shows significant ethnic and income disparities.

Table 15.3 Clinical recommendations for sealant placement in the pit and fissure system. Prerequisites are to employ caries risk assessment and to maintain a dry field during the procedure

Sealant placement	
• In primary or permanent teeth of children, adolescents, or adults, when it is determined that the tooth or the patient is at risk of developing caries • On noncavitated caries lesions to reduce disease progression	
Recommended	**Not recommended**
Resin-based sealants	Self-etching bonding agents
Four-handed delivery	Routine mechanical preparation of enamel
Glass-ionomer sealants as an interim when moisture control is an issue	
Monitor and re-apply sealants as needed	
Source: Adapted from Beauchamp et al.[38]	

Conclusion

There is no doubt that sealants are **effective** in reducing the caries burden. They are a simple, cost-effective means of preventing unnecessary suffering, and for preventing the start of the patient's downward spiral of fillings, crowns, root canal therapy, and finally extraction of teeth. Clinical recommendations (**Table 15.3**) should be integrated with the practitioner's professional judgment and the patient's needs and preferences.[38]

SUMMARY

- Sealing is a cost-effective way of preventing new lesions, and to halt progression of noncavitated lesions.
- Sealants can be placed in a simple manner, for a relative low cost, by any skilled member of the dental team, to various populations, under widely different conditions, and yet achieve the effect of reducing caries rates.
- Careful attention needs to be paid to details during sealant procedures, mainly to methods of cleaning, and to complete moisture control.
- Sealant placement should be based on case-selective, risk-based assessment of both the tooth surface and the individual.
- Mechanical removal of (carious) enamel is not recommended as a routine before sealant placements.

REFERENCES

1. Cueto EI, Buonocore MG. Sealing of pits and fissures with an adhesive resin: its use in caries prevention. J Am Dent Assoc 1967;75(1):121–128
2. Black GV. Operative Dentistry. Vol 1: Pathology of the Hard Tissues of the Teeth. Chicago: Medico-Dental Publishing; 1908
3. Hyatt TD. Prophylactic odontotomy – the ideal procedure in dentistry for children. Dent Cos 1936;78:353–370
4. Bodecker CF. The tooth brush in relation to occlusal fissures. Dent Items Interest 1926;48:161
5. Brucker M. Studies on the incidence and cause of dental defects in children. VI. Pits and fissures. J Dent Res 1944;23:89–99
6. Buonocore MG. A simple method of increasing the adhesion of acrylic filling materials to enamel surfaces. J Dent Res 1955;34 (6):849–853
7. Handelman SL, Shey Z. Michael Buonocore and the Eastman Dental Center: a historic perspective on sealants. J Dent Res 1996;75(1):529–534
8. Bowen RL. Crystalline dimethacrylate monomers. J Dent Res 1970;49(4):810–815
9. Macek MD, Beltrán-Aguilar ED, Lockwood SA, Malvitz DM. Updated comparison of the caries susceptibility of various morphological types of permanent teeth. J Public Health Dent 2003;63 (3):174–182
10. Dye BA, Tan S, Smith V, et al. Trends in oral health status: United States, 1988–1994 and 1999–2004. Vital Health Stat 11 2007; 248(248):1–92
11. Carvalho JC, Ekstrand KR, Thylstrup A. Dental plaque and caries on occlusal surfaces of first permanent molars in relation to stage of eruption. J Dent Res 1989;68(5):773–779
12. Carvalho JC, Thylstrup A, Ekstrand KR. Results after 3 years of non-operative occlusal caries treatment of erupting permanent first molars. Community Dent Oral Epidemiol 1992;20(4): 187–192
13. Sheiham A, Sabbah W. Using universal patterns of caries for planning and evaluating dental care. Caries Res 2010;44(2): 141–150
14. Simonsen RJ, Stallard RE. Sealant-restorations utilizing a diluted filled composite resin: one year results. Quintessence Int Dent Dig 1977;8(6):77–84

15. Mertz-Fairhurst EJ, Curtis JW Jr, Ergle JW, Rueggeberg FA, Adair SM. Ultraconservative and cariostatic sealed restorations: results at year 10. J Am Dent Assoc 1998;129(1):55–66

16. Stewart PW, Stamm JW. Classification tree prediction models for dental caries from clinical, microbiological, and interview data. J Dent Res 1991;70(9):1239–1251

17. Bossert WA. The relation between the shape of the occlusal surfaces of molars and the prevalence of decay. J Dent Res 1933;13:125–128

18. König KG. Dental morphology in relation to caries resistance with special reference to fissures as susceptible areas. J Dent Res 1963;2:461–476

19. Ekstrand KR, Bjørndal L. Structural analyses of plaque and caries in relation to the morphology of the groove-fossa system on erupting mandibular third molars. Caries Res 1997;31(5):336–348

20. Muller-Bolla M, Courson F, Droz D, Lupi-Pégurier L, Velly AM. Definition of at-risk occlusal surfaces of permanent molars—a descriptive study. J Clin Pediatr Dent 2009;34(1):35–42

21. Gillings B, Buonocore M. Thickness of enamel at the base of pits and fissures in human molars and bicuspids. J Dent Res 1961;40:119–133

22. Ekstrand KR, Westergaard J, Thylstrup A. Organic content in occlusal groove-fossa-system in unerupted 3rd mandibular molars: a light and electron microscopic study. Scand J Dent Res 1991;99(4):270–280

23. Rohr M, Makinson OF, Burrow MF. Pits and fissures: morphology. ASDC J Dent Child 1991;58(2):97–103

24. Galil KA, Gwinnett AJ. Three-dimensional replicas of pits and fissures in human teeth: scanning electron microscopy study. Arch Oral Biol 1975;20(8):493–495

25. Juhl M. Three-dimensional replicas of pit and fissure morphology in human teeth. Scand J Dent Res 1983;91(2):90–95

26. Hirano Y, Aoba T. Computer-assisted reconstruction of enamel fissures and carious lesions of human premolars. J Dent Res 1995;74(5):1200–1205

27. Fejerskov O, Melsen B, Karring T. Morphometric analysis of occlusal fissures in human premolars. Scand J Dent Res 1973;81(7):505–509

28. Awazawa Y. Electron microscopic study on the hypomineralized enamel areas descending from the floors of occlusal fissures toward the amelo-dentinal junctions. J Nihon Univ Sch Dent 1966;8(1):33–44

29. Burrow JF, Burrow MF, Makinson OF. Pits and fissures: relative space contribution in fissures from sealants, prophylaxis pastes and organic remnants. Aust Dent J 2003;48(3):175–179

30. Tay FR, Frankenberger R, Carvalho RM, Pashley DH. Pit and fissure sealing. Bonding of bulk-cured, low-filled, light-curing resins to bacteria-contaminated uncut enamel in high c-factor cavities. Am J Dent 2005;18(1):28–36

31. Kolavic Gray S, Griffin SO, Malvitz DM, Gooch BF. A comparison of the effects of tooth brushing and handpiece prophylaxis on retention of sealants. J Am Dent Assoc 2009;140(1):38–46

32. De Craene GP, Martens C, Dermaut R. The invasive pit-and-fissure sealing technique in pediatric dentistry: an SEM study of a preventive restoration. ASDC J Dent Child 1988;55(1):34–42

33. Burrow MF, Burrow JF, Makinson OF. Pits and fissures: etch resistance in prismless enamel walls. Aust Dent J 2001;46(4):258–262

34. Shapira J, Eidelman E. The influence of mechanical preparation of enamel prior to etching on the retention of sealants: three-year follow-up. J Pedod 1984;8(3):272–277

35. Beiruti N, Frencken JE, van't Hof MA, van Palenstein Helderman WH. Caries-preventive effect of resin-based and glass ionomer sealants over time: a systematic review. Community Dent Oral Epidemiol 2006;34(6):403–409

36. Ahovuo-Saloranta A, Hiiri A, Nordblad A, Mäkelä M, Worthington HV. Pit and fissure sealants for preventing dental decay in the permanent teeth of children and adolescents. Cochrane Database Syst Rev 2008;4(4):CD001830

37. Frencken JE, Wolke J. Clinical and SEM assessment of ART high-viscosity glass-ionomer sealants after 8-13 years in 4 teeth. J Dent 2010;38(1):59–64

38. Beauchamp J, Caufield PW, Crall JJ, et al. American Dental Association Council on Scientific Affairs. Evidence-based clinical recommendations for the use of pit-and-fissure sealants: a report of the American Dental Association Council on Scientific Affairs. J Am Dent Assoc 2008;139(3):257–268

39. Mejàre I, Stenlund H, Zelezny-Holmlund C. Caries incidence and lesion progression from adolescence to young adulthood: a prospective 15-year cohort study in Sweden. Caries Res 2004;38(2):130–141

40. Richardson PS, McIntyre IG. Susceptibility of tooth surfaces to carious attack in young adults. Community Dent Health 1996;13(3):163–168

41. Eklund SA, Ismail AI. Time of development of occlusal and proximal lesions: implications for fissure sealants. J Public Health Dent 1986;46(2):114–121

42. Pereira AC, Eggertsson H, Martinez-Mier EA, Mialhe FL, Eckert GJ, Zero DT. Validity of caries detection on occlusal surfaces and treatment decisions based on results from multiple caries-detection methods. Eur J Oral Sci 2009;117(1):51–57

43. Oong EM, Griffin SO, Kohn WG, Gooch BF, Caufield PW. The effect of dental sealants on bacteria levels in caries lesions: a review of the evidence. J Am Dent Assoc 2008;139(3):271–278, quiz 357–358

44. Griffin SO, Oong E, Kohn W, et al. CDC Dental Sealant Systematic Review Work Group. The effectiveness of sealants in managing caries lesions. J Dent Res 2008;87(2):169–174

45. Hitt JC, Feigal RJ. Use of a bonding agent to reduce sealant sensitivity to moisture contamination: an in vitro study. Pediatr Dent 1992;14(1):41–46

46. Choi JW, Drummond JL, Dooley R, Punwani I, Soh JM. The efficacy of primer on sealant shear bond strength. Pediatr Dent 1997;19(4):286–288

47. Mascarenhas AK, Nazar H, Al-Mutawaa S, Soparkar P. Effectiveness of primer and bond in sealant retention and caries prevention. Pediatr Dent 2008;30(1):25–28

48. Griffin SO, Gray SK, Malvitz DM, Gooch BF. Caries risk in formerly sealed teeth. J Am Dent Assoc 2009;140(4):415–423

49. Griffin SO, Jones K, Gray SK, Malvitz DM, Gooch BF. Exploring four-handed delivery and retention of resin-based sealants. J Am Dent Assoc 2008;139(3):281–289, quiz 358

50. Simonsen RJ. Retention and effectiveness of dental sealant after 15 years. J Am Dent Assoc 1991;122(10):34–42

51. Jodkowska E. Efficacy of pit and fissure sealing: long-term clinical observations. Quintessence Int 2008;39(7):593–602

52. Hevinga MA, Opdam NJ, Bronkhorst EM, Truin GJ, Huysmans MC. Long-term performance of resin based fissure sealants placed in a general dental practice. J Dent 2010;38(1):23–28

53. Ahovuo-Saloranta A, Hiiri A, Nordblad A, Worthington H, Mäkelä M. Pit and fissure sealants for preventing dental decay in the permanent teeth of children and adolescents. Cochrane Database Syst Rev 2004;3(3):CD001830

54. Mejàre I, Lingström P, Petersson LG, et al. Caries-preventive effect of fissure sealants: a systematic review. Acta Odontol Scand 2003;61(6):321–330

55. Gooch BF, Griffin SO, Gray SK, et al; Centers for Disease Control and Prevention. Preventing dental caries through school-based sealant programs: updated recommendations and reviews of evidence. J Am Dent Assoc 2009;140(11):1356–1365

56. Deery C. The economic evaluation of pit and fissure sealants. Int J Paediatr Dent 1999;9(4):235–241

57. Griffin SO, Griffin PM, Gooch BF, Barker LK. Comparing the costs of three sealant delivery strategies. J Dent Res 2002;81(9):641–645

58. Quiñonez RB, Downs SM, Shugars D, Christensen J, Vann WF Jr. Assessing cost-effectiveness of sealant placement in children. J Public Health Dent 2005;65(2):82–89

59. Leskinen K, Salo S, Suni J, Larmas M. Practice-based study of the cost-effectiveness of fissure sealants in Finland. J Dent 2008;36(12):1074–1079

60. Bertrand E, Mallis M, Bui NM, Reinharz D. Cost-effectiveness simulation of a universal publicly funded sealants application program. J Public Health Dent 2011;71(1):38–45 10.1111/j.1752-7325.2010.00200x

61. Selwitz RH, Winn DM, Kingman A, Zion GR. The prevalence of dental sealants in the US population: findings from NHANES III, 1988–1991. J Dent Res 1996; 75(Spec):652–660

62. Beltrán-Aguilar ED, Barker LK, Canto MT, et al. Centers for Disease Control and Prevention (CDC). Surveillance for dental caries, dental sealants, tooth retention, edentulism, and enamel fluorosis—United States, 1988–1994 and 1999–2002. MMWR Surveill Summ 2005;54(3):1–43

63. Clarkson JE, Turner S, Grimshaw JM, et al. Changing clinicians' behavior: a randomized controlled trial of fees and education. J Dent Res 2008;87(7):640–644

64. Centers for Disease Control and Prevention (CDC). National Oral Health Surveillance System. Dental sealants. http://apps.nccd.cdc.gov/nohss/IndicatorV.asp?Indicator=1. Updated January 4, 2011. Accessed September 22, 2011

65. Ekstrand KR, Martignon S, Christiansen ME. Frequency and distribution patterns of sealants among 15-year-olds in Denmark in 2003. Community Dent Health 2007;24(1):26–30

66. Agustsdottir H, Gudmundsdottir H, Eggertsson H, et al. Caries prevalence of permanent teeth: a national survey of children in Iceland using ICDAS. Community Dent Oral Epidemiol 2010;38(4):299–309

67. Kervanto-Seppälä S, Pietilä I, Meurman JH, Kerosuo E. Pit and fissure sealants in dental public health – application criteria and general policy in Finland. BMC Oral Health 2009;9:5

68. Virtanen JI, Forsberg H, Ekman A. Timing and effect of fissure sealants on permanent molars: a study in Finland and Sweden. Swed Dent J 2003;27(4):159–165

69. Micheelis W, Schiffner U. Vierte Deutsche Mundgesundheitsstudie – (DMS IV): neue Ergebnisse zu oralen Erkrankungenprävalenzen, Risikogruppen und zum zahnärztlichen Vorsorgungsgrad in Deutschland 2005. Institut der Deutschen Zahnärzte (IDZ). IDZ Materialreihe Band 31. Köln: Deutscher Ärzte-Verlag; 2006

70. Splieth CH, Ekstrand KR, Alkilzy M, et al. Sealants in dentistry: outcomes of the ORCA Saturday Afternoon Symposium 2007. Caries Res 2010;44(1):3–13

Sealing of Approximal Surfaces

Stefania Martignon, Kim Ekstrand

16

The general decrease in caries experience among children and adolescents in the past 30 years[1] is based on a marked decrease in the most susceptible sites (occlusal surfaces), however, with a relative increase of lesions in the approximal and smooth surfaces.[2,3] Studies on young Swedish and Danish adults have shown that, even under strict preventive community measures, slow but continuous progression of approximal caries lesions from enamel into dentin can still be observed.[4,5] In a Swedish cohort of 11- to 13-year-olds proportion of those without radiographically apparent caries lesions increased from 28% to 71% within 8 years.[4] Also, in young adults in Denmark, approximal caries progressed. Over a 6-year period in 57% out of 73 young male adults, approximal lesions initially located in the enamel and extending up to the outer third of the dentin progressed or were restored.[5]

Thus, it seems that if approximal caries has developed it will progress, but slowly. One of the main reasons for this is the lack of patients' adherence in using dental floss.[6] It might be advisable to do some kind of more invasive treatment at some point. However, due to the impaired access to approximal caries lesions, not only their detection but also their restorative treatment is difficult. Often the removal of large amounts of sound enamel and dentin is necessary to "treat" the caries lesions. Owing to this unfavorable ratio for sound fissures, it is desirable to postpone the first invasive intervention for as long as possible and to arrest lesion progression by microinvasive measures, such as **approximal sealing**.

This chapter will cover in detail:
- The transfer of the sealing technique from the occlusal to the approximal surface
- Clinical procedures and dental materials to conduct approximal sealing
- Up-to-date knowledge on the efficacy and indication of approximal sealing

Transfer of the Sealing Technique from the Occlusal to the Approximal Surface

Three recent developments have led to the transfer of sealing techniques from occlusal to approximal surfaces:
- The perception that conventional noninvasive measures alone may not be capable of preventing lesion progression of approximal caries lesions in every individual.[7–11]
- The growing evidence on the efficacy of sealants to arrest caries progression on occlusal surfaces (see Chapter 15). Thus, for some years now, it has been widely recommended to seal initial carious lesions on occlusal surfaces, involving caries lesions with a radiographic severity from deep enamel lesions to lesions into the outer part of the dentin.[9–16]

- The third incentive for introducing sealing techniques for approximal caries lesions has been the prospect of better feasibility, by adopting tooth separation techniques from orthodontics. Hereby, lesion characteristics can be more easily assessed,[17] and materials used for sealing can be satisfactorily applied to the approximal surfaces.

These aspects led to the implementation of the sealing technique for approximal caries lesions, using adhesives or sealants.[18–20] Another method involves the application of an adhesive "patch" onto the enamel surface.[21] More recently, an infiltration method has been developed in particular for approximal caries lesions.[22] This chapter will focus on the sealing methods using either adhesives/sealants or adhesives in combination with the so-called patch.

Clinical Procedure

Which Approximal Lesions Should Be Sealed?

Diagnosis is an important first step before the treatment decision (see Chapters 5–9). As the visual–tactile accessibility of the approximal surfaces of posterior teeth is impaired, bitewing radiographs are used for the detection and assessment of the lesion depth, which correlate fairly well to the histological extension of the demineralization process[23,24] (see Chapter 3). Three main questions that relate to the decision to seal or not to seal approximal lesions need to be answered (see also Chapter 20).
- Is the lesion too deep or too shallow to be treated by sealants?
  - Shallow approximal lesions (confined histologically to enamel) will most likely be arrested by noninvasive measures only. These lesions can be detected on the radiograph as radiolucencies into the outer enamel.
  - A lesion which has extended radiographically into inner enamel or at maximum up to the outer third of the dentin would be suitable for sealing.
  - For deeper lesions radiographically into the middle third or deeper into the dentin, an invasive treatment should be recommended.[11,14,25,26]
- Is there a way to confirm that no cavity is present?
  - The depth of the radiolucency correlates fairly well with the probability of clinical cavitations being present.[23–25] A visual–tactile assessment of the caries lesion will allow for the detection of a cavity and should reinforce the radiographic assessment. This visual–tactile examination is conducted after a two-day temporary separation of the affected teeth (**Fig. 16.1**) using, for example, the ICDAS visual criteria,[27] or if it is not possible to do this assessment at a second appointment, it can be done by using a thin

probe to evaluate whether there is a clinically detectable surface breakdown.

- If the caries lesion has a white/brown opacity with, at the most, a slight surface breakdown in enamel, and the radiolucency depth extends at maximum into the outer dentinal third, sealing is recommended.[11]
- If there is a surface breakdown or a distinctive cavity with exposition of the dentin and the radiolucency extends the outer dentinal third, then invasive treatment is recommended.[11,26]

• Is it possible to assess if the caries lesion will progress in the future?

- The best predictor for assessing progression of approximal caries lesions would be repeated radiographic assessment over time.[26] At a single appointment several criteria have been proposed for lesion activity assessment that should be followed (see Chapter 5).[28]

Techniques for Approximal Sealing

Sealing Procedure[19]

To gain access to the approximal lesions, an orthodontic band is placed between the teeth for 2 days. In a second appointment, the band is removed and the lesion is cleaned with a solo-brush and dental floss. Cotton rolls are used to ensure relative dryness of the area. A wooden wedge is placed between the teeth to maintain the gained space and to absorb any excess of sealant; the neighboring tooth surface is covered with Teflon tape. Then the following treatment steps are performed (**Fig. 16.2**):

1. Etching of the surface with 37% phosphoric acid for 15 seconds
2. Thorough water-rinsing and air drying
3. Repeating of isolation using the Teflon tape
4. Application of the adhesive with a micro-brush and dental floss
5. Removal of excess material with dental floss

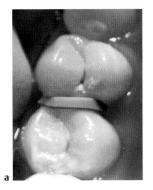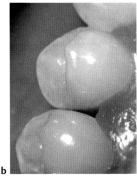

Fig. 16.1a, b Elective temporary separation. (Fig. 16.1a with permission from Schweizer Monatsschrift für Zahnmedizin; Meyer-Lückel H, Fejerskov O, Paris S., Forschung-Wissenschaft-Recherche-Science 2009; 5:454-460.)
a Placement of an elastic band for 2 days.
b Visual/tactile access to an approximal lesion.

6. Re-application of the adhesive
7. 5-second air drying from a distance
8. Light curing from lingual/palatal and from buccal directions
9. Polishing

In a Swedish study approximal sealing was performed quite similarly, also after tooth separation.[20]

Patch Technique[21]

The approximal area is etched using 37% phosphoric acid for 60 seconds after separating the teeth. Afterwards, a bonding agent is applied and the adhesive patch, a thin polyurethane-dimethacrylate foil (not available for sale), is placed on the approximal surface and light cured. Finally, the margins of the patch are polished with discs and strips.

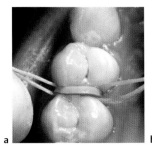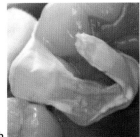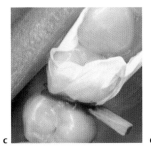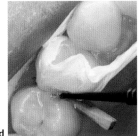

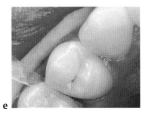

Fig. 16.2a–e Procedure for approximal sealing of a lesion in the distal surface of the first upper right premolar tooth. (Fig. 16.2d with permission from Schweizer Monatsschrift für Zahnmedizin; Meyer-Lückel H, Fejerskov O, Paris S., Forschung-Wissenschaft-Recherche-Science 2009; 5:454–460)
a Elective temporary separation of involved teeth.
b Isolation of neighboring tooth with Teflon tape.
c Etching of lesion's surface.
d Adhesive application.
e Polishing of sealed lesion.

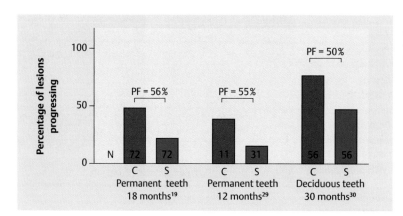

Fig. 16.3 Progression status of sealed (S) and control (C) approximal lesions in three clinical studies.[19,29,30] The preventive fraction (PF) is around 50% in favor for sealing over noninvasive measures alone.

Clinical Evidence

Approximal sealing as described above[19] was tested in a split-mouth design study on 82 young adults, each having at least two approximal caries lesions in posterior teeth with radiolucencies at maximum into the outer third of the dentin. One lesion in each patient was sealed and the other one received no treatment (control). Participants were instructed to floss all surfaces with approximal lesions, including control and test lesions. After 18 months, sealed approximal caries lesions (n=72) showed significantly less caries progression (22%) than the controls (47%) (**Fig. 16.3**). The same trend was seen after 3–4 years. A second study (no split-mouth design) focusing on effectiveness of sealing (OptiBond Solo, Kerr) to arrest noncavitated approximal caries lesions (radiographically up to half of the dentin) in permanent teeth revealed progression of 16% and 36% of the sealed and nonsealed lesions, respectively, after 1 year[29] (**Fig. 16.3**).

Approximal sealing of caries lesions has also been considered in pre-school children.[30] In this age group, the distal surface of the first primary molar is one of the sites where caries lesions may develop. Available data about the caries progression rate in primary teeth suggest that it is at least twice as high compared with that in permanent teeth.[31] Thus, a split-mouth design study was conducted in 91 4–6-year-olds with at least two radiolucencies up to the outer third of the dentin on the distal surface of first primary molars.[30] One lesion was sealed and patients' caregivers received flossing instructions for all interproximal spaces, including those with nonsealed control lesions. The 12-month radiographic evaluation showed dis-

ease progression in 27% of the test lesions and 51% of the control lesions. After 2.5 years (n = 56) corresponding numbers were 46% and 71%, respectively (**Fig. 16.3**). This study included the assessment of the child's behavior and of pain intensity, both at the appointment when the elastic band was positioned as well as when the sealing was performed. Most children (88%) did not report negative feelings at either appointment. Recently, the efficacy of sealing approximal caries lesions was compared to infiltration as well as non invasive treatment alone. The preventive fraction of sealing and infiltration were 42% and 54%, respectively, compared to the third group.[32]

In another sealing study conducted on 50 adolescents with approximal enamel radiolucencies in posterior teeth in one group (n = 17) all enamel caries lesions were sealed.[20] In a second group (n = 7), patients received approximal sealants and fluoride varnish in a split-mouth design; finally, a control group (n = 26) received a standard fluoride varnish treatment. After 2 years disease progression of lesions was found in 7% of the sealed lesions versus 12% in the fluoride-varnish control group, with no statistically significant differences between groups.

The patch technique was also evaluated.[21] Here, 50 patients each with two approximal caries lesions (radiolucency without cavitation) either received the patch using a bonding agent or no treatment (control). Generally, dental flossing and the use of fluoride toothpaste for home care were recommended. The 24-month evaluation (n = 35) showed progression in 6% of both test and control groups and 8% in both groups after 36 months (n = 25). The benefit of the patch approach could not be demonstrated in this study due to the low caries incidence in this population.

Caries Diagnosis and Treatment Decision

The detection of the severity of the lesion should be as precise as possible and should take into consideration aspects such as the caries prevalence and progression rate of the population and the individual caries risk and compliance of the patient. Regarding the first point, the study conducted in preschool children[30] reported a high percentage of progression in both sealed and control lesions after 12 months, which could be explained by the higher progression rate of enamel lesions into dentin in primary teeth in comparison to permanent teeth.[31] So, for primary teeth it seems to be advisable to seal caries lesions that are extended radiographically at maximum up to the enamel–dentinal junction. This also applies to patients with high caries risk.

Clinical Procedure

The two patient appointments needed for allowing the elective temporary separation of the teeth is a disadvantage of this approach in terms of time, even though it adds diagnostic information. Regarding the procedure, an absolute isolation technique with the rubber dam would diminish the possibility of contamination of the dental material. The etching time should be extended to 1 minute, due to the inhomogeneous nature of approximal lesions. Surfaces should be dried with ethanol immediately after etching.[11,14,15]

In conclusion, the sealing of approximal caries lesions is a valuable alternative for preserving sound tooth structure that should be considered in the clinic.

REFERENCES

1. Baelum V, van Palenstein Helderman W, Hugoson A, Yee R, Fejerskov O. A global perspective on changes in the burden of caries and periodontitis: implications for dentistry. J Oral Rehabil 2007;34(12):872–906, discussion 940
2. McDonald SP, Sheiham A. The distribution of caries on different tooth surfaces at varying levels of caries—a compilation of data from 18 previous studies. Community Dent Health 1992;9(1):39–48
3. Ekstrand KR, Carvalho JC, Thylstrup A. Restorative caries treatment patterns in Danish 20-year-old males in 1986 and 1991. Community Dent Oral Epidemiol 1994;22(2):75–79
4. Mejàre I, Källestål C, Stenlund H, Johansson H. Caries development from 11 to 22 years of age: a prospective radiographic study. Prevalence and distribution. Caries Res 1998;32(1):10–16
5. Martignon S, Chavarría N, Ekstrand KR. Caries status and proximal lesion behaviour during a 6-year period in young adult Danes: an epidemiological investigation. Clin Oral Investig 2010;14(4):383–390
6. Frandsen A. Changing patterns of attitudes and oral health behaviour. Int Dent J 1985;35(4):284–290
7. Hujoel PP, Cunha-Cruz J, Banting DW, Loesche WJ. Dental flossing and interproximal caries: a systematic review. J Dent Res 2006;85(4):298–305
8. Autio-Gold J. The role of chlorhexidine in caries prevention. Oper Dent 2008;33(6):710–716
9. Ahovuo-Saloranta A, Hiiri A, Nordblad A, Mäkelä M, Worthington HV. Pit and fissure sealants for preventing dental decay in the permanent teeth of children and adolescents. Cochrane Database Syst Rev 2008;(4, Issue 4):CD001830 10.1002/14651858.CD001830.pub3
10. Hiiri A, Ahovuo-Saloranta A, Nordblad A, Mäkelä M. Pit and fissure sealants versus fluoride varnishes for preventing dental decay in children and adolescents. Cochrane Database Syst Rev 2006;(4, Issue 4):CD003067 10.1002/14651858.CD003067.pub2
11. Splieth CH, Ekstrand KR, Alkilzy M, et al. Sealants in dentistry: outcomes of the ORCA Saturday Afternoon Symposium 2007. Caries Res 2010;44(1):3–13
12. Handelman SL. Therapeutic use of sealants for incipient or early carious lesions in children and young adults. Proc Finn Dent Soc 1991;87(4):463–475
13. García-Godoy F, Summitt JB, Donly KJ. Caries progression of white spot lesions sealed with an unfilled resin. J Clin Pediatr Dent 1997;21(2):141–143
14. Griffin SO, Oong E, Kohn W, et al; CDC Dental Sealant Systematic Review Work Group. The effectiveness of sealants in managing caries lesions. J Dent Res 2008;87(2):169–174
15. Beauchamp J, Caufield PW, Crall JJ, et al; American Dental Association Council on Scientific Affairs. Evidence-based clinical recommendations for the use of pit-and-fissure sealants: a report of the American Dental Association Council on Scientific Affairs. J Am Dent Assoc 2008;139(3):257–268
16. Ekstrand KR, Ricketts DNJ, Kidd EAM. Occlusal caries: pathology, diagnosis and logical management. Dent Update 2001;28(8):380–387
17. Pitts NB, Longbottom C. Temporary tooth separation with special reference to the diagnosis and preventive management of equivocal approximal carious lesions. Quintessence Int 1987;18(8):563–573
18. Ekstrand K, Martignon S. Managing approximal carious lesions: A new non-operative approach. [ORCA abstract] Caries Res 2004;38:361
19. Martignon S, Ekstrand KR, Ellwood R. Efficacy of sealing proximal early active lesions: an 18-month clinical study evaluated by conventional and subtraction radiography. Caries Res 2006;40(5):382–388
20. Gomez S, Uribe S, Onetto JE, Emilson CG. SEM analysis of sealant penetration in posterior approximal enamel carious lesions in vivo. J Adhes Dent 2008;10(2):151–156
21. Alkilzy M, Berndt Ch, Meller Ch, Schidlowski M, Splieth C. Sealing of proximal surfaces with polyurethane tape: a two-year clinical and radiographic feasibility study. J Adhes Dent 2009;11(2):91–94
22. Meyer-Lueckel H, Paris S. Progression of artificial enamel caries lesions after infiltration with experimental light curing resins. Caries Res 2008;42(2):117–124
23. Ekstrand KR, Luna LE, Promisiero L, et al. The reliability and accuracy of two methods for proximal caries detection and depth on directly visible proximal surfaces: an in vitro study. Caries Res 2011;45(2):93–99
24. Ekstrand KR, Ricketts DNJ, Kidd EAM. Reproducibility and accuracy of three methods for assessment of demineralization depth of the occlusal surface: an in vitro examination. Caries Res 1997;31(3):224–231
25. Bille J, Thylstrup A. Radiographic diagnosis and clinical tissue changes in relation to treatment of approximal carious lesions. Caries Res 1982;16(1):1–6
26. Kidd EAM, van Amerongen JP, van Amerongen WE. The role of operative treatment in caries control. In: Fejerskov O, Kidd E, eds. Dental Caries: The Disease and its Clinical Management. 2nd ed. Oxford: Blackwell Munksgaard; 2008:355–366

27. Ismail AI, Sohn W, Tellez M, et al. The International Caries Detection and Assessment System (ICDAS): an integrated system for measuring dental caries. Community Dent Oral Epidemiol 2007;35(3):170–178

28. Ekstrand KR, Martignon S, Ricketts DJ, Qvist V. Detection and activity assessment of primary coronal caries lesions: a methodologic study. Oper Dent 2007;32(3):225–235

29. Abuchaim C, Rotta M, Grande RH, Loguercio AD, Reis A. Effectiveness of sealing active proximal caries lesions with an adhesive system: 1-year clinical evaluation. Braz Oral Res 2010;24(3): 361–367

30. Martignon S, Tellez M, Santamaría RM, Gomez J, Ekstrand KR. Sealing distal proximal caries lesions in first primary molars: efficacy after 2.5 years. Caries Res 2010;44(6):562–570

31. Shwartz M, Gröndahl H-G, Pliskin JS, Boffa J. A longitudinal analysis from bite-wing radiographs of the rate of progression of approximal carious lesions through human dental enamel. Arch Oral Biol 1984;29(7):529–536

32. Martignon S, Ekstrand KR, Gomez J, Lara JS, Cortes A. Infiltrating/Sealing Proximal Caries Lesions: A 3-Year Randomized Clinical Trial. J Dent Res 2012;91:288–292

Caries Infiltration

Hendrik Meyer-Lueckel, Sebastian Paris

17

The microinvasive procedures for occlusal and approximal sealing described in the previous chapters use materials that are familiar from restorative therapy. According to the clinical procedure, the tooth surface is etched with phosphoric acid, then adhesive or fissure sealant is applied which is subsequently light cured.

In this chapter, a microinvasive treatment will be described that was introduced to general dentistry in 2009, namely caries infiltration. In this technique for arresting the progress of caries, a comparatively strong acid (hydrochloric acid 15%) is required to condition the carious tooth surface, and resins with a modified monomer composition, so-called **infiltrants**, are applied. In contrast to adhesives and fissure sealants, these highly liquid resins are able to penetrate the porous structures of the lesion body more deeply and thereby obstruct the diffusion pathways for cariogenic acids. In caries infiltration as opposed to the (occlusal) sealing of caries, the diffusion barrier is created not on but within the caries itself [1–4] (**Fig. 17.1**).

In detail this chapter will cover:
- The development of caries infiltration
- The biological and therapeutic backgrounds of caries infiltration
- The use of caries infiltration to arrest caries progression
- The use of caries infiltration for esthetic reasons

Development of Caries Infiltration

Biological Principles

As described in Chapters 2 and 3, the early-to-intermediate stages of enamel caries manifest a pronounced demineralization of the tooth enamel (lesion body) below an apparently intact surface layer. The elevated mineral loss alters the refraction of light, which gives the lesions their white appearance (white spots). During remineralization, pigments can become incorporated, and the caries lesion assumes a darker color (brown spots). A major portion of these caries lesions that are clearly visible to the dentist (ICDAS 2) is not limited histologically to the enamel. The dentin underneath is also demineralized. Such caries lesions in approximal surfaces (histological extension around the enamel–dentin junction) will be visible in x-ray radiographs as being extended into the enamel only. Thus, the appearance of the caries in the x-ray image under-represents the actual histological extension (see Chapters 5 and 6). Such caries lesions that appear restricted to the enamel in the x-ray photo rarely show cavitated surfaces.

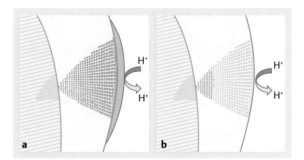

Fig. 17.1a, b   A diffusion barrier is created on the surface by sealing (**a**) a caries lesion. In infiltration (**b**), a low-viscosity resin penetrates the pores of the lesion body and is light cured. Both resins prevent acids as well as substrates for microorganisms from penetrating.

NOTE

Radiographs of enamel lesions (E1 and E2) rarely reveal cavitation. Once the caries has advanced up to the first third of the dentin as shown in the x-ray (D1), cavitation is clinically detectable in approximately one-third of lesions.[5,6]

In contrast to cavitated lesions, noncavitated caries lesions only manifest a few bacteria in the area of the lesion body, and there is no established biofilm.[7] Cavitated caries lesions are more difficult to clean, which is why there is a greater probability that they will progress.[8]

BACKGROUND

Pioneering Work on Penetration of Resins in Caries Lesions

The possibility of penetrating caries with resins was first described in the 1970s, by using artificial enamel caries with a surface layer that was less mineralized than natural carious enamel. Natural lesions are difficult to penetrate with the adhesive that was employed.[9] The progress of caries in artificial lesions was demonstrably halted by applying a low-viscosity resin. However, the material that was used in this study, resorcinol formaldehyde, was highly unsuitable for clinical use due to its toxic properties.[10] The observations of using adhesives for penetrating caries lesions were confirmed in a few subsequent investigations.[11–17] These authors generally described a seal that essentially covers the surface using commercially available adhesives which leaves a surface layer of material. It was revealed that multiple applications of the sealant improved the penetration of the resins.[16] This causes a comparatively strong reduction in the pore volume.[10,15] Generally, in these studies any excess resin on the surface was left, it is assumed, to at least partially block the access of acids to any remaining pores in the lesion body.[10,15] The positive association of penetration depth with application time was also dem-

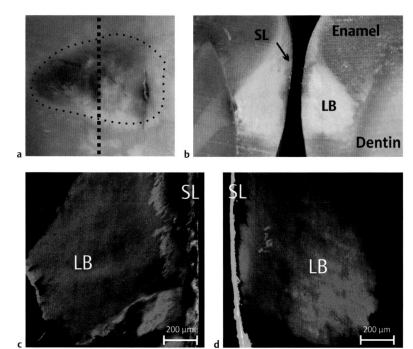

Fig. 17.2a–d This approximal caries lesion (**a**) has some areas that can be identified as *inactive* (brown) and *active* (whitish, opaque surface) (dashed line = cut). The section surface (**b**) reveals the histological correlation between the *thickness of the surface layer* and the clinically identified *activity*. Active areas (bottom lesion area) have a thinner surface layer (SL) than inactive areas. The lesion body (LB) in the enamel extends up to the enamel–dentin junction. The left and right halves of the lesion were etched with hydrochloric and phosphoric acid, respectively, and adhesive was applied. In the confocal microscopic images, it can be seen that etching with hydrochloric acid (**c**) enables the resin to penetrate slightly deeper (diffuse, dark portion + green area) into the lesion body (LB; red) than when phosphoric acid is used for etching (**d**).

onstrated by removing the excess from the surface of artificial lesions.[18] Furthermore, the employed adhesives and fissure sealants inhibited caries to different degrees depending on the application time and homogeneity of the created resin layer within the lesion body.[19]

Development of Caries Infiltration

Even after the tooth surface is etched for 2 minutes with phosphoric acid, the adhesives have difficulty penetrating natural caries lesions.[20] This is due to the relatively low pore volume of the surface layer which prevents deeper penetration, and the inadequate physical properties of available adhesives.[20] Etching the tooth surface for 2 minutes with hydrochloric acid gel (15%) specifically erodes the surface layer[21] and enables the adhesive to penetrate at maximum ca. 100 µm into natural caries lesions[20] (**Fig. 17.2**). On the other hand, monomers of low viscosity may penetrate the demineralized enamel, which can be viewed as a system of minute capillaries much more easily. The penetrating properties of a liquid are described by the **Washburn equation**,[22] where the term in parentheses represents the **penetration coefficient** (PC).[23,24]

$$x^2 = \left(\frac{\gamma \times \cos\theta}{2\eta} \right) r \times t$$

The higher the PC, the faster a liquid will flow through the capillary of radius r over time t to traverse the path x. The PC and the components that determine it are temperature dependent.[23,25]

First, the PCs of a few combinations of monomers were determined,[26] and some of these materials were investigated with regard to their penetrating[27] and caries-

inhibiting[28] properties using artificial caries lesions. The penetration depth of the monomers correlates with the root of the product of the PC and the application time. This means that the penetration coefficient of the monomer mixture is a good predictor of its penetrating and caries-inhibiting ability. Materials with a penetration coefficient above 50 cm/s were consequently termed **infiltrants**.[27,28]

Penetration experiments using the infiltrants on natural lesions revealed results comparable with those for artificial lesions. In an initial study, it was found that the penetration depth of an infiltrant was significantly higher than that of the adhesive used in previous experiments.[29] In particular, infiltrants with a PC above 200 cm/s almost completely penetrated enamel lesions with an average depth of ca. 900 µm.[30,31] The infiltrated lesions were then stored in a demineralization solution to induce the further progress of caries. In contrast to untreated controls, the progress of caries was almost completely stopped by the infiltrants after 400 days of storage in a demineralizing environment at pH 4.95.[32] The relatively long application time of 5 minutes used in these experiments could apparently be shortened to 3 minutes.[31] Treating the tooth surface once with ethanol to dry it directly before applying the infiltrant was not inferior to using acetone.[33]

An initial study of the efficacy of preventing the progress of caries was performed in situ. Ten test subjects wore removable appliances in this experiment. Enamel samples containing artificial caries were placed in these. One part of the lesions was treated before the in situ phase with an infiltrant, and another part served as an untreated (negative) control. Enamel samples with artificial

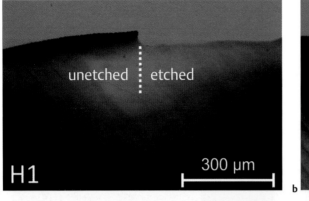

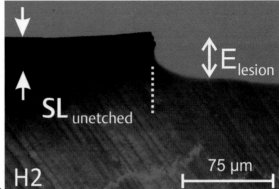

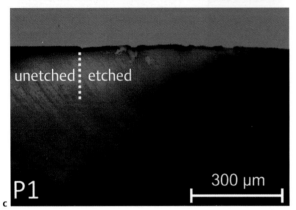

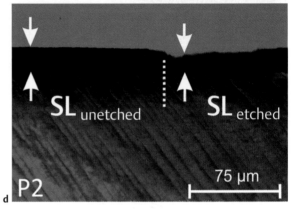

Fig. 17.3a–d Before infiltration with the resin, the caries lesion is etched for 2 minutes with hydrochloric acid gel (**a**, **b**). In contrast to etching with phosphoric acid (**c**, **d**), this significantly reduces the surface layer (SL) to provide access to the pores of the lesion body by erosion (E). (Reproduced with kind permission of Elsevier GmbH from Paris S, Dorfer CE, Meyer-Lueckel H. Surface conditioning of natural enamel caries lesions in deciduous teeth in preparation for resin infiltration. J Dent 2009;38: 65–71.)

caries to which a layer of fissure sealant was applied served as a positive control. The infiltrated areas and positive controls manifested an insignificant amount of caries progression after being worn for 100 days, whereas the untreated areas progressed ca. 100%.[34] These positive results served as a foundation for clinically testing the efficacy of infiltration.

NOTE

The principle of caries infiltration is based on the penetration of a low-viscosity resin (infiltrant) into the lesion body of the caries. After it hardens, the infiltrant seals the pores of the lesion and therefore offers a diffusion barrier to acids and fermentable carbohydrates.

Principle of Caries Infiltration

The relatively strongly mineralized surface layer of caries prevents resins from penetrating the lesion body.[20] Consequently, the surface should first be specifically eroded with a **hydrochloric acid gel.** This cannot be achieved with a phosphoric acid gel even after a long exposure time[21,35] (**Fig. 17.3**). After the surface has been sufficiently etched and is **fully dry**, the **infiltrant** is able to penetrate natural caries lesions up to a few hundred micrometers[29,30] (**Fig. 17.4**). After it hardens, the resin seals the caries internally to prevent the further progression of caries.[32,34,36]

As a positive side-effect, the enamel areas of caries lesions lose their whitish appearance after infiltration. These carious areas are therefore visually similar to healthy enamel. This **masking effect** is based on a modification of the light refraction within the enamel lesion. Healthy enamel has a refractive index (RI) of 1.62. The microporosity within enamel caries is either filled with an aqueous medium (RI: 1.33) or air (RI: 1.0). The different **refraction indices** cause light to scatter at the boundary surfaces which gives these lesions a whitish opaque appearance, particularly when dry.[37] The micropores of the infiltrated lesions are in contrast filled with resin (RI: 1.52) which cannot evaporate like the aqueous medium. Due to the relatively slight difference between the refraction indices of the infiltrated pores and that of the surrounding

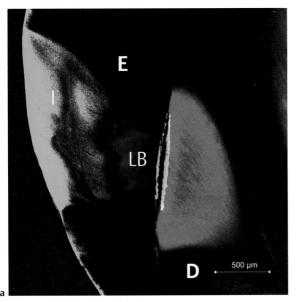

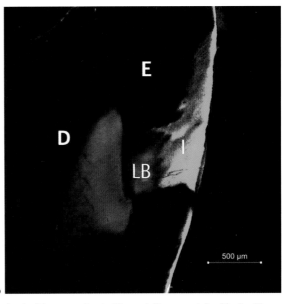

Fig. 17.4a, b Confocal microscopic photographs of two approximal caries lesions that were treated for 3 minutes with the infiltrant (I; green) after being etched with HCl (15%) for 120 seconds. The remaining pores in the lesion body (LB) of the enamel caries (E) and dentin (D) were stained with a red, fluorescent dye [the healthy enamel (E) and dentin (D) are black]. These images illustrate that the infiltrant can penetrate nearly the entire enamel portion of a lesion extending into the dentin.

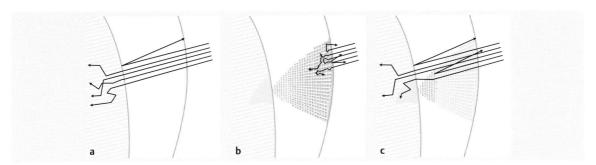

Fig. 17.5a–c Optical phenomena play a role in the masking of esthetically relevant caries lesions. Healthy enamel (refraction index [RI] = 1.62) is almost transparent to light (**a**). If there is a caries lesion, the light scatters at the boundary surface between the pores and mineral (**b**). Since the media in the pores (saliva [RI = 1.3], or air [RI = 1] after drying) have a comparatively low refractive index, the light is reflected more strongly, and the nondiscolored caries lesion therefore appears white (**b**). The refractive index of the infiltrant is 1.52; consequently, after this material has penetrated, it visually matches the surrounding healthy enamel. To optimize the appearance of the caries lesion, it should be infiltrated as deeply as possible (**c**).

healthy enamel, the caries appears much less white than before infiltration[38] (**Fig. 17.5**).

> **NOTE**
>
> The masking of caries by means of infiltration is based on the change in the refraction index of the caries lesion.

Infiltration to Prevent Caries Progression

Due to the strong epidemiological relevance of approximal caries (see Chapter 8) and the few therapeutic options available (either surveillance plus use of fluorides, or filling), caries infiltration was chiefly developed to prevent the progression of caries in these surfaces. Other smooth surfaces (especially of the anterior and buccal teeth) can be infiltrated to stop the progression of caries, especially in patients with a high risk of caries. However, one should avoid overtreating, and microinvasive treatments have to be balanced against noninvasive forms of intervention. In most patients with low or moderate risk for caries, buccal

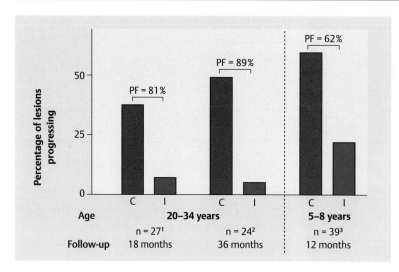

Fig. 17.6 Overview of the percentage progression of approximal caries lesions in control (C) and infiltrated (I) teeth in the two clinical split-mouth studies that have been published (left: Paris et al.[36]; Meyer-Lueckel et al.[39] right: Ekstrand et al. [40]). PF: preventative fraction = relative reduction of the risk of caries by infiltration.

lesions remineralize as a result of enhanced oral hygiene or altered nutritional habits. Consequently, caries infiltration is rarely indicated for these smooth surfaces, which are easily accessible to oral hygiene (Chapter 20).

Clinical Efficacy of Infiltrating Approximal Surfaces

In a clinical study of 20–34-year-olds in Germany, caries lesions in approximal surfaces of posterior teeth were treated. In the radiographs, the lesions extended at a minimum into the inner half of the enamel (E2), and at a maximum into the first third of the dentin (D1). Each patient was assigned one test lesion (infiltration) and one control caries (split-mouth design). Using digital subtraction radiography, it was found that 37% of the control lesions and only 7% of the infiltrated lesions had progressed after 18 months of observation.[36] After 3 years of observation, 46% of the control lesions and 4% of the infiltrated caries lesions had progressed[39] (**Fig. 17.6**). Another clinical study of caries infiltration was performed on deciduous molars in 5–8-year-olds with relatively high caries risk. In addition to infiltration treatment, fluoride varnish was applied to the control and infiltrated lesions every 6 months. The radiographs revealed that 62% of the control lesions and 23% of infiltrated lesions (both mainly D1 at baseline) had progressed after 12 months[40] (**Fig. 17.6**).

The infiltration technique as it is used today has certain limits. Particularly for patients with a high caries risk, lesions that have progressed radiographically into the first third of the dentin should only be referred to caries infiltration with caution. The probability that these caries lesions already show microcavitations that cannot be completely filled with the infiltrant might be increased, which sets the lesion at a higher risk for progression. However, in general the clinical data on sealing approximal caries lesions support the thesis that tightly sealing

caries enamel and dentin halts the advance of caries ("seal and heal," see Chapters 15 and 20).

At present, there are no clinical studies on the progression of post-infiltrated caries in other smooth surfaces besides approximal smooth surfaces. Up to now, existing infiltrants have not been optimized to treat fissure caries efficaciously.

Indications for Approximal Caries Infiltration

To determine whether approximal caries infiltration is indicated:
- The extent of the caries lesion must be assessed radiographically.
- The presence of a clinically relevant cavitation of the lesion surface needs to be assessed as well.
- The probability of caries progression needs to be evaluated.

Patient-related factors also influence the choice of therapy such as the individual's caries risk (Chapters 7–9, 20).

As noted earlier, caries lesions restricted radiographically to the enamel generally represent only a small proportion (< 5%) of **clinically detectable cavitations**[5,6] (**Fig. 17.7**). Consequently, invasive therapy is rarely indicated in this case for approximal caries. Since a significant percentage of enamel lesions progress, especially when the relevant surface is insufficiently cleaned,[8] caries infiltration is recommended as an alternative procedure to noninvasive treatment in caries-active patients when the approximal caries lesions are in the advanced enamel stage (revealed by bitewing x-rays).

When radiographs reveal that the approximal caries extends to the outer third of the dentin, clinically identifiable cavitation of the lesion surface exists in about one-third of such cases.[5,6] However, this means that two-thirds of radiographically determined D1 lesions do not show clinically relevant cavitations (**Fig. 17.8**), which explains why these lesions do not always progress.[8,41]

Presently available infiltrants do not sufficiently fill microcavities (**Fig. 17.9**), and they do not fill large enamel cavities at all. It can therefore be assumed that the progress of lesions with (micro)cavities is arrested less successfully by infiltration than is the progress of lesions without cavitation.[42] Consequently, before infiltration, the presence of **cavitation** should be investigated with a **thin probe** (such as a cowhorn-ended explorer) so that lesions with large cavitation can be excluded from infiltration treatment. It is preferable to restore such cavities (**Fig. 17.10**).

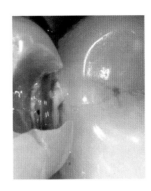

Fig. 17.7   After the neighboring tooth was prepared to insert a filling, a clinically relevant cavity in the adjacent tooth is clearly visualized. The remaining carious portion of the enamel could be infiltrated, but the macroscopic cavity will not be filled.

NOTE

Approximal caries infiltration is indicated for progressive caries lesions which extend radiographically at most into the outer third of the dentin without clinically identifiable cavitation (**Table 17.1**).

To increase the accuracy of the caries evaluation in bitewing x-rays, it is recommended to use the individualizable x-ray film holders presented in Chapter 6 (see also Chapter 25 Case 1). Given the reduced thickness of the approximal surfaces of deciduous molars (Chapter 22), caries infiltration is indicated even when the caries lesions are limited to the outer enamel in the radiograph.[40]

To maximize the efficacy of caries infiltration, the technique should only be used in the situations listed in **Table 17.1** according to our present knowledge. In addition, a few basic contraindications and other current restrictions to use can be specified (**Tables 17.2** and **17.3**).

Table 17.1   Caries infiltration options

Location	Clinical signs	Deciduous teeth	Permanent dentition
Approximal	Noncavitated	√	√
Other smooth surfaces (indication: caries)	Noncavitated	High caries risk	High caries risk
Vestibular/anterior (indication: esthetic)	Noncavitated; possibly in combination with a filling	No	√

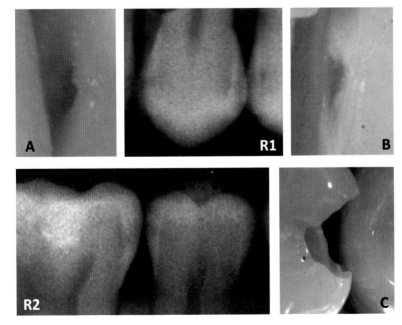

Fig. 17.8   The 26-year-old female patient has four approximal lesions in teeth 24 (mesial/distal) and 25 (mesial) (see R1) as well as 45 (distal) and 46 (mesial) (see R2) that extend into the dentin according to the x-ray image. Only the lesion in 24 mesial has a visible cavitation (**A**). The noncavitated yet active caries lesion in tooth 25 mesial (white-to-brown and opaque) is clearly visible after the cavity in tooth 24 distal was prepared (**B**). The distal surface of tooth 45 appears nearly unchanged in a clinical setting (**C**). When teeth are in approximal contact, the visual detection is much more difficult, but the lesions can at least be evaluated by probing (see **Fig. 17.10**).

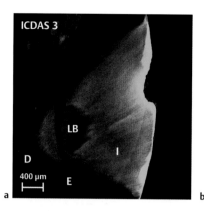

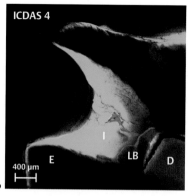

Fig. 17.9a, b The confocal microscopic pictures illustrate that the lesion body (LB, red) is penetrated by the infiltrant (I, green) both in the case of an approximal ICDAS 3 lesion and an ICDAS 4 lesion. However, it is not assured that the cavitation will be filled E: enamel, D: dentin). (With permission from John Wiley & Sons, from Paris S, et al., European Journal of Oral Sciences 2011;119(2):182–186)[42]

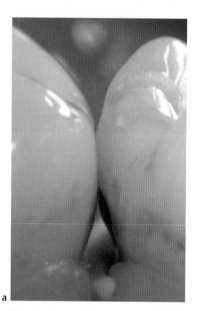

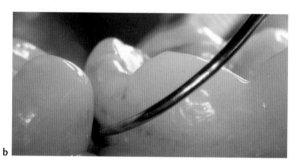

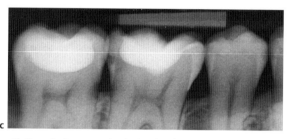

Fig. 17.10a–c This cavitation is hardly visible with the naked eye, even after displacing the papilla downward using a wedge and with high magnification (**a**). Cavitation is clinically detectable when checked with a thin probe (**b**). On the radiograph, the caries lesion at the distal surface of tooth 46 extends into the outer third of the dentin (**c**).

Table 17.2   Contraindications for caries infiltration

ICDAS 4, 5 and 6 and/or radiologic stage >D1
Nonprogressive caries lesions (indication: caries)
Root caries (dentin)
Erosion

Table 17.3   Diseases for which caries infiltration should be applied with caution[a]

Nonprogressive caries lesions (indication: Esthetic)
Caries lesions in fissures and grooves
Molar-incisor hypomineralization, Amelogenesis imperfecta
Fluorosis
Developmental changes in the enamel resulting from trauma

[a]The efficacy of these treatments has not yet been scientifically confirmed. In particular, caries infiltration is frequently unsuccessful in treating esthetically relevant developmental defects.

Clinical Use of Approximal Caries Infiltration

Another important consideration is the clinical feasibility of sealing or infiltrating approximal lesions. The contact between teeth can be sufficiently separated with orthodontic rubber rings,[43–45] making it easier to access the lesion. The separation time is up to two days, however, which needs to be taken into consideration when planning the sealing. For the most part, patients apparently tolerate this procedure for improving the diagnosis of approximal caries, even when used several times[44]; however, it is can be assumed that repeated use is not very practical.

As mentioned in the previous chapter, the teeth to be treated with approximal caries sealing have to be separated for a few days.[46] For infiltration, the corresponding teeth are only separated a few micrometers by flattened wedges, and the materials (hydrochloric acid gel and infiltrant) are applied sequentially with a special application tool. The neighboring teeth are protected from accidental contamination by an application device. The treatment only takes a single session (see Chapter 26). Another significant advantage of approximal caries infiltration over conventional sealants is that the excess material is removed before the tooth surface is light cured. There is therefore no excess material with edges that can retain cariogenic plaque.

CLINICAL PEARL

Infiltration of approximal caries can be accomplished in a single session; tooth separation for a period of days is not necessary.

Follow-up for Approximal Caries

The depth of penetration of the infiltrant cannot be determined after treatment, at least with today's technology, due to the resin's lack of radio-opacity. Neither is a second x-ray image taken directly after infiltration recommended, especially given the necessity of restricting exposure of the patient to ionizing rays. After infiltration therapy, the progression of the caries should be monitored using bitewing radiography at intervals appropriate for each individual, ranging from 6 to 48 months[47] (see Chapter 6) so that the caries lesions can be treated invasively in a timely manner if they enlarge (e.g., if the caries progresses to the middle third of the dentin). When the x-rays are taken, make sure that no overlapping of the approximal surfaces occurs, so that the stage of the caries can be determined with sufficient precision. In addition, make sure that the film and central beam are aligned in the same manner in relation to the teeth to avoid misinterpreting the progression or regression of caries owing to differences in the projection. (Chapter 25, Case 1).

NOTE

The only way to measure the success of approximal caries infiltration over the medium and long term is to determine in radiographs if the progression of the caries has been prevented or slowed, as is the case with the regular monitoring of caries or fissure sealants.

To keep sealed or infiltrated surfaces from being treated prematurely after changing dentists, the patient is given a "treatment booklet" in which the radiographic depth of the treated teeth is noted. This booklet also makes it easier for the subsequent dentist to request existing radiographs and the individualized x-ray holder from the previous dentist.

Infiltration for Primarily Esthetic Reasons

In addition to approximal surface application, infiltration of the enamel parts of caries is useful for esthetic reasons (especially vestibular surfaces). Caries lesions in these surfaces frequently arise after wearing orthodontic brackets, since some patients do not sufficiently clean the associated tooth surfaces.[48,49] After the brackets are removed, very superficial caries lesions frequently **remineralize** completely due to improved oral hygiene, although this rarely occurs with deeper caries lesions. Such lesions remain noticeable as inactive white or brown spots. These generally do not represent a cariological problem, but they are frequently an **esthetic impairment**[49] (**Fig. 17.11a** and **Fig. 17.12a**). The infiltrant has a visual appearance similar to healthy enamel (see above). Noncavitated caries lesions can therefore be masked by infiltration[38] (**Fig. 17.11b** and **Fig. 17.12b**).

Scientific Studies

Brushing abrasion of infiltrated lesion areas is similar to that of healthy enamel.[50] In addition, infiltrated lesions that are polished in vitro show similar resistance to staining as healthy teeth.[50] Existing case reports on clinical efficacy in terms of esthetic improvement have been positive.[38] In an initial clinical study, ca. 65% of **caries lesions** were fully masked, and 35% were partially masked. In contrast, only a few **developmentally related** white enamel changes were completely masked[52] (**Fig. 17.13**).

ERRORS AND RISKS

Caution: Developmentally related whitish enamel will not be sufficiently masked by caries infiltration in many cases.

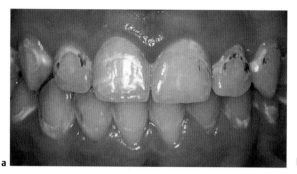

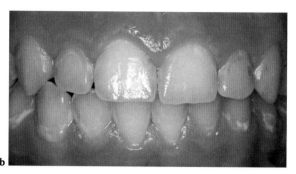

Fig. 17.11a, b During orthodontic treatment with a fixed, orthodontic appliance, adjacent enamel may demineralize (in particular cervical to the brackets). Patients might see these as an esthetic impairment, as seen after bracket removal (**a**). Four weeks later, the upper front teeth were infiltrated. Even 1 year afterward a satisfying esthetic result is still apparent (**b**). Superficial discolorations as seen partially on tooth 22 can be removed by polishing. Most notably, after 1 year those caries lesions in the lower jaw that were not infiltrated, but accessible for remineralization, did only slightly assimilate with the adjacent sound enamel.[38]

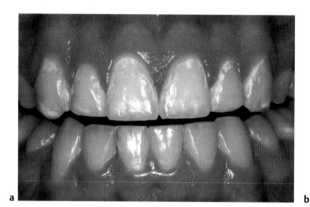

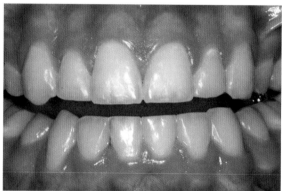

Fig. 17.12a, b   Postorthodontic caries lesions are clearly visible on the upper front teeth (**a**). These can be satisfactorily masked by caries infiltration (**b**).

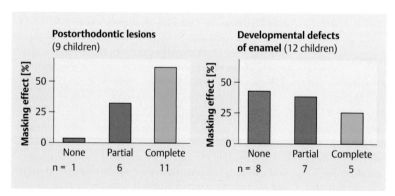

Fig. 17.13   Clinical data on the infiltration of esthetically relevant postorthodontic caries lesions and developmental defects reveal that caries can be at least partially masked almost all the time, whereas defects in the enamel that arise during maturation cannot be fully masked.[51]

Indication

Infiltration should accordingly be used for esthetically relevant, noncavitated carious tooth surfaces (especially of the anterior teeth and premolars) that cannot be improved by noninvasive measures. The general **contraindications** noted in the discussion of approximal caries infiltration (**Table 17.2**) and current restrictions of use (**Table 17.3**) also apply to caries infiltration for merely esthetic reasons. Few hard data exist on the infiltration of developmental (noncarious) defects to the white enamel; the infiltration of these lesions should be performed with caution.

More invasive therapeutic options such as **enamel microabrasion** are available alternatives to caries infiltration. The superficial part of the lesion is abraded with a mixture of hydrochloric acid and pumice.[53,54] Unfortunately, a substantial amount of enamel must be sacrificed when this technique is used to improve esthetics.[55] Restorations with, for example, ceramic veneers or composite fillings, which may be indicated in severe cases, frequently re-

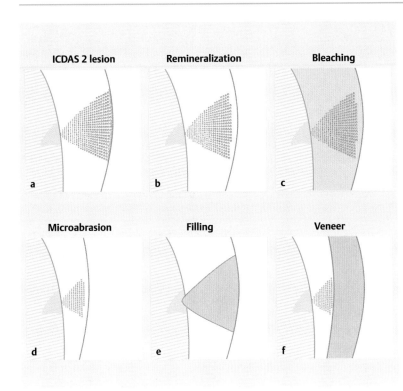

ICDAS 2 lesion **Remineralization** **Bleaching**

a   b   c

Microabrasion **Filling** **Veneer**

d   e   f

Fig. 17.14a–f Diagrams of the histological situation (cross-section) when various methods are used to treat esthetically relevant caries lesions. By means of remineralization, the surface layer of esthetically relevant enamel lesions can be reinforced, although the unsightly appearance (see **Fig. 17.11**) is mostly not altered. Bleaching the surrounding healthy enamel can somewhat attenuate the appearance, but this approach only works when the differences are minor. When microabrasion is used, both healthy enamel and carious enamel are removed until the appearance of the tooth surface is acceptable. With this technique, a significant amount of enamel is removed as is the case with composite or veneer restorations. With caries infiltration (see **Fig. 17.5**), the lesion is stabilized and thereby masked (see **Figs. 17.11** and **17.12**).

quire the removal of even more enamel (**Fig. 17.14**). It is quite possible to combine caries infiltration with composites, especially since composites adhere to infiltrant material in essentially the same way as to enamel adhesive.[56] Noncavitated areas can be infiltrated and cavities can be filled without having to use additional adhesive for the enamel. There should be separate dentin adhesion, however (**Table 17.1**).

CLINICAL PEARL

The basic steps are the same as those used for approximal caries infiltration. Separation is of course not required. It is advantageous, however, to know a few tricks to achieve a satisfactory result. Especially when the caries lesions are inactive, multiple etching may be recommended to completely remove the relatively thick pseudo-intact surface layer. The efficacy of etching is demonstrable by the speed at which the carious defect in the healthy enamel absorbs water or ethanol (see moistening test, **Fig. 17.15** and Chapter 25, Case 4). If the water or ethanol can penetrate the lesion within about 3–5 seconds and this significantly improves the appearance of the tooth, it is highly probable that the infiltrant can accomplish the same thing after an exposure time of 3 minutes.

NOTE

The infiltration of esthetically relevant caries is a nondestructive alternative that can produce attractive results within a reasonable treatment time.

In addition, final **polishing** is important, and similar to polishing a composite filling, to avoid staining of superficial unpolymerized resin components within a short period. Unesthetic unevenness in the tooth surface is eliminated, as well. Frequently, the esthetic appearance can be significantly enhanced in this manner within a relatively short treatment period.

Follow-up

The infiltrated areas only need to be visually inspected during routine examinations. If discoloration arises, the surface can be repolished. The bleaching of deeper discolorations which may arise after a while has not been studied so far but seems to be possible.

This chapter is based on the following articles:

- Meyer-Lueckel H, Fejerskov O, Paris S: Neuartige Therapiemöglichkeiten bei approximaler Karies. Schweiz Monatsschr Zahnmed 2009; 119: 454–461[1;]
- Meyer-Lückel H, Paris S: Kariesinfiltration in der Kinder- und Jugendzahnheilkunde. Oralprophylaxe und Kinderzahnheilkunde 2010; 32: 113–121[2;]

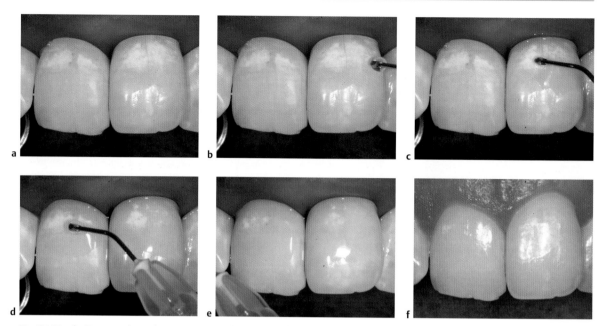

Fig. 17.15a–f To assess the esthetic outcome of infiltration of relevant caries lesions (**a**) during the procedure (before the infiltrant is applied), water is applied onto the etched and dried lesions (**b–d**) to assess whether these are satisfactorily masked within 5 seconds (**e**). If not, a highly mineralized surface layer could be causative. In this case lesions should be etched again using hydrochloric acid or micro-abraded (e.g., abrasive paste + Icon etch) removing superficial enamel. After checking that a substantial and quick masking effect can now be observed, one should apply the infiltrant. In this way a satisfactory esthetic outcome can be achieved in most cases (**f**).

and has been partially published in Meyer-Lückel, H., Paris, S. Kariesinfiltration, Zahnmedizin up2date, Thieme, Stuttgart;2011:232–246.[3]

SUMMARY

At present, caries infiltration is primarily indicated for two locations: **approximal** and **esthetically relevant caries**. The infiltration of *occlusal lesions* has not been researched and is therefore not recommended with the existing treatment set. It is not possible to infiltrate *root caries* by means of the present therapy since the affected dentin contains a great deal of water.

In view of existing clinical results, caries infiltration is recommended for progressive approximal lesions in the posterior region (deciduous and permanent teeth) when the lesions extend radiographically into the outer third of the dentin at a maximum. Lesions should not have any palpable or visible cavitation of the surface. This microinvasive therapy allows for a low-pain, non-destructive treatment of approximal caries lesions, which have mainly been treated with minimally invasive therapies to date. If caries infiltration is performed properly, the initial treatment of the affected tooth with a restoration can at least be delayed. The caries progression should be checked at regular intervals using high quality bitewing x-rays, so that invasive treatment can be pursued in a timely manner if the lesions become enlarged. Infiltration accordingly fills a gap in the treatment of approximal caries. The anticipated clinical data from more extended observations will provide additional insight into the efficacy of caries infiltration. The range of indications may be expanded in the future to cavitated caries lesions following the development of materials and techniques in enamel (ICDAS 3) and fissure caries.

In addition, the infiltration of **other smooth surfaces** being more accessible for oral hygiene is possible. This primarily relates to the treatment of esthetically relevant caries lesions in anterior teeth that can be masked due to the optical properties of the infiltrant. In children and adolescents at high caries risk, caries infiltration may supplement invasive therapy of other smooth surfaces. Developmental changes in the enamel, such as **fluorosis** or **molar-incisor hypomineralization (MIH)**, can at least be partially masked. However, expectations should not be set too high; other studies have yet to provide information about the use of infiltrants for these defects.

REFERENCES

1. Meyer-Lueckel H, Fejerskov O, Paris S. Novel treatment possibilities for proximal caries. [Article in German] Schweiz Monatsschr Zahnmed 2009;119(5):454–461

2. Meyer-Lückel H, Paris S. Kariesinfiltration in der Kinder- und Jugendzahnheilkunde. Oralprophylaxe & Kinderzahnheilkunde 2010;32:113–121

3. Meyer-Lückel H, Paris S. Kariesinfiltration, Zahnmedizin up2date. Stuttgart: Thieme; 2011:232–246

4. Phark JH, Duarte S Jr, Meyer-Lueckel H, Paris S. Caries infiltration with resins: a novel treatment option for interproximal caries. Compend Contin Educ Dent 2009;30(Spec No 3):13–17

5. Pitts NB, Rimmer PA. An in vivo comparison of radiographic and directly assessed clinical caries status of posterior approximal surfaces in primary and permanent teeth. Caries Res 1992;26(2):146–152

6. Hintze H, Wenzel A, Danielsen B, Nyvad B. Reliability of visual examination, fibre-optic transillumination, and bite-wing radiography, and reproducibility of direct visual examination following tooth separation for the identification of cavitated carious lesions in contacting approximal surfaces. Caries Res 1998;32(3):204–209

7. Thylstrup A, Qvist V. Principal enamel and dentine reactions during caries progressions. In: Thylstrup A, Leach SA, Qvist V, eds. Dentine and Dentine Reactions in the Oral Cavity. Oxford: IRL Press; 1987:3–16

8. Mejàre I, Stenlund H, Zelezny-Holmlund C. Caries incidence and lesion progression from adolescence to young adulthood: a prospective 15-year cohort study in Sweden. Caries Res 2004;38(2):130–141

9. Davila JM, Buonocore MG, Greeley CB, Provenza DV. Adhesive penetration in human artificial and natural white spots. J Dent Res 1975;54(5):999–1008

10. Robinson C, Hallsworth AS, Weatherell JA, Künzel W. Arrest and control of carious lesions: a study based on preliminary experiments with resorcinol-formaldehyde resin. J Dent Res 1976;55(5):812–818

11. Rodda JC. Impregnation of caries-like lesions with dental resins. N Z Dent J 1983;79(358):114–117

12. Goepferd SJ, Olberding P. The effect of sealing white spot lesions on lesion progression in vitro. Pediatr Dent 1989;11(1):14–16

13. Donly KJ, Ruiz M. In vitro demineralization inhibition of enamel caries utilizing an unfilled resin. Clin Prev Dent 1992;14(6):22–24

14. Garcia-Godoy F, Summitt JB, Donly KJ. Caries progression of white spot lesions sealed with an unfilled resin. J Clin Pediatr Dent 1997;21(2):141–143

15. Robinson C, Brookes SJ, Kirkham J, Wood SR, Shore RC. In vitro studies of the penetration of adhesive resins into artificial caries-like lesions. Caries Res 2001;35(2):136–141

16. Gray GB, Shellis P. Infiltration of resin into white spot caries-like lesions of enamel: an in vitro study. Eur J Prosthodont Restor Dent 2002;10(1):27–32

17. Schmidlin PR, Zehnder M, Pasqualetti T, Imfeld T, Besek MJ. Penetration of a bonding agent into De- and remineralized enamel in vitro. J Adhes Dent 2004;6(2):111–115

18. Meyer-Lueckel H, Paris S, Mueller J, Cölfen H, Kielbassa AM. Influence of the application time on the penetration of different dental adhesives and a fissure sealant into artificial subsurface lesions in bovine enamel. Dent Mater 2006;22(1):22–28

19. Paris S, Meyer-Lueckel H, Mueller J, Hummel M, Kielbassa AM. Progression of sealed initial bovine enamel lesions under demineralizing conditions in vitro. Caries Res 2006;40(2):124–129

20. Paris S, Meyer-Lueckel H, Kielbassa AM. Resin infiltration of natural caries lesions. J Dent Res 2007;86(7):662–666

21. Meyer-Lueckel H, Paris S, Kielbassa AM. Surface layer erosion of natural caries lesions with phosphoric and hydrochloric acid gels in preparation for resin infiltration. Caries Res 2007;41(3):223–230

22. Buckton G. Interfacial Phenomena in Drug Delivery and Targeting. Chur: Harwood Academic Publishers; 1995

23. Fan PL, Seluk LW, O'Brien WJ. Penetrativity of sealants: I. J Dent Res 1975;54(2):262–264

24. O'Brien WJ, Fan PL, Apostolides A. Penetrativity of sealants and glazes. The effectiveness of a sealant depends on its ability to penetrate into fissures. Oper Dent 1978;3(2):51–56

25. Haas U. Physik für Pharmazeuten und Mediziner. Stuttgart: Wissenschaftliche Verlagsgesellschaft; 2002

26. Paris S, Meyer-Lueckel H, Cölfen H, Kielbassa AM. Penetration coefficients of commercially available and experimental composites intended to infiltrate enamel carious lesions. Dent Mater 2007;23(6):742–748

27. Paris S, Meyer-Lueckel H, Cölfen H, Kielbassa AM. Resin infiltration of artificial enamel caries lesions with experimental light curing resins. Dent Mater J 2007;26(4):582–588

28. Meyer-Lueckel H, Paris S. Progression of artificial enamel caries lesions after infiltration with experimental light curing resins. Caries Res 2008;42(2):117–124

29. Meyer-Lueckel H, Paris S. Improved resin infiltration of natural caries lesions. J Dent Res 2008;87(12):1112–1116

30. Meyer-Lueckel H, Paris S. Infiltration of natural caries lesions with experimental resins differing in penetration coefficients and ethanol addition. Caries Res 2010;44(4):408–414

31. Meyer-Lueckel H, Chatzidakis A, Naumann M, Döfer CE, Paris S. Influence of application time on infiltrant penetration into natural enamel caries J Dent 2011;39(7):465–469

32. Paris S, Meyer-Lueckel H. Infiltrants inhibit progression of natural caries lesions in vitro. J Dent Res 2010;89(11):1276–1280

33. Paris S, Soviero VU, Schuch M, Meyer-Lueckel H. Pretreatment of natural caries lesions after penetration depths in vitro. Clin Oral Invest 2012;16 (in press)

34. Paris S, Meyer-Lueckel H. Inhibition of caries progression by resin infiltration in situ. Caries Res 2010;44(1):47–54

35. Paris S, Dörfer CE, Meyer-Lueckel H. Surface conditioning of natural enamel caries lesions in deciduous teeth in preparation for resin infiltration. J Dent 2010;38(1):65–71

36. Paris S, Hopfenmüller W, Meyer-Lueckel H. Resin infiltration of caries lesions: an efficacy randomized trial. J Dent Res 2010;89(8):823–826

37. Kidd EAM, Fejerskov O. What constitutes dental caries? Histopathology of carious enamel and dentin related to the action of cariogenic biofilms. J Dent Res 2004;83 Spec No C(Spec.):C35–C38

38. Paris S, Meyer-Lueckel H. Masking of labial enamel white spot lesions by resin infiltration—a clinical report. Quintessence Int 2009;40(9):713–718

39. Meyer-Lueckel H, Bitter K, Paris S. Randomized controlled clinical trial on proximal caries infiltration. Caries Res 2012;46 (in press)

40. Ekstrand KR, Bakhshandeh A, Martignon S. Treatment of proximal superficial caries lesions on primary molar teeth with resin infiltration and fluoride varnish versus fluoride varnish only: efficacy after 1 year. Caries Res 2010;44(1):41–46

41. Mejàre I, Källest I C, Stenlund H. Incidence and progression of approximal caries from 11 to 22 years of age in Sweden: A prospective radiographic study. Caries Res 1999;33(2):93–100

42. Paris S, Bitter K, Naumann M, Dörfer CE, Meyer-Lueckel H. Resin infiltration of proximal caries lesions differing in ICDAS codes. Eur J Oral Sci 2011;119(2):182–186

43. Pitts NB, Longbottom C. Temporary tooth separation with special reference to the diagnosis and preventive management of equivocal approximal carious lesions. Quintessence Int 1987;18(8): 563–573

44. Rimmer PA, Pitts NB. Temporary elective tooth separation as a diagnostic aid in general dental practice. Br Dent J 1990;169(3-4): 87–92

45. De Araujo FB, Rosito DB, Toigo E, dos Santos CK. Diagnosis of approximal caries: radiographic versus clinical examination using tooth separation. Am J Dent 1992;5(5):245–248

46. Alkilzy M, Berndt C, Meller C, Schidlowski M, Splieth C. Sealing of proximal surfaces with polyurethane tape: a two-year clinical and radiographic feasibility study. J Adhes Dent 2009;11(2): 91–94

47. Pitts NB. The use of bitewing radiographs in the management of dental caries: scientific and practical considerations. Dentomaxillofac Radiol 1996;25(1):5–16

48. Staudt CB, Lussi A, Jacquet J, Kiliaridis S. White spot lesions around brackets: in vitro detection by laser fluorescence. Eur J Oral Sci 2004;112(3):237–243

49. Mattousch TJ, van der Veen MH, Zentner A. Caries lesions after orthodontic treatment followed by quantitative light-induced fluorescence: a 2-year follow-up. Eur J Orthod 2007;29(3): 294–298

50. Belli R, Rahiotis C, Schubert EW, Baratieri LN, Petschelt A, Lohbauer U. Wear and morphology of infiltrated white spot lesions. J Dent 2011;39(5):376–385

51. Paris S, Keltsch J, Dörfer CE, Meyer-Lueckel H. Visual assimilation of artificial enamel caries lesions by resin infiltration in vitro. [ORCA abstract 41] Caries Res 2010;44:171–248

52. Kim S, Kim EY, Jeong TS, Kim JW. The evaluation of resin infiltration for masking labial enamel white spot lesions. Int J Paediatr Dent 2011;21(4):241-248

53. Croll TP, Cavanaugh RR. Enamel color modification by controlled hydrochloric acid-pumice abrasion. I. technique and examples. Quintessence Int 1986;17(2):81–87

54. Waggoner WF, Johnston WM, Schumann S, Schikowski E. Microabrasion of human enamel in vitro using hydrochloric acid and pumice. Pediatr Dent 1989;11(4):319–323

55. Tong LS, Pang MK, Mok NY, King NM, Wei SH. The effects of etching, micro-abrasion, and bleaching on surface enamel. J Dent Res 1993;72(1):67–71

56. Wiegand A, Stawarczyk B, Kolakovic M, Hämmerle CH, Attin T, Schmidlin PR. Adhesive performance of a caries infiltrant on sound and demineralised enamel. J Dent 2011;39(2):117–121

How Much Caries Do We Have to Remove?

David N. J. Ricketts

18

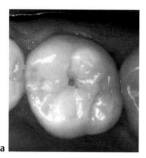
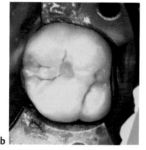
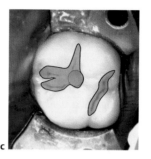

a   b   c

Fig. 18.1a–c Upper molar tooth with occlusal caries just into dentin (**a**) and when all caries has been removed (**b**). The superimposed outline (**c**) indicates the extent of the cavity if the fissures were to be "run out," consistent with "extension for prevention."

Today, the cavity (middle of tooth) would simply be restored with composite and the remaining fissure would be fissure-sealed (the preventive resin restoration).

So far, this book has covered the mode of action, effectiveness, and also the implementation, of noninvasive and microinvasive treatment options. As described in Chapters 1 and 2, the carious process is ubiquitous and common to us all; for many, the subclinical changes that occur at the crystal level do not manifest themselves at the clinical level. This is because the carious process is a dynamic process of demineralization, which is capable of arrest and even remineralization, depending upon the environmental conditions (presence of plaque biofilm, sugar substrate, fluoride, etc.). Once a lesion is detectable at its earliest possible stage, the lesion and patient should be managed from a preventive (non-invasive) perspective—this cannot be emphasized enough. Nonetheless, micro-invasive options should be considered when applicable (see Chapters 15–17). But invasive intervention should only be considered if these more conservative options are suspected to have failed and/or a lesion has progressed to such a degree that caries removal and restoration are indicated.

Unfortunately, the painless non- and microinvasive techniques do not work in every patient, for every caries lesion, or for a whole lifetime. However, ironically, dental caries is one of the most common diseases of mankind and yet there is little evidence to suggest where, along the continuum of the disease process from early white spot lesion to frank cavitation, invasive intervention should be considered. This is reflected in the great variation in caries detection, especially on the approximal and occlusal surfaces, the diagnostic threshold for invasive intervention and, in turn, on the number of plans for restorative care among dentists.[1–3] While great variation exists, the decision to operatively intervene is critical, as restorations cannot be regarded as permanent, as a large proportion of a dentist's time is spent re-restoring teeth, and the decision to do so is equally as idiosyncratic as the decision to restore primary caries in the first instance[4] (see Chapter 20). The more restorations a patient has, the more re-restoration will take place, and the extent to which carious enamel and dentin is removed varies considerably between dentists, as well. Each time a restoration is replaced the cavity gets larger, compromising the tooth. The decision as to when and how to restore a caries lesion and

so enter the **restorative cycle** is therefore an important one.

This chapter will cover in detail:
- Criteria to be used in deciding when to restore a caries lesion
- The histopathology of dentin caries and its relationship to appropriate caries removal
- The microbiology and pulp–dentin complex reactions associated with dentin caries and how these can be exploited in the future to enable the management of caries to move from a surgical approach to one based upon the microbiology and histopathology of the lesion
- The stepwise excavation technique to reduce the risk of pulp exposure

Historical Perspective

One of the first dentists to comprehensively describe cavity preparation in relation to dental caries was G. V. Black (1836–1915).[5] He was able to do this through meticulous study and research of teeth, their morphology, where carious lesions mainly occurred, and the histopathological spread of the disease. G. V. Black also mapped out tooth surfaces into those which were particularly susceptible to caries and those which appeared to be immune. Following caries removal, further preparation of tooth tissue was recommended to extend the cavity margins into immune areas; the so-called G. V. Black's philosophy of "**extension for prevention**."

This had a particular impact on cavity preparation for occlusal and approximal surfaces. On the occlusal surface once all of the carious dentin had been removed at a specific site, it was recommended that the entire fissure system should be prepared with a bur so that the remaining susceptible fissure could also be restored (**Fig. 18.1**). Fissures were also frequently excised in sound teeth and restored as a caries preventive measure, the so-called **prophylactic odontotomy**. For the approximal lesion, once caries had been removed, the cavity on the approximal surface was further extended buccally and lingually into the cleansable embrasure space, and subgingivally into a caries immune area. Once the approximal box was complete, extension into the occlusal fissure system was performed not only for retention and resistance form, but also for "prevention" (**Fig. 18.2**).

With regard to the question of "how much caries do we need to remove?" G. V. Black believed that "generally when the cavity has been cut to form, no carious dentin will remain." Not only would no carious tooth tissue remain, but considerable sound tooth tissue removal would have taken place, leading to the classic angular and often extensive cavities.

There was little change in cavity preparation until this was reviewed by Elderton in 1984.[6] Emphasis was placed on gaining access to caries and its removal, but no longer was extension-for-prevention thought to be necessary, bearing in mind the extensive removal of sound tooth tissue and the short-lived nature of many restorations. Sound pits and fissures could now be protected with fissure sealants and retention to approximal boxes could be achieved with buccal, lingual, and gingival grooves. The advent of adhesive restorative materials also precluded the need for further cavity preparation for retention; more conservative preparations with rounded outlines were the result (**Fig. 18.2**).

> **NOTE**
>
> The extension-for-prevention philosophy was established by G. V Black when no sealant procedure and/or adhesive restorations could be performed. This meant that margins of a restoration were placed in areas where no caries should occur.

When to Remove Caries?

Enamel Lesion

An enamel lesion is the reflection of the carious process taking place in the biofilm on the surface of the tooth and therefore should be treated noninvasively, by disrupting the biofilm with regular oral hygiene procedures in the presence of fluoride (Chapters 9–13). Where enamel caries is concerned, G. V. Black wrote that microorganisms from the biofilm "never enter the tissue until the rods are loosened and fall out. The enamel is a solid into which micro-organisms cannot penetrate." More recent evidence suggests that microorganisms can penetrate non-cavitated enamel lesions; however, their numbers within the tooth tissue are unlikely to have an impact on caries progression alone.[7] A noncavitated enamel lesion therefore does not require caries removal unless it is for esthetic reasons.

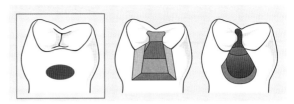

Fig. 18.2 Diagram of a premolar tooth with approximal caries into dentin (left) and when all caries has been removed and the cavity has been extended according to G. V. Black (middle) and when no extension-for-prevention has been performed, according to Elderton (right).

Enamel–Dentin Junction

The enamel–dentin junction (EDJ) is an important threshold for those investigating caries detection devices and in determining disease prevalence in a population—however, while it would be a convenient threshold upon which to base invasive intervention, it is not a logical one. The majority of coronal lesions extending up to the EDJ and into the outer dentin will be noncavitated and can still be managed non- or microinvasively (see Chapters 9, 17, and 20).

> **NOTE**
>
> Numbers of microorganisms within noncavitated enamel lesions are low and only play a minor role with respect to caries progression.

Cavitation

Frank cavitation is an obvious disease state in which invasive intervention could be justified, as cariogenic bacteria can readily invade the tooth structure and, hidden from conventional oral hygiene procedures, can proliferate to a critical mass of biofilm to facilitate lesion progression. Apart from the approximal surfaces, cavitation can readily be detected by examination of clean, dry teeth. While the radiograph is important in the detection of approximal caries, it is often not possible to determine whether the lesion is cavitated or not. For occlusal and approximal lesions it is well established that the actual depth of the lesion will be greater than it appears radiographically. Bearing this in mind only 8%–47% of those approximal lesions with a radiolucency up to the EDJ (and deeper clinically) will be cavitated,[8,9] and in some studies even as few as 35% with a radiolucency into the outer half of dentin were found to be cavitated.[8] A radiolucency up to the EDJ or just into the dentin alone should not therefore prompt invasive intervention for approximal surfaces on the assumption that they are cavitated.

Predicting whether a radiographically visible approximal lesion will be cavitated or not is difficult. High caries risk and gingival inflammation of the interdental papilla may help, as they are associated with a higher risk of

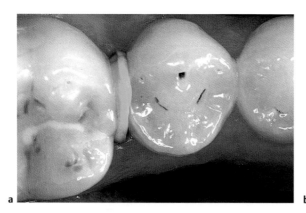
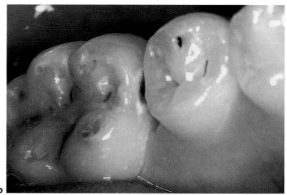
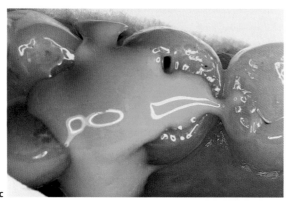
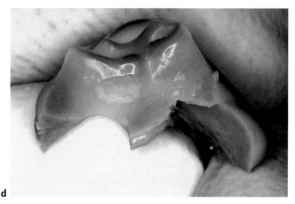

Fig. 18.3a–d Orthodontic tooth separator in place (**a**) to allow direct visualization of the approximal surfaces of teeth (**b**). While this lesion is clearly cavitated, an impression in light bodied silicone can be used to confirm any break in the surface integrity (**c, d**).[62] (**Fig. 18.3 d** reprinted with permission from Quintessence Publishers Ltd., from Christiansen J. Non-operative Caries Treatment. In: Splieth, C ed. Revolutions in Pediatric Dentistry. London: Quintessence Publ;2011:21–35)

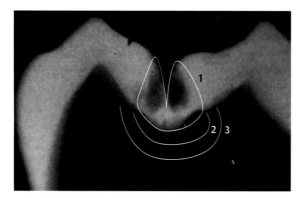

Fig. 18.4 Radiograph of a section through an occlusal fissure showing bilateral enamel lesions on its wall. If prevention fails the lesion will spread as outlined by lines 1, and coalesce beneath the base of the fissure enamel and then deepen as depicted by lines 2 and 3.

cavitation.[10,11] If in doubt the clinician could separate the teeth with orthodontic separators for direct visual–tactile assessment (**Fig. 18.3**) or use a thin probe (cow-end probe or briault probe) without separation.

Microbial Invasion of Dentin

The invaginated anatomy of the occlusal surface of the tooth means that the initial enamel lesions occur at the entrance to the pits and fissures and within its walls. These lesions spread laterally into dentin and coalesce beneath the base of the fissure, eventually spreading into dentin on a wide front. Some professionals think that fluoride makes the occlusal enamel harder and more resistant to collapse and as such cavitation occurs at a late stage in the carious process (**Fig. 18.4**). Throughout the carious process **demineralization precedes bacterial invasion** of the tooth tissues. Therefore at some stage between the occlusal lesion spreading into dentin and becoming frankly cavitated, the lesion in dentin becomes heavily infected and it is thought that this is the factor that should prompt invasive intervention. But what features will predict infection of the dentin?

In a clinical microbiological study, pits and fissures deemed as being carious to various degrees and in need of invasive intervention were investigated by a single operator.[12] The visual appearance of the investigation site was scored on a basic visual scoring system that was acceptable at the time, and bitewing radiographs were scored as to whether a radiolucency was present or not, and if so, how deep. Under rubber dam isolation the

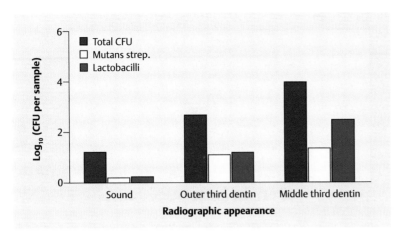

Fig. 18.5 Relationship between the radiographic appearance of occlusal lesions and the level of infection determined by the total $\log_{10}$ colony forming units (CFU), mutans streptococcus, and lactobacillus counts (taken from Ricketts et al.[12]).

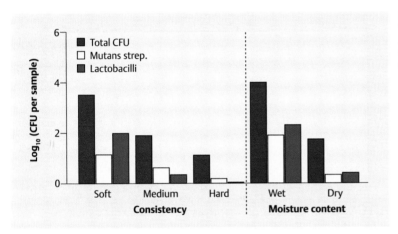

Fig. 18.6 Relationship between the consistency and moisture content of the dentine and the level of infection determined by the total $\log_{10}$ colony forming units (CFU), mutans streptococcus, and lactobacillus counts (taken from Ricketts et al.[12]).

enamel above the dentin lesion was carefully removed and the dentin assessed for color, consistency, and moisture content. Demineralization of the dentin was determined with a caries detector dye and a dentin sample was taken for microbial analysis. While the visual appearance of the pits and fissures was found not to be a good predictor of infected dentin, lesions visible as a radiolucency in dentin were heavily infected compared with those that were not radiographically visible, and the deeper the lesions appeared on the radiograph the heavier the bacterial load[12] (**Fig. 18.5**). Interestingly, the color of the dentin at cavity preparation had no relationship with the bacterial infection, whereas those lesions that were hard to a probe and dry harbored significantly fewer bacteria than those that were soft to the probe and wet (**Fig. 18.6**). This finding will have a significant bearing during caries removal.

NOTE

The appearance of a radiolucency into dentin on the occlusal surface seems to be the single best predictor of the need for operative intervention based upon microbial invasion.

Dentin Caries

No discussion of how much caries should be removed is possible without reviewing the work by Fusayama and colleagues on dentin caries. If infection of the dentin is a factor that should prompt invasive intervention, it would seem logical that all the **infected dentin** should be removed during cavity preparation. In the mid-sixties Fusayama et al.[13] were concerned about the prolonged viability of organisms left in residual caries beneath restorations. As such they performed an experiment to determine the relationship between several variables and **bacterial invasion**. They found that softening of the dentin, by bacterial acids diffusing deeper into the dentin, was followed by discoloration of the dentin and then by bacterial invasion. In slowly progressing lesions the discolored area was generally harder than in rapidly progressing lesions.

In a series of further studies two layers of carious dentin were described that could be differentiated by using a basic fuchsin dye.[14–18] The first layer was the outermost layer closest to the EDJ. The carious dentin of this layer was severely demineralized and the collagen fibers were denatured with irregular inorganic crystals randomly scattered throughout. This layer was found to be heavily infected with bacteria, hence the frequently quoted term **infected zone of carious dentin**, and was incapable of remineralization. The second layer of carious dentin was described at the advancing front of the lesion, closest to the pulp and was found to be demineralized, but not to the same extent as the first layer, and the collagen fibers were sound with more cross-linkages and apatite crystals bound to them. This layer, often termed the **caries affected zone**, was not found to be infected and was capable of remineralization. The basic fuchsin dye (caries detector) was found to stain only the first layer of carious dentin and its use during cavity preparation would ensure that all of the infected dentin caries was removed, in fact "excavation guided by this staining method was always deeper than the bacterial invasion."[17] It was also found that the difference in excavation depth and the depth of bacterial invasion was greater in more active rapidly progressing lesions than less active chronic lesions.

NOTE

Fusayama et al. distinguished between the infected and affected zones in dentin caries. They promoted a "caries detector" that was supposed to stain the infected zone for clinical caries removal.

Conventional Caries Removal

Conventional cavity preparation has therefore involved gaining access to dentin caries by removing superficial enamel, usually with a high speed bur, and then to render the periphery of the cavity (at the EDJ or outer 1–2 mm of dentin if involving the root) completely caries-free by removing all soft and/or stained dentin with a slow round bur. Following on from this, careful removal of pulpal caries is performed with an excavator until hard dentin is reached. It has long been accepted that in deep cavities, hard but stained dentin can be left pulpally, based on the findings that staining precedes bacterial invasion.[13] This can then be lined with a calcium hydroxide lining forming the so-called **indirect pulp cap** (in deep cavities). Some clinicians still advocate the use of caries detector dyes to ensure complete removal of all infected carious dentin. Because of the potential carcinogenicity of basic fuchsin, it is no longer used and has been replaced with 1% acid red in propylene glycol and other protein dyes.

This conventional caries removal and cavity preparation has been performed for more than a century is still done today in dental clinics worldwide; however, there is rapidly growing evidence that questions numerous aspects of this time-honored approach.

NOTE

Classical caries removal in dentin usually terminates at hard but stained dentin. In addition, a caries detector dye is advocated occasionally to check that infected parts are removed thoroughly.

Caries Removal at the Enamel–Dentin Junction

The first series of questions of relevance to caries removal concerns the EDJ:
- Do we actually remove all caries from the EDJ during conventional cavity preparation?
- What happens to residual caries left at the EDJ?
- Is complete caries removal, as guided by caries detector dyes at the EDJ, necessary?
- Should the EDJ be rendered stain-free?

Do We Actually Remove All Caries from the EDJ during Conventional Cavity Preparation?
Two separate studies were performed in the mid to late 1980s that looked at cavities that were prepared by dental students in vivo and deemed to be caries free at the EDJ by both student and supervising tutor.[19,20] In these studies a caries detector dye was applied to the completed cavities and it was found that more than half of the cavities had dye stained dentin at the EDJ (57%–59%). According to Fusayama's work, this would have indicated infected carious dentin and should have been removed.

What Happens to Residual Caries Left at the EDJ?
Concerns over the issue of residual caries at the EDJ following cavity preparation led to a laboratory study which aimed to determine its fate.[21] Cavities were prepared on freshly extracted teeth in a manner similar to that of the clinical study[20] until apparently caries-free at the EDJ. The teeth were restored with amalgam and then thermocycled in tea and chlorhexidine. The amalgam restorations were then carefully dissected out to allow examination of the EDJ. Areas of the EDJ were found to have picked up the stain and these areas corresponded to demineralized dentin when histologically examined. Clinically it was suggested that this could lead to misdiagnosis of secondary caries and lead to unnecessary restoration replacement. Both studies suggested that if complete caries removal at the EDJ was thought to be important, then use of a caries detector dye might be sensible.

Is Complete Caries Removal Guided by Caries Detector Dyes at the EDJ Necessary?
Leaving residual caries at the EDJ after cavity preparation would seem to be commonplace but what implications this would have was less certain. In a further clinical

study[22] cavities were prepared until the EDJ was caries-free based upon the fact that it was hard to a probe and stain-free, and then the caries detector dye was applied. As in the previous study, 52% of the cavities showed some dye staining at the EDJ. Dentin samples taken at the EDJ of dye-stained sites and stain-free sites were then sent for microbial analysis. The results showed that low levels of organisms were recovered from both sites and that there was no significant difference between the two.

CLINICAL PEARL

It appears that visual–tactile confirmation of stain-free and hard dentin is sufficient to assess the EDJ following cavity preparation and use of the caries detector dye could lead to over preparation and larger cavities.

Should the EDJ Be Rendered Stain-free?

It is intriguing that dentists are happy leaving hard stained carious dentin close to vital pulp but are uneasy about leaving such dentin at the EDJ. A series of studies led by Kidd have looked at the consistency (soft/hard), moisture content (wet/dry), and color of dentin (light/dark) at the EDJ during cavity preparation and related them to the level of infection following microbial analysis. Pooled data from these studies have allowed evaluation of over 564 cavities.[23] It was found that hard dentin, whether stained or not, harbored significantly fewer bacteria than soft dentin. Where hard dentin was concerned, stained dentin harbored more bacteria than stain-free dentin, and while this was statistically significant, the numbers of bacteria involved were thought not to be clinically significant. The only caveat to this is when placing **tooth-colored restorations** where a discolored shadow might lead to a poor appearance and make follow-up assessment difficult. In these situations further caries removal to stain-free dentin can be justified.

NOTE

It is suggested that while all soft dentin at the EDJ should be removed, caries removal to hard and stain-free dentin might not be necessary.

Contemporary Caries Removal

To summarize, while various methods have been used to aid caries removal (e.g., Carisolv, air abrasion, sono abrasion, lasers) and guide caries removal (dyes, fluorescence techniques) to ensure all infected carious dentin is removed, the **tactile sensation** of hard dentin to a probe and the judicious use of a sharp **hand-excavator** to remove all soft caries still remains the most appropriate method for caries removal.[24] This ensures that a cavity is not over-prepared, reducing the cavity size and weakening remaining tooth structure. Use of a slow handpiece and bur, while quicker, can lead to over-preparation of the tooth which is important to avoid, especially pulpally.[24]

NOTE

Tactile sensation of hard dentin to a probe and the judicious use of a sharp hand-excavator to remove all soft caries still remains the most appropriate method for caries removal.

Pulp–Dentin Complex

The carious process and its invasive management cannot be looked at in isolation as they have a major impact on the pulp–dentin complex. During the carious process in dentin, bacterial by-products and products from the demineralized dentin itself can diffuse toward the pulp and stimulate pulp–dentin complex reactions (see Chapter 3). These responses will vary depending on the severity of the stimulus.[25] In a slowly progressing caries lesion where the stimulus is mild and the odontoblasts remain healthy, the stimulus simply upregulates the odontoblasts to produce more tertiary dentin, which in this situation is best referred to as **reactionary dentin**. With milder stimuli the reactionary dentin has dentinal tubules and structure comparable to primary dentin. With a more intense stimulus the reactionary dentin becomes less regular with fewer tubules and with cellular inclusions. Where the stimulus is mild, tubular sclerosis also takes place and these pulp–dentin complex reactions are aimed at reducing the permeability of the dentin to the bacteria and their injurious by products. This is in contrast to the situation when the stimulus to the pulp is so severe that odontoblast cells die. In this situation, stem or progenitor cells from within the pulp differentiate into odontoblastlike cells which lead to reparative dentinogenesis and **reparative dentin** formation in the form of a calcific bridge.[26]

Deep Caries

A balance therefore exists between the severity of the carious process on one hand and the pulp's ability to respond on the other. In deep lesions this balance is critical as caries removal during cavity preparation can leave a thin layer of **remaining dentin thickness**. This has been shown to be one of the most critical variables that can influence the health of the dental pulp and a successful outcome to invasive intervention.[27] If the rate of caries progression is such that it outstrips the pulp's ability to produce reactionary dentin, then the pulp can easily be exposed during cavity preparation. In symptomless teeth carious exposures are often managed with a **direct pulp cap** using calcium hydroxide or Mineral Trioxide Aggregate.

When radiographically followed for 3 years, the success rate of direct pulp caps following carious exposures was found to be 33% compared with 92% following mechanical exposures.[28] Similarly at 5 years the success rate of direct pulp caps on carious exposures was 37% and at 10 years only 13%.[29]

NOTE

Direct pulp caps are much less successful when used in carious exposures compared with traumatic/mechanical exposures.

The literature is clear: invasive and restorative procedures can affect pulpal health. The vibration and heat generated by a dental drill, chemicals applied to cavities prior to restoration, the restorative material itself, and in particular the remaining dentin thickness have all been shown to cause adverse pulpal reactions. Is it possible, therefore, to manage caries in an alternative way to tip the **caries/pulp balance** in favor of the pulp? The answer to this question lies in several fissure sealant and stepwise excavation studies where caries has been sealed into the tooth for a set period and the lesion re-entered to allow re-evaluation of the dentin and microbial analysis.

Fissure Sealant Studies

It is widely accepted that resin-based fissure sealants are effective in preventing occlusal caries for individuals with high caries risk. They have also been used to deliberately seal cavitated occlusal caries into the tooth (see Chapter 15). In studies where dentin caries has been sealed into the tooth and re-entered after varying time intervals up to 5 years, it has been shown that the dentin consistency is hard, its moisture content is dry, and color dark.[30,31] These properties have been shown to be consistent with lower **levels of microorganisms** when compared with soft wet sites.[23] Indeed, in those studies where dentin lesions were sealed and on re-entry dentin samples were taken for microbial analysis, all have shown a reduction in the number of viable organisms compared with control unsealed teeth.[32-36] In one study, acid etching alone reduced the number of organisms by up to 75%. While the reduction in the number of organisms is most dramatic in the first 2 weeks following sealant placement, continued reduction in organism numbers takes place until 2 years, at which time the lesions become sterile or bacterial counts have fallen to such a level that they are incapable of sustaining lesion progression.[32]

It is interesting to note that the fissure sealant studies cited involved sealed lesions of varying severity or depth, and it is difficult to interpret just how deep the lesions were. However, several studies have clearly stated that the lesions were visible on bitewing radiographs and previous research has indicated these will extend into the middle third of dentin or deeper,[37] and will be heavily infected.[12] Radiographic monitoring of sealed lesions over a period of 1–2 years has shown no evidence of increased lesion depth[32,34] and in one study there was a suggestion of lesion regression and decrease in depth[38] (see Chapter 15).

Stepwise Excavation Studies

Stepwise excavation is a method of removing caries in two stages separated usually by 6–12 months; however, shorter (4–6 weeks) and longer periods (2 years) have been reported. Most studies on stepwise excavation have been performed on teeth with deep dentin lesions, usually thought to be at risk of pulpal exposure if conventional caries removal were to be performed, but having no signs or symptoms of pulp pathology. At the first stage, access to the dentin caries is gained and only peripheral caries is removed. Pulpal dentin caries is removed sufficiently to place an adequate thickness of restorative material only; no attempt is made to remove further soft dentin caries. This is unlike the indirect pulp cap where caries removal at the outset of cavity preparation is aimed at complete removal of the infected layer, but is stopped when there is a real risk of pulpal exposure. This usually leaves firm, stained carious dentin pulpally. In stepwise excavation the cavity is then lined with calcium hydroxide and restored with the chosen material. This restoration is then left for 6–12 months when **re-entry** allows excavation of residual caries. The two stages allow the dentin left at the first stage of excavation to be compared with the dentin at re-entry after it has been sealed into the tooth for some time (**Fig. 18.7** and Chapter 25, Case 5).

Several clinical studies have shown that the dentin becomes harder, drier and darker in color, consistent with a reduction in the activity of the lesion[39-43] and mirroring the findings of the fissure sealant studies. Comparisons of the levels of infection in the dentin left after the first stage of stepwise excavation with those after the lesions had been sealed (restored) for some time again showed a dramatic decline in the total number of viable organisms,[39,40,42-45] including mutans streptococci and lactobacilli.

NOTE

These studies show that once a lesion has been sealed into the tooth (i.e. by restoration), the dramatic and consistent reduction in the number of viable organisms seen in the dentin is due to the organisms being deprived of their main source of nutrient from the oral cavity.

After sealing-in the caries by a restoration, many of the bacteria die and only those that can break down glycoproteins from tissue fluid derived from the pulp are able

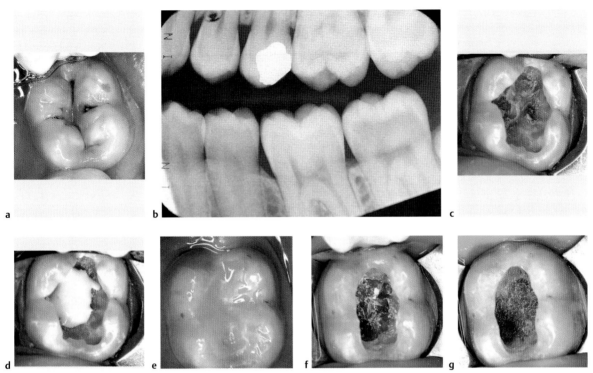

Fig. 18.7a–g Clinical and radiographic images (**a**, **b**) of lower left second molar showing a deep dentin lesion and a large pulp. Complete excavation has an associated high risk of pulpal exposure. This tooth has been managed using stepwise excavation, the appearance of the dentin at the end of the first excavation (**c**), the calcium hydroxide lining (**d**), and completed resin composite restoration (**e**) can be seen. When the lesion was re-entered 8 months later the dentin had become darker, harder, and drier (**f**, **g**).[62] (Fig. 18.7c,e,g reprinted with permission from Quintessence Publishers Ltd., from Christiansen J. Non-operative Caries Treatment. In: Splieth, C ed. Revolutions in Pediatric Dentistry. London: Quintessence Publ;2011:21–35)

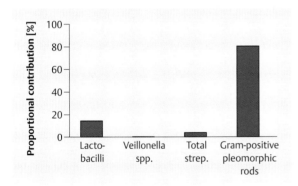

Fig. 18.8 The relative contribution of bacterial species in dentine at the end of the first excavation of stepwise excavation: *Streptococcus*, 8 species; gram-positive pleomorphic rods, *Actinomyces naeslundi*, *A. israelii*, *A. gerencseriae* (taken from Paddick et al.[45]).

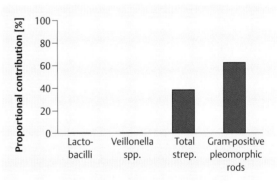

Fig. 18.9 The relative contribution of bacterial species in dentin at the beginning of the second excavation. Lactobacilli have been eliminated, the proportional contribution of streptococci has increased; however, the number of species has fallen from eight to three. Of the gram-positive pleomorphic rods, only *Actinomyces neaslundii* could be cultured once the lesion had been sealed (taken from Paddick et al.[45]).

to survive[45] (**Figs. 18.8** and **18.9**). The bacteria that remain are not associated with an active caries lesion and are in insufficient numbers to allow the lesion to progress. The carious process has therefore been moderated from a microbiological perspective by decreasing the microbial load and microbial diversity, and not by a mechanical excision as in cavity preparation. This tips the caries pulp–dentin complex reaction balance in favor of the pulp; reactionary dentin and tubular sclerosis further restricts the supply of nutrient to the bacteria within.

Three **randomized controlled trials** where stepwise excavation has been compared with complete caries removal have shown that tipping the caries-pulp balance in favor of the pulp can significantly reduce the risk of pulpal exposure when the lesions are re-entered. Leksell et al.[46] and Bjørndal et al.[47] showed that stepwise excavation in permanent teeth reduced the risk of pulpal exposure from 40% to 17.5% and 29% to 17.5%, respectively, and Magnusson and Sundell[48] have shown that in primary teeth the difference is greater, reducing the risk from 53% to 15%. The study of Bjørndal et al.[47] showed an 11.7% greater success rate at 1 year with stepwise excavation compared with complete caries removal, based upon pulpal exposure and maintained pulp vitality.

The evidence to date is compelling: provided a good seal is achieved with a fissure sealant or a restoration, infected, soft caries does not need to be removed. The interesting question now is should stepwise excavation involve the second stage or can caries be sealed permanently into the tooth? One study, where **ultraconservative caries removal** was performed in permanent teeth may provide the answer.[49] In this study, the enamel at the entrance to the fissure was simply beveled to ensure that a composite restoration could bond to sound enamel; no attempt was made to remove any dentin caries. This study was of a split-mouth design with the control tooth having complete caries removal followed by either extension for prevention in the remaining fissure pattern and restoration with amalgam or restoration with amalgam followed by fissure sealing. In the ultraconservative caries removal group the caries sealed into the tooth was radiographically visible and therefore of significant depth and likely to be infected. The composite restorations placed were followed up for 10 years, with no signs or symptoms of pulp pathology and only one failed restoration which could simply be re-restored; the results compared favorably with the control, complete caries removal and amalgam restoration groups.

Systematic Review of the Literature

The strongest evidence is provided in prospective randomized controlled trials. To establish the strength of the evidence for ultraconservative caries removal compared with complete caries removal a systematic review of the literature was performed looking for such trials and was published in 2006.[50] In total only four publications were found to meet the inclusion criteria, two were the two stepwise excavation studies already cited[46,48] and two concerned caries sealed permanently into teeth.[51,52] Clinical studies on Atraumatic Restorative Technique (ART) and indirect pulp caps were not included, as both techniques aim at removing all the infected soft layer of dentin. From the four included studies, data from 538 teeth were available for analysis. No problems were reported in relation to restoration retention or signs of pulp pathology in the two studies of caries sealed permanently into the tooth. The most striking results were those on the incidence of pulpal exposure in the stepwise excavation studies described earlier in this chapter. The systematic

review by Ricketts et al.[50] was currently being updated at the time this book went to press and the subsequent study by Bjørndal et al.[47] has been included and corroborates with the original systematic review conclusions.

It can be argued that the inclusion criteria for such systematic reviews are strict and eliminate important data from observational studies. To address this, Van Thompson et al.[53] performed a further systematic review of the literature, including both randomized controlled trials and observational studies. Their conclusions reinforced those of the original Cochrane review.[50]

> **NOTE**
>
> Cochrane review: "There is substantial evidence that the removal of all infected dentine in deep carious lesions is not required for successful caries treatment—provided that the restoration can seal the lesion from the oral environment effectively."

Is There a Need for Cavity Disinfection?

Several researchers have suggested the disinfection of cavities with chlorhexidine,[54,55] Photo Activated Dye (PAD) techniques,[56,57] gasiform ozone,[58,59] and dentin bonding systems[59] prior to restoration. By far the majority of studies on cavity disinfection have looked at disinfection of root canals in association with endodontic treatment. Those relatively few studies that have looked at disinfection of carious cavities have investigated bacterial counts in vitro and in vivo, postoperative sensitivity, and the effect that some of these disinfectants have on the subsequent bond strength with glass-ionomer and composite resin restorations, often with conflicting results and varying degrees of success.

Compare these disinfection studies with fissure sealant studies, stepwise excavation studies, ultraconservative caries removal studies and now the **Hall technique**,[60] where preformed stainless steel crowns are cemented over carious primary molar teeth with no caries removal. All the latter studies have reported apparent arrest of caries and reduction in sealed bacteria, so the need for cavity disinfection is questionable; a good cavity seal appears to be all that is required. Conventional techniques such as placement of a bacteriocidal lining (e.g., setting calcium hydroxide) and conditioning a cavity with acid etch prior to placement of a resin composite will certainly kill some bacteria, so the added benefit of cavity disinfection is doubtful. Certainly, further research in this area is required.

NOTE

There is no clinical evidence that additional cavity disinfection positively affects either pulp vitality or longevity of a restoration. Thus, phosphoric acid and calcium hydroxide liner seem to be the materials of choice when placing a restoration in deep caries lesions.

SUMMARY

The historical concept that dental caries should be completely excised has been challenged and currently dentists would appear to be comfortable with Fusayama's recommendation that only the outer infected layer of dentin need be removed; excavation to hard stained dentin, especially pulpally, is routine. The concept of leaving hard stained dentin at the enamel–dentin junction rests less comfortably, but there is no logic or evidence to support its removal other than a pragmatic approach to remove it where tooth colored restorations are to be placed for ease of reassessment and optimum appearance. Leaving soft carious dentin during cavity preparation in deep lesions is alien to most dentists,[61] despite the evidence presented. Concerns may lie in problems of bonding resin composites to carious dentin and gap formation,[53] failure of the restoration or tooth, and rapid lesion progression and inability to monitor lesions with time. The second stage of stepwise excavation addresses these insecurities and should be performed in contemporary practices. Leaving the lesions sealed for longer than 1 year may also have added advantages in allowing continued pulp–dentin complex reactions.

Most research on sealed caries has been performed on occlusal lesions where a good seal to the restoration can be achieved; approximal lesions obviously pose unique challenges. Further work on sealed lesions will be required in primary care involving approximal lesions before these techniques are widely accepted by dentists. Sealing caries into teeth is a clinically demanding procedure, as the peripheral seal is critical; such procedures should not be regarded as substandard for those that are clinically inept. Developments in diagnostic techniques such as subtraction radiography may allow lesions to be monitored with time to confirm lesion arrest or progress in rare situations where insidious leakage around restorations could lead to failure. The level of current evidence and continued research in this field will question further how much caries needs to be removed before a permanent restoration is placed without re-entry.

REFERENCES

1. Rytömaa I, Järvinen V, Järvinen J. Variation in caries recording and restorative treatment plan among university teachers. Community Dent Oral Epidemiol 1979;7(6):335–339

2. Kay EJ, Knill-Jones R. Variation in restorative treatment decisions: application of Receiver Operating Characteristic curve (ROC) analysis. Community Dent Oral Epidemiol 1992;20(3):113–117

3. Kay EJ, Nuttall NM, Knill-Jones R. Restorative treatment thresholds and agreement in treatment decision-making. Community Dent Oral Epidemiol 1992;20(5):265–268

4. Elderton RJ. Clinical studies concerning re-restoration of teeth. Adv Dent Res 1990;4:4–9

5. Black GV. Operative Dentistry. Vol 1. Pathology of Hard Tissues of the Teeth: Oral Diagnosis. Vol 3. Treatment of Dental Caries. 7th ed. London: Medico-Dental Publishing; 1936

6. Elderton RJ. New approaches to cavity design with special reference to the class II lesion. Br Dent J 1984;157(12):421–427

7. Parolo CC, Maltz M. Microbial contamination of noncavitated caries lesions: a scanning electron microscopic study. Caries Res 2006;40(6):536–541

8. Hintze H, Wenzel A, Danielsen B, Nyvad B. Reliability of visual examination, fibre-optic transillumination, and bite-wing radiography, and reproducibility of direct visual examination following tooth separation for the identification of cavitated carious lesions in contacting approximal surfaces. Caries Res 1998;32(3):204–209

9. Rugg-Gunn AJ. Approximal carious lesions. A comparison of the radiological and clinical appearances. Br Dent J 1972;133(11):481–484

10. Ekstrand KR, Bruun G, Bruun M. Plaque and gingival status as indicators for caries progression on approximal surfaces. Caries Res 1998;32(1):41–45

11. Ratledge DK, Kidd EA, Beighton D. A clinical and microbiological study of approximal carious lesions. Part 1: the relationship between cavitation, radiographic lesion depth, the site-specific gingival index and the level of infection of the dentine. Caries Res 2001;35(1):3–7

12. Ricketts DN, Kidd EA, Beighton D. Operative and microbiological validation of visual, radiographic and electronic diagnosis of occlusal caries in non-cavitated teeth judged to be in need of operative care. Br Dent J 1995;179(6):214–220

13. Fusayama T, Okuse K, Hosoda H. Relationship between hardness, discoloration, and microbial invasion in carious dentin. J Dent Res 1966;45(4):1033–1046

14. Kato S, Fusayama T. Recalcification of artificially decalcified dentin in vivo. J Dent Res 1970;49(5):1060–1067

15. Fusayama T, Terachima S. Differentiation of two layers of carious dentin by staining. J Dent Res 1972;51(3):866

16. Ogushi K, Fusayama T. Electron microscopic structure of the two layers of carious dentin. J Dent Res 1975;54(5):1019–1026

17. Sato Y, Fusayama T. Removal of dentin by fuchsin staining. J Dent Res 1976;55(4):678–683

18. Kuboki Y, Ohgushi K, Fusayama T. Collagen biochemistry of the two layers of carious dentin. J Dent Res 1977;56(10):1233–1237

19. Anderson MH, Charbeneau GT. A comparison of digital and optical criteria for detecting carious dentin. J Prosthet Dent 1985;53(5):643–646

20. Kidd EA, Joyston-Bechal S, Smith MM, Allan R, Howe L, Smith SR. The use of a caries detector dye in cavity preparation. Br Dent J 1989;167(4):132–134

21. Kidd EA, Joyston-Bechal S, Smith MM. Staining of residual caries under freshly-packed amalgam restorations exposed to tea/chlorhexidine in vitro. Int Dent J 1990;40(4):219–224

22. Kidd EA, Joyston-Bechal S, Beighton D. The use of a caries detector dye during cavity preparation: a microbiological assessment. Br Dent J 1993;174(7):245–248

23. Kidd EA, Ricketts DN, Beighton D. Criteria for caries removal at the enamel-dentine junction: a clinical and microbiological study. Br Dent J 1996;180(8):287–291

24. Banerjee A, Kidd EA, Watson TF. In vitro evaluation of five alternative methods of carious dentine excavation. Caries Res 2000;34(2):144–150

25. Lee Y-L, Liu J, Clarkson BH, Lin CP, Godovikova V, Ritchie HH. Dentin-pulp complex responses to carious lesions. Caries Res 2006;40(3):256–264

26. Smith AJ. Pulpal responses to caries and dental repair. Caries Res 2002;36(4):223–232

27. Murray PE, Smith AJ, Garcia-Godoy F, Lumley PJ. Comparison of operative procedure variables on pulpal viability in an ex vivo model. Int Endod J 2008;41(5):389–400

28. Al-Hiyasat AS, Barrieshi-Nusair KM, Al-Omari MA. The radiographic outcomes of direct pulp-capping procedures performed by dental students: a retrospective study. J Am Dent Assoc 2006;137(12):1699–1705

29. Barthel CR, Rosenkranz B, Leuenberg A, Roulet JF. Pulp capping of carious exposures: treatment outcome after 5 and 10 years: a retrospective study. J Endod 2000;26(9):525–528

30. Jeronimus DJ Jr, Till MJ, Sveen OB. Reduced viability of microorganisms under dental sealants. ASDC J Dent Child 1975;42(4):275–280

31. Mertz-Fairhurst EJ, Schuster GS, Williams JE, Fairhurst CW. Clinical progress of sealed and unsealed caries. Part II: Standardized radiographs and clinical observations. J Prosthet Dent 1979;42(6):633–637

32. Handelman SL, Washburn F, Wopperer P. Two-year report of sealant effect on bacteria in dental caries. J Am Dent Assoc 1976;93(5):967–970

33. Going RE, Loesche WJ, Grainger DA, Syed SA. The viability of microorganisms in carious lesions five years after covering with a fissure sealant. J Am Dent Assoc 1978;97(3):455–462

34. Mertz-Fairhurst EJ, Schuster GS, Williams JE, Fairhurst CW. Clinical progress of sealed and unsealed caries. Part I: Depth changes and bacterial counts. J Prosthet Dent 1979;42(5):521–526

35. Jensen OE, Handelman SL. Effect of an autopolymerizing sealant on viability of microflora in occlusal dental caries. Scand J Dent Res 1980;88(5):382–388

36. Mertz-Fairhurst EJ, Schuster GS, Fairhurst CW. Arresting caries by sealants: results of a clinical study. J Am Dent Assoc 1986;112(2):194–197

37. Ricketts DN, Kidd EA, Smith BG, Wilson RF. Clinical and radiographic diagnosis of occlusal caries: a study in vitro. J Oral Rehabil 1995;22(1):15–20

38. Handelman SL, Leverett DH, Espeland MA, Curzon JA. Clinical radiographic evaluation of sealed carious and sound tooth surfaces. J Am Dent Assoc 1986;113(5):751–754

39. Kreulen CM, de Soet JJ, Weerheijm KL, van Amerongen WE. In vivo cariostatic effect of resin modified glass ionomer cement and amalgam on dentine. Caries Res 1997;31(5):384–389

40. Bjørndal L, Larsen T, Thylstrup A. A clinical and microbiological study of deep carious lesions during stepwise excavation using long treatment intervals. Caries Res 1997;31(6):411–417

41. Bjørndal L, Thylstrup A. A practice-based study on stepwise excavation of deep carious lesions in permanent teeth: a 1-year follow-up study. Community Dent Oral Epidemiol 1998;26(2):122–128

42. Bjørndal L, Larsen T. Changes in the cultivable flora in deep carious lesions following a stepwise excavation procedure. Caries Res 2000;34(6):502–508

43. Maltz M, de Oliveira EF, Fontanella V, Bianchi R. A clinical, microbiologic, and radiographic study of deep caries lesions after incomplete caries removal. Quintessence Int 2002;33(2):151–159

44. Weerheijm KL, Kreulen CM, de Soet JJ, Groen HJ, van Amerongen WE. Bacterial counts in carious dentine under restorations: 2-year in vivo effects. Caries Res 1999;33(2):130–134

45. Paddick JS, Brailsford SR, Kidd EA, Beighton D. Phenotypic and genotypic selection of microbiota surviving under dental restorations. Appl Environ Microbiol 2005;71(5):2467–2472

46. Leksell E, Ridell K, Cvek M, Mejàre I. Pulp exposure after stepwise versus direct complete excavation of deep carious lesions in young posterior permanent teeth. Endod Dent Traumatol 1996;12(4):192–196

47. Bjørndal L, Reit C, Bruun G, et al. Treatment of deep caries lesions in adults: randomized clinical trials comparing stepwise vs. direct complete excavation, and direct pulp capping vs. partial pulpotomy. Eur J Oral Sci 2010;118(3):290–297

48. Magnusson BO, Sundell SO. Stepwise excavation of deep carious lesions in primary molars. J Int Assoc Dent Child 1977;8(2):36–40

49. Mertz-Fairhurst EJ, Curtis JW Jr, Ergle JW, Rueggeberg FA, Adair SM. Ultraconservative and cariostatic sealed restorations: results at year 10. J Am Dent Assoc 1998;129(1):55–66

50. Ricketts DN, Kidd EA, Innes N, Clarkson J. Complete or ultraconservative removal of decayed tissue in unfilled teeth. Cochrane Database Syst Rev 2006;3(3):CD003808

51. Mertz-Fairhurst EJ, Call-Smith KM, Shuster GS, et al. Clinical performance of sealed composite restorations placed over caries compared with sealed and unsealed amalgam restorations. J Am Dent Assoc 1987;115(5):689–694

52. Ribeiro CCC, Baratieri LN, Perdigão J, Baratieri NM, Ritter AV. A clinical, radiographic, and scanning electron microscopic evaluation of adhesive restorations on carious dentin in primary teeth. Quintessence Int 1999;30(9):591–599

53. Thompson VP, Craig RG, Curro FA, Green WS, Ship JA. Treatment of deep carious lesions by complete excavation or partial removal: a critical review. J Am Dent Assoc 2008;139(6):705–712

54. Al-Omari WM, Al-Omari QD, Omar R. Effect of cavity disinfection on postoperative sensitivity associated with amalgam restorations. Oper Dent 2006;31(2):165–170

55. Ersin NK, Candan U, Aykut A, Eronat C, Belli S. No adverse effect to bonding following caries disinfection with chlorhexidine. J Dent Child (Chic) 2009;76(1):20–27

56. Walsh LJ. The current status of laser applications in dentistry. Aust Dent J 2003;48(3):146–155, quiz 198

57. Williams JA, Pearson GJ, Colles MJ, Wilson M. The photo-activated antibacterial action of toluidine blue O in a collagen matrix and in carious dentine. Caries Res 2004;38(6):530–536

58. Noack MJ, Wicht MJ, Haak R. Lesion orientated caries treatment—a classification of carious dentin treatment procedures. Oral Health Prev Dent 2004;2(Suppl 1):301–306

59. Polydorou O, Pelz K, Hahn P. Antibacterial effect of an ozone device and its comparison with two dentin-bonding systems. Eur J Oral Sci 2006;114(4):349–353

60. Innes N, Evans D, Hall N. The Hall Technique for managing carious primary molars. Dent Update 2009;36(8):472–474, 477–478

61. Oen KT, Thompson VP, Vena D, et al. Attitudes and expectations of treating deep caries: a PEARL Network survey. Gen Dent 2007;55(3):197–203

62. Christiansen J. Non-operative Caries Treatment. In: Splieth, C ed. Revolutions in Pediatric Dentistry. London: Quintessence Publ; 2011:21–35

Minimally Invasive Therapy with Tooth-Colored Direct Restorative Materials

Roland Frankenberger, Uwe Blunck

19

Minimally invasive caries therapy with composites has revolutionized restorative dentistry.[1–3] With the help of **composites**, it is possible to restore teeth while maintaining a maximum amount of sound enamel and dentin, so Black's rule **"extension for prevention"** is no longer considered generally valid.[4–8] The fundamental prerequisite for the use of composites is effective adhesion to enamel and dentin (Chapter 14).[9–12] Other materials besides composites are considered of secondary importance in this chapter. Today, composites and compomers are used to an almost equal degree,[13–15] whereas glass-ionomer cements tend to be used for semipermanent restorations.[16]

In the posterior region, amalgams are still the reference against which other materials are compared, owing to their durability, functionality, and role as a basic restoration material[17]; however, amalgam restorations have been superseded for quite a while in dental practices with tooth-colored composite restorations. Attention remains focused on such critical factors as abrasion, secondary caries, and fractures, since these have been the weak areas for decades in posterior composite restorations.[2,11,17–20] Every new development must address these issues. In general, function is the primary consideration in the **posterior region**, that is, clinical performance, with the cofactors of approximal contact, protection of the pulp, and resistance to abrasion and fractures.[5,6,21,22] Esthetics are of secondary importance in this region, since it is mostly not necessary to render posterior fillings invisible to satisfy the patient.

In the **anterior region**, esthetically perfect restorations are generally recommended and explicitly desired by patients. Cutting-edge biomimetic composites are a welcome alternative to conventional, universal composites.

NOTE

Function is paramount in posterior restorations, whereas esthetics is generally the chief consideration for anterior teeth.

In general, a minimally invasive approach involves more than just defect-oriented preparation. If the access in enamel to the cavity is too small to allow for proper application of the adhesive this would jeopardize the whole procedure. The compromised adhesion might result in an untimely renewal of the restoration due to adjacent caries, finally resulting in a rather large restoration. Furthermore, the major advantage of composite materials is that they **can be repaired and corrected**. Since removing all the composite is associated with the hazard of the iatrogenic removal of sound dentin and enamel and exposure of the pulp repair of partially insufficient restorations is a good alternative.[23] The three factors for successful minimally invasive therapy are therefore defect-oriented preparation, permanently adhesive restorations, and reparability.

This chapter addresses the following topics:
- Indications for restorative therapy
- Groups of materials used for direct resin restorations
- The choice of materials for different indications
- Preparation instruments
- The rules of minimally invasive preparations
- Clinical experience with minimally invasive restorative therapy
- Corrections or repairs of existing restorations

Indications for Restorative Therapy

Posterior Teeth

The decision for invasive therapy of approximal caries in posterior teeth is made on the basis of a visual-tactile assessment and radiographic examination of the caries (Chapters 5, 6, 9, and 20). Restoration of an approximal carious tooth surface is indicated when it is cavitated and/or the caries extends radiographically into the middle third of the dentin (**Fig. 19.1**),[24–26] since noninvasive or microinvasive interventions are no longer sufficient to arrest the progress of the caries.

Anterior Teeth

The appearance of anterior teeth is generally very important to an individual's self-image and social acceptance. Carious hard tissues, tooth discoloration, existing restorations, and insufficient margins are generally perceived very quickly by others. Consequently, therapy chiefly needs to focus on **restoring the natural appearance** of the upper anterior teeth in particular. If lesions are diagnosed and treated when they are small, their treatment (e.g. repair) is easier, quicker, and more successful. In addition, restorations may need to be replaced when the discoloration of the surface or margins of existing composite fillings impair the esthetic appearance of the anterior

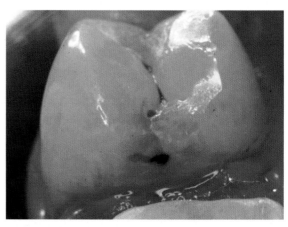

Fig. 19.1 Initial cavitation (ICDAS 3) of approximal caries.

teeth. Such situations can also be remedied by correcting the restoration.

Cervical Area

Manifestations and Causes

Cervical defects have many different manifestations. Some have shell-like configurations, others have the shape of wedges with sharp edges, others are caused by caries, and others manifest different levels of enamel and dentin loss due to wear. All of these lesions can lead to increased sensitivity or esthetic impairment.

Since people are increasingly retaining their teeth, even in advanced age, the cervical area is increasingly becoming a particular problem area. This represents a challenge for dental therapy, since cervical restorations have a much **lower survival rate** than restorations in other areas.[27,28]

Although the appearances of cervical lesions can vary widely, they frequently have the same result: increased sensitivity. As the gingiva recedes, dentin is exposed. The superficial cementum layer wears off relatively quickly, exposing dentin tubules which can result in **hypersensitivity.** Morphological studies have revealed that open tubules are more frequently found in areas of increased dentin sensitivity.[29] Within the tubules, the dentin liquor can be forced to move by osmotic, mechanical, or thermal stimuli. This explanation corresponds to the hydrodynamic theory of Brännström,[30] according to which A-delta fibers are stimulated, which explains the stabbing, sharp pain experienced by the patient. The goal of treating sensitive cervical areas is to seal the tubules and thereby prevent the movement of the dentin liquor by external stimuli.

Dentin hypersensitivity can also arise from the removal of the enamel caused by the (cervical) erosion of the tooth surfaces, for example,[31] which generally also includes a certain amount of mechanical abrasion (Chapters 2 and 3). In combination with occlusal overloading, mechanical abrasion can lead to **wedge-shaped defects** with sharp edges without requiring the effect of acid. The etiological factors are considered to be horizontal brushing and a strong eccentric load on the tooth. It has been proposed

that the tooth bends under the functional load which can contribute to the cervical defect. As photoelastical images reveal, the development of stress is the greatest at the interface between the enamel and cementum when the tooth is under a functional load. The deeper the wedge-shaped defect, the stronger the bending of the tooth.[32,33]

> **NOTE**
>
> Cervical defects in the form of lost dentin and enamel can assume different shapes such as craters or sharp-edged defects. Frequently, patients complain of elevated and sometimes painful sensitivity in the exposed cervical dentin.

There are therefore many reasons apart from caries why cervical defects develop which must each be considered when treating the patient, so that the progress of the lesion can be halted and proper restorative material can be selected (**Fig. 19.2**).

> **NOTE**
>
> Early identification of cervical defects is important so that the patient can be offered early enough instruction regarding appropriate oral hygiene.

Technical Limits to Direct Restorative Materials

Long-lasting reconstructions can be inserted that appear almost natural by combining different opacities and transparencies (**Fig. 19.3**). The appropriateness of laboratory-made veneers increases with the extent of the defect in the labial surface. The extension of veneers passes smoothly to ceramic partial or full crowns.

In the **posterior region,** direct resin restorations tend to be preferred over indirect restorations with, for example, ceramics. Minimally invasive initial restorations of caries lesions are the ideal indication for the direct use of composites; however, nowadays the routine work in restora-

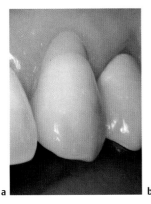 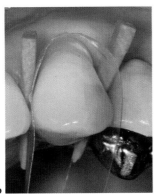 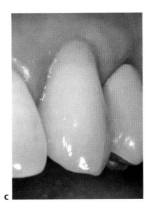

a   b   c

Fig. 19.2a–c Cervical defect of tooth 23, protection of the cavity from contamination with saliva by using a cervical matrix band and after placing composite.

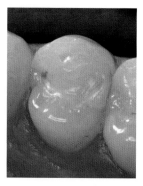
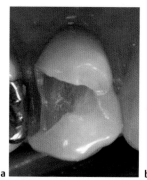
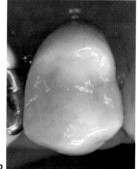
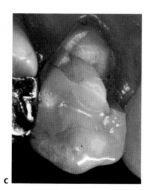

Fig. 19.3 Composite restoration after 17 years.

Fig. 19.4a–c Extremely undermined restoration.
a Cavity.
b Initial situation.
c 11 years afterward.

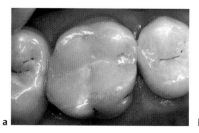
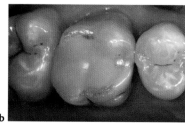

Fig. 19.5a, b Extensive composite restoration, both initially (**a**) and after 6 years (**b**).

tive dentistry mainly includes the replacement of insufficient restorations, which become larger each time, in particular when caries lesions have developed adjacent to the restorations. There are three potential problems or risks associated with direct composite restorations:

1. **Shrinkage during polymerization.** The larger the cavity, the greater the problems associated with the shrinkage of the composite during polymerization.[9,20,34,35] The tension exerted on the enamel structures increases as the support offered by the dentin decreases, which leads to a greater number of cracks that can weaken the dental hard tissues and endanger the overall integrity of the bond to the tooth (**Fig. 19.4**). Horizontal fracture lines are particularly problematic, whereas vertical enamel cracks occur in practically all adhesively restored teeth, especially with greater drying.[4,15,20]

2. **Abrasion behavior.** As long as the occlusion has a certain amount of support in the intact enamel, the occlusal composite will be subject to less load than if there is an extensive composite reconstruction of the masticatory surface.[9,20,36] Whereas minimally invasive composite restorations are protected from being abraded by the enamel components, partial or complete reconstructions of the masticatory surface suffer significantly more abrasion.[3,8,15,21] This does not cause the failure of the restoration; however, the anatomical shape can be slowly lost over time (**Fig. 19.5**).

3. **Time and effort for the dentist.** The shrinkage of the composite is less in small, intracoronal reconstructions with a sufficient amount of residual dentin and enamel; in addition, the amount of effort required by the dentist is limited since the remaining hard tissues in the occlusal area makes it significantly easier to model the composite material and reconstruct the masticatory surfaces.[15] However, if entire occlusal surfaces and cusps need to be reconstructed, the amount of effort required by the dentist is significant.[37] Since occlusion cannot be checked during modeling when using the contamination-sensitive adhesive technique, a great deal of practice and time are required. In addition, there is a certain risk of mislocating in the tip of the cusps as well as important anatomical structures such as central cusp slopes and marginal ridges.

NOTE

Polymerization shrinkage, abrasion, and sensitivity to the technique are the major limitations of resin restorative materials.

Materials for Tooth-colored Direct Restorative Therapy

Overview

Various materials can be used to create tooth-colored resin restorations. In the developmental history of restorations, it was first attempted to adapt classic cements to the color of teeth. From this group of cements, only **glass-ionomer cement** remains relevant in practice, which is easy to process since it independently adheres to the dentin and enamel. In contrast, **composites** can achieve a much more esthetically attractive result. Their translucence approaches the natural appearance of teeth. However, when this group of materials is used, the cavity must be pretreated with adhesive systems, which is relatively time-consuming.

For this reason, there have been several efforts to modify conventional glass-ionomer cements. One of these modifications is **resin-modified glass-ionomer cements**, another is **compomers**.

Glass-Ionomer Cements

Glass-ionomer cements are made of a mixture of **powdered glass** and **polyalkene acids**. They are also termed polyacrylic acids and typically contain carboxylate groups. The primary advantage of this group of materials is their **release of fluoride,** the clinical efficacy of which is a subject of controversy. In comparison to composites, the cavity is relatively easy to pretreat. Glass-ionomer cements adhere chemically to enamel and dentin trough the ion bonds of the carboxylate groups. However, the esthetic appearance of glass ionomer cements is less satisfactory as they are usually highly opaque. Furthermore, materials of this group are **less resistant to abrasion** and are very sensitive to drying and contamination with saliva or blood during the setting phase.[38]

NOTE

Glass ionomer cements have the advantage of chemically bonding to the dental hard tissues.

Composites

Products made of composite materials are the most widespread and frequently used for therapy with tooth-colored resin restorative materials. These consist of **monomer systems** that possess at least two methacrylate groups per residue and harden by polymerization. Embedded in this matrix are fillers of different types and sizes that can form chemical bonds with the monomers by means of silanization to improve stability. A categorization of these composites by fillers is shown in **Fig. 19.6**.

Developments in recent years have yielded commercially available composite fillers that have satisfactory physical properties and are generally suitable for use in dental practice. Composite fillers have been continuously refined over the years, since they are responsible for nearly every clinically relevant factor of a system. For example, the composition of the filler and its particle size determine important properties such as the stress arising from polymerization shrinkage, abrasion resistance, fracture toughness, radiopacity, polishability, and adhesion and hence handling by the user.

NOTE

Composites comprise:
- A monomer matrix
- Fillers of various types and sizes
- Silanes which bind the fillers to the matrix

Fillers are now so advanced that any significant reduction of polymerization shrinkage can only be achieved by new approaches in matrix chemistry: The recently introduced **silorans** (Filtek Silorane by 3 MEspe, Seefeld, Germany) represent a step in this direction with their use of ring-opening systems. They offer a product with **shrinkage below 1%.**[39] With classic composites, a linear shrinkage of about 1.5% appears to be a bottom threshold that cannot be reduced any further through innovations in fillers.

Abrasion resistance which can significantly influence the longevity of a restoration that is subject to mastication has been enhanced to a satisfactory clinical level.[40] This also implies that the classical division of indications for the anterior and posterior composites has become outmoded: All commercially available systems are quite ca-

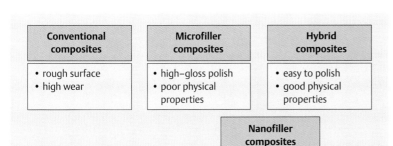

Fig. 19.6 Categorization of dental composite materials by fillers. The nanocomposites combine the positive properties of microfiller and hybrid composites.

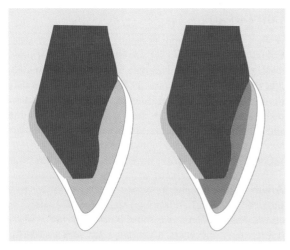

Fig. 19.7 Two-layer (left) and three-layer technique for an anterior restoration (see text below).

pable of satisfying the high physical requirements of abrasion resistance and bending resistance in the posterior region. Practically the only identifiable differences are in polishability.[41]

Since the material properties of the composites have apparently been developed to a level that is difficult to surpass, **classifying composites by filler particles** (**Fig. 19.6**) is important to understand historical development, but no longer helps the practitioner to choose a system for his or her practice. An alternative classification of composite materials according to translucence and opacity can therefore help dentists select the right composite from the broad spectrum of products. A distinction can be made between product lines that offer a single transparency or opacity and those that offer up to three. There are only relatively few composites that offer only one translucency. These provide basic restorations without esthetic considerations, and go so far as to state that they are only available in a single color.

There are two basic types of modern product lines that focus on esthetics. Whereas some manufacturers retain and refine the approach of three opacities/translucencies, other companies focus on the natural anatomy of the tooth. Here only dentin and enamel composites for highly esthetic restorations are available, composites that are consequently limited to two translucencies. These two different approaches determine the layering technique for the specific composites. In general, a distinction can be drawn between the **two-layer** and **three-layer technique** corresponding to the number of translucencies (**Fig. 19.7**).[42]

Composites can therefore be used to create restorations esthetically adapted to the available hard tissue, so that the defects are no longer visible to the naked eye.

Resin-Modified Glass-Ionomer Cements

With resin-modified glass-ionomer cements, **methacrylate groups** were incorporated into the **polyacrylic acid molecule.** This rendered the material light-curable, and adding hydrophilic monomers elevated the fracture toughness of the products in comparison to classic glass-ionomer cements.[43]

Products belonging to this group need to be mixed. In addition to the polymerization of the hydrophilic monomers, the acid/base reaction of polyacrylic acid with the glasses requires water as a medium. Resin-modified glass-ionomer cements therefore have a longer setting time than classic glass-ionomer cements, however, the curing reaction starts immediately on exposure to light. Their curing time is therefore less than that of classic glass-ionomer cements.

Compomers

The name of this group of materials suggests that it consists of a mixture of glass-ionomer cements and composite. These are essentially polyacrylate-modified composites, since **carboxylate** groups are added to the **diacrylate** monomer in this group of materials.[44] The subsequent absorption of water causes the reaction with the glasses (fillers). **Release of fluoride**, although to a much lesser extent than with glass-ionomer cements, is measurable. Nonetheless, there exists some uncertainty as to whether the release of fluoride is clinically relevant.[45]

In any case, products in this group of materials have a higher abrasion resistance than glass-ionomer cements.[46] On the other hand, compomers do not independently adhere to the dentin and enamel, and they must be used together with an adhesive system to achieve gap-free margins.

Choosing Materials for Different Indications

Posterior Region

Whereas glass-ionomer cements are generally used for semipermanent restorations,[16] **composites** allow permanent restorations to be inserted.[5–7,20,37] The range of indications for direct composites extends from minimally invasive restorations to the replacement of cusps.[3,8,22,37]

Anterior Region

Esthetically satisfying restorations in the anterior region can be reliably achieved with composite materials. Clinical studies have demonstrated, however, that compomers can produce satisfactory results for a period of more than two years.[48,49] Over the long term, the surface gloss and color stability of **composite** materials are better.[50]

Cervical Defects

Owing to their potential release of fluoride, the use of glass-ionomer cements is recommended for patients with high caries risk. Resin-modified glass-ionomer cements are also suitable in such instances. It is better to treat erosion and abrasion with an acid- and abrasion-resistant material such as composites. Compomers can also be used. Compomers are recommended for wedge-shaped defects, since they have a low modulus of elasticity and the material can follow the flexure of the tooth under a functional load. Composites have also been successfully used for this type of cervical defect. Given their color, translucency, opacity, and polishability, **composites** can be recommended as a standard material.

In some cases, glass-ionomer cements have the advantage of independently adhering to the dental hard tissue by the formation of ion bonds. It can therefore be occasionally helpful to use glass-ionomer cements in situations where contamination in the form of saliva, blood, and sulcus fluid is difficult to control in order to exploit more efficiently the relatively small time-window of a contamination-free environment. Contrastingly, compomers and composites can only be used together with an adhesive system. Depending on the adhesive system (Etch&Rinse or a self-etching system, see also Chapter 14), more time is required.

NOTE

In general, composites are used in combination with an adhesive system to restore cervical defects.

Preparation Instruments

Preparation instruments for adhesive restorations should enable cavities to be created in a **minimally invasive** manner. However, this does not automatically mean that only the smallest grinding and drilling instruments can be used. Extensive preparation may be necessary when the carious defects are large.

Excavation

Rose-head steel burs for excavating caries are still not outmoded. These burs are easy to use, easy to sterilize, and effective.[51–53] It is preferable to use burs with a larger diameter, if applicable, and to apply low pressure. Zirconium oxide round burs are also effective. However, it is not possible to utilize them to selectively remove caries, since the hardness of the zirconium drills is greater than that of dentin.[54] **Polymer burs** can be advantageous since their reduced hardness causes them to wear once harder dentinal parts within the lesion are reached.[55] After several unsuccessful attempts with related materials, this type of drill was again introduced into the market in 2011. These instruments are intended for single applications and are unsuitable for routine caries excavation. For cautious excavation close to the pulp, these are an (expensive) alternative to **hand excavators** (Chapters 3 and 18).

Rotating Preparation

Diamond burs are suitable for opening cavities in the occlusal surface, for creating an outline form, and refining accessible areas. In the interproximal region, there is a substantial danger of **injuring the neighboring tooth.** Therefore these areas should be protected, for example, by using a steel matrix band.

Oscillating Preparation

Oscillating preparation tools are helpful for the difficult access to the interproximal region, since one side is non-abrasive, which makes them harmless to the neighboring tooth.[1,56–58] There are basically two types of oscillating preparation, the SonicSys system and bevel-shape files (**Fig. 19.8**).[56]

NOTE

Oscillating preparation is one of the cornerstones of the minimally invasive adhesive technique.

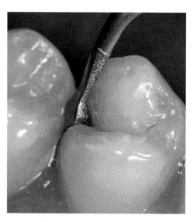

Fig. 19.8 Oscillating preparation tool with a nonabrasive side that protects the neighboring tooth.

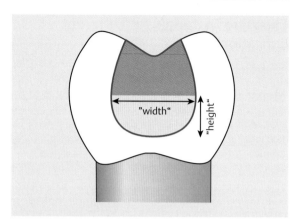

Fig. 19.9 During approximal preparation (vertical slot), the red area indicates sound dental hard tissues that must be sacrificed to reach the caries. The "width" of the lesion area is greater than the "height"

Rules for Minimally Invasive Preparation

General Preparation Rules

In general, Black's preparation rules are not useful for minimally invasive restoration. If the maxim of "extension for prevention" were to be followed, too much hard tissue would be removed.[59] In a modified form, Black's preparation rules (Chapter 20) would run as follows when applied to the adhesive technique:
- **Preventive extension:** Extending the cavity beyond the limits of the carious hard tissues is only recommended if it improves the prognosis of the restoration.
- **Outline form:** Maintaining a certain amount of overall perspective is always necessary with adhesive preparations. Open the cavity until the caries can be reliably excavated.
- **Resistance form:** A resistance form is not necessary. Prepared resistance for the restorative material is superfluous due to adhesion.

Access Forms

Anterior Region

In the anterior region, it is generally recommended to obtain access to the approximal caries lesions from a **palatal direction** to minimize the extension into the visible area.

Posterior Region

Approximal caries in the posterior region can be reached in various ways. **Vertical slot preparation** is most suitable, even if a large amount of the sound marginal ridge needs to be removed.[59] Given the location of the caries, the preparation generally assumes the shape of a double

drop. This means that the prepared cavity looks like a drop from the approximal direction as well as from the buccal/oral direction (imaginary cross-section from mesial to distal). This results from the extent and location of the caries. Viewed from an approximal direction, the caries extends further in a buccal/oral direction ("width") than in a cervical/coronal direction ("height"). If a cross-section of the approximal region is considered (box), the caries in the dentin generally extends further in the cervical direction than in the enamel. Consequently, the dentin at the bottom of the box needs to be removed, but the preparation of the approximal cervical margins is delimited by the enamel.

Slot preparations provide a sufficient overview for the removal of carious dentin. A potential disadvantage is that to reach the actual caries lesion, a considerable amount of the sound dental hard tissues need to be removed in the area of the marginal ridge (**Fig. 19.9**).

It has been suggested that slot preparations may also be prepared at a 90° angle to conventional ones (horizontal).[57] This is possible in principle, but the overview tends to be worse than with conventional slot preparations, given the hidden access from oral or vestibular direction. The incremental technique also becomes more difficult. Injection techniques are preferable using flowable composites.

Tunnel preparation has also been described in the literature.[15,60–63] The idea is to reach the approximal caries from the occlusal fossa (**Fig. 19.10**) and largely bypass the marginal ridge. The approach of tunnel preparation most closely emulates the goal of minimal invasiveness; however, in many cases it is difficult to precisely excavate the caries at the enamel–dentin junction below the marginal ridge, and the fracture resistance of the remaining marginal ridge is also quite low.

Class I (Fissures and Grooves)

The preparation for occlusal composite restorations is simpler than approximal preparation, since there is no danger of harming the neighboring tooth. The occlusal enamel is only removed enough to expose the caries below the fissure and reliably remove it. Beveling of the enamel is not neccessary to increase retention. However, the prepared margins should be modified (rounded, <0.5 mm), since enamel prisms directly next to filling margins could break off which will be clinically visible as white lines.[64] The access cavity should be large enough to ensure adequate excavation of the caries. Overhanging enamel areas do not necessarily need to be removed. Similar principles apply to preparations in the area of grooves in oral or vestibular surfaces.

NOTE

Beveling the enamel is not necessary for increase of retention; rounding the preparation margins, however, is recommended to prevent paramarginal cracks in the enamel.

Class II (Approximal-Occlusal)

Approximal caries lesions are mainly accessed from the occlusal aspect.[57,59,65] Marginal ridges are prepared with a rough diamond bur, preferably without injuring the enamel area directly next to the neighboring tooth. The final fragment is preferably removed by oscillation (e.g., with SonicSys).[60] Always remember that **sonically vibrating preparation** instruments are not preparation instruments per se but rather finishing instruments. Attempts to prepare marginal ridges that are not decayed by using these instruments without previously using rotating instruments will not work well and will wear out the diamond-coated attachment quickly, which is inefficient given its expense. SonicSys instruments as well as bevel-shape files are most suitable for approximal beveling since these instruments significantly reduce the risk of **iatrogenic damage** to neighboring teeth.[1,58]

NOTE

Access to the approximal box is preferably from an occlusal direction. To avoid injuring the neighboring tooth, oscillating finishing instruments that are flat on one side are recommended.

Class III and Class IV (Anterior Tooth)

The preparation for restoring class III cavities (incisally sound) and class IV (edges) involves beveling the margins of the enamel in addition to restricting the cavity to the defect (Chapter 25, Case 3). Depending on the functional

stress on the restoration a bevel of 1.5–2 mm with rotating instruments is prepared. This increases the adhesive surface to provide sufficient retention even under functional loads on incisal margins or edges.[66,67]

In the labial area, it can be useful to make the bevel slightly wavy instead of straight, corresponding to the contour of the labial surface of the upper middle incisors. The bevel is created so that the transition in color from the tooth to the restoration is not noticeable. Deviations from the shape tend to be perceived as different color nuances. Surface structures also help, which imitate the structured surface of the enamel that is, at least, found in children and adolescents. Consequently, when treating lesions in older patients who have generally unstructured, smooth enamel surfaces, it is a greater challenge to create an invisible **color transition** from the enamel to the composite.

NOTE

Depending on the functional load, a sufficiently wide bevel is created which simultaneously helps to make the transition from the restoration to the tooth less obvious.

Class V (Cervical Area)

Generally, after determining the causes of the cervical defects (chemical, mechanical, etc.), **dentin hypersensitivity**, which is what patients generally find the most troubling, is treated first. As mentioned earlier, the goal of treating sensitive cervical areas is to seal the open tubules. This is achieved by applying desensitizing solutions or adhesive systems that seal the tubule systems. The effectiveness of adhesive systems in the treatment of sensitized tooth necks has been demonstrated in various studies.[68–70]

It is obvious that large carious defects need to be treated. Moreover, major wedge-shaped defects should be treated to protect the remaining tooth dental hard tissues and to stabilize the tooth with a restoration. In-vitro studies have not, however, been able to demonstrate the usefulness of restorations for stabilizing a tooth with wedge-shaped defects.[71]

Problems in the Treatment of Cervical Defects

The **gingiva** is a major problem in the treatment of cervical defects since the cervical margin of the lesions is generally near the sulcus. There is the danger of bleeding, and frequently the margin of the cavity extends below the level of the gingiva which renders it uncontrollable, especially in the case of carious defects. In such cases, a gingectomy is the only option in order to reliably restore the lesion.

Independent of the restorative material, **contamination** with saliva, blood, or sulcus fluid should be avoided. This can be done with a dental dam, retraction cords, or transparent cervical matrixes. The latter is a good compromise

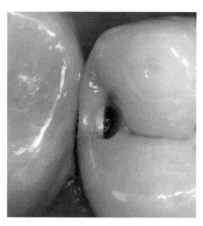

Fig. 19.10 Illustration of the invasive access from the occlusal fossa to treat approximal caries (caries progressiva media).

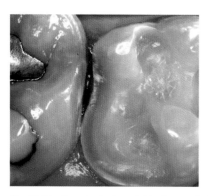

Fig. 19.11 Damage to the neighboring tooth during approximal preparation.

between a cervical dam (the gingiva in the cervical area can be easily traumatized by the clamps) and retraction cords which are not always reliable. The transparent cervical matrix can move the gingiva away from the cervical margin of the cavity and can simultaneously protect it from being contaminated with saliva, blood, and sulcus fluid (**Fig. 19.2**). The long ends of the matrix strip that extend into the oral cavity should be cut to keep patients from displacing the matrix with their tongue.

Another problem associated with applying adhesive systems is **differing dentin structures.** We frequently find sclerotic dentin on the surfaces of cervical defects, which has been exposed to the oral milieu for a long time. The surface layer becomes hypermineralized, and a thin hybrid layer is established only when the adhesive system is applied.[72] This sclerotic dentin can be removed with a round bur, for example. This pretreatment is recommended to increase the efficiency of the adhesive systems.[73,74]

NOTE

In addition to beveling the margins of the cavity in the enamel, it is recommended to abrade the usually hypermineralized dentin of noncarious cervical defects.

Damage to the Neighboring Tooth in Approximal Preparations

If only rotating tools are used to prepare the approximal area, the neighboring tooth may become damaged[75] (**Fig. 19.11**). Of course, it is possible to use interdental wedges with consecutive separation as well as steel matrix bands to protect the intact surface of the neighboring tooth. However, this takes a great deal of time that is avoided if oscillating instruments are used.

Clinical Experience with Minimally Invasive Restorative Therapy

Posterior Teeth

Relevant indicators for the **prognosis of restorative materials** are the median survival rate (the number of years at which 50% of restorations still exist), and the annual rate of failure (the percentage of restorations which fail per year).[5,14,20,35,76] Only after several years of clinical use are restoration changes anticipated, since restorations generally remain functional during the first few years.[3,11,21,76,78,79]

Glass-ionomer cements are semipermanent materials and are not appropriate for the filling of minimally invasively prepared cavities because they generally require a resistance form. They are insufficiently stable, at least at bevelled margins. The annual failure rate in many studies is greater than 10%, which is unacceptable. With conventional glass-ionomer cements, the danger of fractures is usually high,[16] whereas the abrasion resistance of resin-modified glass-ionomers is so low that the anatomical shape cannot be ensured.[77]

To determine the prognosis of composite restorations, several things need to be considered: the age of the study, the use of base materials (e.g. cements), the adhesive system, and quality of the individual dentist. All of these factors influence the probability of clinical success. Older studies which are frequently cited, generally report caries adjacent to restorations as the primary reason for the failure of composite restorations.[2,11,36,76] However, these studies used adhesive systems that are no longer on the market, because they did not work. In addition, conventional phosphate cement or glass-ionomer cement underfillings were used in many older studies. It is now known that the use of **base materials** enhance the danger of fractures to fillings and are consequently not recommended for use in adhesive restorative therapy.[78]

Minimally invasive composite restorations appear to perform outstandingly well when done correctly. All restorations remained intact in a current practice-based study after 6 years of observation.[4,40] However, data from a meta-analysis indicate that the average success rate of direct class I/II restorations was only 9 years for permanent posterior teeth. Indirect restorations, by contrast, have higher success rates due to the decreased polymerization shrinkage due to curing (**Fig. 19.12**).

NOTE

The longevity of composite restorations decreases with the invasiveness of the restoration and the masticatory load.

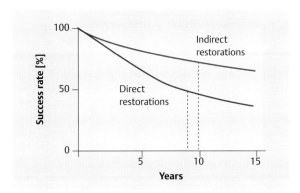

Fig. 19.12 Average success rate (%) of direct and indirect class I/II restorations of permanent posterior teeth (modified according to ref. 27).

Anterior Teeth

A series of factors need to be considered when restoring carious teeth, closing diastemas, and correcting malpositioning and deviant forms of individual teeth[80,81]:

- The color and transparency of the restoration should match that of the natural tooth, if possible.
- The occlusal contacts should be adjusted so that occlusion functions well and the approximal contacts should be sufficiently tight.
- Trauma to the gingiva from the restoration must be avoided.
- The subjective and objective appearance of the restoration should be an improvement over the initial situation.
- The longevity of the restoration must be ensured by appropriately processing the selected composite materials and by the application techniques, layer thicknesses, reliable light curing, finishing and polishing.

In a recently published study of **changes to anterior tooth shape**[81] in which 284 teeth underwent direct composite restorations, a statistical success rate of 80% was observed after 5 years. The advantages of this type of treatment over indirect restorations are:

- Deviations in position and shape can be corrected in a single treatment session.
- Minimally invasive procedure, that is, only a slight amount of dental hard tissue is removed.
- The restoration can be removed if desired, and the tooth can be returned to its original state.
- Good cost effectiveness, since no laboratory work is required.
- More invasive restorations such as veneers or all-ceramic (partial) crowns can easily be inserted later if necessary.

Cervical Area

The clinical experience with treatment of cervical defects using tooth-colored restorative materials such as glass ionomer cement, compomers, and composites is assessed differently in the literature.

The major advantages of **glass-ionomer cements** are the release of fluoride and chemical adhesion to the dental hard tissues. For this reason, glass-ionomers are recommended for treating cervical lesions in patients with a high risk of caries.

Clinical trials have also revealed annual failure rates of ca. 2% over long periods, a statistically significant higher level than all other restorative materials for treating cervical defects.[28] One major disadvantage is that the esthetics of the material are worse than compomers and composites.

Satisfactory cosmetic results can be achieved with **composite materials** which are more transparent. However, the application of the required adhesive system takes longer than pretreating the cavity for glass-ionomer cements. Another advantage of composites is that preparation is minimally invasive since macro-mechanical retention is not required when adhesive systems are used.

The applied composite is subject to **shrinkage during polymerization,** which can be relatively significant due to an unfavorable **C-factor.** The C-factor describes the ratio of the bonded to unbonded surface of the applied composite increments and should be as small as possible to prevent major shrinkage stress. The greater the free surface, the less the shrinkage tension.[82] In class V cavities, the ratio of bonded to free surface can be quite high, depending on the type of preparation, box form, or treatment of shell-shaped erosion defects, and this yields high shrinkage tension.

This problem can be partially remedied by applying **flowable composites.** They possess a lower modulus of elasticity, and a large free surface arises from applying them in a layer. However, this technique takes more time, since several layers have to be applied.

NOTE

Flowable composites are highly suitable for the adhesive restoration of cervical defects.

Repairing Restorations

As outlined, in current daily practice a higher number of restorations are inserted due to **replacement** of old fillings compared with invasive treatment of new caries lesions. This means that each new restoration becomes old after a time and then has to be replaced. Therefore prescribing treatment which is early in relation to the disease stage (such as ICDAS 2 or approximal radiographical E2 lesions) sets into motion the "re-dentistry cycle" with the aforementioned consequences. This cycle starts earlier when noninvasive and microinvasive therapies are implemented (Chapters 15–17 and 20).

When changing a restoration, a substantial amount of dental hard tissue is lost. This is especially the case with tooth-colored restorations such as composite fillings or ceramic inlays.[23] Aggressive indications to completely replace a composite restoration therefore run counter to the goal of minimal interventional treatment. Premature tendencies to create new restorations are often based on an overconfident estimation of the life of dental restorations.

When realistically weighing whether to repair a restoration or insert a new one, the removability of the insufficient restoration always needs to be considered. Hence the reparability of adhesively bonded restorations in particular needs to be assessed, since much effort is required to remove restorations that are well adapted to the dentin, even when magnifying lenses are used. If the required time is not taken, this will undoubtedly mean that an unnecessary amount of dental hard tissue will be lost. The following **recommendations** are therefore made.

- Today, repairs are generally considered preferable and advantageous due to the following:
  - Repairs are cost-effective, especially when a direct application technique can still be used rather than an indirect method (e.g., partial crown)
  - Repairs are acceptable in areas that are esthetically less critical
  - To fill an access cavity
  - For corrections, for example, when the wrong color,

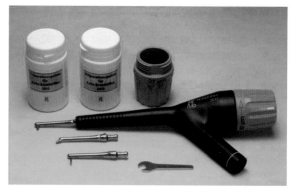

Fig. 19.13   Intraoral sandblaster (Rondoflex, KaVo) connected to the turbine connection of the dental unit. Can be filled with corundum (27 μm or 50 μm) or CoJet sand (27 μm). When blasting using corundum, products bonded to water produce less dust; with CoJet, bonding to water is chemically impossible since intraoral silicatizing only works in dry conditions.

opacity, or translucency was chosen for composite restorations of the upper anterior teeth.

- Contraindications to repairs:
  - Insufficient equipment
  - When untreated bruxism has caused the previous restoration to fail
  - When there probably was a systematic error (e.g., general adhesive failure) with the restoration to be repaired
  - When it is impossible to reliably reconstruct the approximal contact point.

The clinical repair procedure depends on the type and number of surfaces for adhesion, that is, the substrate surfaces to be restored. Repairs are simpler if there are fewer different substrates that have to be dealt with simultaneously.

Repairs are recommended for **cavities bordering composite** only (**Table 19.1**). Earlier, to estimate the success of repairs, the literature only offered analyses of shear bond strength results, which comprised about 65% of the cohe-

Table 19.1   Recommendations for composite repair

	Composite repair (without participation of the enamel and/or dentin)	Composite repair (with participation of the enamel and/or dentin)
Preparation or macroretention	Only to generate direct access Diamond bur (> 80 μm grit) and SonicSys if necessary	Only to generate direct access Diamond bur (> 80 μm grit) and SonicSys if necessary
Microretention	• Silicatizing (such as CoJet, 3M Espe) • Alternative: Sandblasting (PrepStart / Micro-Etcher, Danville; Rondoflex, Kavo, **Fig. 19.13**) • Rotating burs are impractical (danger of damaging the neighboring tooth)	(PrepStart / Micro-Etcher, Danville; Rondoflex, Kavo)
Bonding	Hydrophobic bonding agents (such as Heliobond, Ivoclar Vivadent) + thin layer of flowable composite (0.1–0.5 mm)	Complete adhesive system + thin layer of flowable compound (0.1–0.5 mm)

sive strength of intact composite samples.[83,84] Roughening with green silicon carbide burs, coarse preparation diamond burs, or sandblasting have been considered promising methods.[85,86] Interestingly, it has been shown that intentionally extending the repair cavity into the neighboring enamel is not to be recommended. This situation can be resolved; however, it is easier to only treat one adhesion substrate (composite). The preparation geometry also influences the durability of the bond to old composite restorations. For example, dovetail preparations are not useful since they increase the C-factor, and stress in the composite and hence in the gaps at the composite-to-composite transition also increase. Minimally invasive preparations with an undercut perform best, and lining with flowable composite enhances the marginal quality.[85]

Today, only a small amount of **clinical data** is available that compares new restorations with repairs. Over an observation period of several years, no difference was revealed between repairing, sealing, or replacement for restorations being discolored at their margins.[87]

NOTE

Repairs and corrections instead of new restorations is a clear trend in minimum intervention dentistry. Intraoral repair is now possible for nearly all restorations; the costs and benefits should be weighed, however.

SUMMARY

Tooth-colored resin restorative materials, which are usually inserted with the help of adhesives, are appropriate for restoring defects in the anterior, posterior, and cervical regions. The defects caused by caries lesions can be restored in an esthetically satisfactory and mechanically stable manner. In most situations and locations, composites are preferred over other groups of materials (including compomers and glass-ionomer cements). Because minimally invasive preparation is possible, the use of composites is frequently preferred over direct restorations with the traditional restorative material, amalgam, as well as indirect restorations with gold and ceramics (Chapter 20). Replacement should be weighed against repair of a restoration.

REFERENCES

1. Hugo B. Oscillating procedures in the preparation technic (I). [Article in German] Schweiz Monatsschr Zahnmed 1999; 109(2):140–160
2. Roulet JF. Benefits and disadvantages of tooth-coloured alternatives to amalgam. J Dent 1997;25(6):459–473
3. van Dijken JW. Durability of resin composite restorations in high C-factor cavities: a 12-year follow-up. J Dent 2010;38(6):469–474
4. Krämer N, Reinelt C, Richter G, Petschelt A, Frankenberger R. Nanohybrid vs. fine hybrid composite in Class II cavities: clinical results and margin analysis after four years. Dent Mater 2009;25(6):750–759
5. Manhart J, Chen H, Hamm G, Hickel R. Buonocore Memorial Lecture. Review of the clinical survival of direct and indirect restorations in posterior teeth of the permanent dentition. Oper Dent 2004;29(5):481–508
6. Nikaido T, Takada T, Kitasako Y, et al. Retrospective study of the 10-year clinical performance of direct resin composite restorations placed with the acid-etch technique. Quintessence Int 2007;38(5):240–246
7. Schirrmeister JF, Huber K, Hellwig E, Hahn P. Four-year evaluation of a resin composite including nanofillers in posterior cavities. J Adhes Dent 2009;11(5):399–404
8. van Dijken JW, Pallesen U. Clinical performance of a hybrid resin composite with and without an intermediate layer of flowable resin composite: a 7-year evaluation. Dent Mater 2011;27(2):150–156
9. Ferracane JL. Resin composite—state of the art. Dent Mater 2011;27(1):29–38
10. Frankenberger R, García-Godoy F, Lohbauer U, Petschelt A, Krämer N. Evaluation of resin composite materials. Part I: in vitro investigations. Am J Dent 2005;18(1):23–27
11. Roulet JF. The problems associated with substituting composite resins for amalgam: a status report on posterior composites. J Dent 1988;16(3):101–113
12. Van Meerbeek B, De Munck J, Mattar D, Van Landuyt K, Lambrechts P. Microtensile bond strengths of an etch&rinse and self-etch adhesive to enamel and dentin as a function of surface treatment. Oper Dent 2003;28(5):647–660
13. Frankenberger R, Reinelt C, Petschelt A, Krämer N. Operator vs. material influence on clinical outcome of bonded ceramic inlays. Dent Mater 2009;25(8):960–968
14. Huth KC, Manhart J, Selbertinger A, et al. 4-year clinical performance and survival analysis of Class I and II compomer restorations in permanent teeth. Am J Dent 2004;17(1):51–55
15. Krämer N, García-Godoy F, Reinelt C, Frankenberger R. Clinical performance of posterior compomer restorations over 4 years. Am J Dent 2006;19(1):61–66
16. Frankenberger R, Garcia-Godoy F, Kramer N. Clinical performance of viscous glass ionomer cement in posterior cavities over two years. Int J Dent 2009;10.1155/2009/781462
17. Bharti R, Wadhwani KK, Tikku AP, Chandra A. Dental amalgam: An update. J Conserv Dent 2010;13(4):204–208
18. Burke FJ, Palin WM, James A, Mackenzie L, Sands P. The current status of materials for posterior composite restorations: the advent of low shrink. Dent Update 2009;36(7):401–402, 404–406, 409
19. Ernst CP, Canbek K, Aksogan K, Willershausen B. Two-year clinical performance of a packable posterior composite with and without a flowable composite liner. Clin Oral Investig 2003;7(3):129–134
20. Hickel R, Manhart J. Longevity of restorations in posterior teeth and reasons for failure. J Adhes Dent 2001;3(1):45–64

21. van Dijken JW, Lindberg A. Clinical effectiveness of a low-shrinkage resin composite: a five-year evaluation. J Adhes Dent 2009;11(2):143–148

22. van Dijken JW, Pallesen U. Four-year clinical evaluation of Class II nano-hybrid resin composite restorations bonded with a one-step self-etch and a two-step etch-and-rinse adhesive. J Dent 2011;39(1):16–25

23. Krejci I, Lieber CM, Lutz F. Time required to remove totally bonded tooth-colored posterior restorations and related tooth substance loss. Dent Mater 1995;11(1):34–40

24. Espelid I, Tveit A, Haugejorden O, Riordan PJ. Variation in radiographic interpretation and restorative treatment decisions on approximal caries among dentists in Norway. Community Dent Oral Epidemiol 1985;13(1):26–29

25. Tveit AB, Espelid I, Skodje F. Restorative treatment decisions on approximal caries in Norway. Int Dent J 1999;49(3):165–172

26. Espelid I, Tveit AB, Mejàre I, Sundberg H, Hallonsten AL. Restorative treatment decisions on occlusal caries in Scandinavia. Acta Odontol Scand 2001;59(1):21–27

27. Manhart J, Chen H, Hamm G, Hickel R. Buonocore Memorial Lecture. Review of the clinical survival of direct and indirect restorations in posterior teeth of the permanent dentition. Oper Dent 2004;29(5):481–508

28. Peumans M, Kanumilli P, De Munck J, Van Landuyt K, Lambrechts P, Van Meerbeek B. Clinical effectiveness of contemporary adhesives: a systematic review of current clinical trials. Dent Mater 2005;21(9):864–881

29. Absi EG, Addy M, Adams D. Dentine hypersensitivity. A study of the patency of dentinal tubules in sensitive and non-sensitive cervical dentine. J Clin Periodontol 1987;14(5):280–284

30. Brännström M, Lindén LA, Aström A. The hydrodynamics of the dental tubule and of pulp fluid. A discussion of its significance in relation to dentinal sensitivity. Caries Res 1967;1(4):310–317

31. Lussi A. Dental erosion clinical diagnosis and case history taking. Eur J Oral Sci 1996;104(2(Pt 2)):191–198

32. Piotrowski BT, Gillette WB, Hancock EB. Examining the prevalence and characteristics of abfractionlike cervical lesions in a population of U.S. veterans. J Am Dent Assoc 2001;132(12):1694–1701, quiz 1726–1727

33. Takehara J, Takano T, Akhter R, Morita M. Correlations of noncarious cervical lesions and occlusal factors determined by using pressure-detecting sheet. J Dent 2008;36(10):774–779

34. Garcia-Godoy F, Krämer N, Feilzer AJ, Frankenberger R. Long-term degradation of enamel and dentin bonds: 6-year results in vitro vs. in vivo. Dent Mater 2010;26(11):1113–1118

35. Krämer N, García-Godoy F, Frankenberger R. Evaluation of resin composite materials. Part II: in vivo investigations. Am J Dent 2005;18(2):75–81

36. Drummond JL. Degradation, fatigue, and failure of resin dental composite materials. J Dent Res 2008;87(8):710–719

37. Schmidlin PR, Filli T, Imfeld C, Tepper S, Attin T. Three-year evaluation of posterior vertical bite reconstruction using direct resin composite—a case series. Oper Dent 2009;34(1):102–108

38. Wilson AD, Mclean JW. Glass-ionomer cement. London: Quintessence;Hannover Park 1988

39. Ilie N, Jelen E, Clementino-Luedemann T, Hickel R. Low-shrinkage composite for dental application. Dent Mater J 2007;26(2):149–155

40. Ferracane JL. Is the wear of dental composites still a clinical concern? Is there still a need for in vitro wear simulating devices? Dent Mater 2006;22(8):689–692

41. Da Costa J, Ferracane J, Paravina RD, Mazur RF, Roeder L. The effect of different polishing systems on surface roughness and gloss of various resin composites. J Esthet Restor Dent 2007;19(4):214–224, discussion 225–226

42. Dietschi D. Layering concepts in anterior composite restorations. J Adhes Dent 2001;3(1):71–80

43. Kim Y, Hirano S, Hirasawa T. Physical properties of resin-modified glass-ionomers. Dent Mater J 1998;17(1):68–76

44. McLean JW, Nicholson JW, Wilson AD. Proposed nomenclature for glass-ionomer dental cements and related materials. Quintessence Int 1994;25(9):587–589

45. Millar BJ, Abiden F, Nicholson JW. In vitro caries inhibition by polyacid-modified composite resins ('compomers'). J Dent 1998;26(2):133–136

46. Attin T, Buchalla W, Trett A, Hellwig E. Tooth brushing abrasion of polyacid-modified composites in neutral and acidic buffer solutions. J Prosthet Dent 1998;80(2):148–150

47. Manhart J, Chen HY, Hickel R. Clinical evaluation of the posterior composite Quixfil in class I and II cavities: 4-year follow-up of a randomized controlled trial. J Adhes Dent 2010;12(3):237–243

48. Demirci M, Yildiz E, Uysal O. Comparative clinical evaluation of different treatment approaches using a microfilled resin composite and a compomer in Class III cavities: two-year results. Oper Dent 2008;33(1):7–14

49. Tyas MJ. Three-year clinical evaluation of a polyacid-modified resin composite (Dyract). Oper Dent 2000;25(3):152–154

50. Folwaczny M, Loher C, Mehl A, Kunzelmann KH, Hinkel R. Tooth-colored filling materials for the restoration of cervical lesions: a 24-month follow-up study. Oper Dent 2000;25(4):251–258

51. Banerjee A, Watson TF, Kidd EAM. Dentine caries excavation: a review of current clinical techniques. Br Dent J 2000;188(9):476–482

52. Meller C, Welk A, Zeligowski T, Splieth C. Comparison of dentin caries excavation with polymer and conventional tungsten carbide burs. Quintessence Int 2007;38(7):565–569

53. Neves Ade A, Coutinho E, De Munck J, Van Meerbeek B. Caries-removal effectiveness and minimal-invasiveness potential of caries-excavation techniques: a micro-CT investigation. J Dent 2011;39(2):154–162

54. Dammaschke T, Vesnic A, Schafer E. In vitro comparison of ceramic burs and conventional tungsten carbide bud burs in dentin caries excavation. Quintessence Int 2008;39(6):495–499

55. Dammaschke T, Rodenberg TN, Schäfer E, Ott KH. Efficiency of the polymer bur SmartPrep compared with conventional tungsten carbide bud bur in dentin caries excavation. Oper Dent 2006;31(2):256–260

56. Hugo B, Lussi A, Hotz P. The preparation of enamel margin beveling in proximal cavities. [Article in German] Schweiz Monatsschr Zahnmed 1992;102(10):1181–1188

57. Hugo B, Stassinakis A. Preparation and restoration of small interproximal carious lesions with sonic instruments. Pract Periodontics Aesthet Dent 1998;10(3):353–359, quiz 360

58. Hugo B. Oscillating procedures in the preparation technic (II). Their development and application possibilities. [Article in German] Schweiz Monatsschr Zahnmed 1999;109(3):269–285

59. Wicht MJ, Haak R, Fritz UB, Noack MJ. Primary preparation of class II cavities with oscillating systems. Am J Dent 2002;15(1):21–25

60. Markovic D, Peric T. Clinical evaluation of glass-ionomer tunnel restorations in primary molars: 36 months results. Aust Dent J 2008;53(1):41–45

61. Pyk N, Mejàre I. Tunnel restorations in general practice. Influence of some clinical variables on the success rate. Acta Odontol Scand 1999;57(4):195–200

62. Sundberg H, Mejàre I, Espelid I, Tveit AB. Swedish dentists' decisions on preparation techniques and restorative materials. Acta Odontol Scand 2000;58(3):135–141

63. Wiegand A, Attin T. Treatment of proximal caries lesions by tunnel restorations. Dent Mater 2007;23(12):1461–1467

64. Bortolotto T, Onisor I, Krejci I. Proximal direct composite restorations and chairside CAD/CAM inlays: marginal adaptation of a two-step self-etch adhesive with and without selective enamel conditioning. Clin Oral Investig 2007;11(1):35–43

65. Ernst CP, Buhtz C, Rissing C, Willershausen B. Clinical performance of resin composite restorations after 2 years. Compend Contin Educ Dent 2002;23(8):711–714, 716–717, 720 passim, quiz 726

66. Tan DE, Tjan AH. Margin designs and fracture resistance of incisal resin composite restorations. Am J Dent 1992;5(1):15–18

67. Baratieri LN, Ritter AV. Critical appraisal. To bevel or not in anterior composites. J Esthet Restor Dent 2005;17(4):264–269

68. Prati C, Cervellati F, Sanasi V, Montebugnoli L. Treatment of cervical dentin hypersensitivity with resin adhesives: 4-week evaluation. Am J Dent 2001;14(6):378–382

69. Dondi dall'Orologio G, Lone A, Finger WJ. Clinical evaluation of the role of glutardialdehyde in a one-bottle adhesive. Am J Dent 2002;15(5):330–334

70. Kakaboura A, Rahiotis C, Thomaidis S, Doukoudakis S. Clinical effectiveness of two agents on the treatment of tooth cervical hypersensitivity. Am J Dent 2005;18(4):291–295

71. Osborne-Smith KL, Burke FJ, Farlane TM, Wilson NH. Effect of restored and unrestored non-carious cervical lesions on the fracture resistance of previously restored maxillary premolar teeth. J Dent 1998;26(5-6):427–433

72. Perdigão J. Dentin bonding-variables related to the clinical situation and the substrate treatment. Dent Mater 2010;26(2): e24–e37

73. Kwong SM, Cheung GS, Kei LH, et al. Micro-tensile bond strengths to sclerotic dentin using a self-etching and a total-etching technique. Dent Mater 2002;18(5):359–369

74. Eliguzeloglu E, Omurlu H, Eskitascioglu G, Belli S. Effect of surface treatments and different adhesives on the hybrid layer thickness of non-carious cervical lesions. Oper Dent 2008;33(3):338–345

75. Lussi A. Damage to neighboring teeth during the preparation of proximal cavities. An in-vivo study. [Article in German] Schweiz Monatsschr Zahnmed 1995;105(10):1259–1264

76. Raskin A, Michotte-Theall B, Vreven J, Wilson NH. Clinical evaluation of a posterior composite 10-year report. J Dent 1999; 27(1):13–19

77. Pelka M, Ebert J, Schneider H, Krämer N, Petschelt A. Comparison of two- and three-body wear of glass-ionomers and composites. Eur J Oral Sci 1996;104(2(Pt 1)):132–137

78. Opdam NJ, Bronkhorst EM, Roeters JM, Loomans BA. Longevity and reasons for failure of sandwich and total-etch posterior composite resin restorations. J Adhes Dent 2007;9(5):469–475

79. Krämer N, Reinelt C, García-Godoy F, Taschner M, Petschelt A, Frankenberger R. Nanohybrid composite vs. fine hybrid composite in extended class II cavities: clinical and microscopic results after 2 years. Am J Dent 2009;22(4):228–234

80. Croll TP, Cavanaugh RR. Augmentation of incisor width with bonded composite resin: another look. Quintessence Int 1990; 21(8):637–641

81. Wolff D, Kraus T, Schach C, et al. Recontouring teeth and closing diastemas with direct composite buildups: a clinical evaluation of survival and quality parameters. J Dent 2010;38(12): 1001–1009

82. Feilzer AJ, De Gee AJ, Davidson CL. Setting stress in composite resin in relation to configuration of the restoration. J Dent Res 1987;66(11):1636–1639

83. Saunders WP. Effect of fatigue upon the interfacial bond strength of repaired composite resins. J Dent 1990;18(3): 158–162

84. Swift EJ Jr, Cloe BC, Boyer DB. Effect of a silane coupling agent on composite repair strengths. Am J Dent 1994;7(4):200–202

85. Frankenberger R, Roth S, Krämer N, Pelka M, Petschelt A. Effect of preparation mode on Class II resin composite repair. J Oral Rehabil 2003;30(6):559–564

86. Frankenberger R, Krämer N, Ebert J, et al. Fatigue behavior of the resin-resin bond of partially replaced resin-based composite restorations. Am J Dent 2003;16(1):17–22

87. Gordan VV, Garvan CW, Blaser PK, Mondragon E, Mjör IA. A long-term evaluation of alternative treatments to replacement of resin-based composite restorations: results of a seven-year study. J Am Dent Assoc 2009;140(12):1476–1484

Decision-Making in Managing the Caries Process

Hendrik Meyer-Lueckel, Martin J. Tyas, Michael J. Wicht, Sebastian Paris

20

To arrive at an appropriate, efficient, minimally interventional approach for treating caries, the fundamentals of the **pathogenesis and diagnosis** of caries described in the preceding chapters need to be duly considered (Chapters 1–8). The **synthesis** of these elements was delineated in Chapter 9, and **basic** noninvasive measures which should be complemented by **risk-related noninvasive measures** were described (Chapters 10–13). The fundamentals of **microinvasive and minimally invasive techniques** were also discussed (Chapters 14–19) and will be further explained with reference to patient cases in the practical (second) part of this book (Chapters 24–26).

In addition to the biological limits and the addressed problems of patient compliance with noninvasive measures (Chapter 13), the patient's expectations are also relevant for an adequate caries management. Frequently, invasive procedures are viewed by many of those involved in the health care system, and patients as well, as the appropriate way to manage the caries process. These procedures are consequently honored, be it psychologically (the dentist who drills is a good one, because it is an active response), and/or financially. The "wait and watch" approach of noninvasive therapy, largely based on self-management, is viewed with a certain amount of skepticism, as are microinvasive procedures. Frequently, the patient and even the dentist are afraid of the uncontrollable, rapid progression of caries lesions in the early stages of the process. In addition, dentists fear leaving microorganisms within the tooth after sealing, caries infiltration, or restoration. These considerations often lead the dentist to intervene prematurely with invasive treatment, and extensively excavate the dentin when preparing the cavity (Chapter 18). It is possible, however, to modify the existing treatment philosophy of frequent premature invasive treatment toward a less invasive approach when presented with a thorough diagnosis that reveals the possibilities and limits of the **three basic treatment options**: **noninvasive**, **microinvasive**, and (minimally) **invasive therapy** for the various sites of caries.

This chapter addresses the following topics:
- Fundamentals of evidence-based dentistry
- Fundamentals of shared decision-making
- Changing the treatment philosophy from **"drill and fill"** to **"heal and seal"**
- Limits of noninvasive therapeutic options
- Limits of microinvasive therapeutic options
- Limits of invasive therapeutic options
- Use of decision trees in choosing therapies

Fundamentals of Evidence-Based Dentistry

Therapeutic efficiency was generally evaluated unsystematically well into the 20th century. Valid and reliable assessment criteria for clinical studies based on **good scientific practice** and **evidence-based dentistry** took a long time to become established. In systematic reviews, the available literature was often filtered with a personal bias, and treatment recommendations were based on consensus or the individual opinion of (hopefully) well recognized professionals in their respective fields; initially, medicine and dentistry were more or less "eminence-based."

BACKGROUND

The idea of evidence-based medicine dates back to the concept of "medical arithmetic" developed by British physicians. The expression is found for the first time in an article by the Scottish physician, George Fordyce, published in 1793. One of the first controlled clinical studies was also performed in Great Britain. In 1753, James Lind published the results of his experiment performed on a ship of the British fleet. He investigated how best to treat scurvy, a frequent affliction of seafarers at the time. Today, we know that this disease is caused by a vitamin C deficiency and can be easily avoided and treated. At the time, however, scurvy cost a countless number of seamen their life. James Lind prescribed six different treatment methods to 12 patients. He used the standard therapy of the time (administration of a medication for disinfection) and what can be described as a negative control (one glass of seawater daily). However, the consumption of two oranges and one lemon a day was the most successful since this was the only therapy that contained vitamin C.

In the German-speaking region, the Hungarian physician Ignaz Semmelweis (1818–1865) who worked in Vienna was the first author to recommend the introduction of "systematic clinical observation" in medical research (1848).

The book published in 1972, *Effectiveness and Efficiency: Random Reflections on Health Services* by Archie Cochrane, a British epidemiologist, marks the beginning of current international efforts to pursue evidence-based medicine. His observations during his wartime imprisonment in a German prisoner-of-war camp in Greece contributed to his demand for evidence-based medicine.[1] Many of his fellow prisoners suffered from leg edema, and Cochrane was unaware of how best to treat it. He considered two potential therapies: 2 tablespoons of yeast extract, or 1 vitamin C tablet daily. For the study, 20 volunteers were randomized (according to prisoner number) into two groups. Although the mechanism remained unclear, the edema of the prisoners in the yeast extract group decreased significantly. Later, he described this initial clinical study as the worst yet most successful of his career. His subsequent works led to the increasing acceptance of clinical epidemiology and controlled studies. Today, Cochrane is chiefly known for the international network named after him for the evaluation of efficacy in medicine—the **Cochrane Collaboration.**[2]

Table 20.1 Evidence classes for evaluating the validity of studies

Classes		Requirements for the studies
I	Ia	Systematic review of RCT, perhaps with a meta-analysis
	Ib	At least one high-quality RCT
II	IIa	Evidence from at least one well-designed, controlled study without randomization
	IIb	Evidence from a well-designed, quasi-experimental study
III		Well-designed, non-experimental descriptive studies
IV		Evidence from reports/opinions of circles of experts, consensus conferences, and/or the clinical experience of recognized authorities

RCT: randomized controlled trial.
Source: www.ebm-netzwerk.de/grundlagen/images/evidenzklassen.jpg/image_view_fullscreen (accessed April 19, 2011).

NOTE

Evidence-based medicine or **evidence-based practice** is understood as a systematic medical approach that is based on the best available data to provide the best possible care for patients.

Evidence-based medicine is a standardized, transparent procedure for evaluating data from studies. After collecting the relevant evidence in the medical literature relating to a specific clinical problem, the quality or validity of the evidence is assessed using clinical epidemiological tools, and the magnitude of the effect is evaluated. However, this evidence is only applied to specific patients filtered through the clinical experience of the care provider, who takes into consideration the patient's wishes.[3]

NOTE

"Evidence-based medicine: what it is and what it isn't.— It's about integrating individual clinical expertise and the best external evidence."[4]

The process involves several steps:
- Identify a relevant issue from a clinical case that can be answered.
- Plan and perform a search of the clinical literature.
- Critically evaluate the searched literature (evidence) in regard to validity and usefulness.
- Apply the selected and evaluated evidence to the individual case.
- Evaluate your own efforts.

Source: www.ebm-netzwerk.de (accessed April 19, 2011)

Patients are not treated according to a manual; this would make medicine and dentistry highly impersonal. Rather, the conclusions of the international dental and medical literature that were reached using the aforementioned principles are referenced to choose the best possible therapy (i.e., the therapy with the greatest prospect of healing or stabilizing the disease). The dentist or physician arrives at a therapy together with the patient in a participatory atmosphere.

The relevant literature on a clinical issue is evaluated using **classes of evidence** (Agency for Healthcare Research and Quality). Class Ia studies have the highest class of evidence, and class IV studies have the lowest class of evidence. The higher the evidence class of the recommended therapy, the better the scientific validation (**Table 20.1**).

Treatment Recommendations

Treatments are recommended based on their classes of evidence (source: www.ebm-netzwerk.de). These are categorized as follows:
- **Grade A:** at least one randomized controlled study of generally high quality and consistency that directly relates to the recommendation and was not extrapolated (evidence classes Ia and Ib).
- **Grade B:** well-run clinical trials (excluding randomized clinical trials) that directly relate to the recommendation (evidence classes II or III), or an extrapolation from evidence level I if there is no reference to the specific issue.
- **Grade C:** reports from circles of experts or an expert opinion and/or clinical experience from recognized authorities (evidence category IV), or extrapolations from evidence classes IIa, IIb, or III; this level indicates that high-quality, directly applicable clinical trials were or are not available.
- **Good clinical practice:** when there are no experimental, scientific studies for a specific treatment method, or studies are impossible or are not being pursued yet, the treatment method remains conventional and agreement exists within a consensus group, this method is recommended as **good clinical practice**.

Study Types

Evidence-based dentistry and evidence-based medicine are concerned with the evaluation and assessment of clinical trials and cohort and case-control studies. In dentistry and medicine, numerous other types of studies are used. These also need to be rated to help practicing dentists evaluate therapies and diagnostic methods. In this context, it should be noted that some terms are used synonymously by the industry when marketing medical products and which can give a wrong impression about the level of evidence. This occurs sometimes when data from laboratory studies are used that purportedly demonstrate the **effectiveness** of a therapy or material. Laboratory studies may actually **only indicate the effect** of a material, for example, using so-called surrogates. A "surrogate" is a parameter that is associated with a clinical result. When interpreting such studies, care should be taken to determine whether the measured effect is also clinically significant and not just statistically significant.

Example. In a laboratory experiment with 20 samples per group, the bond strength to the enamel of a new adhesive system is greater by 5 MPa than the bond strength of an earlier system. For example, the bond strength of the older material is 40 MPa, and the bond strength of the new material is 45 MPa. Assuming a standard deviation of 5 MPa, a statistically significant difference between these values exists, given a significance level of $p < 0.05$ and a power of 0.8). Stated more simply, the new system adheres to the enamel significantly better than the older material under laboratory conditions. The question then arises as to whether this statistically-significant higher value of a surrogate parameter is also clinically relevant: does the higher bond strength of the new material result in a longer lasting restoration? This cannot be determined from the above laboratory investigation. Frequently, there is insufficient proof of the surrogate's relevance to the clinical result. This principle also applies to other areas of dentistry, which is why the request for (more) clinical trials is generally justified. Given these facts, laboratory results purportedly demonstrating the superiority of a new product or therapeutic approach need to be considered with a healthy degree of skepticism.

So-called **in-situ studies** provide an initial impression of therapeutic efficacy, or they can be used as more economical substitute methods to obtain clinical surrogate parameters. They cannot, however, replace clinical trials. The same applies to animal studies.

Another type of study, the health economic evaluation, assesses cost as a function of the **efficacy** and **effectiveness** of medical treatment or prevention options, that is, the **cost-effectiveness** or **efficiency** (**Table 20.2**).

Complex studies are performed that usually consider numerous factors. One problem with these studies is that the data are generally based on the assumptions or results of other studies, which must have a sufficient level of evidence. Only a few areas of dentistry possess enough data for them to be used in health economic evaluations.[5,6]

Shared Decision-Making

The **communication between the patient and physician** and importance of models of interaction between **professionals and clients** are becoming increasingly important around the world. In many European and North American countries as well as Australia, an effort is under way to reinforce patient rights and actively include patients in the medical decision-making process.[7] The health care goal is to provide relevant information to enable independent patient decisions that are considered appropriate by both the physician and patient and that are jointly implemented in a spirit of mutual responsibility.

> **NOTE**
>
> In many countries, attempts are under way to influence health care policy to enhance patients' rights and include patients in the medical decision-making process.

Table 20.2 Nomenclature of various conventional types of study

Study type	Question	Term
Laboratory study	Does it work under laboratory conditions?	Effect
Animal study	Can it be duplicated in another species?	Efficacy (under conditions similar to the clinical situation)
In-situ study	Does it work under the conditions that exist in the oral cavity?	Efficacy (under conditions similar to the clinical situation)
Controlled clinical trial	Does it work in a clinical setting?	Efficacy (under clinical conditions)
Practice-based study	Does it work in a clinical environment?	Effectiveness (efficacy under general conditions)
Health economic evaluation	What is the benefit in relation to the cost?	Efficiency/cost-effectiveness

In addition to **giving greater credence to the patient's perspective** and **giving greater respect to the patient's desires**, patient compliance and greater satisfaction of everyone involved in the decision-making process are considered the key advantages of the "responsible patient." In the following, various doctor/patient interaction models will be presented, their advantages and disadvantages will be compared, and the shared decision-making process will be described in detail.

> **NOTE**
>
> In the shared decision-making process, a joint therapeutic decision is reached by the physician and patient.

The Doctor–Patient Relationship

For a majority of doctors and many patients as well, especially of the older generation, including a lay person in a frequently complex decision-making process requires a change in attitude regarding the doctor–patient interaction. Historically, this behavior has been **paternalistic**,[8] that is, the physician has access to the relevant (evidence-based) information and makes decisions for the naïve patient. If the patient is well-informed about his or her illness and potential forms of therapy, and the doctor still makes decisions without involving the patient, the interaction model is one **characterized by dominance**.[9]

> **NOTE**
>
> Historically, the doctor–patient relationship has been paternalistic. The "doctor knows best" principle frequently ignores the patient's perspective and is therefore crisis-prone.

It is a matter of professional responsibility to always consider the patient's well-being and offer the best possible evidence-based therapy. However, the patient's perspective is frequently forgotten, especially when it is believed that we are particularly good practitioners and only seek the best for our patients. For patients, an interaction model characterized by paternalism can be rather pleasant, since they enjoy a passive role and only have to follow explanations and instructions.[8] Paternalistic professionals are frequently felt to be competent, especially when their decision is formulated in a friendly matter and appears plausible to the patient. If the physician is unable to satisfy the patient's expectations or, for example, disregards social or economic factors that can have unforeseeable consequences for the patient's life, the **patient will have problems with acceptance**. The asymmetrical doctor–patient relationship generated by an unequal level of professional knowledge frequently causes communication problems and crises.[10] The asymmetry can cause general dissatisfaction in both doctor and patient, damage trust, lead to a

lack of compliance, or cause the patient to switch to a different physician.[8]

Beyond dominance, classic sociology describes interactive models of **informed choice** and a **consumer attitude**. The models are distinguished according to the location of the decision, whether the person is a physician or patient, and access to and use of relevant information. Informed choice or a consumer attitude is the opposite of the dominant or paternalistic doctor–patient relationship, respectively. In both cases, the patient makes the decision independently. In the first model, the patient collects information beforehand, whereas a consumer more or less uses the doctor as a source of information and makes his or her decision autonomously based on that information.[9]

Including the Patient in the Decision-Making Process

Now that the Internet is available and there is free access to medical knowledge, we are increasingly encountering very **well-informed patients** who do not want to be considered **passive "consumers"** of therapies but rather want to be seen as equal partners involved in health care issues. Neither pure patient autonomy nor physician paternalism allows decision-making on an equal footing. The increased use of dialogue is reflected in **shared decision-making**. The goal of shared decision-making is to include the patient and perhaps his or her relatives in the medical decision-making process so that the patient's individual needs and values are taken into account.[11] By establishing a level of common knowledge, the asymmetry between the doctor–patient relationship is counteracted, the patient is able to understand diagnoses and therapies and **simultaneously assumes responsibility** for all the decisions.

> **NOTE**
>
> Shared decision-making describes an interactive model in which the doctor and patient choose a therapy as partners based on the individual patient's needs.

This interactive model has been well received by both doctors and patients.[12] More than 80% of all adult patients strongly endorse a model of shared decision-making, yet only 45% follow through.[13] Nearly the same percentages are reflected for doctors; frequently a lack of time, missing, or incorrect information, patient fears or poor payment are cited as barriers to implementing shared decision-making in medical and dental offices.[14] Older patients and patients lower on the socioeconomic scale tend to favor physician-based decision-making. There are also cultural and national differences. For example, only 43% of Spaniards want to actively participate in the decision-making process, whereas this is desired by 93% of the Swiss. Originally, shared decision-making was felt to be particularly appropriate in the treatment of **chronic**

diseases or when **alternative therapeutic options** existed. Contrastingly, shared decision-making was not felt to be necessary when clear diagnoses existed and there were no alternative therapies. This may be essentially true; however, shared decision-making represents a style of physician communication as well as an attitude toward the patient and should not degenerate into a dominant or paternalistic form of interaction. Decision-making is of course faster when there are no alternative therapies; however, waiting and observing and refraining from immediate therapy is always an option that should be considered. In **emergencies** and situations in which patients feel **overwhelmed**, shared decision-making may be inappropriate.

> **NOTE**
>
> Shared decision-making is particularly useful when several therapeutic options can be discussed.

The advantages of shared decision-making include[15]:
- Greater patient satisfaction
- Enhanced quality of life
- Improved understanding of the disease
- Control of the situation
- Enhanced patient compliance
- Reduction of fear

Implementing Shared Decision-Making in Practice

There are a few requirements to successfully implement shared decision-making.[16] Since shared decision-making is a professional–client interaction model, at least two parties are needed to participate in the process. It can be very useful to include others in the decision-making process, in addition to the doctor and patient, such as parents, family members, or non-physician medical personnel. It is important to actively include all participating patients and share all relevant information. Once a consensus has been reached, the parties commit to implement the decision and to **jointly bear responsibility**. To employ joint decision-making in a medical practice, the medical provider must possess basic communication skills and be able to carry out a structured medical discussion according to the Calgary–Cambridge Observation Guide (CCOG).[17] Many universities have reacted to the demand to provide social and communication skills, and related content has been incorporated in medical and dental coursework.

The Nine Steps of Shared Decision-Making

Table 20.3 shows the individual steps involved in shared decision-making.[18]

The process starts when the doctor and patient agree that a decision needs to be made (first step). In the second

Table 20.3 The nine practical steps of shared decision-making[18]

Steps in shared decision-making
1. Agreement that a decision needs to be made
2. Offer of shared decision-making
3. Presentation of treatment options
4. Risk/benefit analysis of the individual options
5. Patient response, expectations
6. Which options are preferred?
7. Reasoning and decision-making phase
8. A joint decision is reached
9. Individual commitment to implement the decision

step, the doctor offers his or her patient the option of shared decision-making on an equal footing. It should be emphasized that the treatment option represents a consensus that is reached between doctor and patient, but the patient has the final word. Assuming that the patient accepts the offer of shared decision-making, the information exchange phase begins with a discussion (third step). The physician informs the patient of existing therapeutic options and their benefits, side-effects, cost, etc. The presentation of the different modes of treatment should be as free of judgment as possible and based on the available evidence. The patient informs the doctor of his or her preferences as well as any **reservations, worries, and fears.** The advantages and disadvantages of all potential options are discussed, and the physician assumes the role of the expert who offers information. The patient interprets this information based on his or her own values and chooses a therapy. In describing the individual options, the doctor should make sure in the response phase (fifth step) that the patient has understood all the information before asking for the preferred alternative in the decision-making phase (sixth step). After this phase, both parties can provide the reasons for their perspective; the physician will provide a medical perspective and the patient will probably provide a personal perspective (seventh step). Once all information has been exchanged, the doctor and patient should jointly arrive at a decision (eighth step). It is important for both parties to justify this decision on a medical basis and taking into account all personal considerations. Then the parties commit to **implement the plan of therapy** (ninth step).

Shared decision-making does not mean that the doctor offers potential treatment alternatives to the patient and directly or indirectly influences the patient's choice through the presentation. The frequently asked question of the best therapy cannot be answered without an awareness of the patient's needs. The patient's question "what would you do in my situation?" may indicate a desire for paternalism, but it can also mean that the patient has not been given enough information, or is overwhelmed by the situation, or does not want to deal with it. To help inform the patient, **decision trees** (below) are used that depict all relevant information about a therapy in a patient-appropriate manner, that is, primarily visual information. Some health insurance companies provide their patients with decision trees relating to important issues. In dentistry, decision trees are not very widely used; however, there are some indications that their use makes shared decision-making and evidenced-based dentistry easier.

Decisions, Decisions: Noninvasive, Microinvasive, or (Minimally) Invasive?

When in Rome, Do as the Romans Do

As described in the preceding chapters, noninvasive and microinvasive therapies exist for the treatment of early lesions. These generally do not work for advanced stages of caries, and minimally invasive forms of therapy should be employed. It is difficult to identify the **correct point in time for invasive therapy**. This is illustrated by studies in which dentists were asked at which stage of approximal caries, as assessed on bitewing radiographs, they felt that a restoration was appropriate (**Table 20.4**).

The information provided by the dentists differs from country to country and within a country. In France, a filling is frequently inserted when the radiograph reveals that the caries extends up to the enamel–dentin junction,[19] whereas dentists in Norway tend to be more cautious.[20-22] The approach of Brazilian dentists is similar to that of Scandinavian dentists,[23] whereas dentists sometimes prepare a cavity much earlier in Scotland (older data) and in the United States.[24,25]

> **NOTE**
>
> The choice of invasive therapy for approximal caries differs widely in different parts of the world.

It is similarly difficult to choose an appropriate therapy for occlusal and cervical caries lesions (root caries). One way to escape the dilemma of forecasting the ways in which caries will progress based on the clinical and radiographic characteristics of the lesion is to longitudinally **monitor the caries process**. However, this procedure assumes that:

- Caries is held to be a process which can be arrested at least in its early to medium stages
- The signs and symptoms of caries can be objectively described, and that different points in time in the examination can be compared
- The findings relating to the specific tooth surfaces can be transferred when the patient changes dentists (such as bitewing radiographs or other technologies [e.g., Diagnodent values; Kavo, Germany]) and that no information is lost
- The patient is prepared to undergo regular check-ups

Table 20.4 Selection of studies of dentists' choices of invasive therapy for approximal caries (permanent teeth) depending on the stage of caries assessed radiographically, in several countries[a]

Country	n	Enamel halves External E1	Enamel halves Internal E2	Enamel-dentin junction EDJ	Outer third of dentin D1	Middle third of dentin D2
Sweden [20]	575		2	5	41	52
Norway [21]	640		4	15	62	19
Norway [22]	2375		1	6	56	36
Brazil (students) [23]	346	3	7	29	41	21
Scotland (30 years) [24]	1127	2	18	29		49*
USA (low-risk) [25]	500	2	39	–	54	5
USA (high-risk) [25]		9	66	–	24	1
France [19]	800	20	36	32	11	1

[a]All data given in percentages.
*The progression on the radiograph extends beyond the first third of the dentin but no further than one-half of the dentin.

Economic Consequences of the Time of Therapy

If one compares the frequently low percentage of costs associated with noninvasive therapies with the overall cost of dental interventions in countries with established market economies, such as Germany,[26] it shows that dentistry chiefly focuses on invasive treatment. Invasive measures are very commonly performed by university-trained dentists despite the tendency in recent decades for some restorative measures to be performed by specially trained **dental assistants**, for example, in the Netherlands and Scandinavia. Noninvasive methods contrastingly involve much lower expenses for personnel, infrastructure, and materials, since in many countries they can also be performed by employees without a university degree.[27]

However, the steps required to identify and treat early-stage caries are frequently not reimbursed in many parts of the world today. If at all, support is provided by the national government for adolescents in the form of group and individual dental prophylaxis. Established practice is therefore in conflict with the available knowledge about the possibilities of noninvasive or microinvasive methods for managing the caries process.

NOTE

Noninvasive methods, especially based on groups and populations, are low-cost interventions in comparison to restorative measures that are generally more expensive for both the individual and the public.[27]

However, this awareness should not lead us to believe that invasive methods can be completely avoided just to save money. From an epidemiological perspective, this is certainly not possible (Chapter 8). The practicing dentist needs to remember, however, that the cost to the patient and health care system, that is, the public at large, increases when the initial decision is made to treat caries invasively. By inserting the first filling, the **"death spiral"** of the tooth is initiated.[28] The probability of subsequent tooth loss significantly increases from this point on.[29,30] The familiar saying among English speaking dentists, **"most dentistry is re-dentistry,"** illustrates this fact.

NOTE

The time of the first minimally invasive intervention significantly influences the life expectancy of the tooth as well as a patient's quality of life.

Consequences on Therapy of "Philosophy" in Cariology

Philosophy "Drill and Fill"

Classic invasive caries therapy is based on **Black's understanding of forms of cavities**[31] that is frequently expressed by the term "extension for prevention" (Chapters 18 and 19). According to the classic preparation rules, the goal was to prepare a cavity that offered a sufficient degree of retention for the then-available nonadhesive materials (including cement, amalgam, and gold). The margins of the restoration should lie in areas of the tooth that were easily accessible to oral hygiene to prevent the formation of adjacent caries. This meant that all occlusal fissures were included and that the approximal box should be extended very widely. In addition, "infected dentin" should be completely removed if possible so that the restoration could be placed on supposedly hard, presumably bacteria-free dentin.

ERRORS AND RISKS

Adherence to Black's rules for preparing cavities meant that a substantial amount of sound tooth structure must be removed in the initial treatment.

This philosophy summarized by the expression **"drill and fill"** yielded an invasive treatment strategy that was expensive, possibly painful and, from an epidemiological perspective, resulted in a high DMFT value.

However, is it really necessary to remove all clinical and radiographic signs of caries in its early stages to successfully **control the process of caries**?

A New Philosophy: "Heal and Seal"

Today, it is well accepted that the caries process can be arrested if the factors that promote caries are reduced. In regard to the rate of progression of approximal caries, it was shown that, in most cases, it took several years to even a decade for dentin caries to become detectable on a radiograph.[32] Consequently, there exists a sufficient amount of time to choose the proper moment for minimally invasive therapy. If the tooth surface is easily accessible and the patient is compliant, enamel and dentin caries lesions (root caries) can frequently be arrested by noninvasive measures. The specific measures that are chosen depend on the frequency of use and the patient's risk of caries. The **probability of arresting a caries lesion** solely through noninvasive measures decreases as the extent of the caries and cavitation increases. Correspondingly, a caries lesion tends to progress at a greater rate, usually when it has clinically identifiable cavitation[33] which offers a favorable milieu for microorganisms. Comparable caries-promoting conditions also exist in deep fissures and grooves as well as marginal gaps of restorations.

> **NOTE**
>
> The primary aim of not only noninvasive but also micro- and (minimally) invasive interventions for treating caries and its consequences (restorations) should be to eliminate an unfavorable oral milieu for pathogenic microorganisms/biofilms and permanently keep them from recurring.

The adhesive filling materials and techniques that have been used for decades enable caries to be treated invasively, although with less destruction of enamel and dentin. However, the belief that infected dentin needs to be completely removed remains widespread, although it is becoming increasingly **doubtful whether complete removal of bacteria is possible** or even necessary, especially since radical caries excavation increases the danger of exposing the pulp (Chapter 18).[34] With adhesive fillings, the substrate supply to microorganisms deep within the cavity is inhibited, the access of other microorganisms remains blocked, and the remaining microorganisms are sealed in. At the same time, this therapeutic measure (again) enables the patient to clean the related tooth surface. The influence of the dental biofilm, the driving force behind the caries process, is thereby reduced (Chapter 19).

A similar condition is achieved by sealing plaque-retentive occlusal tooth surfaces that have an elevated risk of caries. In addition to sealing healthy fissures, in particular when the tooth is erupting, it is also recommended to seal initial caries lesions.[35,36] Noncavitated caries lesions on smooth and approximal surfaces can be sealed,[37,38] in principle; however, caries infiltration has certain advantages over sealing in this case (Chapters 15–17).[39,40]

> **NOTE**
>
> A modern caries treatment philosophy, which can be summarized as "heal and seal," seeks to arrest caries with minimum intervention.

The **"heal and seal"** caries treatment philosophy involves the following:
- The patient performing noninvasive basic interventions
- Risk-related noninvasive measures (professionally or self-applied)
- Sealing of occlusal surfaces (both healthy and carious)
- Approximal caries infiltration or sealing
- Pulp-protecting caries excavation
- Adhesive restoration repair
- Minimally invasive adhesive restorative therapy

Limits to Noninvasive Therapies

To identify an appropriate therapy, the many factors which have been presented in the previous chapters need to be considered. A few other considerations can also help dentists in choosing the most appropriate treatment according to the minimal-intervention concept proposed in the book.

Micromorphological Aspects

Under clinical conditions complete remineralization of initial caries lesions to its initial integrity appears possible.[41] Nonetheless, the changes in the surface of the lesions, especially those visible on buccal smooth surfaces which give the appearance of remineralization, are at least partially due to surface abrasion and not to the re-supply of minerals.[42,43] Even though the partial remineralization of the dentin underneath an extensive enamel lesion has been described in the laboratory, it is doubtful that substantial remineralization of a subsurface enamel caries lesion is clinically possible.[38] Rather, the remineralization of the surface can be achieved through the lasting modification of the local milieu. The subsurface lesion exists under a shiny, relatively thick **pseudointact surface layer** which gives the lesion a whitish appearance, and which can become brown after the absorption of pigments. As the thickness of the surface layer increases, further demineralization is prevented, as is the remineralization of the subsurface lesion (see Chapters 2 and 3).

> **NOTE**
>
> The build-up of the mineral content of the surface layer helps to clinically arrest caries. That is, the initial caries lesion remains like a scar but ceases to progress.

Clinical Considerations

To permanently arrest the progress of caries within the tooth by using exclusively noninvasive means, the tooth surface needs to be sufficiently accessible to cleaning. This is largely influenced by the **surface quality** and **extent of the caries**. In addition, the **frequency** at which a **cariogenic biofilm** is regenerated is also important, which especially depends on the surface quality.

Radiographic Extension—Cavitation of the Surface

The degree of cavitation correlates with the radiographic extent of the lesion, that is, there is a greater probability that deeper approximal lesions on a radiograph will be clinically cavitated, compared with early, radiographically detectable lesions. However, to predict the size of the cavitation and the probability of the lesion's progression with an acceptable degree of precision, more is needed than an awareness and interpretation of the extent of the lesion. A clinical investigation of the surface with a fine probe should be performed, especially in areas difficult to access visually (Chapter 5).

To make it easier to detect and assess cavitation resulting from approximal caries, it is useful to know the frequency of occurrence (see Chapter 6). As observed after tooth separation, approximal caries lesions are cavitated in ca. 10% of cases with radiographic extension into the inner half of the enamel (E2), or ca. 30% when they extend radiographically into the outer third of the dentin (D1).[45,46]

In addition to microscopic cavitation, these lesions manifest macroscopic cavitation, which could be termed **clinically relevant cavitation**. However, no standards exist for detecting, assessing, and documenting the different sizes of (micro)cavitation of the surface which are difficult to see and evaluate for the approximal surfaces of an intact dental arch.

NOTE

In addition to identifying the radiographic extent of approximal caries, clinically investigating the extent of cavitation using a cowhorn-ended or binangle explorer (without tooth separation) seems a relatively good method for estimating the probable future progress of approximal caries, requiring only one dental visit.

Cavitation—Biofilm

When a caries lesions is cavitated, it can be assumed that a potentially cariogenic biofilm has become permanently established. Even if the patient regularly flosses, the biofilm will be difficult to remove. Stated simply, it can be assumed that the frequency of generation of a **cariogenic biofilm** depends on the **size of the cavitation** of the enamel or root surface.

Biofilm—Caries Progression

The **frequency of generation of a cariogenic biofilm** obviously influences the probability of the progression of caries. The probability of caries progression is frequently termed the "caries activity" as is the clinical activity of a caries lesion described in Chapter 5, which can lead to confusion.

In regard to detecting and assessing the cariogenicity of plaque (biofilm), one problem is that the visit to the dentist only offers a snapshot. An informed patient tends to be more aggressive about removing plaque before visiting the dentist, and the status of the plaque during the appointment can therefore only yield a conditionally impression of the "truth". Moreover, this is only a quantitative and not a qualitative factor. The frequent establishment of approximal plaque correlates with a **tendency of the gingiva to bleed**. The susceptibility of the gingiva to bleeding is therefore quite a good, but indirect, indicator of the level of a plaque within recent days or weeks, at least in the case of (cervical) smooth surface caries (see also Chapter 5).

NOTE

Increased bleeding of neighboring papillae indicates a higher activity of approximal caries, at least in periodontally healthy patients.[47]

In this context, it cannot be stressed enough that dentists treat patients, and not teeth or tooth surfaces. Nevertheless, specific therapies are chosen primarily based on the tooth surface, or at least the tooth. This (tooth) level is strongly influenced by factors from higher levels (the individual and population), which also need to be taken into consideration. The patient's compliance strongly influences the time span at which the carious process has progressed far enough for more serious measures to be indicated (see Chapter 9).

Speed of Caries Progression

The stage in the caries process at which exclusively noninvasive options may be recommended by the dentist to manage the caries largely depends on knowledge about the probable speed of the caries progression. **Prospective cohort studies** in which the development of caries in patient groups is investigated over several years can provide useful information. In such investigations, it is advantageous to standardize the radiographic technique so that misinterpretation will not arise from different projections of sequential images (see also Chapters 6 and 25, Case 2).

In one of the prospective studies on the progression of caries, the approximal and occlusal surfaces of the anterior teeth were observed. The study was performed in the 1980s and 1990s in Sweden; the DMFT of the 12-year-olds was 3.2 at the time when the study was initiated and hence higher than that which would be expected in most countries today with an established market economy (**Fig. 20.1**).[32]

Age Dependence The caries progression and development rate of new lesions is higher in adolescents than in young adults. The differences in incidence as a function of age are reflected in **Fig. 20.1**. More new approximal caries lesions occur up to 19 years of age than in young adults. This difference is even more pronounced with occlusal lesions. Consequently, starting at age 20 years, approximal lesions increase in frequency in relation to occlusal lesions.[32]

Approximal Surfaces according to the study, the median time of approximal caries (time in years that it takes 50%

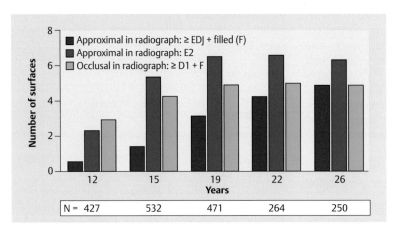

Fig. 20.1 Whereas occlusal lesions requiring invasive treatment (green bar) arose at a young age, approximal lesions in the anterior region were more restricted to the enamel at this stage according to the radiographs (E2; blue). As the age increased, new approximal enamel lesions became detectable. One new approximal caries lesion appears every 3–4 years that at least penetrates the enamel–dentin junction (EDJ) as shown on the radiograph, or has received a filling (F) (red bar).[32]

of the lesions to progress from one stage to the next) from a sound status until it reaches the inner enamel is about 6 years over the ages of 11 to 22 years. The median radiologic progression rate of caries lesions from the enamel–dentin junction (EDJ) into the outer third of the dentin (D1) was approximately twice as high as the rate of progression within enamel (**Fig. 20.2**).[48]

Dependence on the Type of Tooth The median progression time of caries lesions at approximal surfaces of various teeth also differs. To progress from the EDJ up to the first third of the dentin took about 5 years for the distal surface of the first premolars and the mesial surfaces of the lower second molars in the mandible, as well as the distal surface of the upper first molars. The median progression rate was 2–4 years for all other surfaces from the EDJ to D1 (on the radiograph). After 15 years (at 27 years of age), the percentage of healthy distal surfaces of the lower first premolars was substantially higher than that of the distal surfaces of the lower first molars.[48] The progression from radiologic enamel lesion (E2) to radiologic dentin lesion (D1) occurred much more frequently on the distal surface of the lower first molars (**Fig. 20.3**).[32]

Limits to Microinvasive Therapies

Starting at a certain level of tooth destruction, the risk of only treating noninvasively (resulting in consequences such as dental hard tissue fractures or pain) becomes greater than the anticipated benefits (such as lower cost). This means that if invasive measures are not performed, the potential harm is greater than the anticipated disadvantages of treatment. However, if restorative therapy is considered necessary, it needs to be remembered that all restorations age over time. They frequently need to be replaced after a few years with restorations that are usually larger.[49]

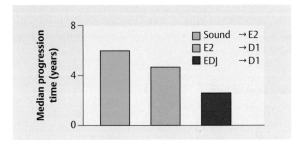

Fig. 20.2 For originally healthy approximal surfaces that were affected by caries later on, it took about 6 years on average to observe radiographic extension into the inner half of the enamel, as studied in a Swedish cohort in the early 1990s. The median times for caries extending into the inner half of the enamel (E2) and caries up to the enamel–dentin junction (EDJ) to progress into the outer third of the dentin were only 5 and 3 years, respectively.[48]

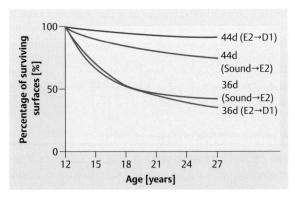

Fig. 20.3 The percentage of remaining (surviving) healthy approximal surfaces is much higher for the distal surfaces of lower first premolars (76%) than for the distal surfaces of the lower first molars (41%). The radiographical progression from enamel (E2) to dentin caries (D1) is more frequent at 44 distal (d) than at 36 d.[32]

Sealants represent a **bridge** between **noninvasive** and **minimally invasive** interventions, and only a slight amount of dental hard tissues needs to be sacrificed during acid etching. The suggested term for this intervention is **"microinvasive therapy"**[50] (see Chapters 9, 15–17).

Avoidance of Overtreatment

To avoid overtreatment, only those caries lesions should be sealed or infiltrated that are expected to progress and have been shown unarrestable by means of noninvasive measures. The assessment of the caries potential progression in just a single session is less valid than the information gleaned from monitoring the lesion over a longer period. **Approximal lesions** that are considered **nonprogressive** do not require (microinvasive) treatment, as is frequently the case with older patients with a low risk of caries. If such a caries lesion were to be infiltrated nevertheless, the risk of lesion progression would not be greater, according to our present knowledge. Especially approximal caries in children (primary molars; 4–10 years of age), and adolescents and adults (14–35 years of age), manifest a relatively high progression rates,[32,49] so the danger of overtreatment in these age groups is therefore considerably less.[51] Occlusal caries lesions that remain stable over a long period also do not have to be sealed. This is frequently the case with older adults and seniors, assuming that the risk of caries has not changed directly before the examination.

The Problem of Undertreatment

It is frequently feared that in **sealing** and **infiltrating**, the true (histological) extent of caries will be underestimated, and accordingly undertreated.

Dentin Involvement

One reason for this concern is that during excavation, approximal caries, which is difficult to identify clinically, frequently extends deep into the dentin. In addition, the fact that discolored or initial carious fissures frequently extend deep into the dentin makes microinvasive techniques seem less appealing. The expression **"hidden caries"** is frequently used in association with approximal caries. This expression was coined at a time when visual–tactile inspection was the primary diagnostic means. However, visual–tactile inspection is not very sensitive in detecting the early and middle stages of approximal caries (only a few of the diseased tooth surfaces are actually identified as such, see Chapter 5). Consequently, approximal caries in initial to medium stages are frequently overlooked, or its extent is underestimated.

Only additional diagnostic tools such as bitewing radiographs or transillumination can detect the early stages of approximal caries and more accurately estimate its extent (Chapter 6). Yet, the actual extent of caries tends to be underestimated, even on radiographs. For many lesions that appear limited to the enamel on the radiograph, the demineralization actually extends into the dentin. However, the histological status of the dentin per se is no indication for a restoration (Chapter 18). As described, the **quality of the lesion surface** is the primary factor in determining the therapy. This means that when D1 lesions are identified on the radiograph and the surface quality of the caries is known, one must judge whether the caries can be arrested by infiltration or sealing. In case of doubt, it can be recommended to choose restorative therapy and not risk the consequences of undertreatment. **However, cavitated caries lesions can also be arrested.** As shown below (**Fig. 20.4**), the proper therapy can only be chosen on an individual basis with a careful risk assessment, and frequently the choice is difficult.

Residual Microorganisms

Noncavitated caries lesions and lesions that are restricted to the enamel generally only contain a few bacteria,[52,53] which cannot form a cariogenic biofilm because of the minimal size of the cavities. It is therefore generally not considered problematic to seal in these bacteria. It should also be remembered that microorganisms remain even in disinfected, "caries-free" fissures. This applies all the more to complete caries excavation (Chapter 18). **One hundred percent sterile conditions are impossible to achieve.** Nonetheless, there are many reservations about sealing or infiltrating noncavitated caries lesions or "incomplete excavation" when preparing cavities, since microorganisms become enclosed in these treatments (Chapters 15–17).

On the basis of presently available data, several authors have concluded that sealing noncavitated caries fissures and adhesive therapy after "incomplete caries excavation" represents a lower-risk alternative to the dogma still held by some, namely techniques of radical caries excavation applied early-on, followed by restoration.[54,55]

Limits to Invasive Therapies

Adhesive filling therapy was discussed in detail in Chapters 14 and 19. Given the correct indication, esthetically attractive and functional restorations can be created using this method. The survival rate of direct restorations (amalgam and resin composite) is an average of about 10 years after insertion in the initial treatment (**Fig. 20.5**). An average 15-year-old person with a life-expectancy of 80 years will therefore need to have the **filling replaced** approximately **six times**.

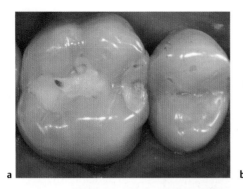
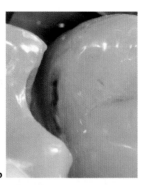

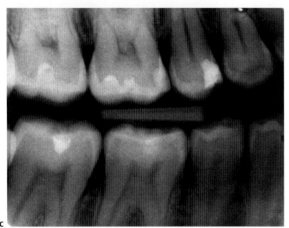
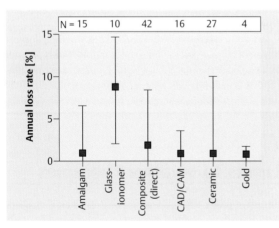

Fig. 20.4a–d An ICDAS 4 lesion can be seen in tooth 25 distally, time point (TP): 10, with a rough surface arising from iatrogenic damage (**a**) while preparing a mesial filling for tooth 26 ten years before (TP: 0) (**b**). On a previous radiograph (TP: 3), 3 years after insertion of the filling in 26, distal, D1 lesions can be found on the distal surfaces of 25 and 26 (**c**). 12 years later, the radiograph shows (TP: 15) that the restorations in 25 and 26 have been replaced, whereas the caries lesions in the other approximal surfaces of these two teeth have not progressed (**d**). This is particularly noteworthy given the roughness (microcavitation) of the distal surface of tooth 25 (**b**).

Each time the filling is replaced, additional dental hard tissue is removed. As the patient grows older, indirect restorations are therefore often inserted which have a greater success rate but cost a great deal more, both fiscally and biologically. The restoration spiral (**Fig. 20.6**) frequently ends in expensive therapies such as crowns, root canals, or even tooth replacement.[28]

NOTE

Slowing or even arresting the progress of caries therefore appears to be a desirable goal in managing the caries process. Given the limited life of restorations and the associated high cost, early invasive treatment should be postponed as long as possible.

Fig. 20.5 Median annual loss (bars = range) of class I/II restorations of permanent posterior teeth (modified according to ref. 49).

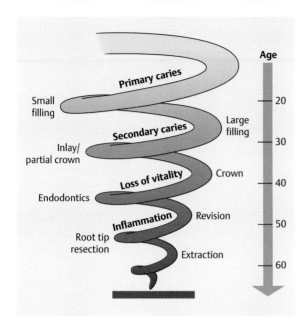

Fig. 20.6 The "death spiral" or restoration spiral illustrates the increased frequency of invasive forms of therapy at the individual ages, starting with the insertion of the initial, small filling (according to ref. 28).

Decision Trees and Choice of Therapy

The above theoretical explanations of the fundamentals of evidence-based medicine and the limits of the three possible therapies (noninvasive, microinvasive, and minimally invasive) for coronal primary caries need to be related to practice. This can be done using decision trees that can also be employed in the **quality management** of clinical settings. In more complex cases, the therapy should be arrived at in a shared decision-making process.

Below are examples of the most important diagnostic criteria for three different locations and situations, and the possible **tooth-related therapeutic options** in the form of decision trees. In addition to these decision trees (for explanations, see **Table 20.5**), the most frequent findings and treatment options are also described in words. Beyond the tooth-related measures cited here, the dentist or patient should also pursue patient-related noninvasive interventions that adequately take into account the risk (Chapters 9–12).

Findings 1: Caries on Occlusal Surfaces and Grooves without a Restoration The following general rules can be applied to this tooth surface (**Fig. 20.7**):
- If the caries is inactive, it should only be monitored (basic prophylaxis).
- Surfaces categorized as ICDAS 0 and active caries of stages ICDAS 1–2 and occasionally 3 should be sealed if there is a higher risk of caries.
- Active caries of stages ICDAS 4–6 should be filled in most cases. If the lesions are very deep, consider stepwise caries excavation technique or incomplete caries removal.

Findings 2: Caries in Occlusal Surfaces and Grooves with a Restoration The following general rules can be applied to this tooth surface (**Fig. 20.8**):
- If the caries lesions are limited to the enamel and/or have small marginal gaps, the restoration should be repaired, if noninvasive measures are not considered enough.
- If it is anticipated that the caries lesion extends up to the pulp and/or if the marginal gap is prominent, replace the restoration.

Findings 3: Caries in Approximal Surfaces of Posterior Teeth without a Restoration The following general rules can be applied to this tooth surface (**Fig. 20.9**):
- In the case of inactive caries of stages ICDAS 1 and 2, basic prophylaxis is sufficient, even given a radiographic extension into the first third of the dentin.
- Active caries of stages ICDAS 1 and 2 with a radiographic extension of E1–E2 should be treated noninvasively (floss, fluoride), if the risk of caries is low.

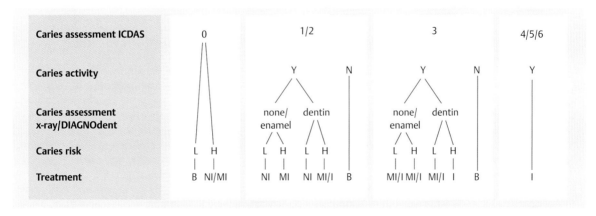

Fig. 20.7 Caries in occlusal surfaces and grooves without a restoration. Y = yes, N = no, L= low, H = high, B = basic prophylaxis, NI = noninvasive (such as fluoride), MI = microinvasive (sealing), I = invasive (filling).

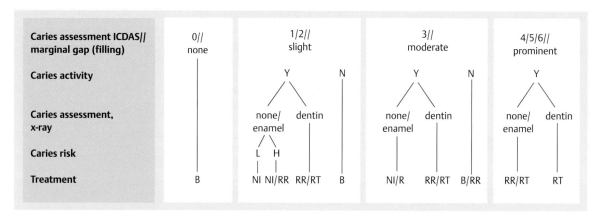

Fig. 20.8 Caries in occlusal surfaces and grooves with a restoration. Y = yes, N = no, L = low, H = high, B = basic prophylaxis, NI = noninvasive (such as fluoride), RR = repair (composite), RT = replacement.

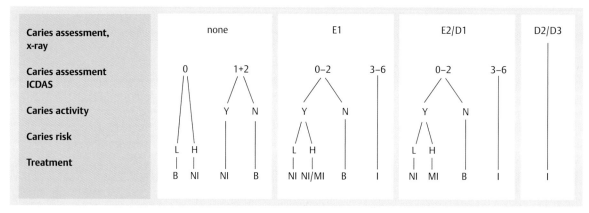

Fig. 20.9 Caries in approximal surfaces of posterior teeth without a restoration. Y = yes, N = no, L = low, H = high, B = basic prophylaxis, NI = noninvasive (such as fluoride), MI = microinvasive (sealing), I = invasive (filling).

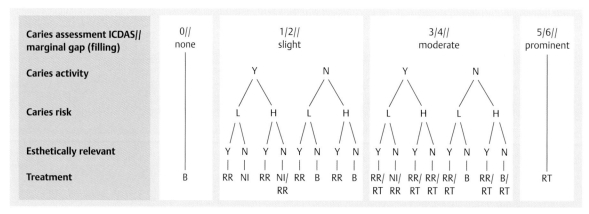

Fig. 20.10 Caries in anterior teeth with a restoration. Y = yes, N = no, L = low, H = high, B = basic prophylaxis, NI = noninvasive (such as fluoride), RR = repair (composite), RT = replacement (filling).

- Active carries of stages ICDAS 1 and 2 with a radiographic extension of E2–D1 should be infiltrated, if the risk of caries is increased.
- Active caries of stages ICDAS 3–6 should be filled in most cases. If the lesions are very deep, consider a stepwise caries excavation technique or incomplete caries removal.

Findings 4: Caries in Anterior Teeth with a Restoration The following general rules can be applied to these teeth (**Fig. 20.10**):
- Initial marginal caries (ICDAS 1 and 2) that is **esthetically irrelevant** and/or with minor marginal gaps rarely requires invasive treatment.

Table 20.5 Explanation of abbreviations and findings for the decision tree

Criterion	Severity	Explanation
ICDAS Criteria	0	Sound
	1	Initial changes in the enamel after drying
	2	Significant changes in the enamel
	3	Breakdown of the enamel
	4	Demineralized dentin that shines through
	5	Small cavity extending into the dentin
	6	Large cavity extending into the dentin
	W0	Sound
	W1	If cavitated then depth of the dentinal cavity <0.5 mm
	W2	Depth of the dentinal cavity ≥0.5 mm
Caries activity, enamel	Yes	Noncavitated: light brown, opaque, rough surface Cavitated: light brown Both: frequent plaque colonization, bleeding of adjacent papilla
	No	Noncavitated: dark brown or somewhat glossy when white, smooth surface on probing Cavitated: dark brown Both: minor plaque colonization, no bleeding of adjacent papilla
Caries activity, root	Yes	Light brown, soft, frequent plaque colonization, gingival bleeding
	No	Dark brown color, hard, minor plaque colonization, no gingival bleeding
DIAGNOdent caries evaluation (occlusal)	None/Enamel	Value <30
	Dentin	Value ≥30
General risk of caries	Low	Value <33% (according to determined caries risk)
	High	Value ≥33% (according to determined caries risk)
Local risk of caries	Low	No anatomical predisposition
	High	Anatomical predisposition
Marginal gap adjacent to restoration	None	Nothing visible or palpable
	Low	No gap for probe
	Moderate	Gap for probe or cavity <0.5 mm
	Prominent	Gap for probe or cavity ≥0.5 mm
Esthetically relevant	Yes	Patient spontaneously is aware of an esthetic impairment
	No	Patient is not spontaneously aware of an esthetic impairment

Table 20.6   Etiology of noncarious dental hard tissue defects

Surface	Location	Etiology
Vestibular (labial/buccal)	Root	Attrition/abrasion/(abfraction)
Vestibular (labial/buccal)	Crown	Erosion/abrasion/(abfraction)
Occlusal	Crown	Erosion/abrasion/attrition
Palatal	Crown (maxilla)	Erosion/attrition

- In the case of **esthetically relevant** caries, minor to moderate marginal gaps and/or caries of stages ICDAS 1–4, consider either repairing or replacing the restoration.
- If it is anticipated that the caries lesion extends to the pulp and/or if the marginal gap is prominent, replace the restoration.

Findings: Noncarious dental hard tissue defects As presented in the initial chapters, noncarious defects are categorized as erosion (chemical: correctly termed "corrosion"), abrasion (mechanical: from a foreign influence), attrition (mechanical: from tooth-to-tooth function), and possibly abfraction (mechanical: cracks and notches in teeth over time), according to the etiology. In practice, the etiology of the change is frequently difficult to assess. In addition to the relevant tooth surface and location (**Table 20.6**), it is helpful to know aspects of the patient's (medical) history (such as bulimia, anorexia, and stress) and relevant but unconscious behaviors (grinding, reflux, tooth brushing technique) when forming a diagnosis.

In therapy, one generally attempts to positively modify the causal factors. In the case of vestibular defects in the root region, the brushing technique should be checked, and the application of less brush pressure and a vertical movement may be recommended. Generalized attrition may be from stress-related bruxism and grinding. It may be useful to recommend a better stress management strategy in difficult situations, or temporary therapy with bite splints. Erosion of the palatal surfaces from bulimia and anorexia, especially in the anterior and premolar regions, requires interdisciplinary therapy. If the patient is experiencing pain and the stability of the tooth and/or vitality of the pulp is endangered, invasive measures are indicated.[56]

SUMMARY

Treatment decision should not be "eminence-based" but should be evidence-based, relying on as much relevant information as possible. Best evidence can be derived from randomized controlled clinical trials. The patient should be informed about the existing evidence level and the treatment being proposed in a participative atmosphere (shared decision-making), where the patient's wishes and needs are also taken into account. For **minimally interventional dentistry**, a regular check-up of the patient's oral condition and hence the carious process is necessary, so that the proper therapy can be chosen. When arriving at a therapy, the tooth-related factors should always be considered together with individual behavioral factors affecting oral health. On a tooth surface level, treatment decision should rely on biological fundamentals of the caries process and the choice of the most minimal interventional treatment option that is indicated. Caries is a ubiquitous, natural process that is difficult to eliminate completely, if at all. If a metabolically active biofilm forms on the tooth surface, apparently only a very few individuals are capable of modifying their behavior over the long term. However, the caries process can be slowed by appropriate measures, and the establishment of extensive caries lesions with cavitation can be counteracted by noninvasive or microinvasive means. Invasive (operative) measures are then no longer necessary, or can at least be postponed. Studies of caries progression, which is generally very slow in most patients, should at least lead to a reconsideration of the practice of early invasive intervention which is established in many countries (from the clinical determination of enamel discoloration without clear discontinuities, or the radiographic extension up to the enamel–dentin junction). The reserved Scandinavian and Australian approach should also lead us to consider offering our patients low-pain treatments that spare the dentin and enamel. Decision trees can help make the range of findings comprehensible and the therapeutic decision-making process understandable to both students and patients.

REFERENCES

1. Cochrane AL. Sickness in Salonica: my first, worst, and most successful clinical trial. Br Med J (Clin Res Ed) 1984;289(6460): 1726–1727

2. Raspe H. Theorie, Geschichte und Ethik der Evidenzbasierten Medizin. In: Kunz R, Ollenschläger G, Raspe H, Jonitz G, Donner-Banzhoff N, eds. Lehrbuch Evidenzbasierte Medizin. Köln: Deutscher Ärzteverlag; 2007

3. Sackett DL. Rules of evidence and clinical recommendations for the management of patients. Can J Cardiol 1993;9(6):487–489

4. Sackett DL, Rosenberg WM, Gray JA, Haynes RB, Richardson WS. Evidence based medicine: what it is and what it isn't. BMJ 1996;312(7023):71–72

5. Källestål C, Norlund A, Söder B, et al. Economic evaluation of dental caries prevention: a systematic review. Acta Odontol Scand 2003;61(6):341–346

6. Oscarson N, Källestål C, Fjelddahl A, Lindholm L. Cost-effectiveness of different caries preventive measures in a high-risk population of Swedish adolescents. Community Dent Oral Epidemiol 2003;31(3):169–178

7. Charles C, Gafni A, Whelan T. Shared decision-making in the medical encounter: what does it mean? (or it takes at least two to tango). Soc Sci Med 1997;44(5):681–692

8. Charles C, Gafni A, Whelan T. Self-reported use of shared decision-making among breast cancer specialists and perceived barriers and facilitators to implementing this approach. Health Expect 2004;7(4):338–348

9. Dierks ML, Seidel G. Gleichberechtigte Beziehungsgestaltung zwischen Ärzten und Patienten – wollen Patienten wirklich Partner sein? In: Härter M, Loh A, Apies C, eds. Gemeinsam entscheiden – erfolgreich behandeln: Neue Wege für Ärzte und Patienten im Gesundheitswesen. Deutscher Ärzteverlag; 2005: 35–44

10. Geisler L. Arzt-Patienten-Beziehung im Wandel – Stärkung des dialogischen Prinzips. Recht und Ethik der modernen Medizin 2002;216–220. Available at http://dip.bundestag.de/btd/14/090/1409020.pdf. Accessed September 10, 2012

11. Härter M. Partizipative Entscheidungsfindung (Shared Decision-Making) – ein von Patienten, Ärzten und der Gesundheitspolitik geforderter Ansatz setzt sich durch. Z Arztl Fortbild Qualitatssich 2002;98:89–92

12. Härter M, Müller H, Dirmaier J, Donner-Banzhoff N, Bieber C, Eich W. Patient participation and shared decision making in Germany – history, agents and current transfer to practice. Z Evid Fortbild Qual Gesundhwes 2011;105(4):263–270

13. Hirsch O, Keller H, Krones T, Donner-Banzhoff N. Acceptance of shared decision making with reference to an electronic library of decision aids (arriba-lib) and its association to decision making in patients: an evaluation study. Implement Sci 2011;6:70 10.1186/1748-5908-6-70

14. Johnson BR, Schwartz A, Goldberg J, Koerber A. A chairside aid for shared decision making in dentistry: a randomized controlled trial. J Dent Educ 2006;70(2):133–141

15. Kriston L, Scholl I, Hölzel L, Simon D, Loh A, Härter M. The 9-item Shared Decision Making Questionnaire (SDM-Q-9). Development and psychometric properties in a primary care sample. Patient Educ Couns 2010;80(1):94–99

16. Kurtz S, Silverman J, Draper J. Teaching and Learning Communication Skills in Medicine. 2nd ed. Oxford: Radcliffe; 2005

17. Scheibler F, Pfaff H. Shared decision-making. Ein neues Konzept der Professionellen-Patienten-Interaktion. In: Scheibler F, Pfaff H, eds. Shared Decision-Making. Der Patient als Partner im medizinischen Entscheidungsprozess. Weinheim: Juventa; 2003: 11–22

18. Scheibler F, Schwantes U, Kampmann M, Pfaff H. Shared decision-making. GGW 2005;5:23–31

19. Doméjean-Orliaguet S, Tubert-Jeannin S, Riordan PJ, Espelid I, Tveit AB. French dentists' restorative treatment decisions. Oral Health Prev Dent 2004;2(2):125–131

20. Mejàre I, Sundberg H, Espelid I, Tveit B. Caries assessment and restorative treatment thresholds reported by Swedish dentists. Acta Odontol Scand 1999;57(3):149–154

21. Tveit AB, Espelid I, Skodje F. Restorative treatment decisions on approximal caries in Norway. Int Dent J 1999;49(3):165–172

22. Vidnes-Kopperud S, Tveit AB, Espelid I. Changes in the treatment concept for approximal caries from 1983 to 2009 in Norway. Caries Res 2011;45(2):113–120

23. Bervian J, Tovo MF, Feldens CA, Brusco LC, Rosa FM. Evaluation of final-year dental students concerning therapeutic decision making for proximal caries. Braz Oral Res 2009;23(1):54–60

24. Nuttall NM, Pitts NB. Restorative treatment thresholds reported to be used by dentists in Scotland. Br Dent J 1990;169(5):119–126

25. Gordan VV, Garvan CW, Heft MW, et al. Restorative treatment thresholds for interproximal primary caries based on radiographic images: findings from the Dental Practice-Based Research Network. Gen Dent 2009; 57(6):654–663; quiz 664–666, 595, 680.

26. Kassenzahnärztliche Bundesvereinigung (KZBV). Aufteilung der Ausgaben für zahnärztliche Behandlung 2005. Köln: Kassenzahnärztliche Bundesvereinigung; 2006

27. Griffin SO, Jones K, Tomar SL. An economic evaluation of community water fluoridation. J Public Health Dent 2001;61(2):78–86

28. Qvist V. Longevity of Restorations – "The Death Spiral". In: Fejerskov O, Kidd EAM, eds. Dental Caries: The Disease and its Clinical Management. 2nd ed. Oxford: Blackwell Munksgaard; 2008:443–456

29. Elderton RJ. Overtreatment with restorative dentistry: when to intervene? Int Dent J 1993;43(1):17–24

30. Luan W, Baelum V, Fejerskov O, Chen X. Ten-year incidence of dental caries in adult and elderly Chinese. Caries Res 2000; 34(3):205–213

31. Black GV. Operative Dentistry. Vol 1. Chicago: Medico-Dental Publishing; 1908

32. Mejàre I, Stenlund H, Zelezny-Holmlund C. Caries incidence and lesion progression from adolescence to young adulthood: a prospective 15-year cohort study in Sweden. Caries Res 2004;38(2):130–141

33. Hintze H, Wenzel A, Danielsen B. Behaviour of approximal carious lesions assessed by clinical examination after tooth separation and radiography: a 2.5-year longitudinal study in young adults. Caries Res 1999;33(6):415–422

34. Bjørndal L, Reit C, Bruun G, et al. Treatment of deep caries lesions in adults: randomized clinical trials comparing stepwise vs. direct complete excavation, and direct pulp capping vs. partial pulpotomy. Eur J Oral Sci 2010;118(3):290–297

35. Stosser L, Heinrich-Weltzien R, Hickel R, Kühnisch J, Bürkle V, Reich E. Leitlinie Fissurenversiegelung. Köln: Zahnärztliche Zentralstelle Qualitätssicherung; 2005

36. Splieth CH, Ekstrand KR, Alkilzy M, et al. Sealants in dentistry: outcomes of the ORCA Saturday Afternoon Symposium 2007. Caries Res 2010;44(1):3–13

37. Gomez SS, Basili CP, Emilson CG. A 2-year clinical evaluation of sealed noncavitated approximal posterior carious lesions in adolescents. Clin Oral Investig 2005;9(4):239–243

38. Martignon S, Ekstrand KR, Ellwood R. Efficacy of sealing proximal early active lesions: an 18-month clinical study evaluated by conventional and subtraction radiography. Caries Res 2006; 40(5):382–388

39. Meyer-Lueckel H, Paris S. Improved resin infiltration of natural caries lesions. J Dent Res 2008;87(12):1112–1116

40. Paris S, Hopfenmuller W, Meyer-Lueckel H. Resin infiltration of caries lesions: an efficacy randomized trial. J Dent Res 2010; 89(8):823–826

41. Von der Fehr FR, Löe H, Theilade E. Experimental caries in man. Caries Res 1970;4(2):131–148

42. Mannerberg F. The incipient carious lesion as observed in shadowed replicas ('en face pictures') and ground sections ('profile pictures') of the Same Teeth. Acta Odontol Scand 1964;22:343–363

43. Backer-Dirks O. Posteruptive changes in dental enamel. J Dent Res 1966;45:503–511

44. ten Cate JM. Remineralization of caries lesions extending into dentin. J Dent Res 2001;80(5):1407–1411

45. Pitts NB, Rimmer PA. An in vivo comparison of radiographic and directly assessed clinical caries status of posterior approximal surfaces in primary and permanent teeth. Caries Res 1992; 26(2):146–152

46. Hintze H, Wenzel A, Danielsen B, Nyvad B. Reliability of visual examination, fibre-optic transillumination, and bite-wing radiography, and reproducibility of direct visual examination following tooth separation for the identification of cavitated carious lesions in contacting approximal surfaces. Caries Res 1998; 32(3):204–209

47. Ekstrand KR, Bruun G, Bruun M. Plaque and gingival status as indicators for caries progression on approximal surfaces. Caries Res 1998;32(1):41–45

48. Mejàre I, Källest I C, Stenlund H. Incidence and progression of approximal caries from 11 to 22 years of age in Sweden: A prospective radiographic study. Caries Res 1999;33(2):93–100

49. Manhart J, Chen H, Hamm G, Hickel R. Buonocore Memorial Lecture. Review of the clinical survival of direct and indirect restorations in posterior teeth of the permanent dentition. Oper Dent 2004;29(5):481–508

50. Meyer-Lueckel H, Fejerskov O, Paris S. Novel treatment possibilities for proximal caries. [Article in German] Schweiz Monatsschr Zahnmed 2009;119(5):454–461

51. Meyer-Lueckel H, Dörfer CE, Paris S. Welche Risiken und Chancen birgt die approximale Kariesinfiltration? Dtsch Zahnarztl Z 2010;65:556–561

52. Seppä L. A scanning electron microscopic study of early subsurface bacterial penetration of human molar-fissure enamel. Arch Oral Biol 1984;29(7):503–506

53. Kidd EAM. How 'clean' must a cavity be before restoration? Caries Res 2004;38(3):305–313

54. Noack MJ, Wicht MJ, Haak R. Lesion orientated caries treatment—a classification of carious dentin treatment procedures. Oral Health Prev Dent 2004;2(Suppl 1):301–306

55. Ricketts DN, Kidd EA, Innes N, Clarkson J. Complete or ultra-conservative removal of decayed tissue in unfilled teeth. Cochrane Database Syst Rev 2006;3:CD 003808

56. Lussi A, ed. Dental Erosion. From Diagnosis to Therapy. Basel: Karger; 2006

How to Maintain Sound Teeth: an Individualized Population Strategy for Children and Adolescents

Kim R. Ekstrand

21

Based on the previous chapters, the focus here is on how to control the caries disease in children and adolescents by timely application of noninvasive and microinvasive treatments. These include *any measure undertaken toward the individual patient, aiming to prevent visible sign of caries and arrest ongoing caries, without resorting to minimally invasive treatment.*[1]

This chapter will elaborate on:
- The multifactorial concept of caries
- Relevant epidemiology
- A program related to dental age and caries risk
- Documentation of caries experience in Denmark

Then Chapter 22 will focus on microinvasive and, in particular, minimally invasive treatment possibilities toward the individual patient in pediatric dentistry.

The Multifactorial Concept of Caries

Figure 21.1 shows one way to visualize the multifactorial concept of the caries disease.[2] The following five factors in this model are considered necessary for the development of caries:
- the **tooth structure** (1);
- **microorganisms** adhering to the teeth (2), particularly when situated in
- **plaque stagnation areas** (PSA) (3)
- **fermentable carbohydrate** (4), which comes from the dietary intake and from the saliva in the form of glycoproteins; and
- **time** (5)

Apart from the tooth structure, the other necessary factors are presented in bold type (**Fig. 21.1**).

Facultative or strictly anaerobic bacteria in the plaque produce lactic acid if a sufficient amount of fermentable carbohydrate is accessible,[3] resulting in pH drops that may demineralize the dental hard tissues over time. In **Fig. 21.1** this is illustrated by the pH going up and down. If little or no fermentable carbohydrate is available, the bacteria in the plaque produce other types of weak acids[3] which are not harmful to the dental hard tissues. The factors next to the teeth indicate the many **biological determinants** influencing the caries process at the tooth surface level, while the more **external determinants** (income, etc.) act at the individual/population level.

However, none of the determinants influencing the caries progression rate are in themselves capable of either initiating or arresting caries. From **Fig. 21.1** it is obvious that if one of the necessary factors (e.g., the microorganisms or plaque) is eliminated, no caries can develop, or an already established lesion will arrest. Thus, the most realistic way to control the caries disease is to disturb or to remove the biofilm trying to adhere to teeth on a regular basis by means of tooth brushing and dental flossing. The

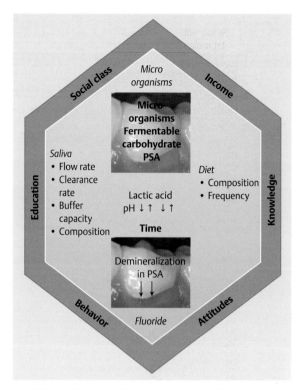

Fig. 21.1   Model to describe the caries disease. The tooth structure, microorganisms, fermentable carbohydrate, plaque stagnation areas (PSA), and time are all considered to be necessary factors for caries to develop. The biological determinants decreasing or increasing the caries progression rate are in italics. In the outer perimeter are the external determinants. (Modified after Fejerskov and Manjii.[2])

tooth brushing should be performed with fluoride toothpaste (influences one of the biological determinants). In the dental office this can be combined with dietary advice on reducing the intake of fermentable carbohydrate (influences one of the necessary factors). Finally, the dentist can effect professional plaque removal (influences one of the necessary factors), apply a high concentration of fluoride (influences one of the biological determinants), or apply sealants (influences several of the necessary factors)—the latter two measures are only effective locally (at the tooth surface level). All individuals need the same type of noninvasive interventions to control the caries disease, but some people need certain treatments more often than others, according to individual needs.[4] The best term for this is **"individualized population strategy,"**[4,5] which is in contrast to both **strict population** and **strict individual strategies** (Chapter 13).

NOTE

Individualized population strategy within cariology: All people require the same types of noninvasive intervention, but some people need certain interventions more often than others, according to individual needs.

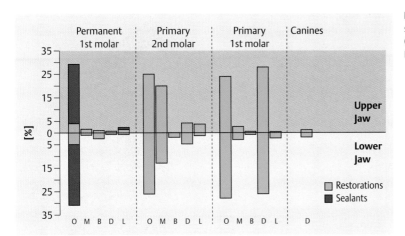

Fig. 21.2 The distribution of filled and sealed surfaces in 9-year-olds in Denmark.[6] O: occlusal; M: mesial; B: buccal; D: distal; L: lingual.

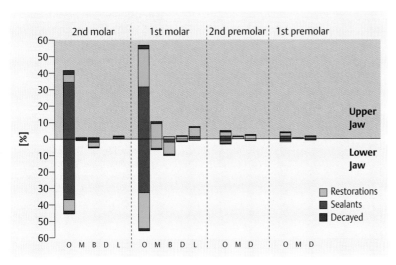

Fig. 21.3 The distribution of decayed, filled, and sealed surfaces in 15-year-olds in Denmark.[10] O: occlusal; M: mesial; B: buccal; D: distal; L: lingual.

Relevant Epidemiology

Chapter 8 dealt with the epidemiology of caries disease worldwide. This section goes into more detail about **caries risk surfaces** in relation to age, how long it takes for caries to penetrate the enamel in deciduous (primary) and in permanent teeth, and the length of eruption periods of different teeth at risk of caries.

Caries in the Primary Dentition

Data from Denmark[6] show that the prevalence of **early childhood caries** (defined as caries in children less than 3 years of age, see Chapter 8) in cavitated stages is as low as 2% of the child population at age 3 years. In other countries, early childhood caries is a bigger problem.[7,8] Data from several countries[6,8,9] show that the primary first molars, in particular the distal surfaces, are the most often restored, followed by the occlusal surfaces of both primary first and second molars, followed by the mesial surfaces of primary second molars (**Fig. 21.2**). Detailed analyses[6] disclosed that 52% of **9-year-olds** in Den-

mark in 2005 had one or more filled approximal surfaces in primary molar teeth.

Caries in the Permanent Dentition

From the ages of around 6–15 years the most caries-affected tooth in the permanent dentition is the permanent first molar. In one study from Denmark (**Fig. 21.3**) dealing with 15-year-olds,[10] 25% of all occlusal surfaces of permanent first molars were restored, followed by the mesial and buccal surfaces (8%) for the same teeth. In addition, more than one-third of the occlusal surfaces in permanent first molars were sealed. This was also the case for the occlusal surfaces of permanent second molars, indicating that this tooth surface can be considered as being at a higher risk as well. Very few occlusal surfaces of premolar teeth were sealed or restored.

Caries Progression Rate through the Enamel

Radiographically, studies show that the median time for caries to penetrate the enamel of primary molar teeth was 2.5 years.[11] Studies from Sweden[12] revealed that the median time for caries penetration through the enamel in permanent premolar and molar teeth was double (5 years) that of primary teeth. However, it was also found that 10% of the lesions penetrated into dentin within 2.5 years. In both dentitions the progression rate in dentin was faster than in enamel (Chapter 20). Studies also show that the progression rate seems faster just after the eruption of the tooth than after the tooth has been in the mouth for a couple of years.[12] In one Swedish study the median time for caries penetrating through the enamel was 4 years at the age of 10–11 years versus more than 7 years for 17–22-year-olds.[13]

Eruption Time for Teeth in the Two Dentitions

The times for tooth emergence in the oral cavity for the individual teeth in the primary dentition[14] and for the permanent teeth[15] were described in Chapter 1 (see **Fig. 1.2a, b**). Two other pieces of information are of interest in the perspective of caries initiation and eventual control of caries in the child population.[16,17]

First, the primary second molar erupts at the age of about 2 years. On average, it takes about 1 year before firm approximal contact with the primary first molar is established.[16] This means that the chance of developing approximal caries distally on primary first molars and mesially on the primary second molars increases by about the age of 3 years. If the progression rate through the enamel is estimated to be around 2.5 years (see above), the child can have approximal dentin caries at the age of about 5.5 years, occasionally even earlier.

Besides, data shows that the time for emergence of permanent first molars varies greatly from an age of less than 5 years to around 8 years. Similarly, the time for emergence of permanent second molars varies from an age of about 8 to 14 years.[15] This variation in emergence time was confirmed in a more recent study,[17] which also disclosed that the time it takes from the emergence of the permanent first molar until firm occlusal contact with the antagonist is on average 1 year. However, some children get contact after 4 months, while in others it can be after 32 months.[17] Corresponding data for the permanent second molars are 24 months to reach firm contact with a variation of 8–48 months.[17] These long-lasting eruption periods of the permanent molar teeth are a predominant risk factor for caries of their occlusal surfaces.[18–21] In contrast, the eruption time to full occlusion for permanent premolar teeth is relatively short.

Diagnostics of Caries in the Child Population

Even under the best clinical conditions for examining clean and dry teeth,[22,23] dentists and dental hygienists overlook many lesions if the visual-tactile examination is not supplemented by radiographic examination on a regular basis.[24] This occurs in both the primary and permanent dentitions. Thus, bitewing radiographs should be an integrated adjunct to the visual–tactile examination of the child's teeth. However, bitewing radiographs should be timed to give as much relevant information as possible. As it is known that the progression rate through the enamel of primary teeth on average is about 2.5 years, and more than 50% of the children eventually get primary molars restored in countries with low caries progression rate such as Denmark, it would be relevant to take bitewing radiographs at the dental age when approximal contact between primary first and second molars and between primary second and permanent first molars have been established for around 1.5 years. As it is known that it takes about 5 years for caries to penetrate permanent enamel, it seems relevant, if we wish to detect enamel lesions early on, to take bitewing radiographs at the dental ages when the approximal contact between permanent first and second molars has been established for about 1.5–2.0 years.

Individualized Population Strategy

Table 21.1 shows a flowchart example of an **individualized population strategy program** for the child population with visits or examinations related to dental ages. The program can be used both in community services and in private practice. The program begins with a visit when the child is

Table 21.1 Caries-related visits/examinations related to dental age

Age	Visit/examination	Date (dental age)	Additional appoint-ment[1]
0 years			
↓	1st visit	First teeth erupt	X?
↓	2nd visit	Primary 1st molar erupts	X?
↓	3rd visit	Primary 2nd molar erupts	X?
↓	Clinical examination	Firm approximal contact between primary 1st and 2nd molars	X?
↓	Clinical and radiographic examination	1.5 years after approximal contact between primary 1st and 2nd molars	X?
↓	Clinical examination	Permanent 1st molar erupts	X?
↓	Clinical and radiographic examination	1.5 years after approximal contact between primary 2nd and permanent 1st molars	X?
↓	Clinical examination	Permanent 2nd molar erupts	X?
↓	Clinical and radiographic examination	1.5–2.0 years after approximal contact between permanent 1st and 2nd molars	X?
↓	Clinical and radiographic examination	Final examination	
18 years			

[1]The "X" marks indicate whether additional visits are needed between two dental ages.

about 8 months old, as this is the time for emergence of the first primary teeth. This visit should focus on **health education** toward the parents, including information about caries as a localized diseased, advice about diet and breast-feeding, fluoride policy, and instructions on how to brush the baby's teeth. The two following suggested visits, timed for when the primary first and second molars erupt, should reinforce the information given at the first visit. In addition, at these visits the parents are instructed on how to brush the primary molar teeth. To avoid dental fluorosis, the parents are advised to brush their child's teeth (from 8 months to full contact of adjacent primary molars) using fluoride toothpaste with ca. 1000 ppm F⁻. However, the amount per day should not exceed the size of the fingernail of the child.[25] If the child is under the influence of "systemic fluoridation" either by using fluoride-containing tablets, living in areas where the water is high in fluoride, or using fluoridated salt, this has to be taken into account. This may result in the dental professional recommending the use of toothpaste with less fluoride (250–500 ppm F⁻).

The first real clinical examination (clean and dry teeth) should be performed at the dental age when the child gets contact between adjacent primary molars (ca. 3.0–3.5 years). Caries on the approximal surfaces around the contact points between primary molars may start at this time.

Instructions to parents on tooth brushing perpendicularly to the contact point, now using regular fluoride toothpaste 1450 ppm F⁻ (amount per day corresponding to the fingernail of the child) should be given. The next, thorough clinical examination at 1.5 years after contact has been established between primary first and second molars should include bitewing radiographs to identify enamel lesions on the approximal surfaces and dentin caries on the occlusal surfaces of the primary molars. Further, information concerning the nonerupted permanent premolars and molars can be obtained on these bitewing radiographs. If superficial caries lesions are detected, reinforcement of earlier given information, supplemented by local application of 2% NaF solutions or fluoride varnish, is mandatory.

The next important dental age is when the permanent first molar erupts, but its emergence time varies a lot.[17] Again, the focus of attention is to instruct the parents in how to brush these and the other teeth. Intervals for recalls (e.g., not longer than 4 months) should be short during the eruption period of the permanent first molars.[18–21] It might even be necessary to seal the occlusal surfaces, if adequate home-based plaque control cannot be established. About 1.5 years after approximal contacts have been established between primary second and permanent first molars, the clinical examination should again

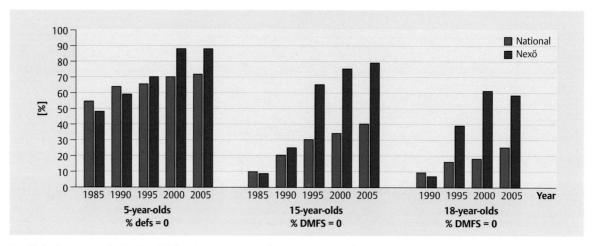

Fig. 21.4   Percentage distribution of defs index = 0 or DMFS index = 0 in 5-, 15-, and 18-year-olds in Nexö and on a national level in Denmark from 1985 to 2005.[27]

include bitewing radiographs not only for identifying approximal caries in the primary molar teeth and mesially in permanent first molars, but also to identify occlusal caries on permanent first molars. As for the eruption period of permanent first molars, the same comprehensive care is given during the eruption period of permanent second molars, including short recall intervals.

Now, the focus of attention toward the parents is replaced by giving the necessary information and the responsibility for oral health to the child. About 1.5–2.0 years after approximal contact has been established between permanent first and second molars, the clinical examination is again supplemented by bitewing radiographs, to indentify early approximal lesions, as well as occlusal caries on molar teeth. A period of 1.5–2.0 years initially may seem a little early, if the median time of 5 years for caries to penetrate enamel is accepted. However, the caries progression rate is faster just after the tooth has erupted than when the tooth has been in the mouth for years.[13] Further, it is important to identify lesion formation in its early stages (outer enamel) to perform effective noninvasive treatment to control for further progression.

The "X" marks in **Table 21.1** are used to indicate whether additional visits are needed between two dental ages. This relates to caries risk assessments done at the previous examination. For example, prolonged breast-feeding many times at night might provoke extra recalls between visits 2 and 3. Thus the population strategy is then supplemented with risk-related treatment in accordance with individual needs and thus becomes an individualized population strategy. As it takes on average between 1.0 and 2.5 years for permanent first and second molars, respectively, to reach full occlusion, extra examinations are necessary during these (caries prone) dental ages.

Documentation of Caries Experience

The flowchart in **Table 21.1** is based on the achievements obtained by means of a program for the whole population of children used in the Public Dental Health Service in the Nexö municipality in Denmark since the end of the 1980s[4–6,26](see also Chapter 8). To conclude this chapter some results obtained by that program are shown.

Comparing caries data for children and adolescents from Nexö with data at the national level from 1985 to 2005, it becomes obvious that in Nexö caries prevalence (**Fig. 21.4**) and caries experience (**Fig. 21.5**) are rather low. It appears that with this individualized population strategy program, much better results, in particular in the permanent dentition, were obtained in the dental service of Nexö compared with national standards.

In 2004, the mean DMFS among 15-year-olds in Nexö was 0.56 and 79% had a DMFS = 0. Analyses disclosed that Nexö was a positive outlier, meaning that relevant background variables such as socioeconomic data, fluoride concentration in drinking water, etc. could not explain the good results in Nexö. Further, the costs for oral health care per child per year were at the national level.[26]

Since 2008, the individualized population strategy described here has been in full-scale use in the Child Dental Health Service in Greenland, a country unfortunately known for very high caries incidence in children and adolescents. So far the strategy[28] has managed to reduce caries significantly in primary dentition from a mean defs of 9.5 (11.8) in 9-year-olds in 2008 (who have not followed the strategy) to 7.8 (9.3) in 9-year-olds in 2011, who had followed the program (see **Table 21.1**).[28]

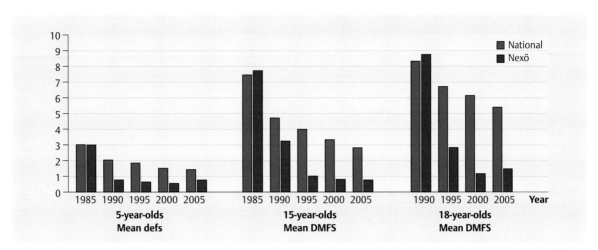

Fig. 21.5   Mean defs or DMFS indexes of 5-, 15-, and 18-year-olds in Nexö and on a national level in Denmark from 1985 to 2005.[27] For a definition of defs/DMFS indexes see Chapter 8, page 122.

SUMMARY

Dentists and hygienists know where caries develops and also when. To maintain teeth sound or in the dental world avoid fillings due to caries, it is important to be ahead of the caries disease. One way to do this is to call-in children and their parents to the clinic according to eight dental ages during childhood. At each visit or examination, oral health education is given first to parents, then to parents and the child, and later only to the child. Health education is followed by noninvasive and microinvasive therapies, when needed. As all children (and parents) get the same information, but some families need it more often, according to their needs the program can be classified as an individualized population strategy. Excellent results in terms of maintaining teeth without fillings have been obtained by following this strategy during a 25-year period in the Child Dental Health Service of Nexö, Denmark.

REFERENCES

1. Christiansen J. Non-operative caries treatment. In: Splieth C, ed. Revolutions in Pediatric Dentistry. London: Quintessence; 2011: 21–35

2. Fejerskov O, Manji F. Risk assessment in dental caries. In: Bader J, ed. Risk Assessment in Dentistry. Chapel Hill: University of North Carolina Dental Ecology; 1990:215–217

3. Geddes DA. Acids produced by human dental plaque metabolism in situ. Caries Res 1975;9(2):98–109

4. Ekstrand KR, Christiansen MEC. Outcomes of a non-operative caries treatment programme for children and adolescents. Caries Res 2005;39(6):455–467

5. Ekstrand KR, Christiansen MEC. Nexø-metoden set I et sundhedsfremmende perspektiv. Tandlaegebladet 2008;112:112–123

6. Ekstrand KR. Kan den kommunale tandpleje gøre det endnu bedre? Tandlaegebladet 2006;110:788–799

7. Kaste LM, Drury TF, Horowitz AM, Beltran E. An evaluation of NHANES III estimates of early childhood caries. J Public Health Dent 1999;59(3):198–200

8. Ballantyne H. Identification of Infants at High Risk to Developing Dental Caries Using Microbiological and Social Factors [PhD Thesis]. Dundee: University of Dundee; 2000

9. Kuzmina IN, Kuzmina E, Ekstrand KR. Dental caries among children from Solntsevsky—a district in Moscow, 1993. Community Dent Oral Epidemiol 1995;23(5):266–270

10. Ekstrand KR, Martignon S, Christiansen ME. Frequency and distribution patterns of sealants among 15-year-olds in Denmark in 2003. Community Dent Health 2007;24(1):26–30

11. Shwartz M, Gröndahl H-G, Pliskin JS, Boffa J. A longitudinal analysis from bite-wing radiographs of the rate of progression of approximal carious lesions through human dental enamel. Arch Oral Biol 1984;29(7):529–536

12. Mejàre I, Stenlund H, Zelezny-Holmlund C. Caries incidence and lesion progression from adolescence to young adulthood: a prospective 15-year cohort study in Sweden. Caries Res 2004;38(2): 130–141

13. Mejàre I, Källest I C, Stenlund H. Incidence and progression of approximal caries from 11 to 22 years of age in Sweden: A prospective radiographic study. Caries Res 1999;33(2):93–100

14. Lysell L, Magnusson B, Thilander B. Time and order of eruption of the primary teeth. A longitudinal study. Odontol Revy 1962;13: 217–234

15. Helm S, Seidler B. Timing of permanent tooth emergence in Danish children. Community Dent Oral Epidemiol 1974;2(3): 122–129

16. Kurol J, Rasmussen P. Occlusal development, preventive and interceptive orthodontics. In: Koch G, Poulsen S, eds. Pediatric Dentistry. A Clinical Approach. Copenhagen: Munksgaard; 2001: 321–349

17. Ekstrand KR, Christiansen J, Christiansen MEC. Time and duration of eruption of first and second permanent molars: a longitudinal investigation. Community Dent Oral Epidemiol 2003;31(5): 344–350

18. Carvalho JC, Ekstrand KR, Thylstrup A. Dental plaque and caries on occlusal surfaces of first permanent molars in relation to stage of eruption. J Dent Res 1989;68(5):773–779

19. Carvalho JC, Ekstrand KR, Thylstrup A. Results after 1 year of non-operative occlusal caries treatment of erupting permanent first molars. Community Dent Oral Epidemiol 1991;19(1):23–28

20. Carvalho JC, Thylstrup A, Ekstrand KR. Results after 3 years of non-operative occlusal caries treatment of erupting permanent first molars. Community Dent Oral Epidemiol 1992;20(4): 187–192

21. Ekstrand KR, Kuzmina IN, Kuzmina E, Christiansen ME. Two and a half-year outcome of caries-preventive programs offered to groups of children in the Solntsevsky district of Moscow. Caries Res 2000;34(1):8–19

22. Möller IJ, Poulsen S. A standardized system for diagnosing, recording and analyzing dental caries data. Scand J Dent Res 1973; 81(1):1–11

23. Ekstrand KR, Zero DT, Martignon S, Pitts NB. Lesion activity assessment. Monogr Oral Sci 2009;21:63–90

24. Mejàre I. Bitewing examination to detect caries in children and adolescents—when and how often? Dent Update 2005;32(10): 588–590, 593–594, 596–597

25. Bruun C, Thylstrup A. Dentifrice usage among Danish children. J Dent Res 1988;67(8):1114–1117

26. Ekstrand KR, Christiansen ME, Qvist V, Ismail A. Factors associated with inter-municipality differences in dental caries experience among Danish adolescents. An ecological study. Community Dent Oral Epidemiol 2010;38(1):29–42

27. Ekstrand KR. Faculty of Health Sciences, University of Copenhagen, School of Dentistry, Department of Cariology and Endodontics. A Non-Operative Caries Treatment Program NOCTP (Nexodent – The Nexø Method). http://www.nexodent.com. Accessed August 9, 2011

28. Senderovitz F, Ekstrand KR, Christiansen J, Christiansen MEC. Caries strategy Greenland for 5–9-year-olds with focus on risk dental ages: Principles and results. Caries Res 2012;46:305 (abstract)

Individualized Caries Management in Pediatric Dentistry

Christian H. Splieth, Mohammad Alkilzy

22

Apart from the previous chapter, this book has mainly dealt with caries management in permanent dentition. Deciduous teeth, however, exhibit fundamental differences from permanent teeth with respect to anatomy, epidemiology, and function. These differences have distinct consequences for the success of non-, micro- and minimally invasive interventions in children and adolescents.

This chapter will cover in detail:

- Differences between the deciduous and permanent dentition with regard to histology, epidemiology, caries progression, and function
- Treatment concepts in the deciduous dentition in individualized settings
- Treatment concepts in the permanent dentition in children and adolescents in individualized settings

Deciduous versus Permanent Teeth

Anatomy

Deciduous teeth possess a much smaller enamel and dentin thickness than permanent teeth (**Fig. 22.1**). Together with the lower mineral density and more voluminous dentinal tubules this leads to a relatively fast caries progression compared with permanent teeth.[1] Moreover, occlusal and/or approximal pulp processes will be reached and affected by the caries process much faster than in permanent teeth.[2]

As a consequence, the "treatment window" for non-, micro-, or minimally invasive techniques in deciduous teeth is narrower in comparison to permanent teeth. Especially deep dentin caries (ICDAS 5 and 6) is often accompanied by pulpal complications and, therefore, pediatric dentists sometimes even prefer a **"preventive" pulpotomy** over less invasive approaches. This ensures a rather high success rate as subsequent pulp necrosis is almost avoided. More conservative, minimally invasive options run a higher risk of further caries progression and subse-

quent pulpal necrosis, often acute pain, abscess, or a fistula, which result in an extraction as the final outcome.

Epidemiology

Caries epidemiology has been described thoroughly in Chapter 8 and certain aspects for pediatric dentistry are emphasized in Chapter 21. Some statements, being important for this chapter, are made below.

- Early Childhood Caries (**Fig. 22.2**) seems to be a rising problem in many places around the globe.[3–7]
- Since 1970, DMFT levels dropped by about 90% in 12-year-olds.[2,8–13]
- During the past 30 years, caries reduction in deciduous teeth was less pronounced in many countries and has decreased by 40%–50%.[9,12]
- Caries experience is somehow "polarized," meaning that a small proportion of children is severely affected.[14]
- In contrast to the fast progression through outer and inner enamel in deciduous teeth, caries progresses much more slowly in permanent teeth, especially in older age groups.[15]

Not only inter-individual differences can be observed in young children. Also on the tooth and surface levels, caries progression shows different rates compared with those in the permanent dentition. Due to excellent follow-up possibilities using bitewing radiographs, this is best examined for approximal surfaces.[15] As pointed out above, caries progresses much more slowly in permanent teeth, especially in older age groups (**Table 22.1**).

Function and Longevity

Primary teeth are deciduous and have a very limited time of function. On the one hand children are often afraid of dental treatment and prefer the most invasive interventions; on the other hand, it is mostly irrelevant in what condition a primary tooth exfoliates, as long as the space for its successor is retained and no pain or distress was caused. Thus, the pediatric dentist has a difficult decision to make, between less invasive approaches which often

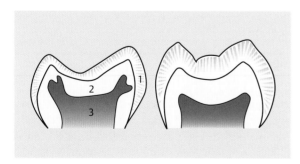

Fig. 22.1 Differences between deciduous (left) and permanent teeth: Enamel thickness (1) is smaller in deciduous teeth and almost uniform. Voluminous pulp horns (3) protrude far into the relatively little dentin (2).

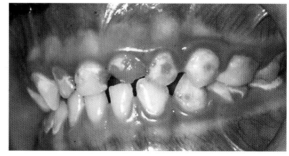

Fig. 22.2 Early Childhood Caries seems to be an increasing problem which, at first sight, does not allow for a non- or minimally invasive approach.

Table 22.1 Caries progression through enamel in approximal surfaces

	Outer enamel	Inner enamel	All enamel
Deciduous tooth	1 year	1 year	2 years
6-year molar (10-year-old)	2 years	3.5 years	5.5 years
6-year molar (17-year-old)	3.5 years	4.5 years	8 years
Source: ref. 15			

require increased preventive efforts by the patients and their parents or, alternatively, more aggressive restorative options. Nonetheless, restored primary teeth are not the beginning of a life-long restorative cycle as in "permanent" teeth, but an adequate, temporary solution until exfoliation and the eruption of the caries-free successors.[14]

Erupting Permanent Teeth

Permanent teeth are supposed to have a much longer period of function. During that course of time they change considerably with age, especially during eruption and the first years thereafter. Due to alternating de- and remineralizing episodes, surface enamel matures post-eruptively. Hereby, mineral quality is improved and solubility is lowered.[16] Due to the life-long activity of the odontoblasts, the pulp recedes, the dentin tubules obliterate and dentin also acquires a higher degree of mineralization. Thus, caries progresses faster in enamel and dentin of newly erupted permanent teeth in children and adolescents than in adults.

Treatment Concepts in Deciduous Teeth

As has been said, the decrease in caries prevalence and experience over the last decades has been accompanied by a polarization of the caries distribution. In conjunction with the fast progression rate of caries lesions in the primary dentition, children either show severe oral destruction or their deciduous teeth are "caries-free," meaning that no cavitated caries lesions are detectable. In addition, cooperation is suboptimal in most kindergarten children, which results in a polarization of the treatment strategies into either:

- comprehensive oral rehabilitation (often under general anesthesia), or
- mostly noninvasive caries therapy with few micro- and minimally invasive therapies.

If unavoidable, dental treatment under **general anesthesia** needs to be performed that requires predictable outcomes and favors **pulpotomies**, full tooth coverage with stainless

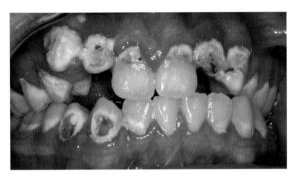

Fig. 22.3 Severe caries experience in the primary or permanent dentition often offers a wide range of lesion extensions, which allow for non-, micro- and minimally invasive treatment early on, to gain cooperation of the patient.

steel crowns, and last but not least, extractions and space-maintainers. Leaving questionable lesions in these children with high caries risk is not advisable as caries progression will result in treatments under general anesthesia.

Most children with early childhood caries and even adolescents with high caries levels present with a wide range of lesions at all stages due to the different eruption times and caries progression rates of the various surfaces (**Fig. 22.3**). These lesions are most suitable to be treated minimal- and micro-invasively in the first dental visits. When sufficient cooperation is reached, more invasive treatments such as pulpotomies and extractions can be performed. This step-by-step introduction of dental procedures from noninvasive to microinvasive and finally restorative treatments is a valuable strategy to get children acquainted with dental practice and to avoid general anesthesia.

Buccal Surfaces

Generally, in most children, initial noninvasive interventions including oral health education are needed to reduce caries risk. For smooth-surface caries lesions mostly developing adjacent to the gingival margin, arrest can be quite easily accomplished by brushing with fluoride toothpaste, whereby the cariogenic biofilm is removed and remineralization in enamel is enhanced. The former chalky white caries lesions appear shiny and hard again, and signs of gingivitis will disappear (**Fig. 22.4**). Later

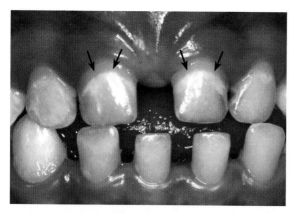

Fig. 22.4 Simple tooth brushing with fluoride toothpaste results in inactivation of buccal lesions (arrows).

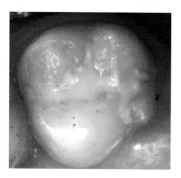

Fig. 22.5 Micro-invasive, pain-free procedures such as sealing offer a chance to introduce more invasive procedures to noncooperative children later. Light-cured glass-ionomer cements reduce the need for etching, spray, and high-speed suction.

these caries lesions will be situated ca. 1–2 mm above the gingival margin, since the inflammation process in the marginal gingiva is now under control and the gingiva has subsequently recessed.

Occlusal Surfaces

In contrast to the easily accessible buccal surfaces, pits and fissures of occlusal surfaces (see Chapter 1) are much harder to clean; approximal surfaces cannot be reached with a toothbrush easily. Preventive sealants can be applied to healthy occlusal surfaces using the air-water syringe, high-speed suction, and light curing for a completely painless procedure (**Fig. 22.5**). If the spray and suction are still too ominous for the child, a resin-modified glass-ionomer might be used for sealing without etching, spraying, and suction, although dryness of the area is still necessary, otherwise retention of the glass-ionomer cement will be lower than adhesive resins. In children with poor cooperation and no other indication for general anesthesia, initial lesions on occlusal surfaces in deciduous molars might be completely sealed without caries removal.[17,18]

Approximal Surfaces

As tooth brushing has been severely neglected in many high-risk patients, flossing (even by parents) is often not a viable option to arrest carious lesions. Other noninvasive approaches are also likely to fail due to the low adherence to oral home care. In addition, remineralizing strategies in the primary dentition bear a higher risk of undertreatment because of the lower mineralization and enamel thickness as described above.

The noninvasive interventions such as brushing instructions and professional tooth cleaning can be used to train the children to cooperate in dental treatment. If parents and their children show adherence to the proposed noninvasive interventions, microinvasive techniques such as approximal sealing and infiltration can be offered to the patients (see Chapters 15–17). In cases of doubt, if these techniques will arrest lesion progression efficaciously, minimally invasive treatment should be done. When a cavity needs to be prepared, hand excavation of caries in easily accessible areas is a feasible method. If no signs of **irreversible pulp** changes (spontaneous or persistent pain, gingival swelling, abscess, fistula, sensitivity) are present, carious dentin close to the pulp might be left (Chapter 18). The additional support of a chemical component such as Carisolv® reduces the need for applying force with the excavator.

NOTE

Non-, micro- or minimally invasive approaches carry a greater risk for failure in the primary than in the permanent dentition. Therefore, these options should be selected with care, as failure might result in pulpal complications and subsequent extractions. If in doubt, the choice of more invasive options seems to be preferable in primary teeth to ensure a maximum success rate at the expense of tooth substance until "exfoliation of the problem."

Minimum Intervention in Permanent Teeth in Children and Adolescents

If children or adolescents show a caries lesion, this has most probably developed within a shorter period compared with adults showing a similar lesion extension. Thus, the caries progression rate for the child is relatively higher. Dental professionals are confronted with the dilemma of having to choose either a minimally invasive approach with minimal additional loss of hard tissues but a higher risk of caries for the remaining enamel, or "extension for prevention" which "costs" additional hard tissue, but leaves margins in self-cleaning areas or tries to "hide them" under the gingiva.

In the primary dentition all restorative approaches will fail if the caries risk is not reduced. Therefore, micro- or minimally invasive approaches have to be accompanied by intensified primary and other secondary preventive measures.

Epidemiological data for the permanent dentition of children and adolescents clearly point out that occlusal surfaces in molars (including buccal and palatal pits) have the highest incidence of caries, followed by approximal surfaces.

Occlusal Surfaces

During the relatively long eruption periods of permanent molars, occlusal brushing in mesial to distal direction and/or self-cleaning during chewing is impaired and plaque removal is most often inadequate. Thus, caries lesions are likely to develop. Initial ones (ICDAS 1 and 2) should be "treated" noninvasively, whereby lesion progression may be reduced or even avoided. Initial lesions are easily inactivated and arrested by oral home care with a toothbrush and fluoride toothpaste (see Chapters 10 and 12). In erupting teeth this can be accomplished by the cross-tooth brushing technique (**Fig. 22.6**); for example, for the first permanent molar this may be better performed by the parents, as 6-year-olds mostly do not comply sufficiently.

If caries cannot be inactivated by non-invasive measures, sealing is indicated. Fissure sealants are widely applied for caries prevention: well-examined and recent systematic reviews provide evidence for their effectiveness in controlling initiation and progression of caries lesions.[17–22] The indication for sealing seems to have shifted in European dental schools from a primary to a secondary preventive measure for initial caries lesions,[18] as oral health programs are well established and caries risk is mostly low (see Chapter 15).

As resin-based sealants require sufficient moisture control, these are difficult to apply properly during eruption (e.g. overlapping gingiva), which is the most critical phase for caries initiation and progression. Glass-ionomer sealants (**Fig. 22.5**) are a suitable alternative, because they are less sensitive to moisture.[23,24] In addition, the fluoride released from glass-ionomers is supposed to promote remineralization and reduce future demineralization.[23,24] If the caries risk remains high after eruption, a conventional resin sealant can replace the glass-ionomer sealant.

For more advanced initial lesions (ICDAS 3 and 4) on occlusal surfaces, a minimally invasive restoration seems to be the best choice, since sealants will in particular not be as effective when a caries lesion is cavitated.

If advanced dentin caries (ICDAS 4 and 5) is present, it should be removed and a small composite filling placed (**Fig. 22.7**). Sealing in cavitated caries lesions without preparation of enamel and dentinal caries by excavation,

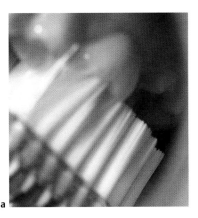
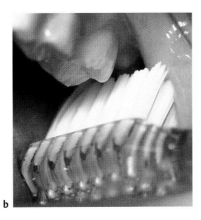

Fig. 22.6a, b Erupting teeth are not cleaned with conventional occlusal brushing (**a**). The cross-brushing technique can be used to avoid or arrest noncavitated caries lesions (**b**).

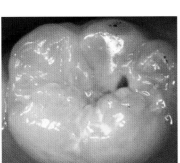
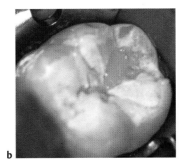
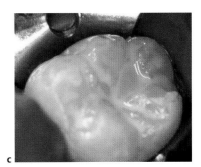

Fig. 22.7a–c Small occlusal defects (**a**) can easily be filled with composite (**b**) and the remaining fissures should be protected with a sealant (**c**).

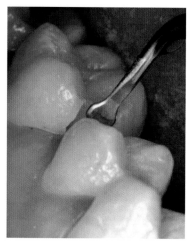

Fig. 22.8 Oscillating files allow the cutting of approximal cavities without damaging the neighboring surface.

which is a viable alternative in deciduous teeth of uncooperative children, is not an appropriate option in the permanent dentition, where caries removal is more feasible due to the increased age and cooperation of the patients.

Sealants for Individuals at High Risk of Caries

Numerous initial caries lesions in a child can be seen as a clear sign of a relatively high caries risk. In these high-risk individuals sealants might not work as well as in lower-risk children. In a 3-year observational study on preventive sealants in first permanent molars, children where followed from ages 12 to 15 years. Besides an overall 30% reduction in caries incidence for sealed occlusal surfaces compared with unsealed equivalents, sealants in children with high baseline caries levels were less effective.[21] In consequence, **preventive and therapeutic sealants** on initial caries lesions should be accompanied by intensified noninvasive interventional efforts.[22]

Approximal Surfaces

Approximal caries poses a serious problem for pediatric dentists, as interproximal plaque removal is hard to achieve, especially in children. Other noninvasive interventions and oral health education may not be implemented sustainably, due to the insufficient adherence of the patients and their parents. In addition, a lesion radiologically at the enamel–dentin junction of a first permanent molar in a 10-year-old reveals a much higher progression rate than the same lesion in a 27-year-old (see above). Therefore, noninvasive interventions as a sole option to arrest caries progression should be chosen with care in children and adolescents. Microinvasive techniques such as an approximal infiltration (Chapter 17) or sealing (Chapter 15) offer an additional safe option. Both techniques have a high risk of failure, if the caries risk is

not reduced. In contrast to adults with a fully erupted permanent dentition, approximal sealants and infiltration are technically more complex to perform in children, as the gingival level is often very high. In addition, the first and second permanent molars, which have the highest caries risk, are the most distal teeth. Thus, rubber dam isolation, separation, and application of the approximal sealant or infiltrant have to be performed on the same tooth which is sometimes challenging. Nonetheless, the same holds true when placing a restoration.

If the approximal lesion is well into dentin on the radiograph, the outer surface most likely exhibits a visible cavitation, which indicates insertion of a filling. Conventional cavity preparation with rotating instruments is strongly associated with the risk of damaging the neighboring approximal surface. Therefore, the additional use of oscillating files is highly recommended (**Fig. 22.8**).

This minimally invasive approach includes a restriction of the preparation to a an approximal slot without an occlusal "dove-tail" or even the whole occlusal surface; the box-only preparation with automatic undercuts due to the caries process offers enough retention even for nonadhesive filling materials (see Chapter 19).

Minimally invasive preparation and restoration require a higher degree of dedication by the dental professional than do the standard Black's type cavities, as:

- Access for preparation, caries removal, and filling application are restricted
- The margins of the restorations are in areas which are difficult to clean
- The application of approximal adhesive restorations is especially technique-sensitive

The selection of the filling material for small approximal cavities is an interesting point of discussion. Nowadays, many dentists would automatically choose composites and adhesive techniques, although amalgams seem to be more durable.[25,26] Research on the longevity of restorations shows clearly that caries adjacent to restorations is the most important reason for the failure of restorations. It has to be kept in mind that the imbalance of de- and remineralizing factors leads to the caries lesion in need of a restoration. This fact will not be changed by the restoration in itself. Therefore, intensified primary and secondary preventive efforts are a prerequisite for the success of minimally invasive techniques.

SUMMARY

Caries management in the deciduous dentition is not quite the same as dentistry in the permanent dentition, owing to smaller teeth with a shorter lifespan. Anatomical, epidemiological, and functional differences lead to a rather dichotomized treatment concept for younger children. This means that the small proportion of children having a high caries risk need more invasive treatments in addition to the reduction of their caries risk, whereas the majority of children needs instead noninvasive interventions and oral health education (see Chapters 13 and 21). As with any dichotomization a "gray zone" cannot be neglected. This means that 20%–30% of children do neither have severe decay (e.g., early childhood caries) nor completely sound dental hard tissues. These children may exhibit caries lesions that need to be treated by the whole spectrum of non-, micro- and minimally invasive dentistry.

In the permanent dentition, caries follows a similar pattern/distribution in children as in young adults Therefore, treatment concepts outlined throughout this book are generally appropriate for adolescents, as well. However, the same degree of demineralization and decay will have happened over a much shorter time compared with adults, which indicates a higher caries progression rate and might result in a more invasive treatment strategy, if noninvasive efforts as a sole treatment are likely to fail.

REFERENCES

1. Sønju Clasen AB, Ogaard B, Duschner H, Ruben J, Arends J, Sönju T. Caries development in fluoridated and non-fluoridated deciduous and permanent enamel in situ examined by microradiography and confocal laser scanning microscopy. Adv Dent Res 1997;11(4):442–447

2. Marthaler TM. Changes in dental caries 1953–2003. Caries Res 2004;38(3):173–181

3. Jin BH, Ma DS, Moon HS et al. Early childhood caries: prevalence and risk factors in Seoul, Korea. J Public Health Dent 2003;63(3): 183–188

4. Robke FJ, Buitkamp M. Häufigkeit der Nuckelflaschenkaries bei Vorschulkindern in einer westdeutschen Großstadt. Oralprophylaxe 2002;24:59–63

5. Postma TC, Ayo-Yusuf OA, van Wyk PJ. Socio-demographic correlates of early childhood caries prevalence and severity in a developing country—South Africa. Int Dent J 2008;58(2):91–97

6. Kaste LM, Drury TF, Horowitz AM, Beltran E. An evaluation of NHANES III estimates of early childhood caries. J Public Health Dent 1999;59(3):198–200

7. Livny A, Sgan-Cohen HD. A review of a community program aimed at preventing early childhood caries among Jerusalem infants—a brief communication. J Public Health Dent 2007; 67(2):78–82

8. World Health Organization (WHO) Collaborating Centre for Education, Training and Research in Oral Health. Oral Health Database. Oral Health Country/Area Profile Project (2010). http://www.whocollab.od.mah.se. Accessed August 9, 2011

9. Deutsche Arbeitsgemeinschaft Jugendzahnpflege V (DAJ). Begleituntersuchungen zur Gruppenprophylaxe 2004. Bonn: Deutsche Arbeitsgemeinschaft Jugendzahnpflege; 2005

10. Bratthall D. Introducing the Significant Caries Index together with a proposal for a new global oral health goal for 12-year-olds. Int Dent J 2000;50(6):378–384

11. Institut der der deutschen Zahnärzte (IDZ). Vierte Deutsche Mundgesundheitsstudie (DMS IV). Köln: Dtsch Ärzteverlag; 2006

12. World Health Organization (WHO). The World Oral Health Report. Geneva: World Health Organization; 2003

13. Bolin AK. Children's dental health in Europe. An epidemiological investigation of 5- and 12-year-old children from eight EU countries. Swed Dent J Suppl 1997;122(Suppl.):1–88

14. Heinrich-Weltzien R, Kühnisch J, Goddon I, Senkel H, Stösser L. Dental health in German and Turkish school children—a 10-year comparison. [Article in German] Gesundheitswesen 2007;69(2): 105–109

15. Shwartz M, Gröndahl HG, Pliskin JS, Boffa J. A longitudinal analysis from bite-wing radiographs of the rate of progression of approximal carious lesions through human dental enamel. Arch Oral Biol 1984;29(7):529–536

16. Fejerskov O, Nyvad B, Kidd EAM. Enamel reactions during eruption. In: Fejerskov O, Kidd EAM, eds. Dental Caries. The Disease and its Clinical Management. 2nd ed. Oxford: Blackwell Munksgaard; 2008

17. Mejàre I, Lingström P, Petersson LG, et al. Caries-preventive effect of fissure sealants: a systematic review. Acta Odontol Scand 2003;61(6):321–330

18. Splieth CH, Ekstrand KR, Alkilzy M, et al. Sealants in dentistry: Outcomes of the ORCA Saturday afternoon symposium 2007. Caries Res 2010;44(1):3–13

19. Ahovuo-Saloranta A, Hiiri A, Nordblad A, Mäkelä M, Worthington HV. Pit and fissure sealants for preventing dental decay in the permanent teeth of children and adolescents. Cochrane Database Syst Rev 2008;4(4):CD001830

20. Mertz-Fairhurst EJ, Curtis JW Jr, Ergle JW, Rueggeberg FA, Adair SM. Ultraconservative and cariostatic sealed restorations: results at year 10. J Am Dent Assoc 1998;129(1):55–66

21. Heyduck C, Meller C, Schwahn C, Splieth CH. Effectiveness of sealants in adolescents with high and low caries experience. Caries Res 2006;40(5):375–381

22. Low T. The combined application of topical fluoride and fissure sealant—results after 2 years. J Oral Rehabil 1982;9(1):1–5

23. Beiruti N, Frencken JE, van't Hof MA, van Palenstein Helderman WH. Caries-preventive effect of resin-based and glass ionomer sealants over time: a systematic review. Community Dent Oral Epidemiol 2006;34(6):403–409

24. Poulsen S, Laurberg L, Vaeth M, Jensen U, Haubek D. A field trial of resin-based and glass-ionomer fissure sealants: clinical and radiographic assessment of caries. Community Dent Oral Epidemiol 2006;34(1):36–40

25. Mjör IA, Moorhead JE. Selection of restorative materials, reasons for replacement, and longevity of restorations in Florida. J Am Coll Dent 1998;65(3):27–33

26. Levin L, Coval M, Geiger SB. Cross-sectional radiographic survey of amalgam and resin-based composite posterior restorations. Quintessence Int 2007;38(6):511–514

Future Trends in Caries Research

Brian Clarkson, Agata Czajka-Jakubowska

23

Over the past three decades, the terms tissue engineering, nanotechnology, genetic engineering, probiotics, genomics, and proteomics have become increasingly familiar in the scientific literature. Cariology research has been somewhat slow in adapting these new technologies and techniques for preventing and treating what is one of the most ubiquitous of human diseases. However, "times they are a-changin'" in the world of cariology as we move away from the focus on invasive care (restorations) to one of caries control and its prevention. Our understanding of the etiology of caries has been expanded by using genomic strategies to probe the genetic contribution to caries susceptibility. The genetic engineering of noncaries-producing "cariogenic" bacteria and antibodies against cariogenic bacteria offers solutions to prevent acid production from plaque and the colonization by cariogenic bacteria. The ability to stimulate new dentin formation for repair of this tissue and the use of nanotechnology to manufacture synthetic enamel and smart materials will aid in the treatment of caries. Finally, proteomics and fluorescent images may help us solve the last great mystery in cariology: when is a carious lesion active?

Thus, in this chapter, promising approaches that in the future might be useful in the prevention and management of caries will be expanded upon and will cover:

- Genetic susceptibility to caries
- Carious lesion activity
- Regeneration and repair of the dentin/pulpal complex
- Antibacterial strategies
- New restorative materials

Genetic Approaches

Genomics—Caries Susceptibility

Although the environmental and host factors which contribute to the risk of caries in individuals have been known for many years, there are still individuals who are more or less susceptible to this disease. Much of the evidence for a **genetic contribution to the risk of caries** has come from studies of twins reared apart. Dental caries has been examined in twin populations since early in the 20th century. In 1927, an evaluation of 301 pairs of twins was undertaken, of which 130 were monozygotic and 171 were dizygotic. The results of the study demonstrated that monozygotic twins had a similar caries incidence, but the dizygotic twins did not. This was later confirmed by other investigators, that the risk of caries in monozygotic but not dizygotic pairs of twins was similar.[1]

It has been estimated that the genetic contribution to the disease is about 40%. Dental caries is a complex disease, and like other complex diseases such as diabetes, osteoporosis, and cleft lip and palate, the knowledge gained from the human genome project does allow us to study genetics. Thus, the approach taken to identify the genetic contribution to an individual's risk for caries has been similar to those used for other complex diseases. There are ongoing studies using DNA samples from caries-resistant and caries-prone siblings to detect SNPs (single-nucleotide polymorphisms) showing an association with caries resistance and caries susceptibility. The most likely candidate genes being pursued are those involved in enamel development and mineralization, salivary protein expression (especially the acidic-rich proteins), and dental hard tissue colonization by bacteria.

Probiotics—Replacement Therapy with non-Acid-Producing Bacteria

Our ability to genetically engineer bacteria makes it possible to "infect" tooth surfaces with bacteria that have the positive characteristics of metabolizing refined carbohydrates into urea rather than organic acids, and thus can fill the ecological niche at caries-susceptible sites with virulent but harmless bacteria. This may have greater implications when one considers the concept of the maternal fidelity of organisms, particularly mutans streptococci, during their passage from mother to offspring. This has intriguing possibilities in terms of prevention.

For example, if the mother were infected or reinfected with a "harmless" mutans streptococcus, which is non-acid-producing, and with the virulence to occupy the caries-susceptible sites, it would then be passed onto her child. It may, however, be difficult to convince the general public to accept a genetically engineered bacterium as a "cure" for a non-life-threatening disease. Therefore, naturally occurring bacteria that compete with cariogenic bacteria for the same ecological niche have been tested for **probiotic therapy**.[2–4]

Gene Therapy—Repairing Salivary Glands

The importance of saliva in the origin of caries is demonstrated most easily by the aggressive progression of the disease in its absence. Recent work, using gene therapy to repair salivary glands, will no doubt reap dividends in the future. It is important to understand that a gland has to be competent even if at a very low level. If it has been destroyed by disease or radiation, it cannot be rescued by gene therapy. This pioneering work has now progressed into human clinical trials, the results of which are eagerly anticipated. As yet, however, there is no easy solution to xerostomia, and the likely chance of it increasing in aging populations is significant, as older people will probably continue to make even greater use of drugs that have salivary flow-limiting side effects.[5]

Proteomics

Antibody Engineering— Bacterial Adherence

Recently, local passive immunization has aroused interest as a safe procedure in prevention of dental caries. New technologies for antibody engineering make possible the production of immunoglobulins in animals and transgenic plants (plantibodies). The murine IgG1 has been isolated and was effective against the streptococcal cell surface adhesion (SAI/II) protein, which mediates bacterial attachment to the salivary pellicle. This IgG1 antibody has been successfully evaluated in humans. After antibody therapy, the incidence of mutans streptococci was very much reduced. High-molecular-weight secretory immunoglobulin against mutans streptococci surface fibrillar adhesins (AgI/II) was produced by introducing cloned genes encoding the chains of monoclonal antibody against AgI/II, a murine J-chain and a rabbit secretory component, into a transgenic tobacco system (*Nicotiana tabacum*). The efficacy of this plant secretory antibody was studied on a small group of human volunteers and it was proven that the antibody was active for up to three days in the human oral cavity (two days longer than murine IgG antibody) and stimulated specific protection in humans against colonization by *Streptococcus mutans* for at least four months.

Enzyme Recognition—Caries Activity Assessment

As our ability to detect caries becomes more sensitive and more precise, then a greater percentage of the population will be declared not to be "caries free." The myriad of detection systems ranging from electrical resistance, to laser fluorescence, transillumination, etc., will lead to earlier detection of the caries lesion and hopefully to earlier application of preventive programs to control the progression of the lesions, and not to earlier restoration of a potential cavity. Unfortunately, being able to detect a lesion only tells the clinician half of the story, that is, whether there is or is not a lesion. It does not tell the clinician the other half of the story, namely whether the **lesion is active or not**. Apart from the part played by genetics in caries susceptibility, this is perhaps the most important question to be answered in cariology today.

There is a tool used in the leather industry which may help us diagnose active root caries lesions. The probe is used to test the resilience of leather that is the give (softness) of the leather. Perhaps this could be adapted to test the surface softness, a cardinal sign of activity, of a root caries lesion. Further, matrix metalloproteinases participate in the breakdown of the organic matrix of dentin. Human versions of these enzymes designated mm-2, mm-8, and mm-9 have been detected in carious dentin and are activated at low pH (4.5). Maybe these can be used as identifiers of carious activity in dentin. In terms of enamel caries, the enzyme glucansucrase/glucosyltransferase is responsible for converting sugars in food into sugar chains that can act as a glue. Both lactobacillus and mutans streptococcus have this enzyme. Its detection in plaque after a sucrose rinse could indicate a potentially active cariogenic plaque. Lactate dehydrogenase oxidizes lactic acid to pyruvate in plaque and its detection would indicate an active, pathogenic plaque, assuming the plaque pH drops below a critical pH (which may be different in different individuals), so as to cause enamel demineralization.

Tissue Engineering

The Dentin–Pulpal Complex

Tissue engineering is a reality in medicine, especially for skin and bone repair and regeneration. Work in the late 1980s on the regeneration of dentin using growth factors, the morphogenic proteins (BMPs), may still pave the way for the treatment of deep carious lesions. In animal experiments, a collagen gel containing the BMPs was applied, which stimulated the pulp to completely replace the medicament with dentin. In human clinical trials, the results were ambiguous because of the inflammation caused by the breakdown products from the collagen carrier. Our ability now to functionalize dendrimers (nano-polymers) with both a BMP and an antiinflammatory, make this nanotherapeutic an ideal choice with which to repeat these experiments.[6]

Further work in our laboratory has shown our ability to turn dental pulp stem cells (DPSCs) into odontoblastlike cells by treating with a dentin extract and a mineralizing stimulating solution.[7] These DPSCs have now been grown on synthetic enamel-like films (**Fig. 23.1**). This brings closer a practical regeneration of the entire coronal pulpal complex, but the regeneration of a tooth root remains to be solved.

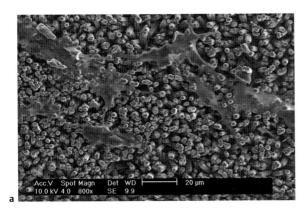

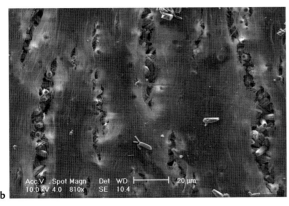

Fig. 23.1a, b Dental pulp stem cells grown on well aligned fluorapatite crystal surfaces.
a After 3 days.
b After 3 weeks.

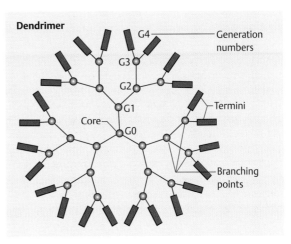

Fig. 23.2 Schematic structure of a generation 4 dendrimer (artificial protein) with a central stem and branches which can be functionalized.

Nanotechnology

Dendrimers—Antimicrobials/ Antiadherents

Nanotechnology has also offered us dendrimers which can be used as **nanotherapeutics** (**Fig. 23.2**). The "beauty" of these artificial proteins is that they are very, very small (3–10 nm in size), which allows them to penetrate into cells and they can also be functionalized. In other words, you can attach to one dendrimer, an antimicrobial, an antimetabolite, an anti-inflammatory, etc. Then, depending on the charge on the dendrimer (and this can be manipulated), the dendrimer will also attach to apatite surfaces. The advantages of using these dendrimers to modify surfaces, either by changing the surface charge or by acting as an antibacterial agent, are obvious. By modifying the enamel/dentin surfaces with these molecules, it will be possible to discourage the attachment of certain oral bacteria and, perhaps encourage the attachment of others.

Cost and toxicity are always issues when talking about new therapies. The dendrimers are inexpensive but, at this moment, expensive to functionalize. They are already

being used in animal trials for targeted drug delivery, especially anticancer drugs.

Antibacterial Nanoemulsions

An inexpensive and nontoxic new anticaries therapy could be the **nanoemulsions**, which are produced by expelling oil through a fine nozzle under pressure to produce nano-droplets of oil which have high energy and remain suspended in the water phase. When these droplets contact bacteria, they attach, give up their energy, and kill the bacterial cells—no antibiotic resistance or sensitivity is involved, it is only oil! It is not clear if this emulsion will be effective on bacteria embedded in biofilms, so the biofilm may have to be disrupted before applying the emulsion. The research performed on these emulsions has shown that they do not harm mammalian cells. Thus, in the future, these emulsions may be available as oral antiseptics.

Degradable Microspheres— Remineralizing Agents

The interaction of saliva, bacteria, food, and microbial products in the production and maintenance of biofilms on the tooth surfaces is an integral part of the etiology of caries and its prevention. It is known that plaque is a **biofilm** that is composed of a polysaccharide matrix, like all biofilms.[3] The discovery of channels passing from the surface of plaque to the tooth surface[8] underscores a need to re-evaluate the structure of this biomass and the importance of these channels in caries formation and its prevention. For example, one might use degradable microspheres which can penetrate the channels in plaque and release bactericidal agents or antimetabolites to either kill the plaque bacteria or disrupt their adherence.

The large surface area provided by the oral mucosa makes it ideal to be used as a reservoir for drug delivery,

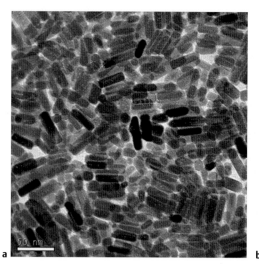
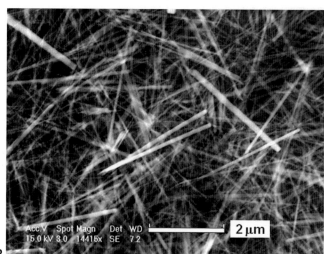

Fig. 23.3a, b Synthetic enamel-like fluorapatite crystals.
a Produced under ambient conditions.
b Produced under hydrothermal conditions.

although the adhesion mechanisms which exist in this area make this ability limited. For this reason, some bioadhesive formulations have been developed to improve drug delivery and allow localized release over an extended period. The mucoadhesion drug delivery systems available use synthetic (chitosans, carbopols, carbomers) and natural polymers (plant lectins) which adhere to the mucosal surface. The first systems used relatively large macromolecules. The latest innovation of the system proposes the use of micro-particles of average diameter about 0.1–10 µm. These can act as platforms (e.g., biodegradable [micro] spheres) for the sustained release of fluoride, calcium, and phosphorus, producing the optimum remineralization conditions. This can be achieved by having some of the spheres contain the phosphorus and fluoride, and the others the calcium, thus preventing any calcium and fluoride interaction prior to their release into the oral cavity. It is also possible to use these bioadhesives as controlled-release systems to deliver other biologically active ingredients important in caries prevention, such as antiseptics and antibacterial materials that can influence bacterial growth and attachment to the tooth surface.

"Smart" Materials—Responding to Physiological and Nonphysiological Changes in the Oral Cavity

In medicine, "smart" materials have been developed to release a variety of molecules or ions depending on the changes in the physiological condition of the body. Fabricated composite materials that react to changes in the plaque pH are a reality. It has been shown that as the pH drops, these materials can release fluoride; and when the pH rises to near neutral the fluoride release stops. This reaction to the oral environment allows fluoride to be released when it is needed rather than being released passively all the time, eventually causing degradation of the restorative material.

Synthetic Enamel

In the age of tissue regeneration, gene therapy, and **nanotechnology**, it is the latter that might offer the least expensive technology to prevent and treat caries. Already, nano/micro composite materials are available that offer advantages as fillers over those that are conventionally used. Using nanotechnology, nano/micro crystals of fluorapatite have been synthesized and these may be the next generation of fillers for composite restorations (**Fig. 23.3**). They have the added advantage of releasing calcium, phosphate, and fluoride when the pH drops under plaque, thus producing the perfect remineralization solution at the plaque/composite interface. This release then stops as the pH is reversed; in a way acting like a "smart" material.

Nanotechnology has also allowed these crystals to be vertically aligned and self-assembled into a prismatic-like structure, resembling natural, human enamel surfaces (**Fig. 23.4**). These films can then be layered on one another and bonded together to produce a laminate 3-D structure which could be used to fabricate veneers (**Fig. 23.5**) or crowns using the CAD/CAM technology.[9]

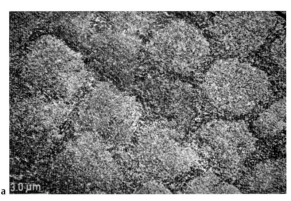
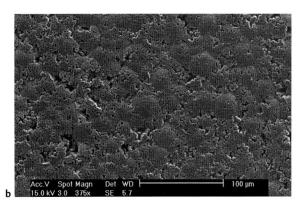

a 3.0 μm
b Acc.V Spot Magn Det WD ⊢————⊣ 100 μm
15.0 kV 3.0 375x SE 5.7

Fig. 23.4a, b Surface prismatic structure of apatite structures.
a Human enamel.
b Synthetic fluorapatite.

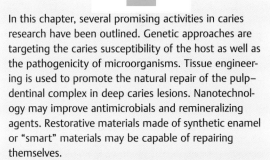

Fig. 23.5 Fluorapatite films removed from the metal plates on which they were grown.

SUMMARY

In this chapter, several promising activities in caries research have been outlined. Genetic approaches are targeting the caries susceptibility of the host as well as the pathogenicity of microorganisms. Tissue engineering is used to promote the natural repair of the pulp–dentinal complex in deep caries lesions. Nanotechnology may improve antimicrobials and remineralizing agents. Restorative materials made of synthetic enamel or "smart" materials may be capable of repairing themselves.

It is often stated that 80% of the caries occurs in 20% of the population, which are generalized as the lower socioeconomic groups. What are presented here are contemporary technologies that could be used to reduce caries in all populations, but because of cost will initially be targeted at the 80% of the population with 20% of the caries. However, this is highly unlikely. It would seem logical, if not practical, to make wealthier the 20% of the population with 80% of the caries. Therefore, the less expensive treatments to reduce caries rates in this less fortunate population should be vigorously encouraged.

REFERENCES

1. Bacharach FH, Young M. A comparison of the degree of resemblance in dental characters shown in pairs of twins of identical and fraternal types. Br Dent J 1927;48:1293–1304

2. Näse L, Hatakka K, Savilahti E, et al. Effect of long-term consumption of a probiotic bacterium, Lactobacillus rhamnosus GG, in milk on dental caries and caries risk in children. Caries Res 2001;35(6):412–420

3. Caglar E, Kavaloglu SC, Kuscu OO, Sandalli N, Holgerson PL, Twetman S. Effect of chewing gums containing xylitol or probiotic bacteria on salivary mutans streptococci and lactobacilli. Clin Oral Investig 2007;11(4):425–429

4. Stecksén-Blicks C, Sjöström I, Twetman S. Effect of long-term consumption of milk supplemented with probiotic lactobacilli and fluoride on dental caries and general health in preschool children: a cluster-randomized study. Caries Res 2009;43(5):374–381

5. He X, Goldsmith CM, Marmary Y, et al. Systemic action of human growth hormone following adenovirus-mediated gene transfer to rat submandibular glands. Gene Ther 1998;5(4):537–541

6. Rutherford RB, Wahle J, Tucker M, Rueger D, Charette M. Induction of reparative dentine formation in monkeys by recombinant human osteogenic protein-1. Arch Oral Biol 1993;38(7):571–576

7. Liu J, Jin T, Chang S, Ritchie HH, Smith AJ, Clarkson BH. Matrix and TGF-beta-related gene expression during human dental pulp stem cell (DPSC) mineralization. In Vitro Cell Dev Biol Anim 2007;43(3-4):120–128

8. Wood SR, Kirkham J, Nattress B. Architecture and matrix composition of intact human plaque revealed. [Abstract 107] J Dent Res 1998;77:645

9. Chen H, Tang Z, Liu J, et al. Acellular synthesis of a human enamel-like microstructure. Adv Mater (Deerfield Beach Fla) 2006;18:1846–1851

Part 2 Caries— Clinical Practice

Diagnostics, Treatment Decision, and Documentation

Sebastian Paris, Rainer Haak, Hendrik Meyer-Lueckel

24

The theoretical fundamentals of modern caries diagnosis and therapy were discussed in the preceding chapters. In the following chapters which deal with practical application, the implementation of this knowledge will be illustrated with reference to **clinical cases** and **individual treatments**. This introductory chapter will therefore present standard forms for documentation and findings tailored to risk assessment, dental diagnostics, and treatment planning. These forms will also be used in the subsequent clinical cases.

When describing clinical cases, several treatments will be described step by step in the following chapters:

- Fissure sealing (adult): Chapter 25, Case 1, **Fig. 25.7**, Page 344
- Fissure sealing (child): Chapter 26, Case 1, **Fig. 26.9**, Page 380
- Composite restoration (molars): Chapter 25, Case 1, **Fig. 25.8**, Page 345
- Composite restoration (anterior teeth): Chapter 25, Case 3, Page 361
- Composite restoration (primary molars): Chapter 25, Case 2, **Fig. 25.21**, Page 356
- Infiltration (arresting caries, permanent): Chapter 26, Case 3, **Fig. 26.26**, Page 391
- Infiltration (arresting caries, primary molars): Chapter 26, Case 1, Page 374
- Infiltration (masking caries): Chapter 25, Case 4, Page 367
- Stepwise caries excavation (adult): Chapter 25, Case 5, Page 371

Caries Diagnostics at the Patient Level

As presented in Chapters 7 and 9, the goal of caries risk analysis is to estimate the patient's risk of experiencing new caries lesions in the future followed by an assessment of the patient's need for risk-related interventions, and to initiate noninvasive or microinvasive therapy with those methods which are most beneficial for this particular patient to lower his or her risk. In addition, the **general caries risk** should also be taken into consideration for the diagnosis of caries at the tooth level. If the patient is assessed as being at high risk, the probability that his or her questionable lesions are progressing is higher than if the risk were assessed as low.

For reasons of practicality, the caries risk should be assessed as quickly and simply as possible. It is therefore recommended to concentrate on easy-to-determine risk factors with a high predictive value. Several factors or predictors that are useful in assessing the caries risk were cited in Chapter 7. Software programs such as the Cariogram[1] that can be downloaded free of charge from the Internet are useful for summarizing and weighting the various risk factors (**Fig. 24.1**). If a computer is not available at the site of treatment, the caries risk can also be determined using a simple form. **Figure 24.2** shows a form for assessing the caries risk which is based on the **Cariogram software**.

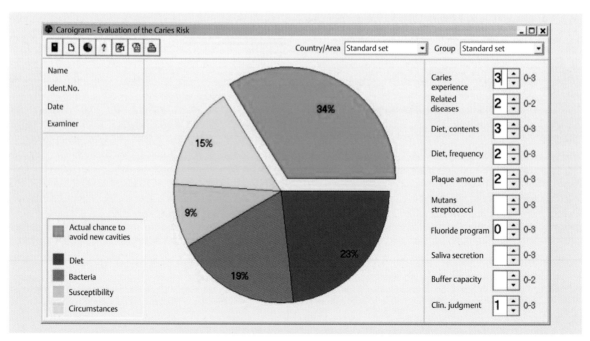

Fig. 24.1 Estimation of the caries risk using the Cariogram software program. The software calculates the future "chance to avoid new cavities" (caries risk = 100%-chance to avoid new cavitation), and it also weights the various risk factors and depicts them as a pie chart

Determining the Risk Factors

The form shown in **Fig. 24.2** is restricted to **four parameters relating to patient history, and two to three clinical parameters** for determining the caries risk. Generally, it takes no more than three minutes to fill out the form, and this can be done by the assistant. In the following, the assessment of the various risk factors will be addressed.

Caries Experience

The patient's **DMFT value** (taken from the examination form) is entered and weighted based on the patient's age. From the diagram, we can determine whether the patient's DMFT is appropriate for his or her age, or whether it is higher or lower than average for the age group. For children up to 13 years of age the number of initial caries lesions (only visual-tactile assessment) plus restorations and teeth extracted due to caries in deciduous ($d_1$mft) and permanent (D_1MFT) teeth is used instead of DMFT (see also Chapter 8).

Sugar Consumption

The patient is asked about the frequency at which he or she consumes **fermentable carbohydrates** (sugar). Ask about hidden sugars in foods and beverages of which the patient is frequently not aware (see Chapter 11).

Frequency of Food Consumption

Here the patient is asked how many **meals and snacks** (including sweetened beverages) he or she consumes over the course of the day. By asking specific questions, many patients become aware for the first time how many snacks they consume daily that may contain hidden carbohydrates. The estimated average number of snacks is documented.

Oral Hygiene

The patient's oral hygiene is evaluated using an easy-to-determine plaque index. In the presented form sheet the **Approximal Plaque Index (API)** is used. The buccal and oral interproximal regions are checked for the presence of plaque in two quadrants using a probe without staining the plaque beforehand, and the percentage of plaque-covered approximal surfaces is calculated. If other, more detailed plaque or gingiva indexes are utilized during prophylaxis sessions, these can be used as alternatives (Chapter 10).

Fluoride Sources

This item is used to identify and document the **different sources of fluoride** to which the patient is exposed and to evaluate if additional fluoridation methods should be used for caries prevention. It is important to ask specific questions to determine whether patients are exposed to certain sources of fluoride of which they might not be aware (such as fluoridated table salt, water fluoridation, etc.) to avoid overdosage (Chapter 12).

Salivary Flow

The salivary flow rate normally only has an appreciable effect on the individual caries risk in extremes (e.g., patients with hyposalivation). Since it is comparatively time-consuming to evaluate the salivary flow rate, this item might only be filled out in the case of suspected hyposalivation (dry mucosa, xerostomia, medications, radiation therapy). In this form, generally the stimulated **saliva flow rate (SSFR)** is determined. The patient chews on a paraffin pellet for a specific period (e.g., 5 minutes). The amount of saliva produced is collected, measured, and the amount of saliva produced per minute (SSFR) is calculated.

Calculating the Caries Risk and Consequences

The different risk factors that are recorded have different predictive values and therefore need to be weighted differently. A "risk value" is assigned corresponding to the different weighting of each risk factor. The different risk values are then added up, and a percentage caries risk is calculated. The calculated number does not equal the specific probability of whether the patient will experience new caries lesions over a specific period; rather, this value provides a **rough estimation of the general caries risk**, and the patient is categorized as having a small, average, or great need of risk-related non- and microinvasive intervention. Depending on the dentist's experience, it may be useful to correct the calculated value upward or downward based on the personal, subjective estimation of the caries risk. The Cariogram software program also provides a similar function.

In the table in the lower part of the form sheet (see **Fig. 24.2**), the individual examination interval as well as intervals for various noninvasive interventions can be determined from the patient's caries risk. The periods can be individually adapted according to the treatment philosophy and the approach of the dental practice. In any case, this categorization helps you select reasonable, demand-oriented **follow-up intervals**.

When selecting the risk-related intervention, the different weighting of the various parameters ("risk value" in the form sheet) should be taken into consideration. In the example in **Fig. 24.2**, recommendations regarding nutrition and the optimization of oral hygiene are especially useful to lower the patient's risk of caries.

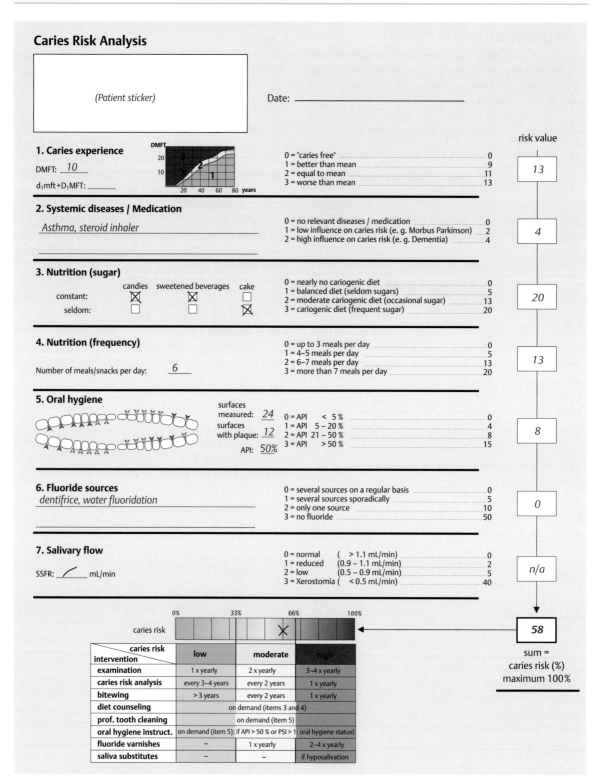

Caries Risk Analysis

Fig. 24.2 Estimation of the caries risk using a form sheet. The different historical and clinical parameters are determined and quantified as described in the text. This yields a "risk value" from the different weightings for each risk factor. In the present example, the amount of saliva was not measured for practical reasons since there was no indication of xerostomia or hyposalivation in the patient's history and examination. The sum of the risk values yields the individual caries risk. The individual follow-up interval for examina-tions and risk assessment as well as the required noninvasive ther-apeutic measures can be derived from the table in the bottom section of the form. The individual need for risk-related interven-tions depends on the individual weighting of the various risk factors. (Modified from Cariogram: Bratthall D, Hansel Peterson G. Cariog-ram—a multifactorial risk assessment model for a multifactorial disease. Commun Dent Oral Epidemiol 2003;33(4):255–264.) n/a = not applicable

It is useful to determine the caries risk of the patient so that the noninvasive therapy can be adapted to the individual risk factors. Moreover, the intervals of the patient's follow-up examinations can be adapted to the individual caries risk. In terms of quality management, the follow-up interval can be rationally identified on the basis of individual need.

Caries Diagnostics at the Tooth Level

The patient's teeth can be examined either before or after determining their individual risk of caries (afterwards the caries risk can be estimated immediately). Since a range of tools are available to assist dentists with the diagnosis of caries, the findings need to be clearly documented. The examination (hereafter, exam) form in **Fig. 24.3** is organized in a similar way to classical dental exam forms. That is, the clinical findings are recorded in a schematic diagram representing the different tooth surfaces. In addition, there are fields above or below the individual teeth for documenting additional diagnostic information (radiographic, laser fluorescence, transillumination). That way, all of the relevant information is presented in a clearly laid-out manner, and the various findings can be combined and weighted to form an appropriate diagnosis (see Chapter 9).

To retain an overview of the various pieces of information, it has become standard practice to assign colors to the visual–tactile findings (including the activity status). In the presented exam form, stoplight colors are used to provide an intuitive system orientating on the subsequent (probably) selected therapy. As with classical dental exam forms, caries lesions that will probably require invasive therapy according to the visual–tactile examination (IC-DAS 3–6 and/or x-ray D2/D3, active) are marked in red (**Table 24.1**). In addition, lesions that will probably require none- or microinvasive therapy (ICDAS 1–2 and/or x-ray E1, E2, D1, active) are colored yellow (or orange for improved visibility). Inactive caries lesions that do not require intervention or only need to be monitored are colored green. Existing restorations in this sheet are colored blue (**Fig. 24.3**)

In addition to marking caries lesions, the stoplight colors can be used to label the quality of restorations or root canal fillings (see **Table 24.1**). In addition, healthy surfaces that are temporarily exposed to an increased caries risk (such as the occlusal surfaces of erupting molars) can be colored yellow to indicate that these surfaces require special noninvasive or microinvasive intervention.

According to the stoplight color scheme, all inactive lesions should be colored **green** on the exam form. Particularly with older patients, this may mean that quite a few surfaces are colored green. This causes one to lose the general overview, and the necessity of monitoring the green surfaces appears less important when a large number of surfaces are green. Consequently, one may decide not to document **inactive lesions**. However, for educational purposes, it may be recommended in training centers to note inactive lesions. This indicates to students that they not only need to detect caries lesions, but they also need to assess caries activity. Furthermore, it is useful to mark inactive lesions green to document the course of therapy (such as the inactivation of active lesions through noninvasive therapy).

Even though the colors that are used for the documentation of visual–tactile examinations already point toward appropriate therapeutic options (**Fig. 24.3**), it is important to note that additional diagnostic measures beyond the visual–tactile examination are frequently necessary to come to a reliable diagnosis. The colors in the exam form should therefore be understood as the visual–tactile findings but not as definitive diagnosis. The diagnosis is only documented later in the form of a table (**Table 24.2**).

Visual–Tactile Examination

The visual–tactile examination forms the basis of caries diagnosis, during which the teeth are normally examined sequentially proceeding from 18 to 28 and from 38 to 48. Generally, **clean teeth** are examined so that all of the tooth surfaces can be assessed. In individual cases, however, it can be useful to examine uncleaned teeth to enable a better evaluation of the plaque, and hence the caries activity, on individual tooth surfaces.

Primary Caries

Once the dentist has detected caries and excluded other diseases in a differential diagnostic process, he/she assesses the caries severity and activity. To document the findings, the dentist generally communicates to the assistant the related tooth, the affected surface, the disease and, in the case of caries, the activity and stage (such as the ICDAS caries code). The assistant enters the code for the caries stage in the corresponding field and marks the relevant surface in the tooth diagram with the corresponding color (see **Table 24.1** and **Fig. 24.4**).

Caries Adjacent to Restorations

When existing restorations are being examined, the dentist first communicates to the assistant the restored tooth surfaces, the type of restoration, and the material used. This information is noted on the exam form. Then the

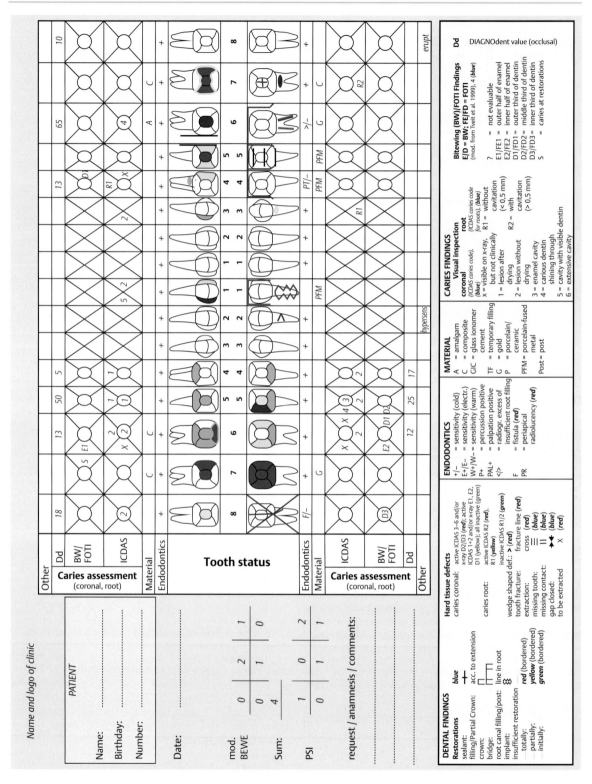

Fig. 24.3 An example of a filled-out dental examination form. A legend is in the bottom part of the form; FOTI: fiberoptic transillumination.

Table 24.1 Meaning of color code in the exam form. It should be noted that the colors in the exam form only indicate a (probable) diagnosis and therapy. Nonetheless they need not be identical with the column chosen in the diagnoses and treatment plan (**Table 24.2**) for a certain tooth.

	Green	**Yellow/orange**	**Red**
Meaning of the color	Monitor closely	Indicates non-invasive or micro-invasive therapy	Indicates (minimally) invasive therapy
Caries	Inactive	Aktive, ICDAS 1–2	Active, ICDAS 3–6
Healthy	–	Insufficient local caries risk	–
Restorations (circled)	Suspect	Insufficient but repairable	Insufficient and requiring replacement
Wedge-shaped defect	–	Requiring desensitization	Requiring restoration
Root canal fillings	Suspect	–	Requiring revision

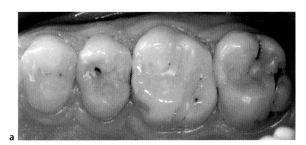

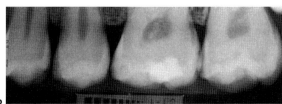

Fig. 24.4a–c Example of documented clinical findings. The visual–tactile findings (**a**) e.g., primary caries and restorations are entered in the examination form (**c**) (see the legend in **Fig. 24.3**). If primary caries is detected (such as 25 occlusal), the stage (ICDAS, caries code) is entered in the "ICDAS" field corresponding to the affected surface. If the caries is inactive, it is noted as green in the teeth diagram. If the lesion is active, it is noted as yellow (ICDAS 1–2) or red (ICDAS 3–6). If there are several findings for one tooth surface, it is preferable to document the more serious finding in the tooth status. For example, occlusal surface 27 has active caries (ICDAS 4, D1) in the disto-palatinal fissure in addition to a composite filling requiring renewal. However, the active caries is not noted,

since both diagnoses will be treated at the same time with a new restoration. In the fields above and below the illustrated teeth, the results of additional diagnostic measures are noted such as radiographic findings (**b**). The radiographically identifiable caries in the mesial surface in tooth 26 (E2) is clinically clearly inactive due to its position and surface characteristics (ICDAS 2, inactive) and is therefore colored green. The radiographically detected distal caries in tooth 24 (D1) cannot be assessed visually (marked with 'x'). However, the adjacent papilla bleeds upon probing. Consequently, the corresponding surface in the illustrated tooth is colored yellow. DIAGNOdent values are entered in the column "Dd."

dentist examines the restoration in greater detail and tells the assistant if the restoration needs to be monitored, for example, due to discolored margins (green), requires correction (yellow), or needs to be replaced (red).

Additional Diagnostic Tools

Frequently, a visual–tactile examination alone is insufficient to arrive at a definite diagnosis. Consequently, additional diagnostic tools often need to be used, especially for locations that are difficult to access visually.

Bitewing Radiographs and Fiberoptic Transillumination

When bitewing radiographs are taken, the findings for the respective surface (E1, E2, D1, D2, D3) are documented in the corresponding fields (Chapter 6). In practice, it is recommended to re-examine lesions detected with radiographs that were not discovered in the former visual–tactile examination. For example, a more precise inspection or temporary separation of the teeth may reveal the condition of the surface (activity, cavitation) more pre-

Table 24.2 Documentation of diagnoses and treatment plan. The various diagnoses for individual tooth surfaces are listed under "tooth surface" in the three color-coded columns. Next to the tooth and surface the chosen therapy is listed (examples are shown). If the therapy is completed for a certain surface this can be documented with a check mark. o = occlusal, v = vestibular, m = mesial, d = distal, or = oral.

Diagnosis	Caries	Caries non-progressiva (CNP)		Caries progressiva superficialis (CS)			Caries progressiva media (CM) et profunda (CP)		
	Restorations	Restauratio insufficienta initialis (RII)		Restauratio insufficienta partialis (RIP)			Restauratio insufficienta totalis (RIT)		
	Sound surfaces	–		Sanus majoris periculi (SMP)			–		
Treatment		Particular surveillance		Noninvasive or microinvasive/repair			(Minimally) invasive		
		Tooth + Surface	Diagnosis	Tooth + Surface	Diagnosis	Therapy	Tooth + Surface	Diagnosis	Therapy
		11 v	CNP	17 o	SMP	FS ✔	46 o	CM	FC ✔
				16 o	CS	LF + CB ✔	36 o	CP	FC + EW ✔
				27 o	RIP	POL	37 mod	RIT	C–P

LF   local fluoridation
CB   cross brushing (molars)
OH   local oral hygiene training
FS   fissure sealing
INF   caries infiltration
POL   polishing
REP   repair

FC   composite filling
FA   amalgam filling
GIZ   glass-ionomer filling
I   inlay (G: gold; P: porcelain [ceramic])
PC   partial crown (G: gold; P: porcelain)
C   full crown (G: Gold; P: porcelain; PFM: pocelain-fused metal)
SW   stepwise excavation
RCT   root canal treatment
POST   post (G: gold; F: fiber)
Ex   extraction
!   examine adjacent surface during preparation

cisely. Since an individual x-ray image is informative about the depth but not the activity of a lesion, it is recommended to consider gingival inflammation (only recommended when probing depth is less than 5 mm) and plaque stagnation as criteria of caries activity (see Chapter 5). If the adjacent papilla is not inflamed (no bleeding in response to careful probing), the related tooth surface is marked green in the tooth diagram. If, in contrast, the papilla is inflamed, the related tooth surface is marked yellow (E1, E2, D1) or red (D2, D3) (**Fig. 24.4**).

If fiberoptic transillumination is used instead of, or in addition to, bitewing radiographs, the related findings are entered in the same field. In this case, an "F" is entered before the abbreviation indicating the extent of the lesion.

Laser Fluorescence

If occlusal caries is suspected as a result of a clinical or radiologic examination, laser fluorescence can be used as an additional diagnostic tool to assess lesion depth (Chap-

ter 6). However, using laser fluorescence for screening of all occlusal surfaces is not recommended due to potential increase in false-positive values that this would provoke (see Chapter 9). The maximum value per tooth (peak) is noted in the related field in the exam form (**Fig. 24.4**).

Endodontic Findings

The exam form can also be used to document endodontic findings. In addition to sensitivity (to cold, heat, electricity), fistulas, sensitivity to percussion, etc. can be noted in the relevant fields.

Additional Diagnostics

In addition to caries, other diseases of the oral cavity are also diagnosed and treated in dental practices such as periodontitis, noncarious dental hard tissue defects, and diseases of the oral mucosa. Since not every patient is affected by such diseases, an extensive examination is not needed in every case. For this reason, various **screening indexes** have become established which help identify periodontopathies and noncarious dental hard tissue defects (erosion, abrasion, attrition) early on, and allow the quick identification of patients suffering from these diseases without an extensive examination. If pathological changes are suspected in the screening examination, additional, more detailed exam forms are used to obtain a more thorough diagnosis. In the presented exam form, the periodontal screening index (PSI) to screen for periodontal diseases[2] is used along with the modified basic (erosive) wear examination (modified BEWE) index[3] to screen for noncarious hard tissue defects in the permanent dentition. The modified BEWE differs from the original index in that other, noncarious, hard tissue defects such as attrition or wedge-shaped defects are also recorded in addition to erosive defects. The maximum PSI and BEWE values for the respective sextants are entered in the table. Based on the maximum value of each sextant (PSI and mod. BEWE) or the sum of the values for all sextants (mod. BEWE), the general individual risk of periodontal and noncarious hard tissue defects can be estimated, and additional diagnostic measures can be pursued. These measures can be found in the related reference works for periodontology and erosion.

Diagnosis and Planning a Therapy

Not only for forensic reasons, it is necessary to collect the various findings and form a specific diagnosis that will serve as the basis of subsequent therapy. As noted in Chapter 9, the only diagnoses which are relevant are those that relate to the available therapeutic options. The stoplight colors used to document the visual–tactile examination can be used to link the various lesions to their diagnosis and assign the various interventions in a treatment plan. **Table 24.2** shows a **combined diagnosis and therapy plan**. The various diagnoses are documented, and their severity is indicated by color. Then the planned therapy is determined and entered. The same form can be used later to note therapeutic measures that have been taken and thereby provides an overview of the course of therapy.

REFERENCES

1. Bratthall D. Cariogram Software. http://www.mah.se/fakulteter-och-omraden/Odontologiska-fakulteten/Avdelning-och-kansli/Cariologi/Cariogram. Accessed January 22, 2013

2. Ekanayaka AN, Sheiham A. A periodontal screening index (PSI) to assess periodontal treatment needs. Odontostomatol Trop 1980; 3(1):11–19

3. Bartlett D, Ganss C, Lussi A. Basic Erosive Wear Examination (BEWE): a new scoring system for scientific and clinical needs. Clin Oral Investig 2008;12(Suppl 1):S65–S 68

4. Tveit AB, Espelid I, Skodje F. Restorative treatment decision on approximal caries in Norway. Int Dent J 1999;49(3):165–172

Minimal Interventional Treatment of Caries in the Permanent Dentition: Clinical Cases

Hendrik Meyer-Lueckel, Sebastian Paris, Christian A. Schneider, Leandro A. Hilgert, Soraya Coelho Leal

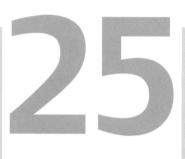

Case 1: A 30-year-old Woman with Low-to-Medium Caries Risk

Hendrik Meyer-Lueckel, Sebastian Paris

Anamnesis

Gender: female
Age: 30 years
First visit: October 2010
Last visit: February 2011
Follow-up visit: October 2011

The patient was referred to the university clinic by a private practitioner, since a routine check-up had revealed several caries lesions as detected by radiographic examination. She had been informed that these caries lesions might be treated by caries infiltration (Chapter 17), but the dentist was not sure whether the technique would be adequate for the stages of caries present. No general health issues were reported by the patient.

Clinical Findings (Tooth Level)

Clinical examination revealed a permanent dentition with first bicuspids and third molars having been extracted for orthodontic reasons. Signs of gingivitis as well as tooth stain and calculus were observed; the oral mucosa was healthy. Modified BEWE index was assessed as score 2 for both anterior sextants (incisal abrasion), the sum was 5. No frank cavities, but some restorations could be detected at a first glance (**Fig. 25.1**).

Caries detection was based on visual–tactile (**Fig. 25.1**) and radiographic (**Figs. 25.2** and **Fig. 25.3**) examinations as well as DIAGNOdent measurements (see **Fig. 25.4**). In general, only four restorations (all first molars), for the upper first molars including the respective mesial approximal areas were detected clinically. The central fissure of the fourth first molar (tooth 46) had been sealed, but revealed some darkish area around the sealant. For the occlusal aspects of three second molars (teeth 17, 27, 37), caries lesions with ICDAS 2 were assessed, one of them being scored as active (tooth 17), the two others as being inactive (teeth 27, 37). Tooth 47 showed remnants of fissure sealant and an adjacent ICDAS 2 lesion (**Figs. 25.1** and **25.5**). The D$_3$MFT was counted as 5, including the fissure-sealed tooth 47 with adjacent active caries in need of restoration.

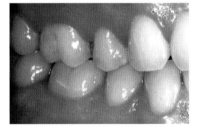
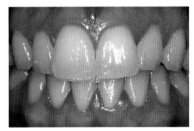
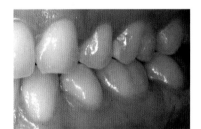

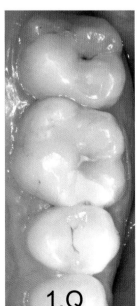
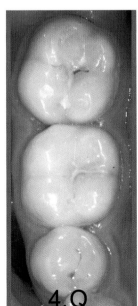
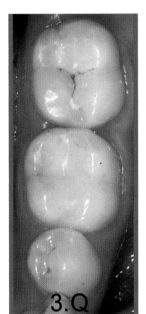
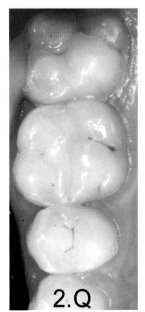

Fig. 25.1 Clinical aspect of the vestibular as well as occlusal aspects of the upper and lower jaws at the first visit. Q = quadrant

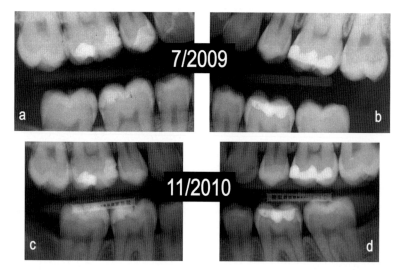

Fig. 25.2a–d Bitewing radiographs taken in July 2009 by the previous dentist (**a, b**) and in November 2010 by the authors (**c, d**) reveal caries lesions on several approximal surfaces of the posterior teeth. Although detailed comparison of caries lesion extension and radiolucency between 2009 and 2010 is jeopardized by differing angles of the central x-ray beam in relation to the axes of the teeth, it seems that some of the caries lesions have slightly progressed.

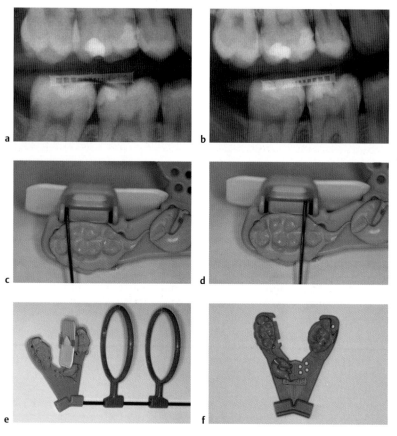

Fig. 25.3a–f A standardizable bitewing holder (TenoLux DMG, Hamburg, Germany) is helpful to obtain optimized and reproducible x-ray angulations with respect to teeth and film. When the central beam does not impinge at low degrees (tangential) to the approximal surface, overlapping approximal areas will be displayed on the x-ray image (**a**). Ideally, most approximal surfaces are situated at 90 degrees in relation to the film, which can easily be controlled by the bite impressions for, in particular, the upper molars, since these are the ones which are the most difficult to display properly (**c, d**). This procedure might not result in null overlapping for every approximal area (**b**), but will reduce this effect. The x-ray tube (not shown) is guided through two rings (**e**), thus a most rigid relationship between x-ray beam, tooth, and film can be established. The film holder can be removed and the relatively flat bitewing holder (**f**) may be stored for later bitewing radiographs in due course (follow-up see **Fig. 25.14**).

Radiographic caries assessment (**Fig. 25.2c, d**) revealed eight D1 lesions and four lesions being visible in enamel only. Thus, except for three approximal surfaces, all of these surfaces—being at a higher risk for caries development (mesial surface of second molar to distal surface of second premolar, first premolars are missing)—either showed a caries lesion or had already been restored.

CLINICAL PEARL

Individualized bitewing holders are of great help to reduce overlapping of approximal surfaces in bitewings and to monitor caries progression/stabilization (**Fig. 25.3a–f**).

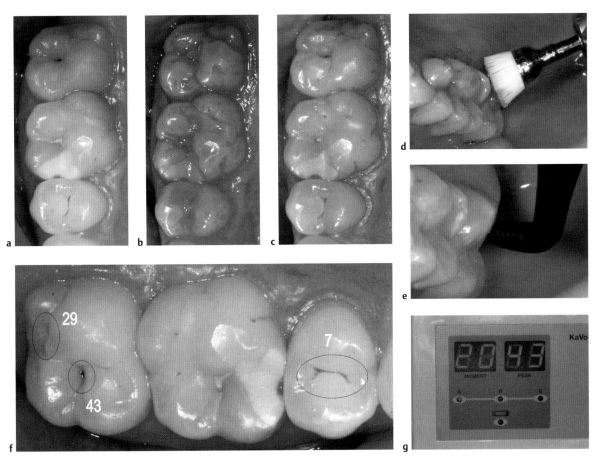

Fig. 25.4a–g DIAGNOdent values (DIAGNOdent, Kavo, Biberach, Germany) were obtained for all molars and premolars, as depicted here for the upper right posterior teeth (**a**). Initially, the dental biofilm, which was visualized by a plaque revelator (not generally necessary) (**b, c**), was removed using a brush and polishing paste (**d**). Measurements were performed in fissure and grooves (**e–g**) and the highest value for each tooth recorded (see **Fig. 25.5**). Tooth 17 revealed a maximum value of 20 and 43 in the distal and central fissures, respectively (**f, g**).

Diagnodent measurements were performed on all suspect occlusal surfaces of the posterior teeth as shown for the upper right posterior teeth. Fissure sealants as in the central fissure of tooth 16 might have given false-positively high values. Therefore, no measurement was performed in this case (**Fig. 25.4**).

Detailed information about the findings for each tooth surface is available from the dental exam form (**Fig. 25.5**). The treatment decisions will be discussed for each quadrant of an arch separately.

Caries Risk Assessment (Individual Level)

Caries risk was assessed as shown in Chapters 7 and 24. Caries experience (DMFT = 5) was in the lower range for the respective age group for a German population, where no water fluoridation is established. Medium, but regular consumption of sweetened food and beverages was reported. Oral hygiene was fair (API: 50%). The patient reported use of fluoride toothpaste (brushing twice daily) as well as fluoridated salt. She was aware of the benefits of flossing, but seemed not to have included this as a daily habit. Salivary flow rate was neither reported to be reduced by the patient nor considered by as of being below normality, thus no measurements were performed. As a result of integration of all these factors for caries, she was classified to have a low-to-medium caries risk (Risk: 31%). Nonetheless, it was assumed from the numerous approximal caries lesions that caries risk had been higher in previous years.

NOTE

Salivary flow rate should be determined quantitatively if the patient either complains or if the dental professional detects any conspicuous signs and symptoms of xerostomia (dry mouth). In most patients qualitative assessment is sufficient.

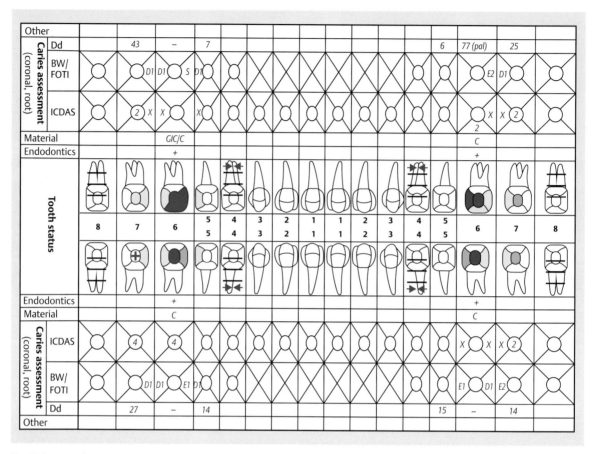

Fig. 25.5 Dental status

Diagnoses and Treatment Plan

Individual Level

The patient was encouraged to proceed with brushing twice daily using regular fluoride toothpaste (1500 ppm F⁻). Advice for more regular use of flossing, including some practical tips on how to handle the floss, was given. As she used fluoride toothpaste and fluoridated salt, no other home-use fluoride products were recommended. The role of sugar consumption on the cariogenicity of the dental biofilm was explained, in particular with respect to sweetened beverages.

Tooth Level

Diagnoses and treatment decisions regarding certain tooth surfaces are summarized in **Table 25.1**. Inactive caries lesions received no current treatment, but were recorded for "particular surveillance." Since the patient revealed a rather high number of approximal caries lesions, the deeper ones (mostly D1) were referred to the infiltration technique. Two fissures were sealed and four restorations placed. A more conservative approach might have favored noninvasive treatment of the caries lesions for a period of time (e.g., local application of fluoride varnish; Chapter 12). However, here the next intervention would have been already the placement of a restoration when the caries lesion exceeded radiographically the outer third of dentin or showed progression. The aim of the current treatment plan was to postpone or even avoid future restorations (see Chapters 17 and 20).

Table 25.1 Diagnoses and treatments at a glance

Diagnosis	Caries	Caries non-progressiva (CNP)		Caries progressiva superficialis (CS)			Caries progressiva media (CM) et profunda (CP)		
	Restorations	Restauratio insufficienta initialis (RII)		Restauratio insufficienta partialis (RIP)			Restauratio insufficienta totalis (RIT)		
	Sound surfaces	–		Sanus majoris periculi (SMP)			–		
Treatment		Particular surveillance		Noninvasive or microinvasive/ repair			(Minimally) invasive		
		Tooth + Surface	Diagnosis	Tooth + Surface	Diagnosis	Therapy	Tooth + Surface	Diagnosis	Therapy
		27o	CNP	17o	CS	FS ✔	16 mo	RIT	FC ✔
		37o	CNP	17m	CS	INF ✔	16 op	RIT	FC ✔
				16d	CS	INF ✔	46o d!	RIT	FC ✔
				15d	CS	INF ✔	47o	CM	FC ✔
				26 d	CS	INF ✔			
				26 p	CS	FS ✔			
				27 m	CS	INF ✔			
				37 m	CS	INF ✔			
				36 d	CS	INF ✔			
				36 m	CS	LF ✔			
				45 d	CS	INF ✔			
				47 m	CS	INF ✔			
				46 m	CS	LF ✔			
				FS fissure sealing INF caries infiltration LF local fluoridation			FC composite filling ! examine adjacent surface during preparation		

Right Upper Jaw (first Quadrant; Fig. 25.6)

Tooth 17. The noncavitated caries lesion in the central fissure was considered as being active, but radiographically no caries lesion extending into dentin could be detected. However, DIAGNOdent measurement revealed a medium (43) and lower (29) value for the central and the distal fissure, respectively. Thus, the decision was to seal all the fissure areas, without any prior excavation/preparation (**Fig. 25.7**). The noncavitated caries lesion on the mesial surface extending radiographically into the outer third of dentin was infiltrated (positive papilla bleeding as single indicator for activity), since it was supposed to progress with noninvasive measures alone (see **Fig. 25.10**).

Teeth 16/15. Both restorations (mesio-occlusal and palatal-occlusal) of tooth 16 were judged as insufficient and renewed using composite (**Fig. 25.8**). The noncavitated caries lesions at the distal surfaces of both 16 and 15 (positive papilla bleeding as single indicator for activity) extending radiographically into the outer third of dentin were infiltrated (**Figs. 25.9** and **25.10**).

CLINICAL PEARL

An unfilled transparent resin material enables further DIAGNOodent measurements of the sealed areas but is much harder to visualize clinically compared with colored sealants.

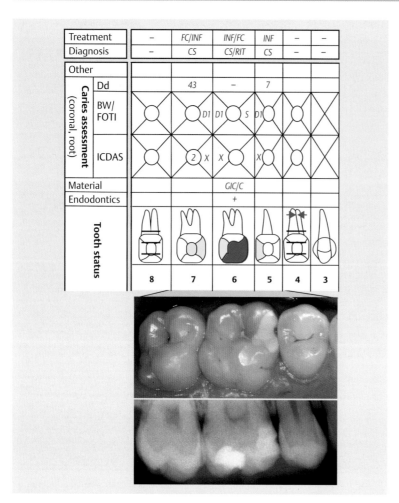

		–	FC/INF	INF/FC	INF	–	–
Treatment		–	CS	CS/RIT	CS	–	–
Diagnosis							
Other							
Caries assessment (coronal, root)	Dd		43	–	7		
	BW/ FOTI	○	○ D1	D1 ○ S	D1 ○		
	ICDAS	○	② X	X ○	X ○		
Material				GIC/C			
Endodontics				+			
Tooth status		8	7	6	5	4	3

Fig. 25.6 Overview of caries detection and assessment as well as the treatment decision for the posterior teeth of the right upper arch (teeth 17 to 15).

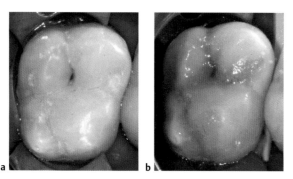 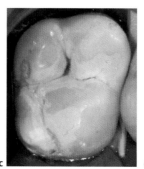

Fig. 25.7a–d The occlusal aspect of tooth 17 was sealed using an unfilled transparent resin. After cleaning with abrasive paste, some remnants of tooth stain that could not be removed without damaging the tooth are visible in the distal fissure parts (**a**). Etching was performed for 60 seconds using 37% phosphoric acid gel (**b**). After rinsing and thoroughly drying (**c**), the resin (Helioseal Clear, Ivoclar Vivadent, Schaan, Lichtenstein) was applied and light cured for 20 seconds (**d**).

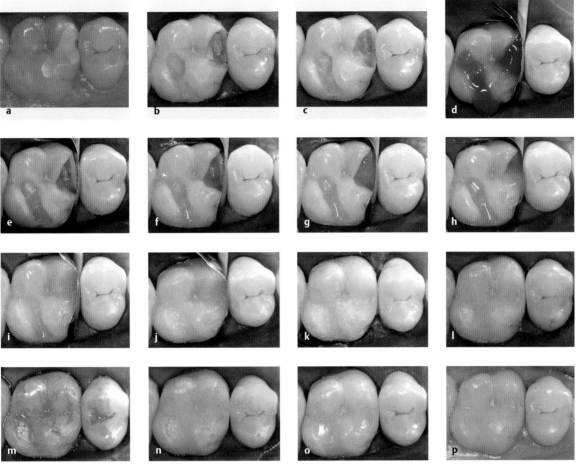

Fig. 25.8a–p Composite restoration of tooth 16. The insufficient glass-ionomer (no contact point to adjacent tooth 15) as well as the composite restoration (ditching at margin) were removed with a diamond bur (**a, b**). However, having done this, it might be argued that repair of the composite restoration would have been sufficient. Deeper parts of the cement were removed with a slow-speed steel bur to avoid pulp exposure. No particular beveling was performed (**c**). Then, a wooden wedge and an anatomic matrix were used to help to form the approximal area. Total etch with 37% phosphoric acid gel for 20 seconds (**d**), etching pattern (**e**), application of a two-step adhesive (Optibond FL, Kerr, West Collins, USA) (**f**), flowable composite (Tetric EvoFlow; Ivoclar Vivadent, Schaan, Lichtenstein) applied at the cervical approximal part of the mesial cavity (**g**), application of composite (Tetric EvoCeram; Ivoclar Vivadent) to palatal part of the mesial cavity (**h**), facial part of the mesial as well as distal part of the disto-palatinal cavity (**i**), mesial part of the disto-palatinal cavity (**j**). After removing the wedge and the matrix and removal of remnants with a scaler, the fissure anatomy in the composite filled areas was shaped by fine-grain diamond burs (**k, l**). At the next appointment a red plaque revelator was applied as an aid to stain adhesive and composite remnants (**m, n**), and to polish without damaging adjacent enamel (**o**). Result after several weeks (**p**).

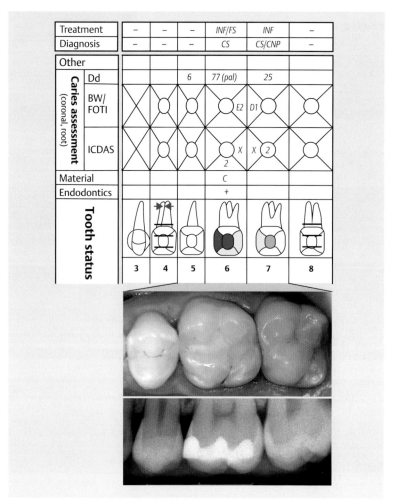

Fig. 25.9 Overview of caries detection and assessment as well as the treatment decision for the posterior teeth of the left upper arch (teeth 26+27).

Left Upper Jaw (2nd Quadrant; Fig. 25.9)

Tooth 27. The noncavitated caries lesion of the occlusal aspect was considered as being inactive (visual–tactile examination). No radiolucency could be found and a medium DIAGNOdent value (25) was assessed. Since the status of the lesion was most likely to be stable (Caries non-progressiva), the decision was to monitor this surface. In comparison to the occlusal "active" caries lesion of tooth 17, where a fissure sealant was applied (**Fig. 25.7**), for tooth 27 a less pronounced discoloration and a lower DIAGNOdent value were assessed. The noncavitated caries lesion on the mesial surface extending radiographically into the outer third of dentin was infiltrated (positive papilla bleeding as indicator for activity).

Tooth 26. The composite restoration was judged as being sufficient. However, the palatal fissure showed an active, noncavitated caries lesion and a DIAGNOdent value of 77 was measured. Nonetheless, this caries lesion was sealed and not filled, since the DIAGNOdent value was judged as being false-positively high (Caries progressiva superficialis). The noncavitated caries lesion on the distal surface extending radiographically into the inner half of enamel was infiltrated (positive papilla bleeding as indicator for activity).

Left Lower Jaw (3rd Quadrant; Fig. 25.10)

Tooth 37. The noncavitated caries lesion of the occlusal aspect was considered as being inactive by visual–tactile examination. No radiolucency could be found and a low DIAGNOdent value (14) was assessed. Thus, it was decided to monitor this surface (Caries non-progressiva). The noncavitated active (positive papilla bleeding as single indicator for activity) caries lesions on the mesial surface extending radiographically into the inner half of enamel were diagnosed as Caries progressiva superficialis. With regard to the relatively high number of approximal caries lesions it was decided to infiltrate and not only fluoridate this area.

Tooth 36. The occlusal composite restoration was judged as being sufficient. The noncavitated caries lesion on the distal surface extending radiographically into the outer third of dentin was infiltrated (activity assessment see above). The shallow, but active (no papilla bleeding, but opaque surface) caries lesion on the mesial surface (Caries

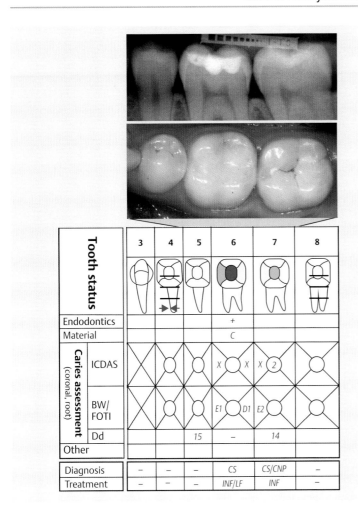

Fig. 25.10 Overview of caries detection and assessment as well as the treatment decision for the posterior teeth of the left lower arch (teeth 37+36).

Tooth status	3	4	5	6	7	8
Endodontics				+		
Material				C		
Caries assessment (coronal, root) — ICDAS		○	○	X ○ X ○	X ②	○
Caries assessment (coronal, root) — BW/FOTI		○	○	E1 ○ D1	E2	○
Caries assessment (coronal, root) — Dd			15	–	14	
Other						
Diagnosis	–	–	–	CS	CS/CNP	–
Treatment	–	–	–	INF/LF	INF	–

progressiva superficialis) was referred to local fluoridation (Duraphat, Gaba, Lörrach, Germany).

Right Lower Jaw (4th Quadrant; Fig. 25.11)

Tooth 47. A noncavitated caries lesion (ICDAS 2) that was assessed as being active was visible adjacent to remnants of fissure sealant. No radiolucency could be found and a Diagnodent value of 27 (adjacent to the sealant) was assessed. It was decided to prepare the central fissure part (minimally invasive filling), since it was thought to be safer to remove the fissure sealant remnants, but leave the intact fissure sealant in the mesial fissure area. The noncavitated caries lesions on the mesial surface extending radiographically into the inner half of the enamel (E2) was infiltrated, since the lesion could be assessed as being active after drilling the distal surface of the adjacent tooth (Diagnosis: Caries progressiva superficialis).

Tooth 46. Although the occlusal composite restoration in the distal fissure area (hardly visible clinically, but detectable on the x-ray image) was judged as being sufficient, it was decided to remove the occlusal restoration to assess the adjacent approximal caries lesion extending radiographically slightly into the middle third of dentin. The fissure sealant showed a dark shadow around it. Therefore, it was also removed and the resulting cavity filled with composite (**Fig. 25.12**). The noncavitated, active (opaque surface and papilla bleeding) caries lesion on the mesial surface (E1) was diagnosed as Caries progressiva superficialis. Since it was rather shallow it was decided to fluoridate (Duraphat).

Tooth 45. The noncavitated caries lesion on the distal surface extending radiographically into the outer third of dentin was infiltrated (papilla bleeding).

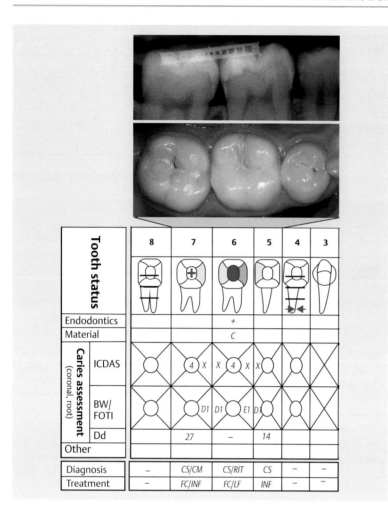

Fig. 25.11 Overview of caries detection and assessment as well as the treatment decision for the posterior teeth of the right lower arch (teeth 45–47).

Clinical Aspect at the End of the Treatment

Several surfaces still showed signs of inactive caries lesions (**Fig. 25.13**). The patient was told to inform any subsequent dentist about the minimal interventional concept of caries management to avoid unnecessary (invasive) treatments. For this purpose a booklet (see Chapter 17) was handed over, in which the radiological stages of the infiltrated approximal as well as the sealed occlusal caries lesions were listed. The standardizable bitewing holder was kept for the follow-up investigation.

Follow-up

According to the caries risk, the patient was supposed to be recalled twice annually. The last appointment of the treatment phase (4 months after initial treatment) was considered as a "first recall." Advice and instruction with regard to flossing was repeated. Thereafter, first clinical, including radiographic, follow-up was performed 8 months after the end of the treatment. No clinical signs of new caries lesions were detected. Instructions for oral hygiene and noncariogenic diet were reinforced, a professional tooth cleaning was performed. Follow-up radiographs revealed no progression or onset of any caries lesion of posterior teeth (**Fig. 25.14a–d**).

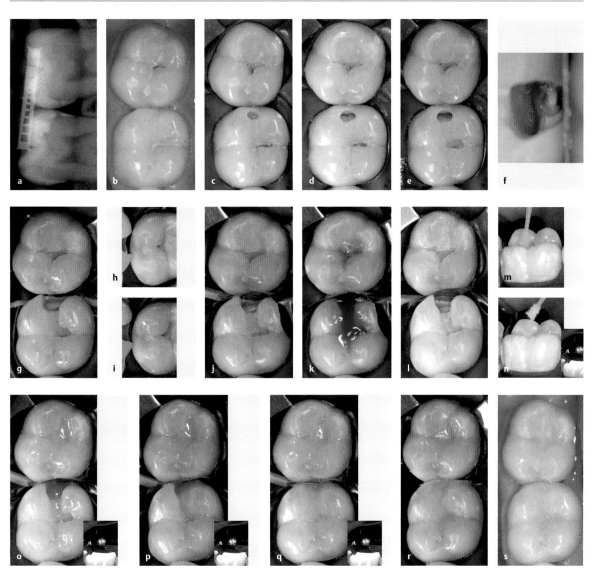

Fig. 25.12a–s Infiltration and restoration of teeth 46 and 47. The radiographic assessment revealed approximal caries lesions extending into dentin for the teeth 46 distal and 47 mesial (**a**). Clinically (**b**), for the occlusal aspect of tooth 46 some dark area could be observed around the remnants of the fissure sealant, on tooth 47 a caries lesion of ICDAS 2 was assessed in parts of the central fissure. The primary preparations using diamond burs were performed as sparingly as possible in the areas where the described caries lesions had been detected (**c**).The carious distal surface of the 1st molar was reached from the occlusal distal fissure, removing the composite restoration partially (**c–g**). Highly demineralized enamel (**e, f**) could be observed on the approximal area below the contact point. The underlying dentin was soft and needed to be removed up to half-way toward the pulp (**g**). Soft dentin was also removed in the central parts of 46 (**e**) and 47 (**j**). For tooth 46, the distal cavity was combined with the central one by removal of the "old" restoration. Margins of all the cavities were rounded with a bur, but no distinct beveling was performed (**g**). Before an adhesive restoration was placed, the noncavitated caries lesion on the mesial surface of tooth 47 was etched (**h**, see etching pattern after using Icon Etch for 2 minutes) and infiltrated (**i**). A wooden wedge and an anatomic matrix were used to help to form the approximal area of 46 distally (**j**). Total etch with 37% phosphoric acid gel for 20 seconds (**k**), etching pattern (**l**), application of primer that was allowed to evaporate its solvent (**m**) before application of the adhesive (**n**) (Optibond FL, Kerr, West Collins, USA) (**m**). A, flowable composite (Tetric EvoFlow; Ivoclar Vivadent, Schaan, Lichtenstein) was applied at the cervical approximal part (**o**), then a composite (Tetric Evo-Ceram; Ivoclar Vivadent) to lingual (**p**) and facial parts (**q**), Remnants were removed using a scaler. The filled areas were shaped by fine-grain diamond burs and polishing strips (cervical approximal), abrasive discs (coronal approximal) as well as a rubber polisher (occlusal) (**r**). Result after several weeks (**s**).

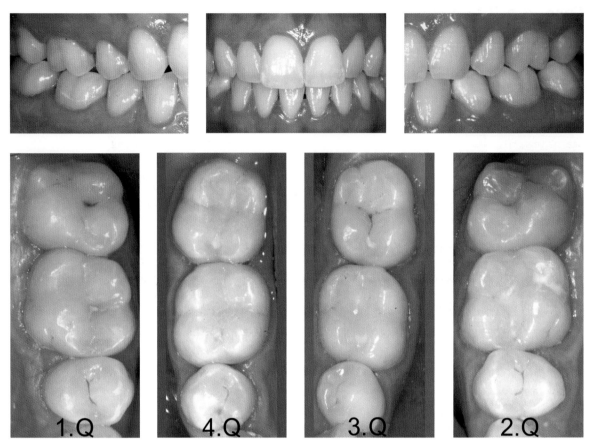

Fig. 25.13 Final clinical aspect at the end of the treatment phase. Q: quadrant.

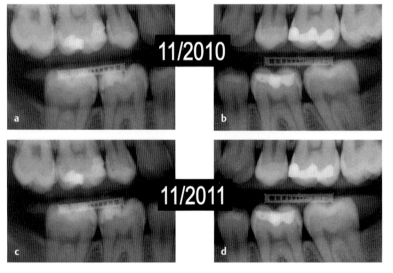

Fig. 25.14a–d Twelve months after the last bitewing radiographs (**a, b**), follow-ups (**c, d**) showed no progression of any infiltrated (mesial 17, distal 16, distal 15, distal 26, mesial 27, distal 36, mesial 37, distal 45, and mesial 47) or noninfiltrated (mesial 26, mesial 37, mesial 36, mesial 46) proximal caries lesions, nor any caries lesions of an occlusal part that were eligible (mainly second molars).

Case 2: A 22-year-old Man with Medium Caries Risk

Hendrik Meyer-Lueckel, Sebastian Paris

Anamnesis

Gender: male
Age: 22 years
First visit: January 2011
Last visit: April 2011
Follow-up visit: October 2011

The patient visited the university clinic because he was concerned about gum bleeding. Regular antimicrobial mouth rinse had been recommended by a private practitioner one year before, but the patient did not notice any improvement. No cause-related noninvasive measures (e.g., professional cleaning or oral health instructions) had been performed. The patient was not aware of any caries lesions being present and was unsure whether bitewing radiographs had previously been taken. No general health issues were reported by the patient.

Clinical Findings (Tooth Level)

Oral examination revealed a permanent dentition with lower third molars being extracted. Signs of gingivitis in particular of the buccal surfaces of the anterior teeth as well as tooth stain and calculus (lower anterior teeth) were observed; the mucosa was healthy. Modified BEWE index was assessed as 0. Only a few restorations at the occlusal aspects of the molars but no deep caries lesions could be detected at first glance (**Fig. 25.15**).

Caries documentation was based on visual–tactile (**Fig. 25.15**), radiographic (**Fig. 25.16a–c**), and laser fluorescence (DIAGNOdent) assessments. In general, five (insufficient) restorations in the molars being restricted to the occlusal surfaces were detected (teeth 17, 16, 26, 36, 46). Remnants of sealants could be detected in three of the molars (28, 37, 47), two others showed active caries lesions (18, 27). Clinically, none of the premolars revealed caries lesions, but a restoration mesially to a developmental defect could be observed on tooth 11.

Radiographic caries assessment of approximal surfaces revealed one E2, five D1 (plus one on tooth 26 being hardly visible) and two D2 lesions. Occlusal radiolucencies underneath restorations/sealants were detected for teeth

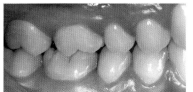
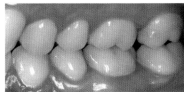
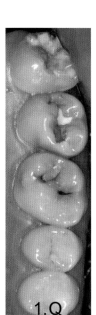
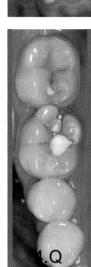
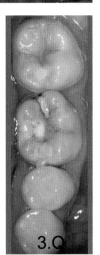
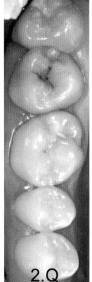

Fig. 25.15 Clinical aspect of the vestibular as well as occlusal aspects of the upper and lower jaws at the first visit. Q = quadrant

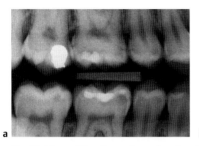 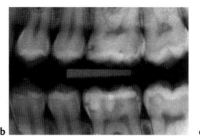 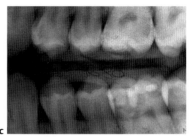

a   b   c

Fig. 25.16a–c Bitewing radiographs taken in January 2011 for both sides (**a, b**). To assess the distal and mesial surface of teeth 26 and 27, respectively, another bitewing radiograph was taken on the left side (**c**). Here the other approximal surfaces are not displayed in sufficient quality for caries assessment. Several approximal caries lesions of the posterior teeth are visible (see detailed assessments in **Fig. 25.17**).

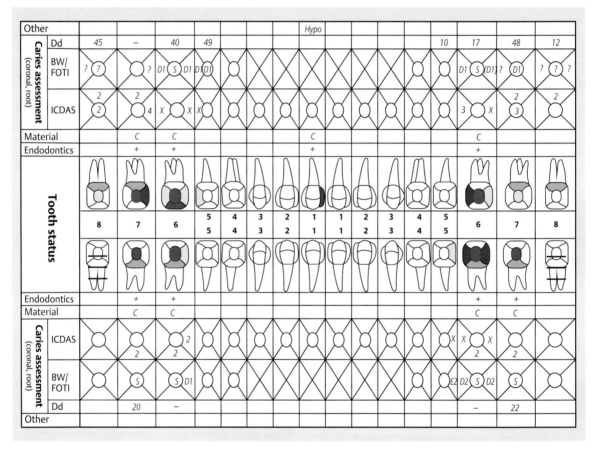

Fig. 25.17 Dental status

16, 26, 37, 36, 46 and 47; tooth 27 showed an occlusal D1 lesion (**Figs. 25.16** and **25.17**).

DIAGNOdent values of the molars and some premolars reflected the clinical and radiographic findings. Detailed information for each tooth surface is available from the dental exam form (**Fig. 25.17**). The diagnoses and treatment decisions will be discussed for each quadrant separately.

Caries Risk Assessment (Individual Level)

Caries experience (DMFT = 9) was in the medium upper range for the respective age group for a German population. Regular consumption of sweetened food and beverages was reported. Oral hygiene was fair (API: 40%). The patient reported use of fluoride toothpaste (brushing twice daily) as well as fluoridated salt. He did not use dental floss on a regular basis. Salivary flow rate was not determined, no relevant general medical issues were reported or observed. According to the integration of all

Table 25.2 Diagnoses and treatment at a glance

Diagnosis	Caries	Caries non-progressiva (CNP)		Caries progressiva superficialis (CS)			Caries progressiva media (CM) und Caries profunda (CP)		
	Restorations	Restauratio insufficienta initialis (RII)		Restauratio insufficienta partialis (RIP)			Restauratio insufficienta totalis (RIT)		
	Sound surfaces	–		Sanus majoris periculi (SMP)			–		
Treatment		Particular surveillance		Noninvasive or microinvasive/repair			(Minimally) invasive		
		Tooth + Surface	Diagnosis	Tooth + Surface	Diagnosis	Therapy	Tooth + Surface	Diagnosis	Therapy
		18b	CNP	18o	CS	FS ✔	17o m!	RIT/CS	FC + FS ✔
		17b	CNP	16d	CS	INF ✔	16o	RIT/CS	FC + FS ✔
		27b	CNP	16m	CS	INF ✔	26m	CM	FC ✔
		28b	CNP	15d	CS	INF ✔	26o d!	RIT	FC ✔
		37b	CNP	15o	CS	FS ✔	27o	CM	FC ✔
		36b	CNP	35d	CS	INF ✔	36 mod	CM	FC ✔
		46b	CNP				37 o	RIT	FC + FS ✔
		47b	CNP				46 o m!	RIT	FC ✔
							47 o	RIT	FC + FS ✔
				FS fissure sealing INF caries infiltration			FC composite filling ! examine adjacent surface during preparation		

these factors a medium risk for future caries development was calculated (Risk: 57%). Nonetheless, it was assumed from the numerous approximal caries lesions that caries risk had been higher in previous years.

Diagnosis and Treatment Plan

Individual Level

The patient was instructed to brush his teeth (with emphasis on the front teeth with gingivitis) twice daily using fluoride toothpaste (1500 ppm F⁻). He was encouraged to floss his teeth at least every second day. Practical advice of how to handle the floss was given and re-evaluated during the forthcoming appointments. For regular fluoride availability, besides fluoride toothpaste and fluoridated salt, weekly brushing with fluoride gel was recommended. The role of sugar consumption frequency on the cariogenicity of the dental biofilm was explained.

Tooth Level

Tooth surfaces with Caries non-progressiva were recorded for particular surveillance. Some of the approximal caries lesions extending radiographically around the enamel–dentin junction (mostly D1) were referred to minimally invasive treatment, while most of these were infiltrated. Occlusally, two teeth were fissure-sealed, while others were restored with composite, if eligible, in combination with a fissure sealant. The aim of the current treatment plan was to postpone or even avoid future restorations (**Table 25.2**).

Right Upper Jaw (1st Quadrant; Fig. 25.18)
Tooth 18. The noncavitated caries lesion in the central fissure was considered as being active. DIAGNOdent measurement revealed a value of 45. Thus, the decision was to seal all fissure areas, without any prior preparation (Diagnosis: Caries progressiva superficialis). The noncavitated caries lesions on the buccal surfaces of both teeth 17 and 18 were assessed as being inactive and diagnosed as Caries non-progressiva.

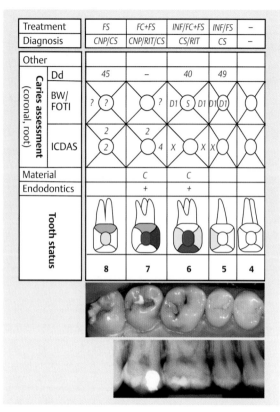

Treatment	FS	FC+FS	INF/FC+FS	INF/FS	–
Diagnosis	CNP/CS	CNP/RIT/CS	CS/RIT	CS	–
Other					
Dd	45	–	40	49	
BW/FOTI	? (?)	?	D1 (S) D1 (D1)		
ICDAS	2 (2)	2	4 X X X		
Material		C	C		
Endodontics		+	+		
Tooth status	8	7	6	5	4

Fig. 25.18 Overview of caries detection and assessment as well as the treatment decision for the posterior teeth of the right upper arch. The mesial surface of tooth 17 shows a dark shadow. Due to overlapping radiograph assessment is not possible for 17 mesial.

Tooth 17. Clinically, the mesial part showed a dark shadow and was therefore judged as ICDAS 4; however, no cavitation could be detected by probing (cow-ended probe) interproximally (**Fig. 25.18**). It was decided to remove the amalgam restoration (desired by the patient), although it might be argued that no clinical or radiographic signs for adjacent caries could be detected. The decision for removal of the adjacent fissure sealant as well as preparation of the mesial surface was postponed until removal of the amalgam restoration. In case of cavitation (mesially) or large extension of the carious dentin these parts were supposed to be integrated in the occlusal cavity where the amalgam was situated so far.

Teeth 16/15. The occlusal restoration of tooth 16 was judged as insufficient and renewed using composite in combination with sealing of the central fissure (DIAGNOdent value = 40). During occlusal treatment it was planned to decide whether or not the noncavitated caries lesion on the adjacent distal surface of tooth 16 extending radiographically into the outer third of the dentin should be filled or infiltrated. The decision was based on the amount of remaining dental hard tissue of the distal ridge after removal of the distal-occlusal restoration. The noncavitated caries lesions (D1) at the mesial and distal surfa-

ces of teeth 16 and 15, respectively, were infiltrated (**Fig. 25.19**), since both were considered as active (predictor assessed was positive papilla bleeding). The occlusal surface of tooth 15 (D1; DIAGNOdent value = 49) was sealed, although a restoration might have also been adequate, if one assumes that this surface was a Caries progressiva media.

CLINICAL PEARL

A dark underlying shadow derived from colored, but hard dentin (no active caries) or metallic restorations cannot easily be distinguished from active caries. The best way to save dental hard tissue is to monitor these lesions clinically (assessment of margins of restorations) and radiographically (radiolucencies).

Left Upper Jaw (2nd Quadrant; Fig. 25.20)

Teeth 28 and 27. The noncavitated caries lesions on both buccal surfaces were considered as being inactive (Caries non-progressiva). The cavitated carious area of the occlusal aspect of tooth 27 (ICDAS 3) was considered as being active by visual–tactile examination. Radiolucency into dentin (D1) as well as a medium DIAGNOdent value (48) could be assessed. Thus, a restoration was placed in the carious fissure part, but no sealant was placed in the other parts of the occlusal surfaces of 27 and 28, since here no signs of (initial) caries could be detected and these surfaces were not considered as being at a higher risk for future caries. The enamel part of the mesial surface of 27 could not be judged radiographically; nonetheless, no radiolucency extending into the outer third of the dentin could be observed. For tooth 28, owing to the minor clinical signs for caries, it was decided not to take an extra x-ray photo.

Tooth 26. The partial occlusal (distal fissure area) composite restoration was judged clinically (imperfect margins) and radiographically (radiolucency underneath) as being insufficient (Restauratio insufficienta totalis). The other fissure parts revealed no signs of caries and a rather low DIAGNOdent value of 17. Thus, only the restoration was renewed and the other fissure areas were not treated. During cavity preparation the extension of the lesion in the direction of the approximal area, where a D1 lesion could be assessed radiographically, was supposed to be examined clinically again. The distal surface was considered for either minimally or microinvasive treatment depending on the cavity status, and the lesion extension was confirmed during the clinical treatment occlusally. The mesial surface (radiographically: D1) showed an active cavitated caries lesion (ICDAS 3) that was in need of a restoration (Caries progressiva media) (**Fig. 25.21**).

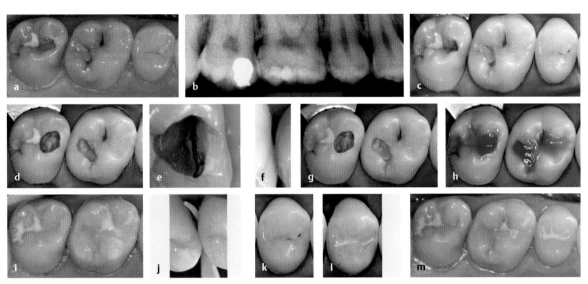

Fig. 25.19a–m Aspects of the right upper posterior teeth at the first examination (**a–c**). As described in the text, the amalgam restoration of tooth 17 was removed to judge the mesial surface. The occlusal surfaces of 16 and 15 were filled and sealed, respectively. After removal of both occlusal restorations of 16 and 17, fairly hard but dark-colored dentin was visible (**d**). Both the sealant of 17 and the palatal restoration of 16 were kept in place. The bottom part of the inner mesial surface of 17 was stained due to the amalgam (**e**), but revealed no cavitation extending to the outer mesial surface (**f**). Some more softened dentin was removed using a slow-speed steel bur (**g**), but it was not considered necessary to prepare approximal slots on either 17 mesial or 16 distal. Total etching of all occlusal parts using 37% phosphoric acid gel for 20 seconds was performed (**h**) and the teeth carefully dried. Both cavities were filled with composite (Tetric EvoCeram; Ivoclar Vivadent) after using a two-step adhesive (Optibond FL, Kerr); nonrestored fissures were sealed (**i**) (Helioseal, Ivoclar Vivadent). The mesial surface of 16 showing a noncavitated caries lesion (**j**) was infiltrated. The fissures of 15 (**k**) were sealed (**l**). Caries infiltration was also performed on the distal surfaces of both 15 and 16 (not shown). After placing the tooth-colored restoration on 17, the discoloration of the mesial surface was hardly visible; the caries underneath the sealant in the central fissure of 16 could still be detected but not diagnosed as being progressive (**m**).

Fig. 25.20 Overview of caries detection and assessment as well as the treatment decision for the posterior teeth of the left upper arch (teeth 26–28).

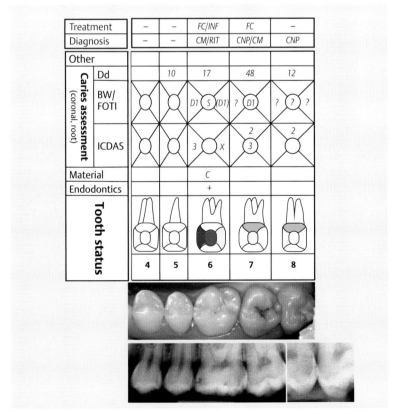

			FC/INF	FC	
Treatment	–	–	FC/INF	FC	–
Diagnosis	–	–	CM/RIT	CNP/CM	CNP
Other					
Dd		10	17	48	12
BW/FOTI	◯	◯	D1 ◯ S ◯ (D1)	? ◯ D1	? ◯ ? ◯ ?
ICDAS	◯	◯	3 ◯ X	2 ◯ 3	2 ◯
Material			C		
Endodontics			+		
Tooth status	4	5	6	7	8

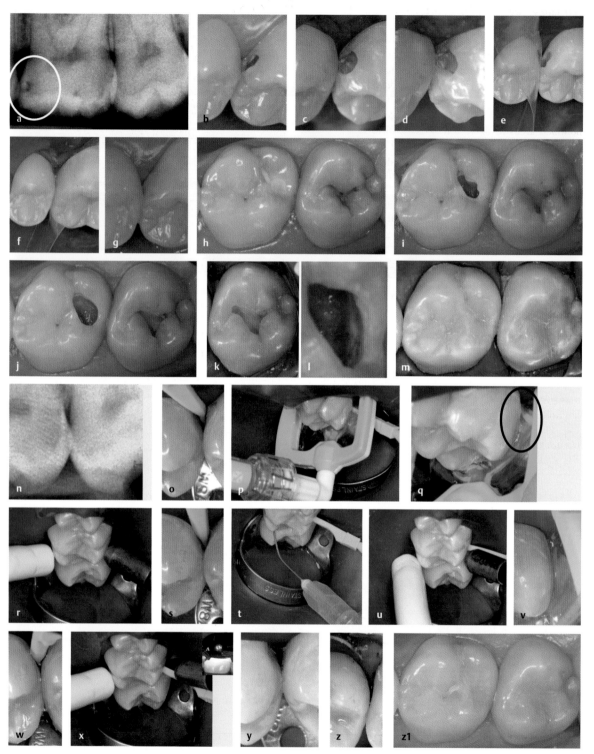

Fig. 25.21 a–z1   The mesial surface of tooth 26 revealed radiologically a D1 lesion (**a**) that was clinically cavitated (**b**). In the enamel, a horizontal slot was prepared as small as possible to get access to the dentin using diamond burs and oscillating preparation tools (**c**). Softened dentin was excavated (**d**). A translucent matrix band was used (**e**) and the cavity filled with flowable composite (**f**). Margins were beveled using abrasive strips as well as disks (**g**). As described thoroughly in the text, teeth 26 (mesial and occlusal) and 27 (occlusal) needed restorations (**h**). Primary preparation was kept as little as possible to get access to the underlying carious dentin (**i, j, k**). During invasive treatment (**l**) it was decided to infiltrate the noncavitated caries lesion on tooth 26 distally (**n, o**) and not to extend the cavity. After cleaning and placing a rubber dam, teeth 26 and 27 were separated (**o**) using a flattened wedge (Icon; DMG, Hamburg). This enabled the application of a foil (**p**). This foil applicator consists of two partially welded double foils, of which only one (green) is perforated. By screwing the respective syringe the etching gel (HCl 15%; Icon Etch) was applied. It was visually determined

Left Lower Jaw (3rd Quadrant; Fig. 25.22)

Tooth 37. Clinically, an aged composite restoration with sufficient margins (no gaps) was observed in the mesial fissure part. Underneath, a radiolucency that could either be a nonradiopaque restorative material or a caries lesion could be detected from the bitewing radiograph. Owing to the unclear assessments, this part of the occlusal surface was diagnosed as Restauratio insufficienta totalis. The nonfilled areas revealed a maximum DIAGNOdent value of 22 and signs of initial caries (ICDAS 2) and was diagnosed as Caries progressiva superficialis. Thus, a composite restoration in combination with a fissure sealant was planned (**Fig. 25.23**).

Tooth 36. The occlusal composite restoration was judged as being insufficient (Restauratio insufficienta totalis). Several radiolucencies into dentin also supported the diagnosis of Caries progressiva media on the mesial, occlusal and distal surfaces. These surfaces needed to be restored (**Fig. 25.23**). The noncavitated caries lesions on the buccal surfaces of both molars were considered as being inactive (Caries non-progressiva).

Tooth 35. The noncavitated caries lesion on the distal surface extending radiographically into the outer third of dentin was infiltrated, since it was considered as being a progressive caries lesion that could not be arrested by noninvasive measures only, although no papilla bleeding was observed. Nonetheless, this area could be seen as a plaque stagnation area, and the generally medium caries risk supported the decision for infiltration.

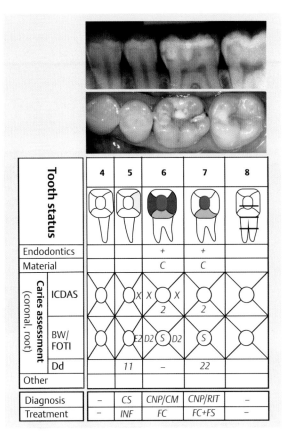

Tooth status	4	5	6	7	8
Endodontics			+	+	
Material			C	C	
Caries assessment (coronal, root) — ICDAS		X X	X 2	2	
Caries assessment (coronal, root) — BW/FOTI		E2 D2 (S) D2		(S)	
Caries assessment (coronal, root) — Dd		11	–	22	
Other					
Diagnosis	–	CS	CNP/CM	CNP/RIT	–
Treatment	–	INF	FC	FC+FS	–

Fig. 25.22 Overview of caries detection and assessment as well as the treatment decision for the posterior teeth of the left lower arch (teeth 35–37).

◄ whether the gel had spread over the whole approximal surface (**q**). After removing the etching gel using water spray (**r**) and subsequent air drying, an opaque appearance of the etched parts could be observed (**s**). By applying ethanol (Icon Dry) residual water was mixed with the ethanol (**t**), and so the lesion was dried out more efficiently (**u**). A new foil applicator for the infiltration step was taken using the wedge for separation again. A constant "film" of infiltrant was supposed to be established between the foil and the teeth (**v**). If this was not the case, further infiltrant was applied (ca. every 30 seconds). After a total application time of 3 minutes,

excess material (**w**) was removed using the dental suction and air (**x**). The area was also cleaned by flossing (not shown) and the infiltrant was light cured for 40 seconds. To compensate for polymerization shrinkage the infiltrant was applied a second time (1 minute) and cleaned as described (not shown). No material surplus (**y**) (which, just in case, can be removed easily with a scaler; **z**) could be detected. Radiographic extension of the caries lesion as well as the date were recorded in a booklet belonging to the treatment kit. The final image shows a clinical view taken several weeks after the treatments (**z1**).

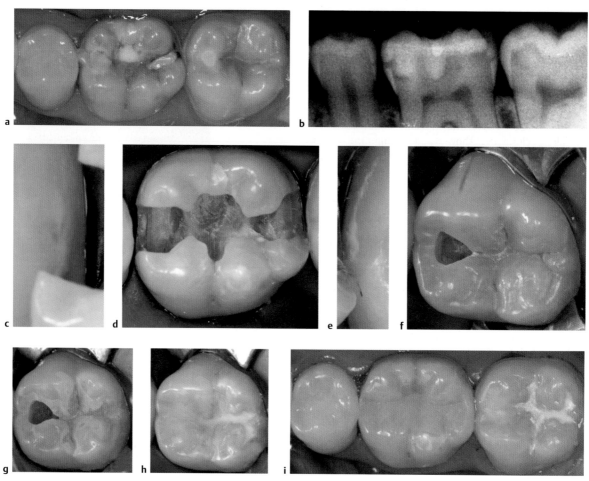

Fig. 25.23a–i   The diagnoses Caries progressiva media and Restauratio insufficienta totalis (**a**, **b**) on teeth 36 (mesial-occlusal-distal) and 37 (mesial part occlusally) indicated invasive intervention. The distal surface of tooth 35 revealed a caries lesion extending into the inner enamel (E2) (**b**) that was clinically noncavitated (**c**), as could be confirmed after removal of the restoration on 36 (**d**) (this lesion was later infiltrated). Also the mesial surface of 37 revealed an inactive caries lesion (no radiolucency) that was noncavitated (**e**). Therefore, no current treatment was considered for the mesial aspect. At the bottom of the occlusal cavity of 37, stained but hard dentin could be found (**f**). The lesion as well as all fissure areas were etched; an adhesive restoration and a sealant were placed, respectively (**h**). The result after several weeks (**i**).

Right Lower Jaw (4th Quadrant; Fig. 25.24)

Tooth 47. Clinically, an aged composite restoration with sufficient margins (no gaps) was observed in the mesial fissure part. Underneath, a radiolucency that could either be a nonradiopaque restorative material or a caries lesion could be detected from the bitewing radiograph. Owing to the unclear assessments, this part of the occlusal surface was diagnosed as Restauratio insufficienta totalis. The nonfilled occlusal parts showed a maximum DIAGNOdent value of 20 and signs of initial caries (ICDAS 2) and were diagnosed as Caries progressiva superficialis. Thus, a composite restoration in combination with a fissure sealant was performed (**Fig. 25.25**).

Tooth 46. The occlusal composite restorations were judged as being insufficient (see margins and radiolucencies underneath; Restauratio insufficienta totalis). Thus, it was decided to remove the occlusal restoration also to assess the mesial caries lesion extending radiographically into dentin from the occlusal aspect. After occlusal preparation the planned infiltration of the active caries lesion (opaque appearance, papilla bleeding) at the mesial surface (Caries progressiva superficialis) was supposed to either be confirmed or changed to an invasive slot restoration (**Fig. 25.25**). The noncavitated caries lesions on the buccal surfaces of both molars were considered as being inactive (Caries non-progressiva).

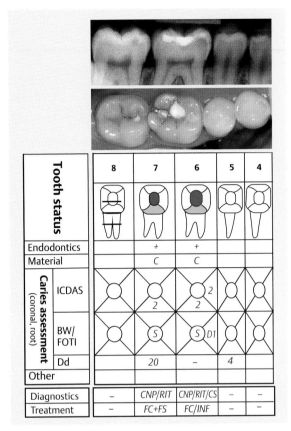

Tooth status	8	7	6	5	4
Endodontics		+	+		
Material		C	C		
Caries assessment (coronal, root) — ICDAS	○	○ 2	○ 2 2	○	○
BW/ FOTI		S	S D1		
Dd		20	–	4	
Other					
Diagnostics	–	CNP/RIT	CNP/RIT/CS	–	–
Treatment	–	FC+FS	FC/INF	–	–

Fig. 25.24 Overview of caries detection and assessment as well as the treatment decision for the posterior teeth of the right lower arch (teeth 47+46).

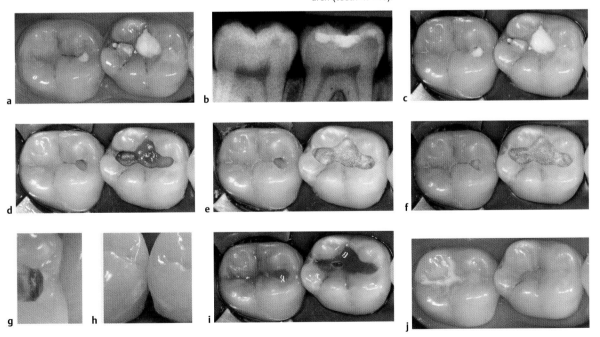

Fig. 25.25a–j Treatments of teeth 46 and 47 (**a**). The radiographic assessment revealed a approximal caries lesion extending into dentin for 46 mesial (**b**). After placing rubber dam (**c**) the primary preparations using diamond burs were performed (**d**). Softened dentin was removed (**e, f**). The noncavitated caries lesion on the mesial aspect of 46 (**g, h**) was connected to the prepared cavity (**g**). Nonetheless, it was decided to save most of the mesial enamel and only infiltrate the carious part from the mesial aspect (not shown in detail). The occlusal parts were restored/sealed using an acid-etch technique (**i**). The result after several weeks (**j**).

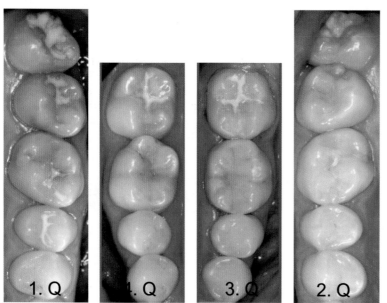

Fig. 25.26 Final clinical aspect at the end of the treatment phase. Q = quadrant

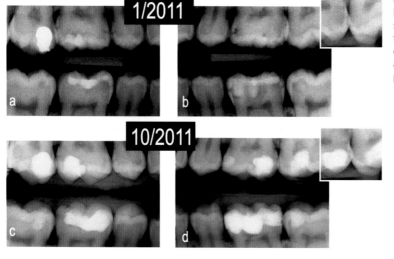

Fig. 25.27a–d Nine months after the last bitewing radiographs (**a, b**), follow-ups (**c, d**) showed no caries progression of any infiltrated teeth (distal and mesial 16, distal 15, distal 26, distal 35 and mesial 46) nor in the area of sealed caries lesions of the occlusal parts (primarily 18, 15).

Clinical Aspect at the End of the Treatment

Several surfaces still showed signs of inactive caries lesions (**Fig. 25.26**). The patient was told to inform any subsequent dentist about the minimal interventional concept of caries management to avoid unnecessary (invasive) treatments. For this purpose a booklet was handed over, in which the stages of the infiltrated and sealed carious lesions were listed.

Follow-up

According to the caries risk the patient was supposed to be recalled three times a year. The last appointment of the treatment phase (3 months after initial treatment) was considered as a "first recall." Advice and instruction with regard to tooth cleaning (brush and floss) and use of fluorides (salt and gel) were repeated.

Six months after the end of the treatment clinical and radiographic follow-up was performed. No clinical signs of new caries lesions were detected. Instructions for oral hygiene and noncariogenic diet were reinforced, and a professional tooth cleaning was performed. Follow-up radiographs revealed no progression or onset of any caries lesion of the posterior teeth (**Fig. 25.27**).

Case 3: Minimally Interventional Anterior Restorations

Christian Andres Schneider, Hendrik Meyer-Lueckel

Anamnesis

The 32-year-old patient presented for the first time in the emergency ward of our clinic with an acute abscess proceeding from tooth 26. The patient was fearful of dentists and stated that he had not visited a dentist for several years owing to a traumatic treatment. Due to the overwhelming symptoms, the patient had become quite aware of the necessity of thorough treatment, and we were able to convince him that he needed treatment involving several departments in our clinic.

His general medical history was unremarkable.

Clinical Findings

In addition to the panoramic film (**Fig. 25.28**) taken in the emergency department, bitewing x-rays and a single-tooth radiograph of tooth 26 were also taken. The intraoral findings revealed an insufficiently cared-for dentition with insufficient restoration and numerous cavitated carious lesions as well as an inflamed periodontum (PSI code 3–4). Teeth 35 and 48 were missing.

Since we wish to illustrate the treatment of caries in the anterior region, we will restrict ourselves in this description to the diagnosis of caries in the anterior maxilla. Along with the treatment of the anterior teeth, the posterior teeth were treated over a period of three months.

In the panoramic film (**Fig. 25.28**) from the emergency ward, distal D2 caries and a mesial filling could be seen in teeth 12 and 22 (Black class III); the filling in tooth 22 manifested significant radiolucency (caries adjacent to the restoration) at the cervical margin.

The anterior teeth without crowns manifested ICDAS 2 white-to-brown caries in the vestibular surfaces (**Fig. 25.29a**). Tooth 12 manifested caries (ICDAS 4) distal and mesial to a three-surface Black class III composite filling with discolored, partially projecting margins (**Fig. 25.29**). The margins of the crowns of teeth 11 and 21 were sufficient. Even though the esthetic appearance of these crowns could be considered optimal, they were left alone since a restoration was not indicated due to a lack of caries. The endodontic tooth cavity in tooth 11 was not quite completely filled with composite (**Fig. 25.29b**). Tooth 22 had a mesial, two-surface, Black class III composite filling with insufficient margins that shadowed through in the area of the restoration (**Fig. 25.29**). Distal ICDAS 4 caries was also documented. Tooth 23 distal showed a cavitated enamel caries lesion (ICDAS 3).

CLINICAL PEARL

Fiberoptic transillumination (FOTI) is particularly suitable for determining the extent of the caries process in the anterior region. This allows one to choose the best access for the preparation in this esthetically sensitive area.

Caries Risk

The patient's DMFT score was 20. He stated that he snacked frequently and regularly consumed sweets and sweetened drinks. There was a generalized presence of plaque with occasional calculus below the gingival margin. Beyond using a toothbrush and fluoride toothpaste, the patient stated that he did not use any additional means of oral care. His salivary flow was normal. His risk of caries was rated as high.

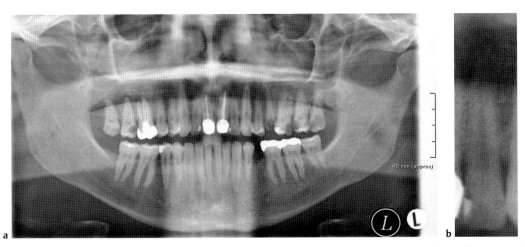

Fig. 25.28a, b The panoramic film reveals dentition requiring extensive treatment and restoration (**a**). Tooth 22 excerpted from the panoramic tomography discloses distal D2 caries and a mesial filling with significant radiotranslucency at the cervical margin (**b**).

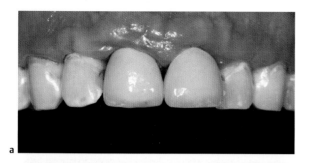

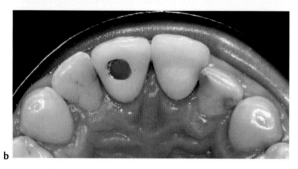

Fig. 25.29a, b
a Vestibular surfaces of the maxillary anterior have experienced initial demineralization (ICDAS 2) and calculus.
b Incisal view: teeth 12 and 22 with clearly visible approximal caries (ICDAS 4), distal in each case. An insufficient composite filling (Black class III) is identifiable in tooth 22 mesially.

Diagnosis and Treatment Plan

The primary goals of treatment were to lower the caries risk, establish a healthy periodontal situation, and treat the caries lesions.

Individual Level

An effort was made to motivate the patient to regularly care for his teeth, and he was instructed on how to brush and floss. The patient was given a thorough, professional tooth cleaning in two sessions to provide a foundation from which to proceed. We explained to the patient the relationship between his eating habits and the status of his teeth, and advised him to reduce the number of snacks and sugar consumption. Advice for use of highly concentrated fluoride toothpaste (5000 ppm) was given.

NOTE

Patients who are fearful of dentists frequently have poor oral hygiene. Due to the gingival inflammation, tooth brushing was frequently experienced as being painful, and the bleeding of the gingiva that this caused was misinterpreted as injury from the toothbrush. It is particularly important to clearly explain the actual situation to break the vicious cycle.

Tooth Level

The diagnosis and therapy for the posterior teeth will not be described. The diagnosis of the anterior teeth that was made is noted in the **Table 25.3**, and the patient underwent therapy.

We will present the restoration of tooth 22 as an example to illustrate the steps involved in filling an anterior tooth (**Fig. 25.30**).

CLINICAL PEARL

If it is difficult to determine a tooth's color due to dark caries shining through or due to a discolored filling, the contralateral tooth can be referenced for the tooth color. Thin, light-cured samples of applied composite can make it easier to identify the correct color.

CLINICAL PEARL

The rubber dam includes the entire anterior region which allows the symmetry of the dental arch to be retained during treatment. The rubber dam is inverted using compressed air and a spatula. If this is insufficient when the cavities extend deeply in a cervical direction, a ligature can be applied with dental floss, or the rubber can be inverted in the sulcus using a cord.

The color was determined using color rings and hardened composite samples. These were applied to the slightly dried tooth without prior etching. The rubber dam was then placed, and the distal caries was exposed from a palatal direction while retaining an enamel lamella (**Fig. 25.31a, b**).

A spherical or pear-shaped diamond-coated bur of an appropriate size is suitable for the primary preparation of small anterior cavities. A fine enamel lamella can initially be left to protect the neighboring tooth. A metal matrix strip or oscillating attachment can also be helpful in minimally invasive preparations (such as the SONICflex).

CLINICAL PEARL

In the case of approximal caries with an associated Black class III preparation, it is easier to work from a vestibular direction; nevertheless, a palatal access retaining significant elements of the vestibular enamel lamella frequently produces the best esthetic results.

The caries was excavated (**Fig. 25.31c**), and the edges of the enamel were beveled (**Fig. 25.32**). In addition, the mesio-palatal composite filling was removed. A slight amount of work with rotating instruments was sufficient since the remainder was successfully released with a

Table 25.3 Diagnosis and treatment plan of the anterior of the maxilla. In addition, the buccal surfaces of a few anterior teeth were infiltrated for esthetic reasons

Diagnosis	Caries	Caries non-progressiva (CNP)		Caries progressiva superficialis (CS)			Caries progressiva media (CM) et profunda (CP)		
	Restorations	Restauratio insufficienta initialis (RII)		Restauratio insufficienta partialis (RIP)			Restauratio insufficienta totalis (RIT)		
	Sound surfaces	–		Sanus majoris periculi (SMP)			–		
Treatment		Particular surveillance		Noninvasive or microinvasive/repair			(Minimally) invasive		
		Tooth + Surface	Diagnosis	Tooth + Surface	Diagnosis	Therapy	Tooth + Surface	Diagnosis	Therapy
				12m	CS	POL ✔	12 d	CM	FC ✔
							22 m	RIT	FC ✔
							22 d	CM	FC ✔
							23 d	CM	FC ✔
				POL polishing			FC composite filling		

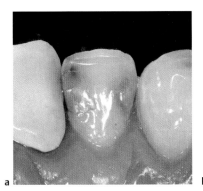 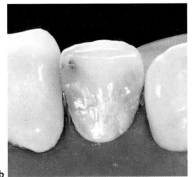 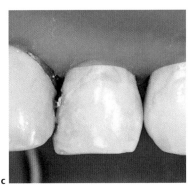

Fig. 25.30a–c Initial situation of tooth 22 from a palatal direction (**a**), with rubber dam (**b**), and a vestibular view with the rubber dam in place (**c**).

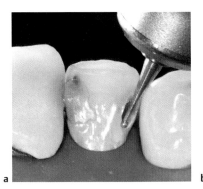 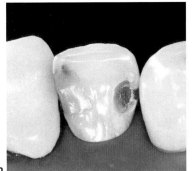 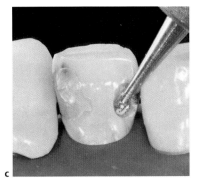

Fig. 25.31a–c Tooth 22 primary cavity preparation retaining an enamel lamella (**a**), the exposed caries with local enamel degeneration below the contact point (**b**), and excavation (**c**).

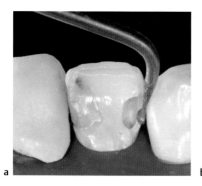
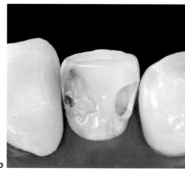

Fig. 25.32a, b
a Distal beveling of the enamel edges with a SONICflex attachment (KaVo, Biberach, Germany).
b Finished distal beveling, and mesial exposure of the caries under the old composite filling.

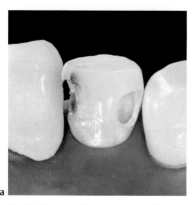
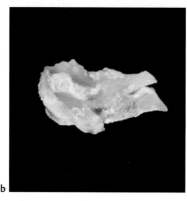
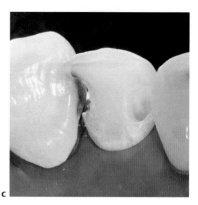

Fig. 25.33a–c The mesial cavity after removing the composite filling (**a**), a fragment of composite easily prised off due to the lack of adhesive bond (**b**), and discolored preparation marks from the previous dentist in the ceramic of the crown on tooth 21 (**c**).

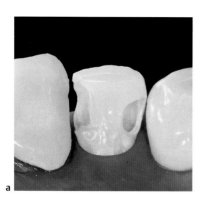
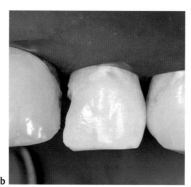

Fig. 25.34 Finished cavities before conditioning with visible preparation marks from the previous dentist in the ceramic of the crown on tooth 21 from a palatinal (**a**) and vestibular (**b**) direction.

probe due to the lack of an adhesive bond. During removal, discolored preparation marks were revealed from the previous dentist on the ceramic of the crown of tooth 21 (**Fig. 25.33**). Since the defect did not impair the function or esthetics, the ceramic was merely polished. After the mesial excavation of tooth 22, the enamel margins were also beveled here as well (**Fig. 25.34**).

The enamel margins were beveled from a vestibular direction with a flame-shaped finishing diamond bur, and from a lingual direction with a button or spherical-shaped finishing diamond bur. The SONICflex attachment is very useful in this case as well (**Fig. 25.32a**).

After 15 seconds of etching (Total Etch) (**Fig. 25.35a**), a two-component adhesive system (Optibond FL; Kerr) was applied (**Fig. 25.35b**). Before light curing, the bonding compound should be thinly blown onto the bevel, especially since the translucency is elevated due to the lack of filler, and the margins of the filling may thereby appear dark.

It is preferable to initially layer on the composite (Venus; Heraeus) to create a "single-surface cavity" which is later filled.

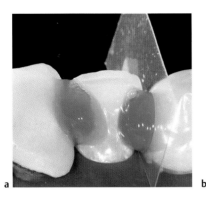
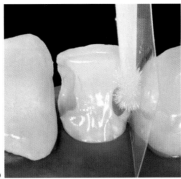

Fig. 25.35a, b Etching (**a**) and bonding (**b**) of the cavities.

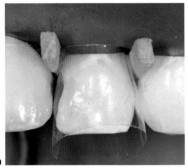
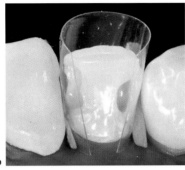
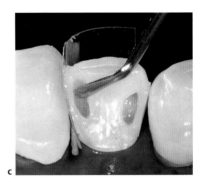

Fig. 25.36a–c Vestibular view of the applied matrix (**a**), palatal view with a modeled distal enamel lamella (**b**), and view while modeling the mesial enamel lamella (**c**).

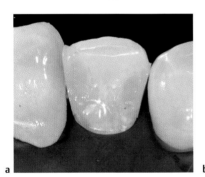
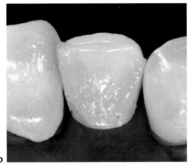
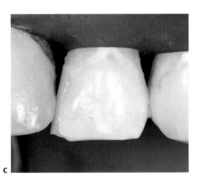

Fig. 25.37a–c Finished dentin cores (**a**); finished filling from a palatal (**b**) and vestibular (**c**) direction.

CLINICAL PEARL

With a Black class IV or a three-surface Black class III preparation, a silicone key of the palatal surface up to the incisal margin can be made before preparation. The silicone key can be made of the intact tooth, the old filling or a mock-up. A palatal enamel lamella is thinly layered against the silicone key (maximum thickness: 0.5 mm). If the composite adheres too strongly to the metal modeling instruments, a microbrush can also be used.

The approximal enamel lamellas were modeled against a transparent plastic strip (a delicate, sharp spatula can be very useful) (**Fig. 25.36**).

CLINICAL PEARL

To make it easier to obtain an anatomical convex shape, the transparent and dual convex Lucifix matrixes (Kerr) are recommended, which were originally developed for posterior teeth (**Fig. 25.36**).

After the approximal enamel lamellas were modeled, the remaining single-surface cavities were filled with dentin composite and then covered with enamel composite (**Fig. 25.37a, b**). To hide the bevel, it is recommended to cover approximately one-third of the bevel with dentin since the margin can otherwise appear dark due to the properties of the enamel composites.

The major residue of the finished filling was carefully removed with a scalpel (**Fig. 25.38a**).

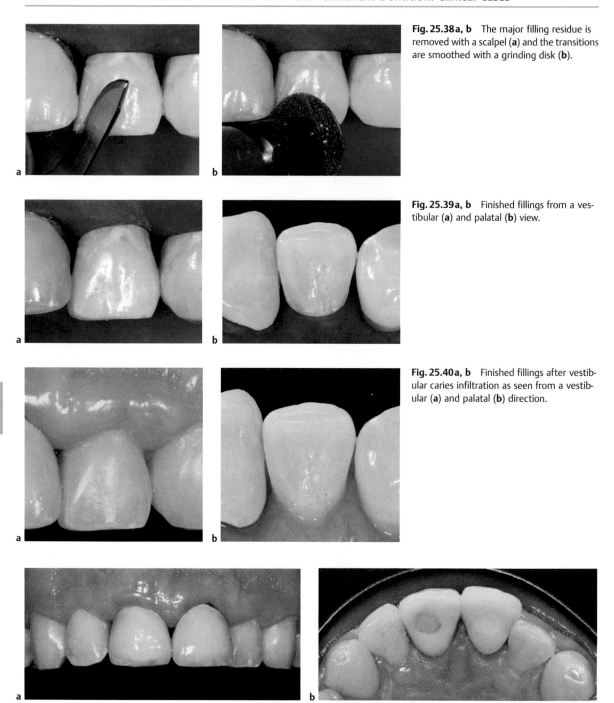

Fig. 25.38a, b The major filling residue is removed with a scalpel (**a**) and the transitions are smoothed with a grinding disk (**b**).

Fig. 25.39a, b Finished fillings from a vestibular (**a**) and palatal (**b**) view.

Fig. 25.40a, b Finished fillings after vestibular caries infiltration as seen from a vestibular (**a**) and palatal (**b**) direction.

Fig. 25.41a, b Final view on both labial and palatal aspects of the maxillary anterior teeth.

NOTE

A scalpel is then used to finalize the composite, and the enamel surface is not touched.

Then the transitions were smoothed out with a finishing disk (**Fig. 25.38b**). When working under dry conditions, the residual filling has white margins at the transitions from the powder generated by processing.

The incisal margins and vestibular surfaces were ground with finishing discs of decreasing grit until they assumed a approximal shape, and then they were polished. Conical silicon polishers were used to polish the concave palatal surfaces (**Figs. 25.39** and **25.40**). Since the matrix yielded a perfectly smooth surface no further finishing was required there. Finally, the planned subsequent therapy of the anterior teeth was performed (see above) (**Fig. 25.41**).

Case 4: Infiltration to Mask Caries Lesions

Leandro Augusto Hilgert, Soraya Coelho Leal

Anamnesis

A 14-year-old female patient had been used to coming to the dental office every six months since she was a baby. Although oral health education had been performed frequently, the patient was not capable of establishing good oral hygiene. In June 2011, she came to the dental clinic for her first consultation after removal of the orthodontic appliances she had worn earlier, searching for a solution for the "white spots" on the buccal surfaces of her anterior teeth. She had finished a 4-year orthodontic treatment about 6 months before the consultation. There were no other complaints or relevant medical information.

Clinical Findings

Oral examination revealed a complete permanent dentition with no visible cavitated caries lesions or restorations. There were sealants on the occlusal surfaces of teeth 26, 46, 37, and 47. Cleaning of all teeth was performed using brushes and prophylactic pastes. Caries lesions (ICDAS 1 and 2) were observed on the buccal surfaces of all anterior teeth (canine to canine) in both jaws. The lesions were located around the areas where the orthodontic brackets had been situated, especially toward the gingival margin. The patient and her mother complained about the esthetics, since the white spots caries lesions could be easily seen when smiling (**Fig. 25.42a–e**). The caries lesions did not present the opaque, rough and chalky appearance that is typical for active lesions. Already 6 months had passed since the removal of the orthodontic appliances. During that time the caries lesions had become inactive, since brushing without the appliances was easier.

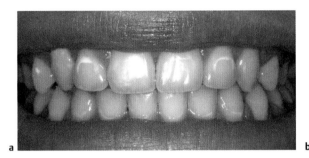

a

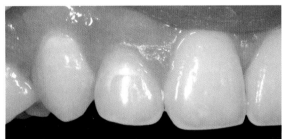

b

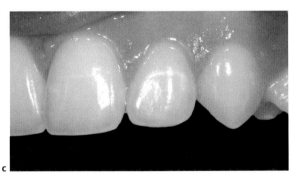

c

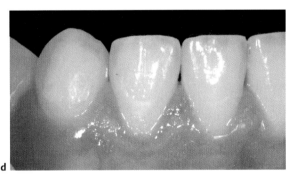

d

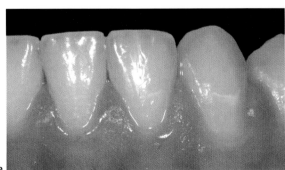

e

Fig. 25.42a–e Initial aspect of the white spot caries lesions on the buccal surfaces of the anterior teeth.
a Smile.
b Upper-right anterior teeth.
c Upper-left anterior teeth.
d Lower-right anterior teeth.
e Lower-left anterior teeth.

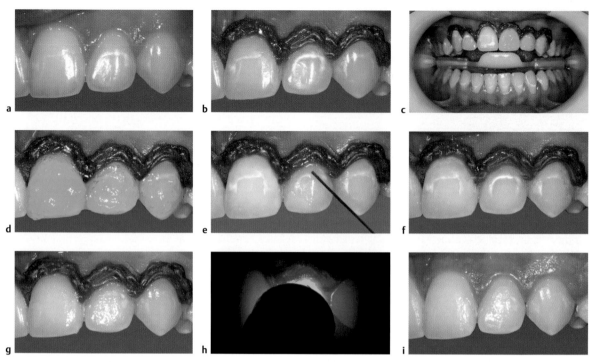

Fig. 25.43a–i First infiltration session to the upper-left anterior teeth.

a Initial aspect of the upper-left anterior teeth.

b Soft tissues were protected using a light-cured resin dam (Top Dam, FGM).

c A lips and cheek retractor (ArcFlex, FGM) was used to grant access and visibility to the teeth.

d Acid etching with Icon Etch for 120 seconds.

e After rinsing and air drying, Icon Dry (ethanol) was applied to observe the "rewetting" effect. Since the caries lesion could still be clearly observed, the acid etching was repeated to promote a better infiltration.

f The area has become thoroughly dry after 30 seconds in contact with ethanol.

g The Icon Infiltrant (low-viscosity resin) was applied for 3 minutes and surplus was removed afterwards.

h The Icon Infiltrant was light cured for 60 seconds. A new 1-minute infiltration was performed followed by surplus removal and 60-second light curing.

i Final situation of the upper-left anterior teeth.

NOTE

Post-orthodontic white spots disappear with time, only if they are shallow. The process involved is much more related to abrasion than to remineralization, since usually only the most superficial layer is remineralized. Deeper white spot lesions are commonly still visible as 'scars', even after many years.

Caries Risk

The patient presented no cavitated caries lesions or restorations that could be included in a DMFT count. There were no medications or health problems that increased caries risk. Sugar consumption was regular, but not extremely frequent. Plaque removal was the most concerning factor of the caries risk assessment, since the patient had a history of deficient oral hygiene and visible plaque accumulation was observed in many sites. Access to fluoride sources was regular (fluoride toothpaste and fluoridated tap water) and salivary flow was normal. The caries

risk assessment result placed the patient in the threshold zone between low and medium risk. However, the use of brackets during the orthodontic treatment along with the patient's poor oral hygiene were related to the development of white spot caries lesions at that time.

Diagnosis and Treatment Plan

The treatment plan focused on the prevention of future caries lesions (individual level) and the microinvasive treatment of the esthetic problem caused by the white spots, which was desired by the patient and her mother (tooth level).

Individual Level

The patient was instructed and motivated to improve her brushing and flossing habits. The dentist explained to her and her mother the direct relationship between lack of oral hygiene and the occurrence of caries lesions. Clinical pictures of more destroyed caries lesions were used to show the evolution of the caries process.

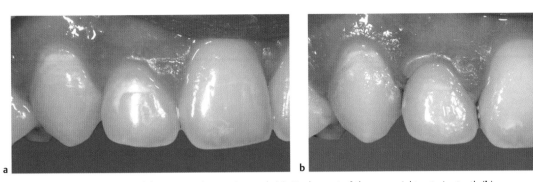

Fig. 25.44a, b Initial aspect of the upper-right anterior teeth (**a**). Final aspect of the upper-right anterior teeth (**b**).

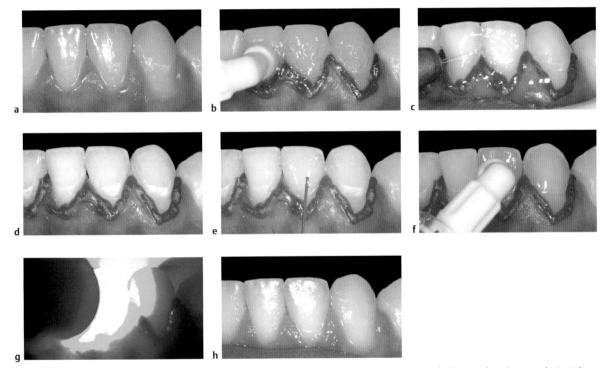

Fig. 25.45a–h Second infiltration session
a Initial aspect of the lower-left anterior teeth.
b Acid etching (2 minutes).
c Rinsing.
d Air drying.

e "Rewetting" using ethanol. Observe that the caries lesion "disappears" with the ethanol application, which means that the acid etching was sufficient and the expected result is promising. After 30 seconds ethanol and air drying.
f The infiltrant is applied for 3 minutes.
g Light cured for 1 minute. The infiltrant is reapplied for 1 minute and light cured again (1 minute).
h Final aspect of the lower-left anterior teeth.

Tooth Level

Since the patient did not present any cavities, the proposed treatment was resin infiltration of the white spot caries lesions on the buccal surfaces of the anterior teeth. The diagnosis was Caries non-progressiva, so no further treatment was indicated from a cariological point of view. Nonetheless, the esthetic impairment and the patient's desire justified the decision for microinvasive treatment. The patient and her mother were informed that caries infiltration might give good results without sacrificing dental structure. If an unsatisfactory result were obtained,

all other more invasive measures could still be performed in the future. Two appointments were scheduled: one for the infiltration of each arch (six teeth to be infiltrated per arch).

The first infiltration session is depicted in **Figs. 25.43a–i** and **25.44a, b**. The second session is presented in **Fig. 25.45a–h**. Resin infiltration (Icon, DMG) was performed using a light-cured resin dam to protect soft tissues as well as a lips and cheeks retractor (commonly used for in-office dental bleaching).

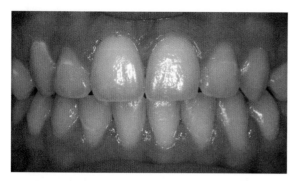

Fig. 25.46 Final clinical aspect of the patient's anterior teeth at the end of the treatment. Although some of the caries lesions were still visible, the patient was satisfied with the esthetic outcome.

The infiltration process started with an acid etching of the whole vestibular surface of the teeth, followed by rinsing and air drying. The next step was application of ethanol to promote desiccation of the lesion. (Note: when the alcohol is applied on the etched and dried surface, it is possible to observe a "preview" of the resin infiltration result, since the alcohol refractive index (1.36) is more similar to the resin (1.52) than the air (1.0) (Chapter 17). If, during this step called "re-wetting," an insufficient reduction of the lesion appearance is observed, the reason might be an incomplete erosion of the pseudo-intact surface layer. In this case the etching can be repeated aiming at better access of the infiltrant in the subsurface porosities of the white spots. After acceptable results during the "re-wetting" with alcohol a thorough air drying was performed. The low-viscosity resin infiltrant was applied, surplus removed and light cured. The infiltrant was then reapplied and once more light cured. Before each light-curing step, resin excesses were removed using dry gauze and floss. Finishing and polishing was performed using flexible abrasive disks (Sof-lex, 3 M ESPE) and silicon carbide impregnated rotating brushes (Jiffy Brush, Ultradent).

Clinical Aspect at the End of the Treatment

The esthetic improvement of the resin infiltration treatment can be easily seen when comparing **Fig. 25.42a** and **Fig. 25.46**. Caries lesions that were smaller (and probably shallower) completely disappeared. Larger and deeper caries lesions (teeth 13, 12, 22, 42) were still visible at the end of the treatment but their area had been reduced and their contrast with the surrounding "sound" enamel had become less apparent. The patient and her mother were very satisfied with the esthetic result, especially because it was obtained without drilling. The patient seemed at the end of the treatment to be more conscious of her responsibility for her smile appearance (better hygiene) and did not request any additional treatment for the white spots that were still visible.

Case 5: Stepwise Caries Excavation

Hendrik Meyer-Lueckel, Sebastian Paris

Figure 25.47a–l, I and II

A 20-year-old patient visited the dental clinic because of pain in the right upper arch while eating and drinking. The visual examination revealed an active ICDAS 4 lesion (**a**; all surfaces affected) for tooth 15 that reacted sensitively to ice spray testing, but not to vertical percussion. A radiograph (taken after the first treatment session) did not reveal any radiolucencies around the apices of the roots or deep caries lesions for any other tooth in the area (not shown). No radiological signs of a periapical lesion could be detected for tooth 15 either (**I**).

After initial preparation (**b**) the large extension of the lesion became visible. A diamond bur was used to remove chalky carious enamel (**b**), and also to gain acceptable access to the carious dentin, which was removed with care to avoid pulp exposure (**c**). Soft dentin (scratching of a probe would have resulted in clear marks) was left alone everywhere, also underneath the cups (**d**), with the idea to save as much dental hard tissue as possible in order to place a partial crown rather than a full crown. If all soft dentin had been removed only enamel laminates would have been left. Most of the soft dentin close to the pulp was protected by $Ca(OH)_2$ (Calxyl, OCO products) and on top a light-curing resin modified glass-ionomer cement (Vitrebond; 3 M Espe) was applied (**e**, **f**). A metal-reinforced glass-ionomer restoration (Ketac silver; 3 M Espe) was placed as an intermediate material (**g**).

After 1 month the rather unstable palatal cusp broke (**h**). Sharp margins were beveled and the tooth kept as seen on the image (**h**) for another 3 months. Four months after initial treatment, the glass-ionomer cement and the lining restorative materials were carefully removed (**i**). All previously soft dentin had become hard. The deepest area was again covered by Calxyl and Vitrebond and all dentin covered with an adhesive subfilling (**j**; TetricCeram; Ivoclar Vivadent). A partial crown was prepared (**k**) and inserted one week later (**l**).

The follow-up radiograph after 12 months revealed no apical radiolucency (II) and the patient showed no signs or symptoms of pulpal infection.

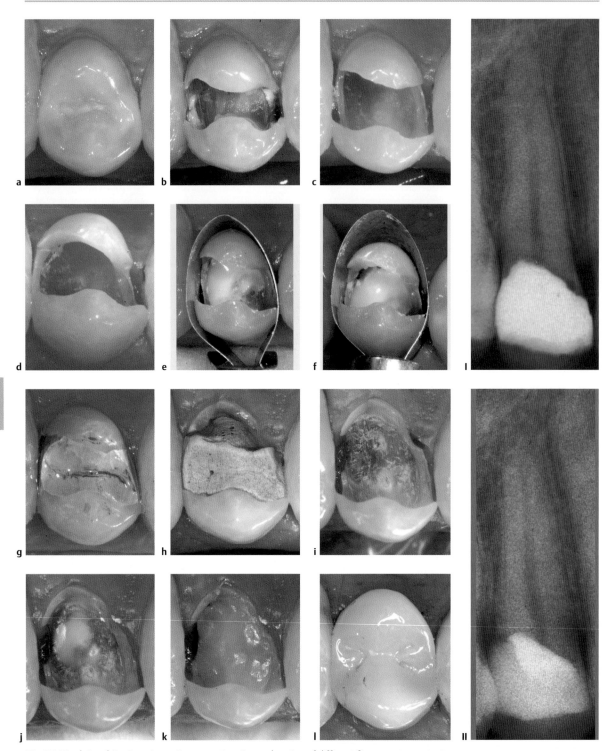

Fig. 25.47a–l, I and II Stepwise caries excavation. For explanation of different figure parts, see text.

Minimal Interventional Treatment of Caries in Young Children: Clinical Cases

Vera Mendes Soviero, Soraya Coelho Leal, Christian Splieth, Mohammad Alkilzy

26

Case 1: A 6-Year-Old Boy with High Caries Risk

Vera Mendes Soviero, Soraya Coelho Leal

Anamnesis

Gender: male
Age: 6 years
First visit: June 2010
Last visit: September 2010
Follow-up visit: May 2011

The patient came to the pediatric dental clinic for his first ever visit to the dentist. Both he and his mother were aware of the presence of cavitated caries lesions in the primary teeth and wanted to have them treated. According to his mother the patient had been complaining of tooth pain earlier, but felt no pain at the moment. No relevant general medical information was reported by the mother.

Clinical Findings (Tooth Level)

Oral examination revealed a mixed dentition with lower permanent central incisors and one upper permanent first molar already having erupted. The mucosa was healthy, the gingiva was inflamed, but no signs of periodontitis could be observed (**Fig. 26.1**). Frank cavities could easily be detected in the upper primary molars.

Caries detection was based on visual–tactile examination combined with bitewing radiographs (**Fig. 26.2**). For extensively carious teeth, radiographs depicting the periapical area were taken to support an eventual treatment decision regarding pulp therapy or extraction (**Fig. 26.3**).

CLINICAL PEARL

Tooth surfaces must be cleaned before caries assessment; otherwise initial caries lesions will not be detected. It does not matter whether the dental biofilm is removed with a rotating instrument or toothbrush. However, if the dental professional uses the toothbrush, it is possible to combine plaque removal with oral hygiene instructions to the patient/parents and to show them how the toothbrush can be as effective as the "professional rotating instrument."

All primary molars were affected by active caries lesions at different levels of severity. Extensive cavitated caries lesions were clearly visible (ICDAS 6) in the upper primary molars (**Fig. 26.1a**). Tooth 55 was the most severely affected; only roots remained in the mouth. In the lower primary molars, approximal caries lesions were detected radiographically (**Fig. 26.2a, b**). An active noncavitated caries lesion (ICDAS 1) was detected in the occlusal surface of the upper permanent first molar. Only the anterior teeth were not affected by caries lesions. The d_1ft count was 8 and the D_1MFT was 1. Detailed information about

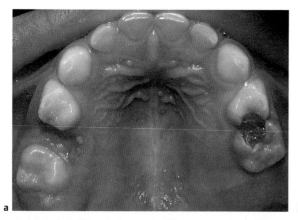
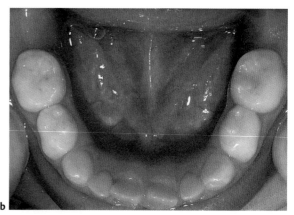

Fig. 26.1a, b Clinical aspect of the upper (**a**) and lower (**b**) jaws at the first examination.

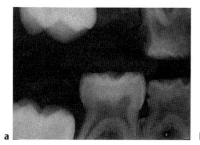
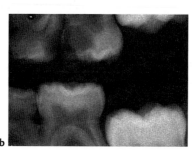

Fig. 26.2a, b Initial right (**a**) and left (**b**) bitewing radiographs. See **Fig. 26.4** for assessment.

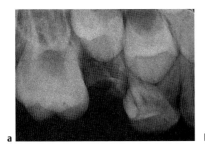 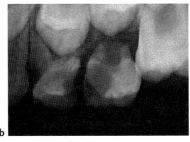

Fig. 26.3a, b Periapical radiographs of upper right (**a**) and left (**b**) molars.

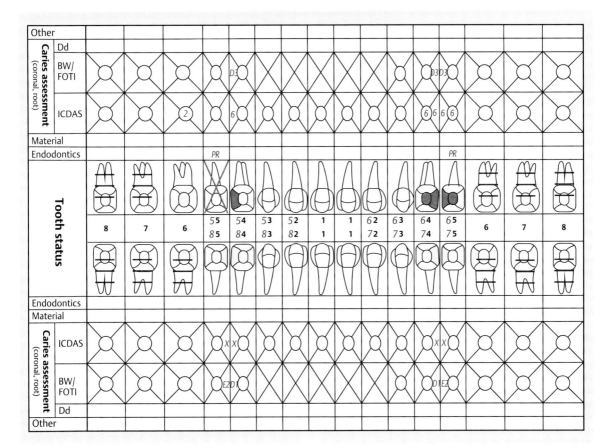

Fig. 26.4 Dental status

each tooth surface is available in the dental examination scheme (**Fig. 26.4**).

Caries Risk Assessment (Individual Level)

Caries risk assessment is based on the evaluation of a series of factors at the individual level, which may influence oral health positively or negatively (see Chapter 7).

Regarding the dietary habits, high and regular consumption of sweetened food and beverages from four to five times daily was reported by the mother. When asked about the frequency of consumption of drinking water, the mother informed us that the child almost never drinks water, but sweetened beverages like juice, tea, or soda.

The family had access to fluoridated water and the child brushed his teeth with fluoridated toothpaste usually twice daily. Dental floss had never been used and tooth brushing was not assisted by an adult. Visible dental biofilm was present in 53% of the approximal sites, specifically at those with an adjacent tooth and an intact contact point. Dental plaque was assessed visually with no disclosing solution. If the dental plaque was not visible in the entrance of the approximal area, a probe was used to confirm the presence or the absence of approximal plaque. The occlusal surface of the permanent first molar was covered by thick biofilm.

The high caries experience ($d_1ft + D_1MFT = 9$), the cariogenic dietary habits, and the presence of a considerable amount of visible biofilm were relevant risk factors in the present case. However, the patient had regular access to fluoride sources (fluoridated water and fluoride toothpaste), did not use any medications, and had normal salivary flow. As a result, he was classified as being medium risk at present (53%), but this would have been higher in previous years.

Diagnosis and Treatment Plan

Based on the minimum interventional treatment concept, the treatment plan was focused on the prevention and arrest of caries, preserving dental tissues as much as possible. After a comprehensive examination and the caries risk assessment, treatment strategies were planned at two levels: the individual level and the tooth/surface level.

Individual Level

Oral Hygiene and Fluoride

The parents were instructed to have their son's teeth brushed twice a day with regular fluoride toothpaste ($1000–1500$ ppm F^-) and flossed once a day. As the child had access to fluoridated water, no other home-use fluoride product was prescribed. As the patient had active caries lesions, topical application of fluoride gel was recommended on a weekly basis. The mother was asked to help the child with tooth brushing once daily to ensure proper plaque control at least once a day, emphasizing that the quality of cleaning is more important than the frequency.

CLINICAL PEARL

Instead of advising that parents should brush their child's teeth before bedtime, let parents decide the best time of the day for them to do it. Explain how important it is to disorganize the dental biofilm once a day, and that a child needs help to do it properly. The chance of a good compliance is increased when the decisions are shared with parents.

Oral hygiene instructions were focused on two main aspects: plaque control in the occlusal surface of the erupting permanent first molar, and flossing the lower primary molars. The mother was shown how to reach the permanent first molar better by positioning the toothbrush transversally to the tooth. At the first visit, the child presented only one permanent first molar, but at the end of the treatment phase one more had partially erupted. The mother was instructed to brush the permanent molars first and then brush the other teeth.

CLINICAL PEARL

Give clear oral hygiene instructions and prioritize what is most important for each case. Dental professionals usually say to the patient/parents, in a generic way, that tooth cleaning should be improved. Be specific: concentrate your explanation on the most important needs. Suggest that tooth cleaning should begin with tooth surfaces at risk of caries development or progression, that is, occlusal surfaces of permanent first molars partially erupted or tooth surfaces with initial enamel caries lesions.

The approximal caries lesions in the lower primary molars visualized on the radiographs were shown to the mother to emphasize the importance of daily flossing. It was mentioned that the extensive caries lesions in the upper teeth clearly started as approximal lesions and that flossing would help to avoid the progression of the noncavitated approximal caries lesions in the lower teeth.

CLINICAL PEARL

Show the tooth surfaces with thick biofilm to the patient/parents. Show the difference between a clean and a dirty tooth surface. Encourage the patient to feel with his or her tongue the smoothness of a clean tooth surface in comparison to the roughness of a dirty one. These are simple and practical ways to make patients able to check the quality of their own tooth cleaning at home.

Dietary Counseling The influence of high frequency of sugar consumption on the cariogenic potential of the dental biofilm was explained to the mother.

CLINICAL PEARL

Explain the association between sugar and dental biofilm with easy and clear words. Patients are usually advised to eat less sugar, because it causes caries. But this association is often not clearly explained. Encourage the patient to perceive in his or her own teeth how dental plaque will be thicker in the end of a day full of sugar, in comparison to another day when much less sugar was consumed.

Table 26.1 Diagnoses and treatments at a glance

Diagnosis	Caries	Caries non-progressiva (CNP)		Caries progressiva superficialis (CS)			Caries progressiva media (CM) et profunda (CP)		
	Restorations	Restauratio insufficienta initialis (RII)		Restauratio insufficienta partialis (RIP)			Restauratio insufficienta totalis (RIT)		
	Sound surfaces	–		Sanus majoris periculi (SMP)			–		
"Treatment"		Particular surveillance		Noninvasive or microinvasive/ repair			(Minimally) invasive		
		Tooth + Surface	Diagnosis	Tooth + Surface	Diagnosis	Therapy	Tooth + Surface	Diagnosis	Therapy
				16 o	CS	FS ✔	55	CP	EX ✔
				75 m	CS	INF ✔	54 od	CP	FC ✔
				74 d	CS	INF ✔	64	CP	EX ✔
				85 m	CS	INF ✔	65	CP	EX ✔
				26 o*	SMP	CB ✔	84 od	CM	FC ✔
				FS fissure sealing INF caries infiltration CB cross brushing			FC composite filling EX extraction		

*Diagnosed during treatment.

The patient was instructed to reduce the consumption of sweetened food and beverages, particularly during the weekdays. It was emphasized that water should always be the first choice to relieve thirstiness instead of sweetened beverages.

CLINICAL PEARL

Suggest some deals between parents and children like: "always have a glass of water before any other beverage."

Tooth Level

Diagnoses and treatment decisions are summarized in **Table 26.1**. To eliminate plaque stagnation areas, the cavity on the distal surface of tooth 54 was temporarily filled with glass-ionomer cement and extractions were planned to be done at the beginning of the treatment.

Due to Caries progressiva profunda, teeth 55, 65, and 64 were extracted (**Fig. 26.5**). Tooth 55 had only roots remaining and teeth 65 and 64 were extensively affected by caries with advanced root resorption, contraindicating pulp therapy. Due to advanced coronal destruction of tooth 55, tooth 16 had drifted mesially, causing loss of space in the arch. As it was necessary to regain space before placing a space maintainer, the patient was referred to the orthodontic clinic after the end of the treatment.

In the lower left side, noncavitated caries lesions were detected radiographically in the distal surface of tooth 74 and in the mesial surface of tooth 75, scored as D1 and E2, respectively (see **Fig. 26.2b**). These lesions were considered as being progressive, although activity could only be affirmed by the local plaque level (no gingival bleeding, other assessments not feasible). Nonetheless, owing to the generally high caries risk, both caries lesions were treated by the infiltration technique (**Fig. 26.6**).

In the lower right side the caries lesion at the distal surface of tooth 84 was cavitated (clearly detectable on the bitewing radiograph) and considered as being active (Caries progressiva media). The mesial surface of tooth 85 had a caries lesion scored radiographically as E2 (**Fig. 26.2a**). On tooth 84, caries was accessed by a vertical slot and the resulting cavity was filled with composite (**Fig. 26.7**). During invasive treatment, cavity and activity status of 85 mesial was assessed thoroughly (**Fig. 26.7b**). The lesion was diagnosed as Caries progressiva superficialis that was not supposed to be hampered in progression by noninvasive measures only and thus was treated by the infiltration technique (alternatively sealing) (**Fig. 26.7c–e**).

When approximal caries lesions extend into dentin the probability of further progression is rather high. This fact supported the decision of infiltrating the approximal caries lesions of the distal surface of tooth 74, scored radiographically as D1. The approximal lesions of both 75 and 85 mesial were scored as E2. The decision for infiltrating

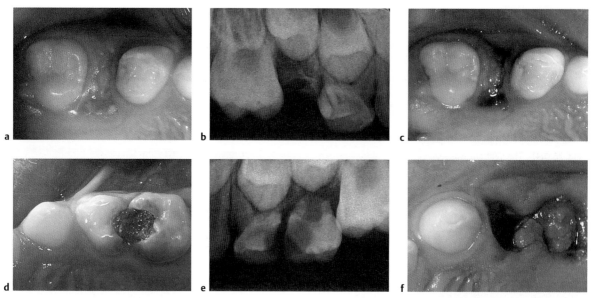

Fig. 26.5a–f   Tooth 55 is extensively destroyed by caries (**a**); periapical radiograph shows only roots remaining of tooth 55 (**b**); clinical aspect directly after extraction of tooth 55 (**c**); teeth 65 and 64 have extensive caries (**d**); periapical radiograph show deep caries in teeth 65 and 64 and pathological reabsorption of tooth 65 (**e**); clinical aspect directly after the extraction of teeth 65 and 64 (**f**).

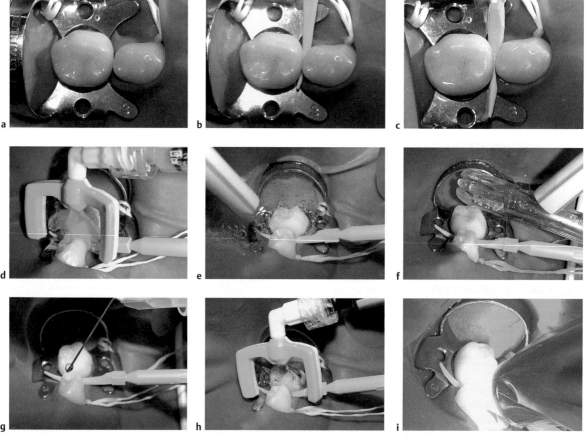

Fig. 26.6a–l   Teeth 75 and 74 after rubber dam placement (**a**); the wedge for immediate tooth separation is inserted (**b**); after 30–60 seconds, enough space is obtained between the teeth (**c**); the foil attached to the acid syringe is placed and the distal surface of tooth 74 is etched with HCl for 120 seconds (**d**); washing for 30 seconds (**e**); air drying for 30 seconds (**f**); application of ethanol for 30 seconds (**g**). After air drying, a new foil attached to the infiltrant syringe is placed between the tooth surface and the wedge and the infiltrant is applied (**h**); after 3 minutes, any excess must be removed with dental floss before light curing for 60 seconds (**i**).

Fig. 26.6j–l   ▷

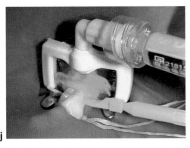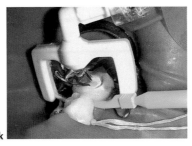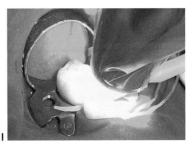

Fig. 26.6j–l The infiltrant was reapplied for 1 minute and light cured for 60 seconds before all steps were repeated for the mesial surface of tooth 75, with etching (**j**); after washing, air drying and ethanol application, the infiltrant is applied (**k**); light curing for 60 seconds, reapplication of the infiltrant for 1 minute and final light curing (**l**).

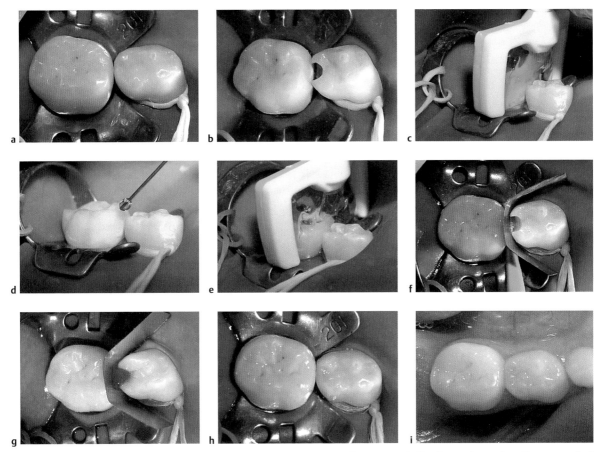

Fig. 26.7a–i Teeth 85 and 84 after rubber dam placement (**a**); after caries removal in the distal surface of tooth 84, the absence of a cavity is confirmed in the mesial surface of tooth 85 (**b**); the foil attached to the acid syringe is placed (it was not necessary to use the wedge in this case) and the mesial surface of tooth 85 is etched with HCl for 120 seconds (**c**); after washing and air drying, ethanol is applied for 30 seconds (**d**); after air drying, the infiltrant is applied for 3 minutes using a new foil (**e**); after light curing for 60 seconds, reapplication for 1 minute, and final light curing of the infiltrant, the cavity (**f**) in tooth 84 is etched with H_3PO_4 (**g**); the finished composite restoration (**h**); the clinical aspect 1 month later (**i**).

these lesions was based on the fact that the patient had advanced caries lesions in many other approximal surfaces and relevant risk factors for caries progression were recorded during caries risk assessment.

On tooth 54 the temporary glass-ionomer was removed with a bur and caries removal in dentin was completed manually (**Fig. 26.8**). In the same session a fissure sealant was applied onto the occlusal surface of tooth 16 (**Fig. 26.9**), which presented an active noncavitated caries lesion scored as ICDAS 1 (more clearly visible in the distal fissure). The decision for sealing this occlusal surface was based not only on the presence of general risk factors for caries progression, but also because the surface was persistently covered by dental biofilm. As the lower permanent first molar was not erupted, the occlusal surface of the antagonist would remain without masticatory attri-

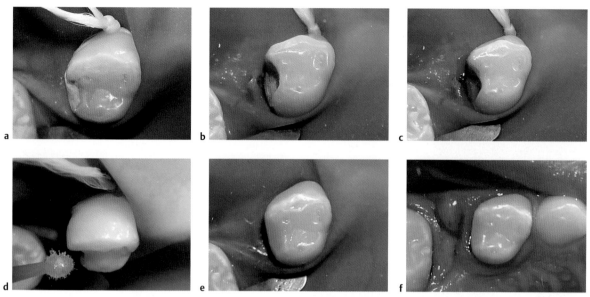

Fig. 26.8a–f Tooth 54 after rubber dam placement (**a**); the temporary filling was removed by bur and the carious dentin was removed by hand excavation (**b**); acid etching with H_3PO_4 (**c**); adhesive application (**d**); composite restoration finished (**e**); clinical aspect directly after rubber dam removal (**f**).

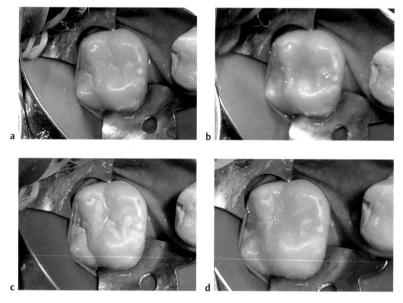

Fig. 26.9a–d Tooth 16 after rubber dam placement. The active caries lesion (ICDAS 1) is more clearly visualized in the distal fossa (**a**); acid etching with H_3PO_4 (**b**); aspect after etching (**c**); fissure sealant light cured (**d**).

tion and therefore susceptible to plaque stagnation for a considerable period of time. Due to the low compliance with brushing in the past, the fissure was referred to sealing rather than cross brushing or fluoridation only.

Clinical Aspect at the End of the Treatment (Fig. 26.10)

Follow-up

Ten months after the end of the treatment no clinical signs of new caries lesions were detected. Instructions for oral hygiene were reinforced, emphasizing the importance of cleaning the occlusal surface of the permanent first molars, with their being partially erupted. Follow-up radiographs were obtained to monitor the infiltrated approximal lesions after 10 months. No caries progression was detected (**Fig. 26.11**). Regarding the management of space loss in the upper arch, the patient continued to be under the surveillance of the orthodontic clinic. The orthodontist was waiting for the upper permanent molars to erupt more, before inserting any orthodontic appliance.

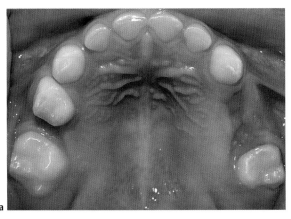
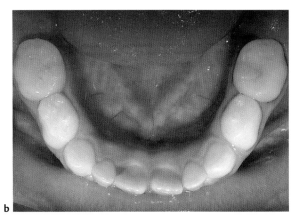

Fig. 26.10a, b Final clinical aspect of the upper (**a**) and lower (**b**) jaws at the end of the treatment.

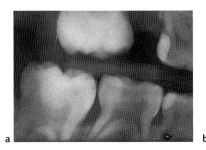
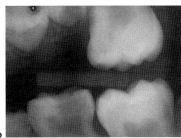

Fig. 26.11a, b After 10 months, follow-up radiographs showed no progression of the infiltrated approximal lesions in the mesial surface of tooth 85 (**a**) or in the distal surface of tooth 74 and mesial surface of tooth 75 (**b**).

Case 2: A 7-Year-Old Girl with Medium Caries Risk

Vera Mendes Soviero, Soraya Coelho Leal

Anamnesis

Gender: female
Age: 7 years old
First visit: August 2010
Last visit: September 2010
Follow-up visit: June 2011

The patient came to the pediatric dental clinic for a routine visit. She first visited the dentist when she was 4 years old, and at that time had some of her primary molars filled under local anesthesia. She has never experienced tooth pain. Her last visit to the dentist was 2 years ago when a dental examination and a topical fluoride gel application were performed. Dental radiographs had never been performed. No relevant general medical information was reported by the mother.

Clinical Findings (Tooth Level)

Oral examination showed mixed dentition, with the permanent first molars and the permanent central incisors partially erupted and healthy soft tissues (**Fig. 26.12**).

Caries detection was based on visual–tactile examination complemented by bitewing radiographs. Clinically, the distal surface of tooth 84 revealed a cavity (ICDAS 5). For the distal and mesial surfaces of tooth 85 and the distal surface of tooth 74, approximal caries lesions were detected radiographically (**Fig. 26.13**). Tooth 85 had an enamel lesion scored as E1 in both the mesial and distal surfaces. Tooth 74 distal showed a dentinal lesion (D1).

The occlusal surfaces of the primary first molars (54, 64, 74, 84) had been restored with composite when the child was 4 years old. The primary second molars (55, 65, 75, 85) had occlusal fissure sealant. The permanent first molars showed no signs of early caries lesions. The lower permanent first molars were almost fully erupted, but the upper ones were partially erupted. The d_1ft count was 5 and D_1MFT was 0 (**Fig. 26.14**).

Caries Risk Assessment (Individual Level)

Medium consumption of sweetened food (up to three times a day) and low consumption of sweetened beverages was reported by the mother. Visible dental biofilm was present in 56% of the approximal sites and on the occlusal surfaces of the erupting permanent first molars (**Fig. 26.15**). For the API index, the plaque was assessed visually in the approximal sites without using disclosing dye. When there was no visible plaque in the entrance of the approximal site, a probe was used to confirm the absence/presence of plaque.

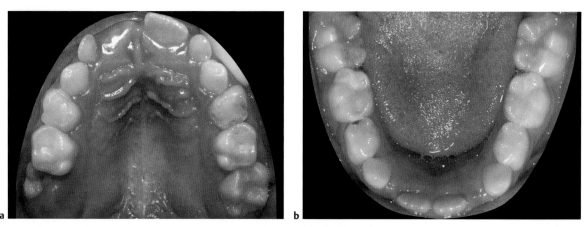

Fig. 26.12a, b   Clinical aspect of the upper arch (**a**) and lower arch (**b**) at the first visit.

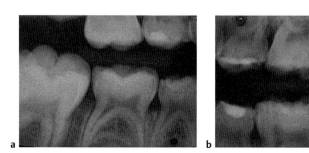

Fig. 26.13a, b   Initial right (**a**) and left (**b**) bitewing radiographs.

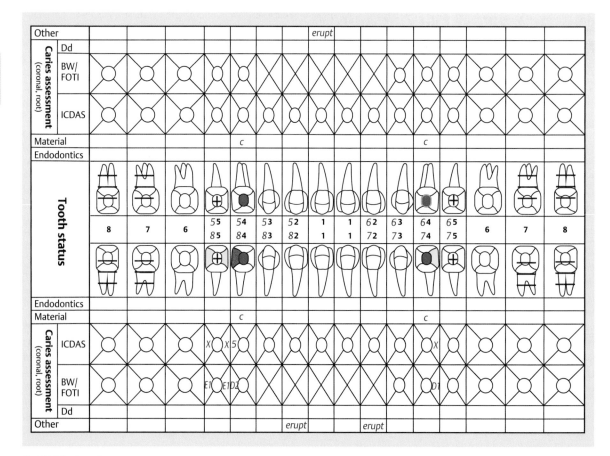

Fig. 26.14   Dental status

The family had access to fluoridated water and the child usually had her teeth brushed with fluoride toothpaste three times a day. Tooth brushing before bedtime was assisted by the mother occasionally. Dental floss had never been used. Although the patient had a relatively high caries experience ($d_1ft = 5$), other risk factors such as sugar consumption were less severe. Besides, she had regular access to fluoride sources, did not use any medications, and had normal salivary flow. According to the current status the patient was classified as low-to-medium risk (33%), but had been at higher risk for caries in earlier years.

Diagnosis and Treatment Plan

The main concern in the present case was to control caries, avoiding invasive treatments as much as possible, and keeping in mind that restorations do not control the carious process by themselves.

Individual Level

Oral Hygiene and Fluoride

Oral hygiene instructions focused on two main aspects: dental flossing and plaque control on the occlusal surface of the permanent first molars, with their being partially erupted. As no signs of initial caries lesions were detected, it was decided not to seal the occlusal surface of the permanent first molars. Besides, the patient and her mother seemed to be motivated to improve oral hygiene. The habit of having her teeth brushed three times a day could be kept, but one of them should be prioritized to ensure proper plaque control at least once a day. The mother was asked to assist the child during the tooth cleaning at bedtime more often, especially with flossing. It was suggested to floss once a day. Regular use of fluoride toothpaste was recommended (1000–1500 ppm F), but no other home-use fluoride was prescribed. One topical professional application of neutral fluoride gel was performed in the whole mouth.

CLINICAL PEARL

Individualize your oral hygiene instructions. Be sure that the mother understands why some tooth surfaces are being prioritized at this moment. If the patient understands clearly why he/she is being asked to do something, the chance of a good compliance is increased.

Dietary Counseling The association between sugar consumption and caries development was explained to the child and her mother. However, exhaustive recommendation to modify dietary habits was avoided, because diet was not the main risk factor for this patient.

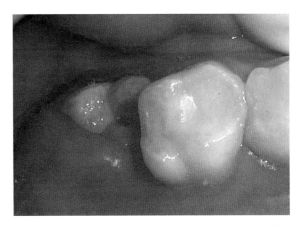

Fig. 26.15 Erupting upper permanent first molar with thick plaque.

Tooth Level

CLINICAL PEARL

Commend the patient for the good habits and make suggestions to change only what is really necessary to change.

Treatment decisions at the tooth surface level are summarized in the treatment plan (**Table 26.2**).

The restorations in teeth 54, 64, 74, and 84 were sufficient, no repair/replacement was necessary. However, restoration in tooth 64 was referred for particular surveillance because a slight radiolucency beneath the composite was detected in the radiography (see **Fig. 26.13b**) and discolored margins were visible clinically (Restauratio insufficienta initialis). In spite of that, it was not replaced because no signs of active lesion were detected along the margins of the restoration and the patient had no complaint of pain or any other discomfort.

CLINICAL PEARL

Before deciding to replace a restoration, stop and think if there is a very good reason to do that. For primary teeth, always take into consideration how much time the tooth will be in the mouth up to exfoliation.

Tooth 84 had an obvious cavity at the distal surface (diagnosis: Caries progressiva profunda). Carious tissue was accessed using a bur and the soft dentin was removed by hand excavation. After caries removal in tooth 84, a cavity was confirmed for the mesial surface of tooth 85, as well (**Fig. 26.16c**). It was "cleaned" by hand excavation, preserving the marginal crista. Both cavities were filled with composite (**Fig. 26.16a–f**).

Table 26.2 Diagnoses and treatments at a glance

Diagnosis	Caries	Caries non-progressiva (CNP)		Caries progressiva superficialis (CS)			Caries progressiva media (CM) et profunda (CP)		
	Restorations	Restauratio insufficienta initialis (RII)		Restauratio insufficienta partialis (RIP)			Restauratio insufficienta totalis (RIT)		
	Sound surfaces	–		Sanus majoris periculi (SMP)			–		
"Treatment"		Particular surveillance		Noninvasive or microinvasive/repair			(Minimally) invasive		
		Tooth + Surface	Diagnosis	Tooth + Surface	Diagnosis	Therapy	Tooth + Surface	Diagnosis	Therapy
		64 o	RII	74 d	CS	INF ✔	84 od	CP	FC ✔
				85 d	CS	LF + OH ✔	85 m*	CM	FC ✔
				LF local fluoridation OH local oral hygiene training INF caries infiltration			FC composite filling		

*Diagnosed during treatment of tooth 84.

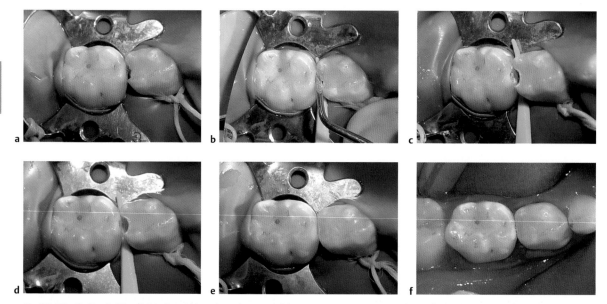

Fig. 26.16a–f Teeth 85 and 84 after rubber dam placement (**a**); removal of carious dentin by hand excavation (**b**); a cavity was confirmed in the mesial surface of tooth 85 (**c**); conservative prep- arations, preserving the marginal crista of tooth 85 (**d**); composite restorations finished (**e**); clinical aspect of the composite restora- tions immediately after removing the rubber dam (**f**).

CLINICAL PEARL

The chance of arresting a cavitated caries lesion in a approximal surface which is in contact with the adjacent tooth is in most cases not to be expected. Cavities in approximal surfaces must be restored.

Noncavitated caries lesions were detected on the bitewing radiographs for the distal surfaces of tooth 74 (D1) and tooth 85 (E1) (see **Fig. 26.13a, b**), and both were diag- nosed as Caries progressiva superficialis, although posi- tive clinical activity status was only based on increased local plaque stagnation. For the approximal lesion classi- fied as E1, the treatment decision was the application of

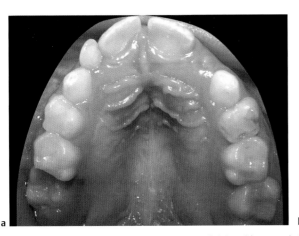
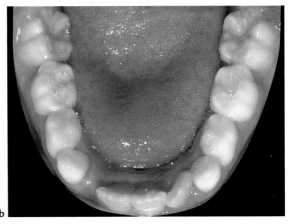

a   b

Fig. 26.17a, b   Clinical aspect of the upper arch (**a**) and lower arch (**b**) after 6 months.

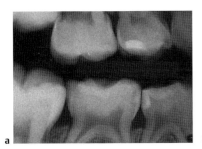
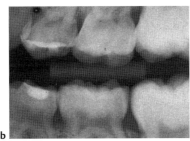

a   b

Fig. 26.18a, b   Follow up right (**a**) and left (**b**) bitewing radiographs after 9 months.

topical fluoride and instruction for daily flossing. One topical application of neutral fluoride gel was performed using dental floss to ensure wetting of the approximal surfaces with the fluoride gel. The D1 lesion on 74 distal was treated by the infiltration technique. As the patient was classified as being of low caries risk in the future, it was decided to infiltrate only the approximal lesion that had reached the dentin.

Follow-up

Nine months after the end of the treatment phase, follow-up interproximal radiographs were performed to monitor the approximal caries lesions treated by noninvasive or microinvasive treatment. No caries progression and no signs of new caries lesions were detected clinically (**Fig. 26.17**) or radiographically (**Fig. 26.18**). Instructions for daily flossing were reinforced. Ectopic eruption of tooth 16 was detected. Tooth separation was the first attempt to solve the problem. The patient continued to be under surveillance.

Case 3: A 6-Year-Old Girl with Very High Caries Risk

Vera Mendes Soviero, Soraya Coelho Leal

Anamnesis

Gender: female
Age: 6 years
First visit: September 2010
Last visit: December 2010
Follow-up visit: June 2011

The patient came to the pediatric dental clinic complaining of tooth pain. It was her first experience in a dental chair. During anamnesis the mother reported that the child suffered from complications related to gastro-esophageal reflux disease (GERD), being mainly chronic respiratory disease and failure to gain weight properly. Ranitidine and meprazole were used orally to relieve the symptoms of GERD. In the last year, due to repeated respiratory infections, antibiotics were used three times.

Clinical Findings (Tooth Level)

Dental examination showed initial mixed dentition with the lower permanent first molars erupted and healthy soft tissues. Extensive carious lesions were clearly visible (**Fig. 26.19**).

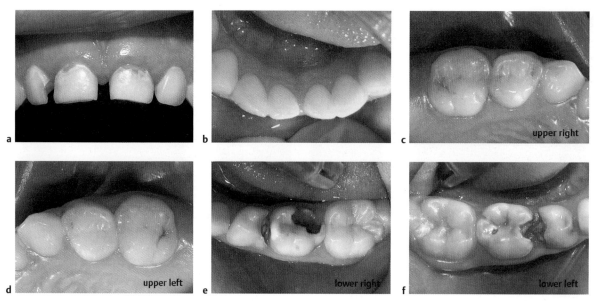

Fig. 26.19a–f Clinical aspect of the upper incisors (**a**), lower incisors (**b**), upper right molars (**c**), upper left molars (**d**), lower right molars (**e**), and lower left molars (**f**) at the first visit.

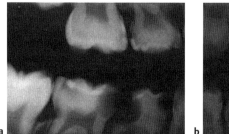 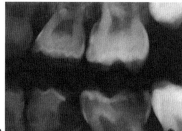

Fig. 26.20a, b Initial right (**a**) and left (**b**) bitewing radiographs. Details see Fig. 26.22.

Caries detection was based on visual–tactile examination combined with bitewing radiographs (**Fig. 26.20**). For the teeth with extensive cavities, radiographs including the periapical area were performed to support an eventual treatment decision between extraction or pulp therapy (**Fig. 26.21**). Active caries lesions at different stages were detected in primary and permanent teeth. Only the lower primary incisors were free of caries lesions.

The lower molars and the upper incisors had obvious cavities clinically scored as ICDAS 5 or 6 (**Figs. 26.19a, e, f**). The occlusal surfaces of teeth 54 and 65 also had cavitated caries lesions scored as ICDAS 5 (**Fig. 26.19c, d**).

ICDAS 4 was assigned to the mesial surface of tooth 55 and to the distal surface of tooth 54, which were confirmed radiographically as D2 caries lesions (**Fig. 26.19c** and **Fig. 26.20a**). More shallow approximal caries lesions were detected in the primary teeth radiographically (**Fig. 26.20a, b**). The presence or absence of cavitation was confirmed clinically after immediate tooth separation. ICDAS 1 was assigned to the occlusal surface of tooth 36 and to the occlusal and buccal surfaces of tooth 46 (see **Fig. 26.25b, f**).

The d_1ft count was 16 and the D_1MFT count was 2. Detailed information about each tooth surface is available in the dental examination form (**Fig. 26.22**).

Caries Risk Assessment (Individual Level)

High consumption of sugar was reported by the mother. The child usually had sweetened food and beverages four- or five-times a day. In addition, the patient had to use medicine for GERD regularly, and used antibiotics for respiratory infections quite frequently. Besides, many of these medicines for children contain sugar and must be taken three-to-four times/day, sometimes for 2–3 weeks. This whole situation contributed to an increase in the caries risk.

The family lived in an area with fluoridated water and the child usually had her teeth brushed once a day with fluoride toothpaste. According to the mother, tooth brushing was not easy because the child was often complaining of pain and gingival bleeding when brushing. She had never used dental floss and tooth brushing was not assisted by an adult. Visible dental biofilm was present in

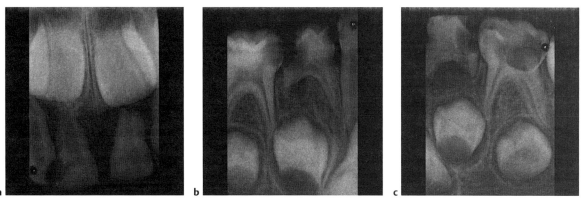

Fig. 26.21 a–c   Periapical radiographs of upper incisors (**a**), right lower molars (**b**), and left lower molars (**c**).

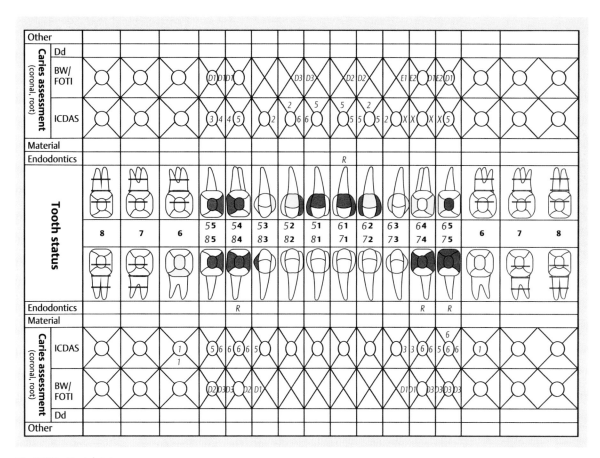

Fig. 26.22   Dental status

90% of the interproximal sites (API index) and also in the occlusal surface of the lower permanent first molars.

The most relevant risk factors for caries development and progression were high caries experience ($d_1ft = 16 / D_1MFT = 2$), high frequency of sugar consumption, and poor oral hygiene. Because of recurrent health problems, oral care was often neglected. The patient was classified as being of high risk to develop caries lesions.

CLINICAL PEARL

When a child is often ill, usually the mother tends to neglect oral hygiene because she is more concerned about the medical problems.

Table 26.3 Diagnoses and treatments at a glance

Diagnosis	Caries	Caries non-progressiva (CNP)		Caries progressiva superficialis (CS)			Caries progressiva media (CM) et profunda (CP)		
	Restorations	Restauratio insufficienta initialis (RII)		Restauratio insufficienta partialis (RIP)			Restauratio insufficienta totalis (RIT)		
	Sound surfaces	–		Sanus majoris periculi (SMP)			–		
"Treatment"		Particular surveillance		Noninvasive or microinvasive/repair			(Minimally) invasive		
		Tooth + Surface	Diagnosis	Tooth + Surface	Diagnosis	Therapy	Tooth + Surface	Diagnosis	Therapy
				55 o	CS	FS ✔	55 m	CM	FC ✔
				63 m/d	CS	LF + OH ✔	54 od	CM	FC ✔
				64 m	CS	LF + OH ✔	52 m	CP	FC ✔
				73 d	CS	LF + OH ✔	51 bd	CP	FC ✔
				64 d*	CS	INF	61#	CM	EX ✔
				65 m*	CS	LF + OH	62 md	CM	FC ✔
							65 o	CM	FC ✔
							75	CP	EX ✔
							74	CP	EX ✔
							83 d	CM	FC ✔
							84	CP	EX ✔
							85 mo	CP	PT/FC ✔
				LF local fluoridation OH local oral hygiene training FS fissure sealing INF caries infiltration			FC composite filling EX extraction PT pulpotomy		

*The first diagnoses were changed to Caries progressiva media during the initial treatment phase, and composite fillings werde placed.
Extraction was indicated due to trauma, not caries.

Diagnosis and Treatment Plan

After a comprehensive examination and caries risk assessment, treatments were planned at two levels: the individual level and the tooth/surface level based on the diagnoses. The main goal was to motivate the patient/parents to improve oral care at home so that the high caries risk could be controlled. It was necessary to improve oral hygiene and to reduce sugar consumption. In addition, noninvasive or invasive strategies were planned according to the diagnoses at the tooth surface level.

Individual Level

Oral hygiene and Fluoride

The patient was instructed to have her teeth brushed twice daily with regular fluoride toothpaste. No additional home-use fluoride product was prescribed. Regular topical applications of highly concentrated fluoride products were planned for the whole mouth.

The mother was asked to assist her child with tooth brushing once a day. To facilitate oral hygiene at home, teeth with extensive cavities were prioritized in the treatment plan at the tooth surface level. Two main aspects were emphasized during oral hygiene instructions: the occlusal surfaces of the permanent first molars should be brushed first and flossing was thought of as being very important for the success of the restorative treatment in the primary teeth. Flossing was recommended once a day.

Dietary Counseling The correlation between the cariogenic potential of dental plaque and high frequency of sugar consumption was explained to the patient and parents. It was suggested to reduce the consumption of sweetened food and beverages, particularly during the weekdays, and to replace sweetened snacks for healthier food. Particular attention should be given to tooth cleaning whenever a sweetened medicine was in use.

Tooth level

Treatment was planned to achieve two main goals: relieve pain and facilitate oral hygiene at home. Pulp therapy and extractions were planned first, followed by sealants and restorations. Diagnoses and treatment decisions were based on lesion severity and activity (**Table 26.3**).

Tooth 85 had deep caries lesions and history of pain from cold stimulus (Caries progressiva profunda, irreversible pulpitis). Pulp was exposed as soon as the caries dentin started to be removed by hand excavation. A pulpotomy with calcium hydroxide was performed, followed by a composite restoration (**Fig. 26.23**).

The extensively carious primary molars 75, 74, and 84 were extracted. Teeth 84 and 74 had extensive periapical radiolucencies and advanced root reabsorption and were undoubtedly indicated for extraction (**Fig. 26.24b, e**). The crown on tooth 75 had been extensively destroyed and caries was reaching the root cement in some areas, making the placement of a restoration or even a stainless steel crown rather complicated (**Fig. 26.24b**; Caries progressiva profunda). A lingual arch was inserted as a space maintainer in the lower arch (**Fig. 26.24a–g**).

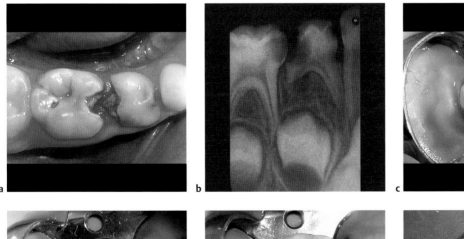
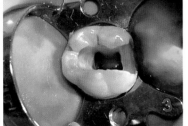
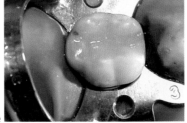
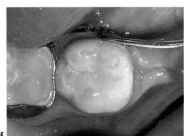

Fig. 26.23a–f Clinical appearance of deep caries in tooth 85 (**a**); bitewing radiographs showing that the carious lesions reached the mesial pulp horn (**b**); exposition of the pulp occurred in the beginning of dentin excavation (**c**); pulp camber after pulp amputation (**d**); resin restoration placed after calcium hydroxide pulpotomy (**e**); clinical aspect of the resin restoration after 6 months (**f**).

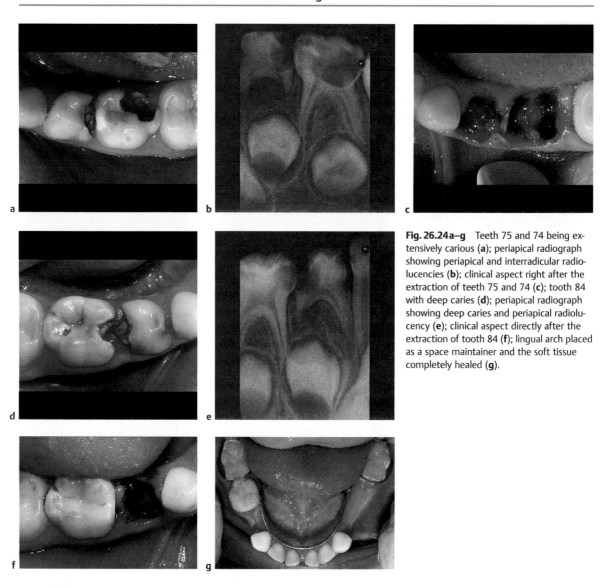

Fig. 26.24a–g Teeth 75 and 74 being extensively carious (**a**); periapical radiograph showing periapical and interradicular radiolucencies (**b**); clinical aspect right after the extraction of teeth 75 and 74 (**c**); tooth 84 with deep caries (**d**); periapical radiograph showing deep caries and periapical radiolucency (**e**); clinical aspect directly after the extraction of tooth 84 (**f**); lingual arch placed as a space maintainer and the soft tissue completely healed (**g**).

Although a significant improvement in the tooth cleaning was noticed, the occlusal surfaces of the permanent first molars were sealed (**Fig. 26.25a–h**), because the initial enamel caries were considered at high risk of progression (Caries progressiva superficialis). Moreover, the upper permanent first molars had not erupted and, in the absence of masticatory attrition, the occlusal surfaces of the lower molars were susceptible areas for plaque stagnation.

The upper primary molars were the next teeth to be treated. The distal surface of tooth 54 (**Fig. 26.26c**) and the mesial surface of tooth 55 (**Fig. 26.26b**) were clearly cavitated, as evident after placing a rubber dam and inserting a wedge. This was not surprising, since both approximal caries lesions had been scored as D1 (see **Fig. 26.20a**). In the occlusal surface of tooth 54, the mesial part of the fissure was cavitated (diagnoses of all surfaces: Caries progressiva media). Minimally invasive cavity preparations were performed and the teeth were filled with composite. The distal fissure of the occlusal surface of tooth 55, although scored as ICDAS 3, was sealed; no radiolucency (Caries progressiva superficialis; **Fig. 26.26a–i**).

On the left side, the approximal lesions in teeth 65 and 64 were not so deep radiologically (E2 and D1, respectively; see **Fig. 26.20b**). Therefore, it was initially assumed that these might be treated non- or microinvasively (Caries progressiva superficialis). However, after the immediate separation with a wedge (**Fig. 26.27b, c**), the presence of cavitation was confirmed in both approximal surfaces, and the diagnoses were changed to Caries progressiva media. Minimally invasive preparations were performed and the teeth were filled with composite (**Fig. 26.27a–i**).

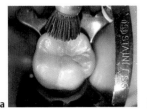
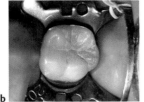
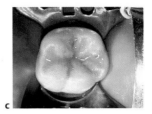
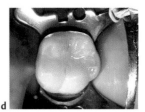

Fig. 26.25a–d   Tooth 36 after rubber dam placement (**a**); after plaque removal and drying the initial enamel lesion is more easily visualized (**b**); acid etching with phosphoric acid (**c**); fissure sealant light cured (**d**).

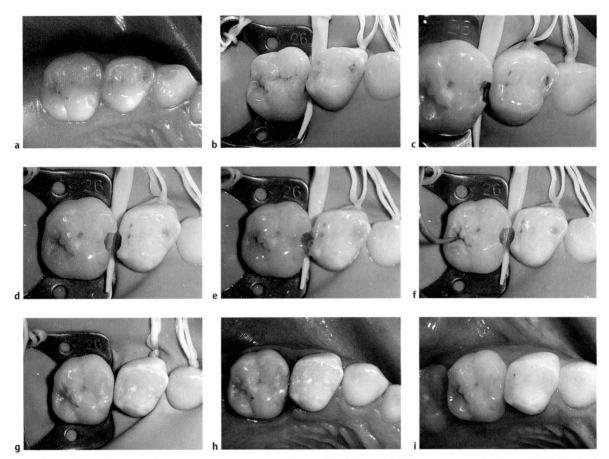

Fig. 26.26a–i   Clinical aspect of teeth 55 and 54 (**a**); a cavity is visible in the mesial surface of tooth 55 (**b**) and in the distal and occlusal (mesial fossa) surfaces of tooth 54 (**c**) after immediate tooth separation; conservative preparations (**d**); acid etching with phosphoric acid (**e**); fissure sealant application in the distal occlusal fossa of tooth 55 (**f**); resin restorations finished (**g**); clinical aspect directly after rubber dam removal (**h**); resin restorations after 5 months (**i**).

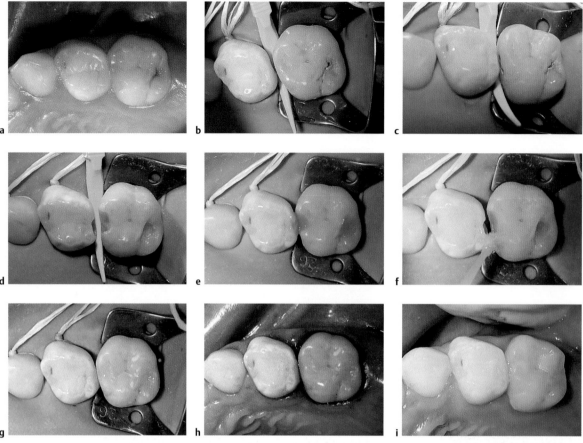

Fig. 26.27 a–i Clinical aspect of teeth 65 and 64 (**a**); space between teeth is visible around 30 seconds after inserting the wedge (**b**); a cavity is visible in the mesial surface of tooth 55 (**c**); minimally invasive preparations (**d**); acid etching with phosphoric acid (**e**); adhesive application (**f**); resin restorations finished (**g**); clinical aspect right after rubber dam removal (**h**); resin restorations after 5 months (**i**).

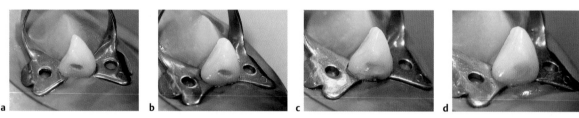

Fig. 26.28 a–d Dentin cavity in the distal surface of tooth 83 (**a**); after the removal of soft dentin by hand excavation (**b**); acid etching with phosphoric acid (**c**); the finished resin restoration (**d**).

CLINICAL PEARL

Direct visual examination of approximal surfaces can be done after tooth separation. Rubber rings can be used to mediate tooth separation, but at least two days are necessary until enough space is obtained. Immediate separation with a wedge can be performed in the same session, particularly if another surface of the tooth has to be restored anyway (e.g., the occlusal surface). Then, the wedge can be inserted after local anesthesia and rubber dam placement.

The distal surface of tooth 83, which showed a cavity into dentin (ICDAS 5; diagnosis: Caries progressiva media), was filled with composite after the removal of soft dentin by hand excavation (**Fig. 26.28**). Although the distal surface of tooth 73 had an enamel discontinuity (ICDAS 3), it was not filled (Caries progressiva superficialis). After the extraction of tooth 74 this tooth surface would be continuously exposed to saliva and easily accessed by the toothbrush. Thus, we believed that this caries lesion would most probably be arrested without micro- or minimally invasive interventions.

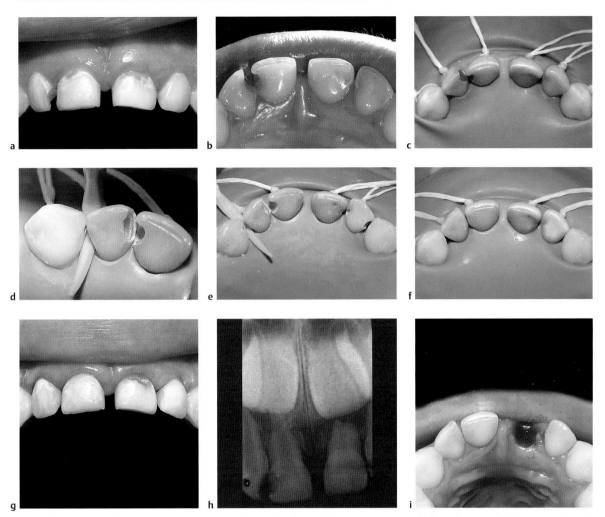

Fig. 26.29a–i Initial clinical aspect of the buccal surfaces (**a**) and lingual surfaces (**b**) of the upper incisors; after rubber dam placement (**c**); a cavity was confirmed in the mesial surface of tooth 53 after tooth separation (**d**); preparations after caries removal mainly by hand excavation (**e**); resin restorations finished (**f**); clinical aspect of the resin restorations by buccal view, tooth 61 was not restored because it was indicated for extraction (**g**); periapical radiograph showing periapical radiolucency and pathological root reabsorption of tooth 61 due to trauma (**h**); clinical aspect directly after the extraction of tooth 61 (**i**).

Finally, the upper anterior teeth were treated (diagnoses: Caries progressiva media et profunda). As many other invasive procedures were necessary, the treatment of these teeth was left to the end, because the local anesthesia in this region is known as being relatively uncomfortable for the patient. Tooth 61 was indicated for extraction (Caries progressiva media) because a significant periapical radiolucency and pathological root reabsorption (consequences of a previous trauma) were detected on the radiograph (**Fig. 26.29h**). The rubber dam was placed from tooth 53 to tooth 63. The frank cavities in teeth 52, 51, and 62 were cleaned by hand excavation to remove only the most demineralized and infected dentin, taking care not to expose the pulp. The cavities of the distal surface of tooth 52 and the mesial surface of tooth 53 (confirmed after tooth separation) (**Fig. 26.29 d**) were accessed by a bur. After the placement of the composite fillings, tooth 61 was extracted (**Fig. 26.29a–i**).

CLINICAL PEARL

Partial removal of carious dentin may be less deleterious to the pulp than vigorous excavation. Infectious dentin left in the bottom of the cavity does not seem to be harmful for the pulp. Once sealed by the restoration, the lesion will be arrested.

Clinical Aspect at the End of the Treatment (Fig. 26.30)

Follow-up

The patient was called for a follow-up examination 6 months after the end of the treatment period. Clinically, no signs of new caries lesions were detected. The patient and her parents were much more motivated toward oral

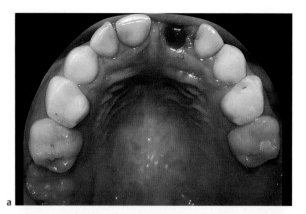

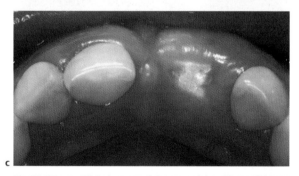

Fig. 26.30a–c   Clinical aspect of the upper (**a**) and lower (**b**) jaws (space retainer) at the end of the treatment period; one month after the extraction of tooth 61, soft tissues were completely healed (**c**).

care than they had been at the first visit. Oral hygiene instructions were reinforced and the patient was commended for her good habits related to oral health. Another interval of 6 months was planned up to the next follow-up visit.

Case 4: An 8-Year-Old Boy with Medium Caries Risk

Mohammad Alkilzy and Christian Splieth

Anamnesis

Gender: male
Age: 8 years
First visit: August 2010
Last visit: October 2010
Follow-up visits: January 2011, April 2011

A healthy, 8-year-old, left-handed boy visited the dental clinic for the semi-annual recall. No relevant general medical information was reported by the mother.

General Findings

Clinical oral examination revealed healthy oral mucosa and tongue. In the mixed dentition, the permanent central lower incisors and permanent first molars had already erupted (**Fig. 26.31**).

Oral Health Indices

Before dental examination is performed, the indices of oral health should be obtained. In younger children, the Quigley Hein Index (QHI) is a useful plaque index. The QHI reflects how much plaque covers the smooth tooth surfaces on a scale from 0 to 5. In older children and adolescents, the Approximal Plaque Index (API) concentrates on the approximal aspect of oral hygiene. This index indicates parent's ability to brush their child's teeth and the use of dental floss. The modified Periodontal Bleeding Index (mPBI) is an easy, dichotomized gingival index that calculates the percentage of positive sites for bleeding on probing; the Periodontal Screening Index (PSI) can document early, destructive forms of periodontitis (**Table 26.4, Fig. 26.32**).

CLINICAL PEARL

Oral health indices are standard parameters to evaluate the recent oral health status and to control the improvement of the patient's oral health. Plaque disclosers help to train and motivate patient and parents for improvement in oral hygiene.

Clinical Findings (Tooth Level)

Plaque removal is important for accurate caries detection and assessment. This can be achieved by professional tooth cleaning with a rotating brush bearing toothpaste, polishing paste, or fluoride gel (**Fig. 26.33**). Interproximal plaque should be removed by flossing.

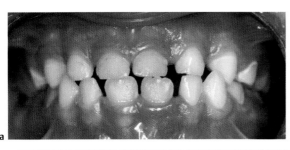

Fig. 26.31 a–c Early phase of mixed dentition, frontal view: eruption of the lower permanent central incisors.
a Healthy gingiva.
b Lower jaw and healthy mouth floor.
c Upper jaw with healthy hard and soft palate.

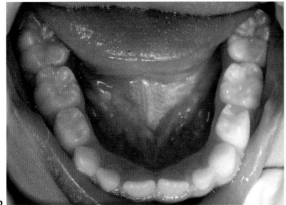

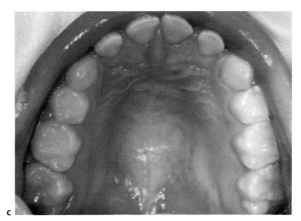

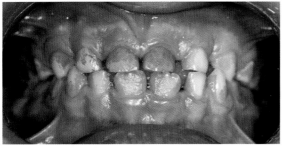

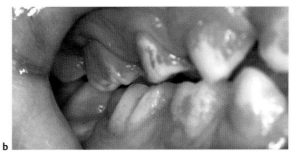

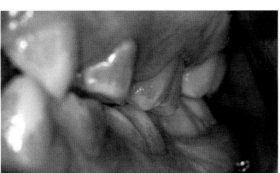

Fig. 26.32 a–c Dental plaque disclosed with Mira-Ton (Hager & Werken): most surfaces colored in pink which indicates 1–2-day-old plaque; very thin line adjacent to gingiva on a few teeth such as 53 and 61 is colored with purple indicating plaque which is more than 2 days old.

Table 26.4 Plaque, gingival and periodontal indices in an 8-year-old boy

Approximal Plaque Index	40%	Periodontal Screening Index (PSI)		
		Teeth	16	11	26
Modified Periodontal Bleeding Index	5%	PSI value	1	0	1
Quigley Hein Index	2	Teeth	46	31	36
		PSI value	1	0	1

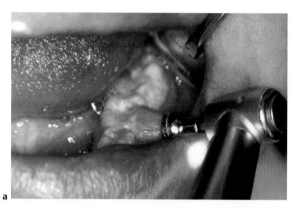
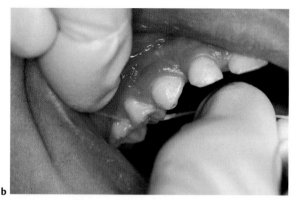

Fig. 26.33a, b Professional tooth cleaning with a brush and paste (**a**), and interproximal flossing (**b**).

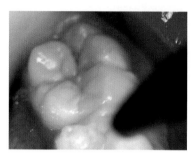
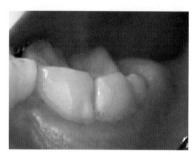
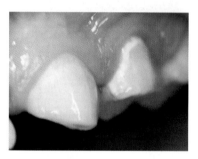

Fig. 26.34   Brown fissures (ICDAS 2) and dark brown localized minimal enamel breakdown in the distal pit of tooth 36 (ICDAS 3).

Fig. 26.35   Enamel hypoplasia in the vestibular fissure of tooth 36 appears chalky and yellow, with clear borders to healthy enamel.

Fig. 26.36   A clearly inactive lesion (shiny) situated 1–2 mm away from the gingiva in the vestibular surface of tooth 63 can be seen, while the lesion on tooth 64 seems be active (both ICDAS 2).

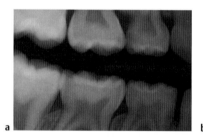
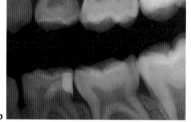

Fig. 26.37a, b   Bitewing radiographs of an 8-year-old boy: Stage D1 caries lesion in the distal surface of tooth 54; note the pulp reaction by the formation of tertiary dentin in the pulp chamber (**a**), and the E2 caries lesion in the mesial surface of tooth 75 (**b**). Stage D1 lesions were also assessed for 64 d and 84 d.

CLINICAL PEARL

Clinical caries detection is a complex, important procedure which needs knowledge about the kinetics (pathology) of dental caries. The use of magnification and drying of the teeth may help to detect initial caries lesions and determine their appearance. Sufficient time should be given and probing the lesion should be avoided to prevent the destruction of the demineralized enamel of initial lesions.

Noncavitated caries lesions were detected in three surfaces clinically. The buccal surfaces of teeth 53, 63, and 64 were scored as ICDAS 2. For the occlusal surface of tooth 36 a caries lesion scored as ICDAS 3 was detected (**Fig. 26.34**) and, buccally, hypomineralized enamel was observed (**Fig. 26.35**). The caries lesions in 36 occlusally and 64 buccally were considered as being active (opaque, dull, and rough on probing) (**Fig. 26.36**).

Tooth 74 (buccal, occlusal, and distal surfaces) had been restored by minimally invasive cavity preparation using glass-ionomer cement some months before. The $d_1$ft count was 5 and the D_1MFT count was 1.

Four approximal caries lesions were detected radiographically (**Fig. 26.37**) and classified as D1 (54 d, 64 d, 84 d) and E2 (75 m). For all these approximal areas plaque scores were high, but no papilla bleeding could be observed.

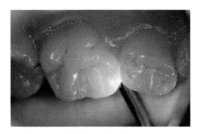
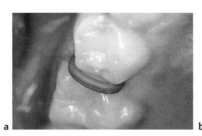
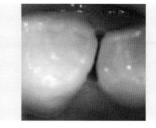

Fig. 26.38   Using FOTI on the interproximal area of teeth 54 and 55 revealed no alterations due to caries.

Fig. 26.39a, b   Separation ring being placed in the interproximal area between teeth 55 and 54 (**a**). After 3–4 days an interproximal space of ca. 1mm for visual and gentle tactile inspection of cavitation in a approximal lesion was gained (**b**).

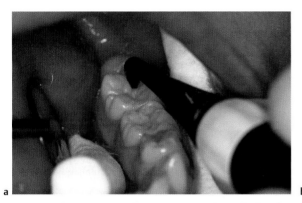
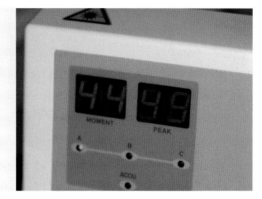

Fig 26.40a, b   Assessment of caries severity in the occlusal surface of tooth 36 using the head A for pits and fissures: DIAGNOdent showed high fluorescence in the distal pit.

CLINICAL PEARL

The detection of approximal caries lesions is enhanced by radiographs. It is reasonable to indicate baseline bitewings for children of 5 years of age, especially if risk factors for caries are present or active caries lesions are detected visually. Even in populations with low caries prevalence, around one-third of the 5-year-olds do have approximal caries which is not detectable by visual examination only (Chapter 21). However, exposure to x-rays must be reduced as much as possible and unnecessary radiographs must definitely be avoided.

Supplementary diagnostic tools were used to support the final diagnosis and then the treatment decision for the approximal caries lesions. On the distal part of tooth 54, no shadow which would indicate a moderately deep dentin lesion was detected by fiberoptic transillumination (FOTI) (**Fig. 26.38**). In addition, the absence of cavitation was confirmed after tooth separation (**Fig. 26.39**).

For the occlusal surface of tooth 36, the higher fluorescence assessed by DIAGNOdent indicated a more advanced demineralization (**Fig. 26.40**).

The dental chart summarizes all the detections and assessment which were performed for this patient with respect to caries and hypomineralized teeth (**Fig. 26.41**).

Caries Risk Assessment (Individual Level)

Caries experience ($d_1ft = 5 / D_1MFT = 1$) and plaque index ($API = 40\%$) as relevant factors for caries prediction were in the medium range. Although the patient was healthy, he had some impairment to movement in his right arm. He used an electric toothbrush once a day and a horizontal brushing technique. His parents controlled tooth brushing irregularly. He had regular access to fluorides (fluoride-reduced toothpaste [500 ppm], fluoridated table salt, and fluoride gel once a week). For the first two years in life he had taken fluoride tablets. His dietary habits were not highly cariogenic and included one snack or piece of chocolate per day, seldom juice, no soft drinks and three meals per day. Due to the evaluation of the determinants for caries risk, this patient showed a **medium caries risk**.

Diagnosis and Treatment Plan

Inactive lesions were supposed to be monitored further, whereas active caries lesions were either referred to noninvasive or microinvasive interventions. On the individual level the improvement of oral hygiene was in this case the main target.

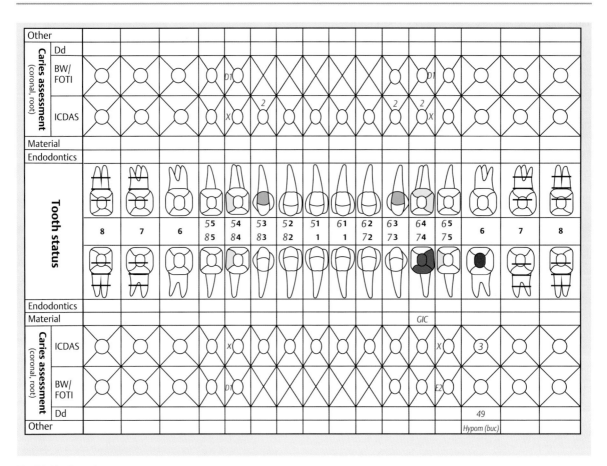

Fig. 26.41   Dental status

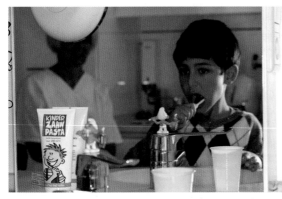

Fig. 26.42   Demonstration and control of tooth brushing by the dental hygienist.

Individual Level

Plaque removal: The clear presence of visible plaque calls for training in tooth brushing and flossing (**Fig. 26.42**). The tooth brushing frequency should be increased to twice per day under parents' supervision while the child is brushing his teeth. In addition, parents should help with difficult areas once per day, especially the permanent first molars.

Flossing once a day under parents' supervision or by the parents is recommended due to the approximal lesions.

Fluoride toothpaste plays a key role in caries prevention. Thus, the toothpaste for children with 500 ppm fluoride concentration should be replaced by fully fluoridated toothpaste of about 1400 ppm F at latest at an age of 6 years. In addition, higher concentrated fluoride gel should be used at home once per week.

Due to the unproblematic **diet**, no further changes were required. In light of the initial lesion on the occlusal aspect of tooth 36, preventive pit and fissure sealants might be considered for all permanent first and second molars, if adherence to noninvasive measures is suboptimal.

Tooth Level

Diagnoses and treatment decisions were based on lesion severity and activity (**Table 26.5**):

- Both buccal surfaces of teeth 53 and 63 were diagnosed as Caries non-progressiva, thus no current treatment was considered necessary.
- For those active noncavitated caries lesions being diagnosed as Caries progressiva superficialis, the generally increased plaque stagnation at the respective surfaces, being an indirect sign of activity, as well as the generally

Table 26.5 Diagnoses and treatments at a glance

Diagnosis	Caries	Caries non-progressiva (CNP)		Caries progressiva superficialis (CS)			Caries progressiva media (CM)		
	Restorations	Restauratio insufficienta initialis (RII)		Restauratio insufficienta partialis (RIP)			Restauratio insufficienta totalis (RIT)		
	Sound surfaces	–		Sanus majoris periculi (SMP)			–		
"Treatment"		Particular surveillance		Noninvasive or microinvasive/repair			(Minimally) invasive		
		Tooth + Surface	Diagnosis	Tooth + Surface	Diagnosis	Therapy	Tooth + Surface	Diagnosis	Therapy
		53 b	CNP	54 d	CS	INF ✔	36 o	CM	FC + FS ✔
		63 b	CNP	64 b	CS	LF + OH ✔			
				64 d	CS	INF ✔			
				75 m	CS	LF + OH ✔			
				84 d	CS	INF ✔			
				36 b	Hypo	FS ✔			
				LF local fluoridation OH local oral hygiene training INF caries infiltration FS fissure sealing			FS fissure sealing FC composite filling		

increased caries risk were taken into account for the decision. Treatments were:

- noninvasive intervention on tooth 64 buccally, with special attention to plaque removal and fluoride use
- noninvasive intervention on tooth 75 mesially (E2) by instruction to floss once a day.
- Caries infiltration of the approximal lesions (D1) at the distal surfaces of teeth 54, 64, and 84.
- Minimally invasive preparation of the distal pit of tooth 36 (localized enamel breakdown). Sealant application was performed here as well as onto the whole pit-and-fissures system including the hypomineralized buccal pit. The other (sound) permanent first molars were not sealed, but monitored.

Monitoring and Recall

An individual recall interval was established for this boy based on his caries risk. After initial controlling of the compliance for improving oral hygiene within the time span between initial visits, the primary recall interval was set at 3 months. With a clear reduction of the caries risk due to better plaque removal, the recalls might be adjusted to 6-month intervals.

Every recall consisted of the following procedures:
- Application of plaque discloser on all teeth
- Recording of plaque and gingival indices
- Motivation of child and parents for maintaining good oral hygiene.
- Instructions and control of tooth brushing by child and parents
- Professional tooth cleaning with subsequent application of high fluoride paste/gel
- Examination of the teeth
- New appointment for the next recall

The intervals between radiographic examinations should be determined individually based on future caries progression and general caries risk. For the presented case, the next appointment for bitewing x-rays will be after two years. Special attention should be given to monitoring the eruption of the permanent teeth and, if indicated, to adapt the tooth brushing technique, to apply topical fluorides, or sealants in pits and fissures.

Appendix

27

The following blank forms can be downloaded
free of charge using the following link:
http://mediacenter.thieme.com/

- Dental examination form
- Caries Risk Analysis
- Treatment plan

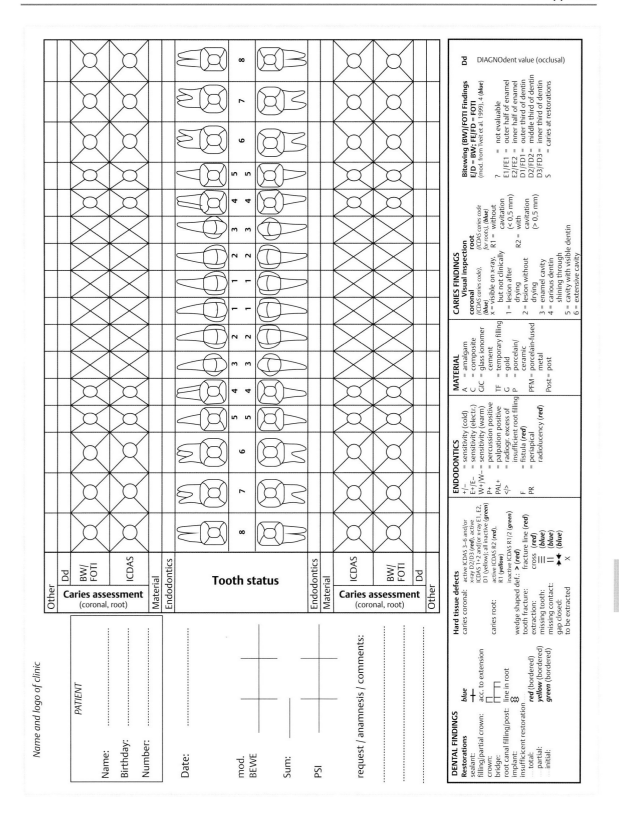

Name and logo of clinic

PATIENT

Name: ....

Birthday: ....

Number: ....

Date: ....

mod. BEWE

Sum:

PSI

request / anamnesis / comments:
....
....
....

Other		
Dd		
BW/FOTI		
Caries assessment (coronal, root)	ICDAS	
	Material	
	Endodontics	

Tooth status

	Endodontics	
Caries assessment (coronal, root)	Material	
	ICDAS	
	BW/FOTI	
	Dd	
	Other	

Tooth numbers shown: 8 7 6 5 4 3 2 1 | 1 2 3 4 5 6 7 8 (upper), 8 7 6 5 4 3 2 1 | 1 2 3 4 5 6 7 8 (lower)

DENTAL FINDINGS

Restorations   *blue*
sealant: ⌒   acc. to extension
filling/partial crown:
crown:
bridge:
root canal filling/post: line in root
implant:
insufficient restoration
...total: *red* (bordered)
...partial: *yellow* (bordered)
...initial: *green* (bordered)

Hard tissue defects
caries coronal: active ICDAS 3–6 and/or x-ray D2/D3 (*red*), active ICDAS 1+2 and/or x-ray E1, E2, D1 (yellow); all inactive (*green*)
caries root: active ICDAS R2 (*red*), R1 *yellow*
inactive ICDAS R1/2 (*green*)
wedge shaped def.: > (*red*)
tooth fracture: fracture line (*red*)
extraction: cross (*red*)
missing tooth: ꞊ (*blue*)
missing contact: ꞊꞊ (*blue*)
gap closed: ⤪ (*blue*)
to be extracted: ✕

ENDODONTICS
+/– = sensitivity (cold)
E+/E– = sensitivity (electr.)
W+/W– = sensitivity (warm)
P+ = percussion positive
PAL+ = palpation positive
</> = radiogr. excess of insufficient root filling
F = fistula (*red*)
PR = periapical radiolucency (*red*)

MATERIAL
A = amalgam
C = composite
GIC = glass ionomer cement
TF = temporary filling
G = gold
P = porcelain/ceramic
PFM = porcelain-fused metal
Post = post

CARIES FINDINGS
Visual inspection
coronal (*ICDAS caries code*), (*blue*)
x = visible on x-ray, but not clinically
1 = lesion after drying
2 = lesion without drying
3 = enamel cavity
4 = carious dentin shining through
5 = cavity with visible dentin
6 = extensive cavity

root (*ICDAS caries code for roots*), (*blue*)
R1 = without cavitation (< 0,5 mm)
R2 = with cavitation (> 0,5 mm)

Dd   DIAGNOdent value (occlusal)

Bitewing (BW)/FOTI Findings
E/D = BW: FE/FD = FOTI (mod. from Tveit et al. 1999), 4 (*blue*)
? = not evaluable
E1/FE1 = outer half of enamel
E2/FE2 = inner half of enamel
D1/FD1 = outer third of dentin
D2/FD2 = middle third of dentin
D3/FD3 = inner third of dentin
S = caries at restorations

Caries Risk Analysis

(Patient sticker)

Date: _____

                                                Risk value

1. Caries experience

DMFT: _____

$d_1mft + D_1MFT$: _____

0 = "caries free"	0
1 = better than average	9
2 = equal to average	11
3 = worse than average	13

2. Systemic diseases / Medication

_____

_____

0 = no relevant diseases / medication	0
1 = low influence on caries risk (e. g. Morbus Parkinson)	2
2 = high influence on caries risk (e. g. Dementia)	4

3. Nutrition (sugar)

	candies	sweetened beverages	cake
constant:	☐	☐	☐
seldom:	☐	☐	☐

0 = nearly no cariogenic diet	0
1 = balanced diet (seldom sugars)	5
2 = moderate cariogenic diet (occasional sugar)	13
3 = cariogenic diet (frequent sugar)	20

4. Nutrition (frequency)

Number of meals/snacks per day: _____

0 = up to 3 meals per day	0
1 = 4–5 meals per day	5
2 = 6–7 meals per day	13
3 = more than 7 meals per day	20

5. Oral hygiene

surfaces measured: ____

surfaces with plaque: ____

API: ____

0 = API < 5 %	0
1 = API 5 – 20 %	4
2 = API 21 – 50 %	8
3 = API > 50 %	15

6. Fluoride sources

_____

_____

0 = several sources on a regular basis	0
1 = several sources sporadically	5
2 = only one source	10
3 = no fluoride	50

7. Salivary flow

SSFR: _____ mL/min

0 = normal (> 1.1 mL/min)	0
1 = reduced (0.9 – 1.1 mL/min)	2
2 = low (0.5 – 0.9 mL/min)	5
3 = Xerostomia (< 0.5 mL/min)	40

Caries risk: 0% — 33% — 66% — 100%

Sum =
Caries risk (%)
maximum 100 %

Caries risk / Intervention	Low	Moderate	High
Examination	1 x yearly	2 x yearly	3–4 x yearly
Caries risk analysis	every 3–4 years	every 2 years	1 x yearly
Bitewing	> 3 years	every 2 years	1 x yearly
Diet counseling	on demand (items 3 and 4)		
Prof. tooth cleaning		on demand (item 5)	
Oral hygiene instruct.	on demand (item 5); if API > 50 % or PSI > 1: oral hygiene status!		
Fluoride varnishes	–	1 x yearly	2–4 x yearly
Saliva substitutes	–	–	if hyposalivation

Treatment plan

(Patient sticker)

Date: _____

Tooth level

Diagnosis	Caries	Caries non-progressiva (CNP)	Caries progressiva superficialis (CS)		Caries progressiva media (CM) et profunda (CP)		
	Restoration	Restauratio insufficienta initialis (RII)	Restauratio insufficienta partialis (RIP)		Restauratio insufficienta totalis (RIT)		
	Sound surfaces	–	Sanus majoris periculi (SMP)		–		
	"Treatment"	Particular surveillance	Noninvasive or microinvasive/repair		(Minimally) invasive		
		Tooth surface / Diagn. CNP	Tooth surface	Diagnosis	Therapy	Tooth surface	Diagnosis	Therapy

(Treatment rows with empty fields and checkboxes in Therapy columns)

CS abbreviations		CP abbreviations	
LF	local fluoridation	FC	composite filling
CB	cross brushing (molars)	FA	amalgam filling
OH	local oral hygiene training	GIC	glas-ionomer filling
FS	fissure sealing	I	inlay (G: gold; P: porcelain [ceramic])
INF	caries infiltration	PC	partial crown (G: gold; P: porcelain)
POL	polishing	C	full crown (G: gold; P: porcelain; PFM: porcelain-fused metal)
REP	repair	SW	stepwise excavation
		RCT	root canal treatment
		POST	post (G: gold; F: fiber)
		Ex	extraction
		!	examine adjacent surface during preparation

Patient level

Procedure	Date of diagnosis/intervention	Next diagnosis/intervention
General findings		
Risk analysis		
Bitewing		
Diet counseling		
Professional tooth cleaning		
Oral hygiene instruction		
Fluoride varnish		
Saliva substitutes		

405

Page numbers in *italics* refer to illustrations or tables

A

abrasion 125
  composite restorations 274, *274*
  prevalence 130
abscess 361
acetic acid 30
acid-etch technique 230
  dentin 209
  enamel 209
  sealant placement 230
  see also etching
acids
  cariogenic challenge 22, 30–32
    Stephan curve 30–32, *31*, *32*
  dental erosion 35–36, 59–61, *61*
  endogenous 35
  exogenous 35
acquired defects 125, 130
  see also abrasion; erosion
activity 295
  assessment 79–80, 137, 322
    caries adjacent to restorations 80
    coronal lesions 79, *79*, *80*, *81*
    root lesions 79–80, *81*
  predictive value 115–116, *115*, *116*
  therapeutic sealant placement
    232–233
  white spot lesions 42–43, *43*
adhesive technology 209
  adhesion–decalcification (AD) concept
    212, *212*
  adhesive classification 210, *211*
  bond degradation mechanisms 219
  clinical performance 220–221, *221*
  dentin bonding 209–221
    carious dentin 220
    obstacles 214, *214*
  enamel bonding strategies 212–214,
    213
  etch-and-rinse technique 210, *211*, *213*,
    214–215, 220, 221
    nanoleakage 217, *217*
    recent developments 217–218
    rewetting 216–217
    shortcomings 215–217, *215*
    wet bonding 216, *216*
  evolution 209–210
  glass-ionomers 210, *211*, 218, 220
  interaction with hydroxyapatite-based
    tissues 212, *212*
  self-etch adhesives 210, *211*, 212, 214,
    214, 218–219, 220
  see also sealants

adolescents
  acquired defects 130
  caries index 123, *123*
  epidemiological trends 126–128, *127*,
    128
  minimum intervention 316–318
  radiography follow-up 123
age distribution 125–126, *126*
age-dependent changes 13–14, *13*
air-drying 71, *71*
amalgams 209, 226, 272
  sealants 225, *225*
ameloblasts 7
amelogenesis 7
ammonia 169
antibody engineering 322
apatites 26
  see also hydroxyapatite
Approximal Plaque Index (API) 331,
  394
approximal surfaces 7
  caries lesion *247*
  caries progression 295–296, *296*
  infiltration 249–253
    caries progression prevention
      249–250, *250*
    clinical efficacy 250, *250*
    clinical use 253
    follow-up 253
    indications 250–251, *251*, *252*
  sealing technique 240–241, *241*
    clinical evidence 242, *242*
    patch technique 241
  therapeutic options 143, *144*
  treatment in children and adolescents
    316, 318, *318*
aprismatic enamel 9, 230
Atraumatic Restorative Technique (ART)
  268
attrition 125
autofluorescence 54–55

B

backscatter electron imaging 47, *47*
bacteria *see* oral microorganisms
basic erosive wear examination (BEWE)
  125, 130
  modified BEWE 337
benzoates 169
biofilm 14, 28, 40
  biological control 156–157
  caries progression relationship 295
  cavitation relationship 295

chemical control 154–156
dental plaque as a biofilm 147–148
drug delivery 323–324
fissures 229–230
  significance for sealant placement
    230
mechanical control 148–154
  interdental hygiene 153–154, *153*
  professional tooth cleaning 154, *154*
  tooth brushing 148–153, *149*, *150*,
    151, *152*
therapeutic measures 140, *141*
see also dental plaque
bitewing radiographs 87, *88*, 91–95, *94*,
  138, 335–336
  bitewing holders 340, *340*
  caries progression probability
    assessment 95
  case studies *340*, *352*, 396–397, *397*
  documentation 93, *94*, 335
  follow-up 95–96, *96*
    children and adolescents 96–97
  occlusal surface evaluation 94
  preparations 91
  radiation exposure 96
  technique 91–92, *92*
  see also radiographic diagnostics
bonding *see* adhesive technology
brown spot lesion 43, 71, *72*
brushite 33

C

C-factor 281
calcium fluoride 28
  formation 183–184
calcium lactate 169
calcium phosphate 26, 33
  solubility 26
  see also hydroxyapatite (HAP)
carbohydrates 162–165, *162*
  conventional sugars 162–163
  intense sweeteners 162, *162*, 168
  metabolism by cariogenic micro-
    organisms 163–164, *163*
    direct phosphorylation 163
    extracellular pathway 164
    glycogen production 163–164
  sugar alcohols 162, *162*, 167–168
  see also sugar ingestion
carbonate-modified hydroxyapatite
  (CHAP) 8
caries
  artificially created lesions 47

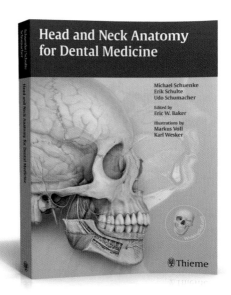
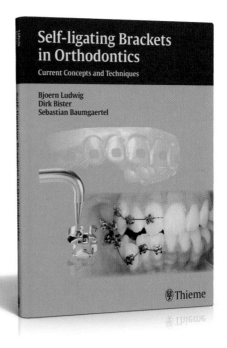
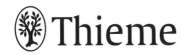

More bestselling dentistry books from Thieme

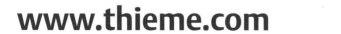 **www.thieme.com**

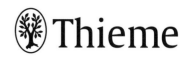 Thieme